Lysosomal Storage Disorders: Molecular Basis and Therapeutic Approaches

Lysosomal Storage Disorders: Molecular Basis and Therapeutic Approaches

Editor

Enrico Moro

MDPI • Basel • Beijing • Wuhan • Barcelona • Belgrade • Manchester • Tokyo • Cluj • Tianjin

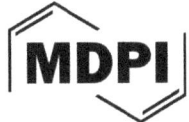

Editor
Enrico Moro
Molecular Medicine
University of Padova
Padova
Italy

Editorial Office
MDPI
St. Alban-Anlage 66
4052 Basel, Switzerland

This is a reprint of articles from the Special Issue published online in the open access journal *Biomolecules* (ISSN 2218-273X) (available at: www.mdpi.com/journal/biomolecules/special_issues/Lysosom_Stor_Disord).

For citation purposes, cite each article independently as indicated on the article page online and as indicated below:

LastName, A.A.; LastName, B.B.; LastName, C.C. Article Title. *Journal Name* **Year**, *Volume Number*, Page Range.

ISBN 978-3-0365-1967-8 (Hbk)
ISBN 978-3-0365-1966-1 (PDF)

© 2021 by the authors. Articles in this book are Open Access and distributed under the Creative Commons Attribution (CC BY) license, which allows users to download, copy and build upon published articles, as long as the author and publisher are properly credited, which ensures maximum dissemination and a wider impact of our publications.
The book as a whole is distributed by MDPI under the terms and conditions of the Creative Commons license CC BY-NC-ND.

Contents

About the Editor vii

Preface to "Lysosomal Storage Disorders: Molecular Basis and Therapeutic Approaches" ... ix

Enrico Moro
Lysosomal Storage Disorders: Molecular Basis and Therapeutic Approaches
Reprinted from: *Biomolecules* **2021**, *11*, 964, doi:10.3390/biom11070964 1

Adenrele M. Gleason, Elizabeth G. Woo, Cindy McKinney and Ellen Sidransky
The Role of Exosomes in Lysosomal Storage Disorders
Reprinted from: *Biomolecules* **2021**, *11*, 576, doi:10.3390/biom11040576 5

Filippo Pinto e Vairo, Diana Rojas Málaga, Francyne Kubaski, Carolina Fischinger Moura de Souza, Fabiano de Oliveira Poswar, Guilherme Baldo and Roberto Giugliani
Precision Medicine for Lysosomal Disorders
Reprinted from: *Biomolecules* **2020**, *10*, 1110, doi:10.3390/biom10081110 19

Naresh K. Meena and Nina Raben
Pompe Disease: New Developments in an Old Lysosomal Storage Disorder
Reprinted from: *Biomolecules* **2020**, *10*, 1339, doi:10.3390/biom10091339 45

Allen K. Murray
The Release of a Soluble Glycosylated Protein from Glycogen by Recombinant Lysosomal -Glucosidase (rhGAA) In Vitro and Its Presence in Serum In Vivo
Reprinted from: *Biomolecules* **2020**, *10*, 1613, doi:10.3390/biom10121613 65

Ken Kok, Kimberley C. Zwiers, Rolf G. Boot, Hermen S. Overkleeft, Johannes M. F. G. Aerts and Marta Artola
Fabry Disease: Molecular Basis, Pathophysiology, Diagnostics and Potential Therapeutic Directions
Reprinted from: *Biomolecules* **2021**, *11*, 271, doi:10.3390/biom11020271 87

Vincenza Gragnaniello, Alessandro P Burlina, Giulia Polo, Antonella Giuliani, Leonardo Salviati, Giovanni Duro, Chiara Cazzorla, Laura Rubert, Evelina Maines, Dominique P Germain and Alberto B Burlina
Newborn Screening for Fabry Disease in Northeastern Italy: Results of Five Years of Experience
Reprinted from: *Biomolecules* **2021**, *11*, 951, doi:10.3390/biom11070951 107

Rosa Manzoli, Lorenzo Badenetti, Michela Rubin and Enrico Moro
Lysosomal Function and Axon Guidance: Is There a Meaningful Liaison?
Reprinted from: *Biomolecules* **2021**, *11*, 191, doi:10.3390/biom11020191 127

Ilaria Tonazzini, Chiara Cerri, Ambra Del Grosso, Sara Antonini, Manuela Allegra, Matteo Caleo and Marco Cecchini
Visual System Impairment in a Mouse Model of Krabbe Disease: The Twitcher Mouse
Reprinted from: *Biomolecules* **2020**, *11*, 7, doi:10.3390/biom11010007 141

Christiane S. Hampe, Jacob Wesley, Troy C. Lund, Paul J. Orchard, Lynda E. Polgreen, Julie B. Eisengart, Linda K. McLoon, Sebahattin Cureoglu, Patricia Schachern and R. Scott McIvor
Mucopolysaccharidosis Type I: Current Treatments, Limitations, and Prospects for Improvement
Reprinted from: *Biomolecules* **2021**, *11*, 189, doi:10.3390/biom11020189 153

Valeria De Pasquale, Michele Costanzo, Rosa Anna Siciliano, Maria Fiorella Mazzeo, Valeria Pistorio, Laura Bianchi, Emanuela Marchese, Margherita Ruoppolo, Luigi Michele Pavone and Marianna Caterino
Proteomic Analysis of Mucopolysaccharidosis IIIB Mouse Brain
Reprinted from: *Biomolecules* **2020**, *10*, 355, doi:10.3390/biom10030355 . . . . **177**

Jarrod W. Barnes, Megan Aarnio-Peterson, Joy Norris, Mark Haskins, Heather Flanagan-Steet and Richard Steet
Upregulation of Sortilin, a Lysosomal Sorting Receptor, Corresponds with Reduced Bioavailability of Latent TGF in Mucolipidosis II Cells
Reprinted from: *Biomolecules* **2020**, *10*, 670, doi:10.3390/biom10050670 . . . . **201**

Giulia Massaro, Amy F. Geard, Wenfei Liu, Oliver Coombe-Tennant, Simon N. Waddington, Julien Baruteau, Paul Gissen and Ahad A. Rahim
Gene Therapy for Lysosomal Storage Disorders: Ongoing Studies and Clinical Development
Reprinted from: *Biomolecules* **2021**, *11*, 611, doi:10.3390/biom11040611 . . . . **221**

Renuka P. Limgala and Ozlem Goker-Alpan
Effect of Substrate Reduction Therapy in Comparison to Enzyme Replacement Therapy on Immune Aspects and Bone Involvement in Gaucher Disease
Reprinted from: *Biomolecules* **2020**, *10*, 526, doi:10.3390/biom10040526 . . . . **263**

Manasa P. Srikanth and Ricardo A. Feldman
Elevated Dkk1 Mediates Downregulation of the Canonical Wnt Pathway and Lysosomal Loss in an iPSC Model of Neuronopathic Gaucher Disease
Reprinted from: *Biomolecules* **2020**, *10*, 1630, doi:10.3390/biom10121630 . . . . **275**

Margarita M. Ivanova, Julia Dao, Neil Kasaci, Benjamin Adewale, Jacqueline Fikry and Ozlem Goker-Alpan
Rapid Clathrin-Mediated Uptake of Recombinant -Gal-A to Lysosome Activates Autophagy
Reprinted from: *Biomolecules* **2020**, *10*, 837, doi:10.3390/biom10060837 . . . . **289**

About the Editor

Enrico Moro

Enrico Moro is Associate Professor of Cell Biology at the Medical School of the University of Padua (Italy). He has been actively working as scientist for almost 25 years in the field of human diseases, including cystic fibrosis, diabetes, cancer, and lately also lysosomal storage disorders. He is expert in zebrafish developmental biology and manipulation and he was the first who developed a fish model for Mucopolysaccharidosis type II. He is currently member of the Scientific Advisory Board for the ISMRD (International Society for Mannosidosis and Related Diseases) and the Italian Sanfilippo Fighters organization.

Preface to "Lysosomal Storage Disorders: Molecular Basis and Therapeutic Approaches"

In the 19th century William Osler, a famous medical doctor wrote: "The good physician treats the disease; the great physician treats the patient who has the disease". Scientists and physicians are aware that basic science and medicine need to intertwine to make the difference. This book collects the precious contribution of distinguished scientists and physicians in the field of lysosomal disorders and offers an original example of how basic science and clinical medicine may integrate for the scientific advancement and the development of potential new therapeutic strategies.

Enrico Moro
Editor

Editorial

Lysosomal Storage Disorders: Molecular Basis and Therapeutic Approaches

Enrico Moro

Department of Molecular Medicine, University of Padova, via U.Bassi 58/b, 35131 Padova, Italy; enrico.moro.1@unipd.it

Keywords: lysosomal storage disorders; biomarkers; gene therapy

Lysosomal storage disorders (LSDs) are a group of 60 rare inherited diseases characterized by a heterogeneous spectrum of clinical symptoms, ranging from severe intellectual disabilities, cardiac abnormalities, visceromegaly, and bone deformities to slowly progressive muscle weakness, respiratory insufficiency, eye defects (corneal clouding and retinal degeneration), and skin alterations [1]. Pioneering biochemical studies between the early 1970s and 1990s attributed the pathogenesis of LSDs to a disrupted catabolic function of lysosomal enzymes and consequent primary lysosomal substrate storage [2]. However, in the past two decades, a wealth of published research expanded this classical view to a more complex scenario, whereby multiple primary defects produced by lysosomal enzyme deficiency concur, leading to a range of cellular abnormalities, including oxidative stress, mitochondrial alterations, cell signaling defects, and calcium dyshomeostasis [3,4]. This Special Issue covered an overview of the current knowledge regarding the pathogenesis of different lysosomal diseases and their therapeutic perspectives. In their work, Hampe and colleagues provided an exhaustive description of therapeutic approaches for Mucopolysaccharidosis type I, including enzyme replacement therapy (ERT) and hematopoietic stem cell transplantation (HSCT). Throughout the paper, the authors claimed that both treatments do not provide full recovery from primary symptoms and suggested that early diagnosis is critical for correct therapeutic management [5]. Meena and Raben discussed similar findings in their review on Pompe disease, covering novel aspects of disease pathogenesis, including the role of autophagic impairment in glycogen storage and therapeutic advances in the field of ERT. In their detailed overview of the different alpha-glucosidase (GAA) formulations developed over the years, the authors pointed out that significant, but still limited, clinical improvements have been achieved in affected patients [6]. Regarding the same topic, Murray described his findings on glycogen-containing carbohydrates masked by an unknown protein derived from the recombinant GAA (rhGAA)-dependent glycogen breakdown outside of the lysosome and the cell. The author proposes the use of these new detected terminal degradation products of rhGAA in the serum as biomarkers for follow-up and treatment protocols [7]. Gragnaniello and collaborators presented their long-term experience on a wide newborn screening for Fabry disease and proposed lyso-Gb3 as a useful biomarker for diagnostic and follow-up protocols [8]. Kok and colleagues collected an exhaustive overview of Fabry disease pathogenesis and treatment, considering the role of neutralizing antibodies against recombinant enzymes, which are responsible for the relapse in plasma lysoGb3 levels after several years of ERT in affected patients. The authors stressed the prompt need to develop alternative therapeutic strategies, of which α-1,4-Galactosyltransferase (A4GALT) inhibitors represent a quite promising approach [9]. In research of the same disease, Ivanova and colleagues described their findings on the role of clathrin-mediated endocytosis of recombinant alpha-galactosidase A (rh-α-Gal A) in different experimental cellular models. Interestingly, they provided limited but clear evidence that rh-α-Gal A uptake was responsible of autophagy induction in their experimental models [10]. Impaired intracellular trafficking was also evoked in the paper by Barnes and colleagues who presented their intriguing data on TGFβ1 missorting and increased sortilin levels in experimental models of mucolipidosis type II (MLII) [11]. In the field of sphingolipidoses, Limgala and Goker-Alpan provided a preliminary description of the measured plasma levels of secreted biomarkers, including osteopontin (OPN), osteoprotegerin (OPG), and chemokine (C-C motif) ligand 18 (CCL18) and percentages of T and B-lymphocytes in Gaucher patients under ERT and SRT [12]. Indeed, Srikanth and Feldman reported a very interesting study on the extracellular Dickkopf-1 (Dkk1)-mediated downregulation of the canonical Wnt pathway in an induced-pluripotent stem cell model of neuronopathic Gaucher disease [13]. Three other elegant reviews also contributed to this Special Issue: the work of Pinto e Vairo and colleagues reported a summarizing overview on the relevance of precision medicine in the field of lysosomal storage disorders [14], while Massaro and colleagues included their comprehensive summary of the currently available and developing gene therapy approaches and clinical trials in the management of lysosomal diseases [15]. Gleason and colleagues reported an excellent collection of data related to the significance of exosomes in the context of lysosomal disorders pathogenesis, but the authors also emphasized the clinical application of exosomes as therapeutic delivery vehicles [16]. In one additional review, Manzoli and colleagues raised an important and puzzling question related to the potential relevance of investigating the axonal guidance-related aspects in lysosomal disorders. The authors provided an extensive list of axon guidance diseases exhibiting clinical features resembling those of lysosomal disorders [17]. Tonazzini and colleagues described through the Twicher (TWI) mouse, the most used model of Krabbe disease, the onset of visual impairment, reduced contrast sensitivity, and neuropathological signs, including astrogliosis and reduced myelination in the early life stages [18]. Finally, De Pasquale and collaborators reported the application of a label-free quantitative proteomic approach in a mucopolysaccharidosis type IIIb mouse model, which enabled the classification of three major clusters of proteins dysregulated in the diseased brain [19].

Altogether, the articles of this Special Issue have broadened our concepts in the field of lysosomal storage disorders, offering a reference cue for the pathogenic aspects and evolving therapeutic approaches related to these rare diseases.

Acknowledgments: The guest editor would like to thank all of the authors for their valuable contributions to this Special Issue and all of the reviewers for their helpful comments during the peer review process.

Conflicts of Interest: The author declares no conflict of interest.

References

1. Platt, F.M.; d'Azzo, A.; Davidson, B.L.; Neufeld, E.F.; Tifft, C.J. Lysosomal storage diseases. *Nat. Rev. Dis. Primers* **2018**, *4*, 36. [CrossRef] [PubMed]
2. Mehta, A.; Beck, M.; Linhart, A.; Sunder-Plassmann, G.; Widmer, U. History of lysosomal storage diseases: An overview. In *Fabry Disease: Perspectives from 5 Years of FOS*; Mehta, A., Beck, M., Sunder-Plassmann, G., Eds.; Oxford PharmaGenesis: Oxford, UK, 2006; Chapter 1.
3. Fiorenza, M.T.; Moro, E.; Erickson, R.P. The pathogenesis of lysosomal storage disorders: Beyond the engorgement of lysosomes to abnormal development and neuroinflammation. *Hum. Mol. Genet.* **2018**, *27*, R119–R129. [CrossRef] [PubMed]
4. Parenti, G.; Medina, D.L.; Ballabio, A. The rapidly evolving view of lysosomal storage diseases. *EMBO Mol. Med.* **2021**, *13*, e12836. [CrossRef] [PubMed]
5. Hampe, C.S.; Wesley, J.; Lund, T.C.; Orchard, P.J.; Polgreen, L.E.; Eisengart, J.B.; McLoon, L.K.; Cureoglu, S.; Schachern, P.; McIvor, R.S. Mucopolysaccharidosis Type I: Current Treatments, Limitations, and Prospects for Improvement. *Biomolecules* **2021**, *11*, 189. [CrossRef] [PubMed]
6. Meena, N.K.; Raben, N. Pompe Disease: New Developments in an Old Lysosomal Storage Disorder. *Biomolecules* **2020**, *10*, 1339. [CrossRef] [PubMed]
7. Murray, A.K. The Release of a Soluble Glycosylated Protein from Glycogen by Recombinant Lysosomal α-Glucosidase (rhGAA) In Vitro and Its Presence in Serum In Vivo. *Biomolecules* **2020**, *10*, 1613. [CrossRef] [PubMed]

8. Gragnaniello, V.; Burlina, A.P.; Polo, G.; Giuliani, A.; Salviati, L.; Duro, G.; Cazzorla, C.; Rubert, L.; Maines, E.; Germain, D.P.; et al. Newborn screening for Fabry disease in North-Eastern Italy: Results of five years of experience. *Biomolecules* **2021**, *11*, 951. [CrossRef]
9. Kok, K.; Zwiers, K.C.; Boot, R.G.; Overkleeft, H.S.; Aerts, J.M.F.G.; Artola, M. Fabry Disease: Molecular Basis, Pathophysiology, Diagnostics and Potential Therapeutic Directions. *Biomolecules* **2021**, *11*, 271. [CrossRef] [PubMed]
10. Ivanova, M.M.; Dao, J.; Kasaci, N.; Adewale, B.; Fikry, J.; Goker-Alpan, O. Rapid Clathrin-Mediated Uptake of Recombinant α-Gal-A to Lysosome Activates Autophagy. *Biomolecules* **2020**, *10*, 837. [CrossRef] [PubMed]
11. Barnes, J.W.; Aarnio-Peterson, M.; Norris, J.; Haskins, M.; Flanagan-Steet, H.; Steet, R. Upregulation of Sortilin, a Lysosomal Sorting Receptor, Corresponds with Reduced Bioavailability of Latent TGFβ in Mucolipidosis II Cells. *Biomolecules* **2020**, *10*, 670. [CrossRef] [PubMed]
12. Limgala, R.P.; Goker-Alpan, O. Effect of Substrate Reduction Therapy in Comparison to Enzyme Replacement Therapy on Immune Aspects and Bone Involvement in Gaucher Disease. *Biomolecules* **2020**, *10*, 526. [CrossRef] [PubMed]
13. Srikanth, M.P.; Feldman, R.A. Elevated Dkk1 Mediates Downregulation of the Canonical Wnt Pathway and Lysosomal Loss in an iPSC Model of Neuronopathic Gaucher Disease. *Biomolecules* **2020**, *10*, 1630. [CrossRef] [PubMed]
14. Pinto E Vairo, F.; Rojas Málaga, D.; Kubaski, F.; Fischinger Moura de Souza, C.; de Oliveira Poswar, F.; Baldo, G.; Giugliani, R. Precision Medicine for Lysosomal Disorders. *Biomolecules* **2020**, *10*, 1110. [CrossRef] [PubMed]
15. Massaro, G.; Geard, A.F.; Liu, W.; Coombe-Tennant, O.; Waddington, S.N.; Baruteau, J.; Gissen, P.; Rahim, A.A. Gene Therapy for Lysosomal Storage Disorders: Ongoing Studies and Clinical Development. *Biomolecules* **2021**, *11*, 611. [CrossRef] [PubMed]
16. Gleason, A.M.; Woo, E.G.; McKinney, C.; Sidransky, E. The Role of Exosomes in Lysosomal Storage Disorders. *Biomolecules* **2021**, *11*, 576. [CrossRef] [PubMed]
17. Manzoli, R.; Badenetti, L.; Rubin, M.; Moro, E. Lysosomal Function and Axon Guidance: Is There a Meaningful Liaison? *Biomolecules* **2021**, *11*, 191. [CrossRef] [PubMed]
18. Tonazzini, I.; Cerri, C.; Del Grosso, A.; Antonini, S.; Allegra, M.; Caleo, M.; Cecchini, M. Visual System Impairment in a Mouse Model of Krabbe Disease: The Twitcher Mouse. *Biomolecules* **2020**, *11*, 7. [CrossRef] [PubMed]
19. De Pasquale, V.; Costanzo, M.; Siciliano, R.A.; Mazzeo, M.F.; Pistorio, V.; Bianchi, L.; Marchese, E.; Ruoppolo, M.; Pavone, L.M.; Caterino, M. Proteomic Analysis of Mucopolysaccharidosis IIIB Mouse Brain. *Biomolecules* **2020**, *10*, 355. [CrossRef]

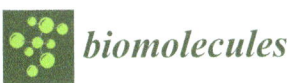

Article

The Role of Exosomes in Lysosomal Storage Disorders

Adenrele M. Gleason, Elizabeth G. Woo ⬤, Cindy McKinney and Ellen Sidransky *

Medical Genetics Branch, National Human Genome Research Institute, National Institutes of Health, Bethesda, MD 20892, USA; adenrele.gleason@nih.gov (A.M.G.); elizabeth.woo@nih.gov (E.G.W.); dr.cmckinney@gmail.com (C.M.)
* Correspondence: sidranse@mail.nih.gov

Abstract: Exosomes, small membrane-bound organelles formed from endosomal membranes, represent a heterogenous source of biological and pathological biomarkers capturing the metabolic status of a cell. Exosomal cargo, including lipids, proteins, mRNAs, and miRNAs, can either act as inter-cellular messengers or are shuttled for autophagic/lysosomal degradation. Most cell types in the central nervous system (CNS) release exosomes, which serve as long and short distance communicators between neurons, astrocytes, oligodendrocytes, and microglia. Lysosomal storage disorders are diseases characterized by the accumulation of partially or undigested cellular waste. The exosomal content in these diseases is intrinsic to each individual disorder. Emerging research indicates that lysosomal dysfunction enhances exocytosis, and hence, in lysosomal disorders, exosomal secretion may play a role in disease pathogenesis. Furthermore, the unique properties of exosomes and their ability to carry cargo between adjacent cells and organs, and across the blood–brain barrier, make them attractive candidates for use as therapeutic delivery vehicles. Thus, understanding exosomal content and function may have utility in the treatment of specific lysosomal storage disorders. Since lysosomal dysfunction and the deficiency of at least one lysosomal enzyme, glucocerebrosidase, is associated with the development of parkinsonism, the study and use of exosomes may contribute to an improved understanding of Parkinson disease, potentially leading to new therapeutics.

Keywords: exosomes; endocytic pathways; neurodegenerative disease; Gaucher disease; Parkinson disease; lysosomes; lysosomal storage disorder

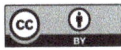

Citation: Gleason, A.M.; Woo, E.G.; McKinney, C.; Sidransky, E. The Role of Exosomes in Lysosomal Storage Disorders. *Biomolecules* **2021**, *11*, 576. https://doi.org/10.3390/biom11040576

Academic Editor: Enrico Moro

Received: 17 March 2021
Accepted: 12 April 2021
Published: 15 April 2021

Publisher's Note: MDPI stays neutral with regard to jurisdictional claims in published maps and institutional affiliations.

Copyright: © 2021 by the authors. Licensee MDPI, Basel, Switzerland. This article is an open access article distributed under the terms and conditions of the Creative Commons Attribution (CC BY) license (https://creativecommons.org/licenses/by/4.0/).

1. Introduction

Cells have several different means of conveying intercellular bioinformation. This may occur by direct cell-to-cell contact, through signaling via secreted soluble molecules, and by small vesicle-packaged molecules [1]. These different **vesicles (see Appendix A for the definitions of terms shown in bold)** include **exosomes, ectosomes, apoptotic bodies,** and **autophagosomes**. Exosomes, the subject of this review, [2,3] were initially described as waste material, encapsulated in small lipid vesicles, captured from the cytoplasm of maturing reticulocytes. However, it subsequently became clear that exosome cargos represent a heterogeneous source of normal or pathological biomarkers that capture a cell's metabolic state at a given point in time. Exosomes are formed from endosomal membranes and their evolution intersects with steps in **autophagy-lysosomal pathways (ALPs)**. As they mature, exosomes become filled with a selected set of sorted biomolecules. These may include lipids, metabolites, **mRNAs, miRNAs,** and proteins. While many important aspects of exosome biology in health and disease remain to be defined, **exosomal cargos** have at least two fates. They may act as intercellular messengers (e.g., paracrine signaling) and/or inter-organ communicators (e.g., metastatic disease). They also carry defined intracellular cargo from interconnected autophagic/lysosomal degradation pathways in the cell. Depending on the cell of origin and the cargo source, the exosomes contribute to homeostatic or metabolic regulation, as well as to disease processes, including viral infection, cancer metastasis, and neurodegenerative diseases [4]. While a better understanding of the role of exosomes in normal physiology is just now emerging, their role in pathological conditions, such as neurodegeneration, has been more rigorously examined.

2. The Biogenesis of Exosomes: A Subclass of Extracellular Vesicles (EVs)

All cells release exosomes, 30–150 nm membrane-bound vesicles that derive from the invagination of endosomal membranes. Exosomes acquire their content both from biosynthetic routes and by **endocytosis**, a form of intracellular trafficking. Endocytosis begins with the invagination of the plasma membrane (PM), which can be **clathrin-coated**. Upon internalization, these vesicles first fuse with the **early endosome** (EE), also described as the sorting endosome. Here, major decisions on the next trafficking route occur. Classically, cargo destined for degradation enter the endosomal-lysosomal system, where the EEs mature and begin to invaginate parts of their membranes. These **intraluminal vesicles** (ILVs) then become part of the **multivesicular bodies** (MVB), organelles comprised of vacuoles delimited by a single membrane [5]. The MVBs host multiple vesicles, and depending on the invagination size, these vesicles range from 50-150 nm in diameter [6]. Two trafficking routes can occur at the MVB. Membrane components and other macromolecules encapsulated in these vesicles can be hydrolyzed after fusing with lysosomes. Enzymes within the lysosomes then degrade the delivered carbohydrates, proteins, fats, and other cellular products into smaller and simpler components that are then recycled as building blocks for new molecules (Figure 1). Alternatively, these vesicles become future exosomes when released from cells, through a process called secretion. In this trafficking step, MVBs fuse with the plasma membrane and release the ILVs as exosomes [7]. The exosome membrane composition is similar to that of the plasma membrane and contains inserted and captured cytoplasmic proteins. The internal cargo within small vesicles is sorted, sometimes as part of protein complexes that assist in moving and/or sorting. This complex of proteins is also known as **endosomal sorting complex required for transport (ESCRT)**-associated pathways [8].

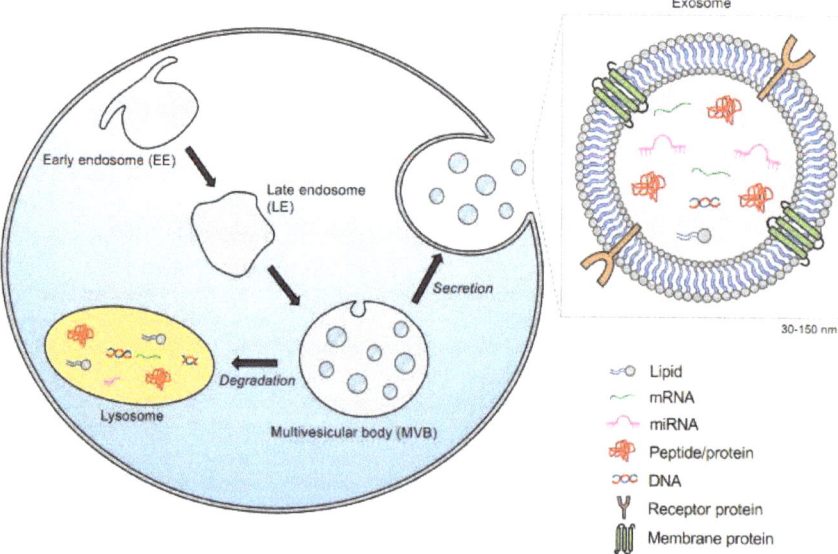

Figure 1. Intracellular biogenesis of exosomes. Exosomes can be formed through the endocytic trafficking pathway. These vesicles are generated by limited inward budding of the late endosome to form the intraluminal vesicles (ILVs). ILVs are components of multivesicular bodies (MVB). Two routes can occur at the MVB: 1. Degradation, resulting from fusion with lysosomes and 2. Secretion, that takes place when multivesicular bodies (MVBs) fuse with the plasma membrane and release their contents into the extracellular space. Secreted exosomes can be captured by nearby or distant cells and regulate the physiological state of the recipient cell.

3. Exosome Cargo and Transport:

The recent explosion of exosome research has been driven by their newly defined role in intercellular vesicular trafficking. This results in the transmission of their signaling cargo by means of secretion at the plasma membrane into the extracellular space, enabling uptake in recipient cells. Characterizing the content of exocargo can provide information about exosome biogenesis, potential effects on the recipient cell, and insights into disease diagnosis, progression, and prognosis, by serving as biomarkers. Exocargo may also be useful in monitoring cellular responses to disease treatments [9]. Depending on the cell of origin, exosomes may contain cargos enriched in proteins (such as TSG101 and Alix) [10,11], miRNAs [12], translatable mRNAs [13], lipids (i.e., ceramide) [14,15], and other bioactive molecules (see Exocarta.org [16] a database of biomolecules reported in exosomes). Surprisingly, the propagation and release of exosomes is conserved across species spanning from fungi to humans, and thus, it is possible that exosomes from other species could communicate signals to humans, e.g., bovine exosomes in milk. Horizontal transfer between species, or between cells of multiple organs in the body, could have either a beneficial or detrimental effect. The exact role that these exoproteins and macromolecules play in external cellular communication is currently under investigation [17,18].

Our knowledge of how the selection and packaging of cargo into exosomes is accomplished is advancing, although many questions remain unresolved. The cargo and membrane content of exosomes differs depending on the on the nature of the parent cell. This suggests that there are mechanisms in the cell directing the sorting of specific molecules [19] and enzymes [20,21], indicating that active processing helps define the content of mature exosomes. Several complexes appear to be involved in sorting and packaging pathways, including Rab family members, p53 and its effector tumor suppressor-activated pathway (TSAP) [22–24]. In the case of miRNA content, it was shown that the internal sequence GGAG at the 3′-end can direct certain miRNAs to ILVs. Similarly, in murine hepatocytes, the GGCU motif located on the 3′-end of miRNAs is recruited to the RNA binding protein SYNCRIP (synaptotagmin-binding cytoplasmic RNA-interacting protein) [25]. This sequence specific interaction directs miRNA sorting into exosomes [25]. Further studies are needed to improve our understanding of how miRNAs are sorted into these membrane-bound exosomes [1]. A better characterization of the cargoes intrinsic to exosomes derived from different cell types will help to clarify the molecular mechanisms governing exosome function and their role in various aspects of biology and disease.

4. Exosomal Signatures: Lessons from the CNS

Most cell types in the central nervous system (CNS) release exosomes, including astrocytes, microglia, oligodendrocytes, and neurons. As potential vectors for intercellular communication, exosomes harbor distinct molecular contents that reflect their donor cell. This section will summarize the signature of exosomes found in the cell types comprising the CNS. This is particularly relevant to specific lysosomal storage disorders, as most have CNS involvement that is only partially understood.

4.1. Exosomes from Astrocytes

It is well established that **astrocytes** influence neuronal function, however the molecular mediators that regulate this process continue to be under intense investigation. To study their effects on neural uptake, differentiation, and maturation, astrocyte-derived extracellular vesicles (ADEVs) were isolated from human primary astrocytes in culture [26]. In this study, the proteomic signature of exosomes derived from astrocytes revealed astrocyte-specific markers including GFAP, excitatory amino acid transporter 1 (SLC1A3/GLAST), and glucose transporter member 1 (SLCA1/GLUT1). In addition, the authors also examined the exocargo of astrocytes treated with the classic pro-inflammatory cytokine interleukin-1 β, termed IL-1β-ADEVs. When compared to controls, the proteomic profile was enriched in proteins characteristic of reactive astrocytes [26]. To examine the physiological consequences of neurons treated with IL-1β-ADEVs, different assays were performed, showing delayed outgrowth and a reduction in neurite length, total surface area, node number, and neuronal firing [26].

Other ex-vivo studies showed that exosomes purified from astrocyte processes freshly prepared from adult rat cerebral cortex participated in signal transmission and could target both near and distant sites. The exosomes were enriched for markers typically found on astrocytes, including GFAP and Ezrin [27], as well as the neuroprotectant protein neuroglobulin (NGB). The released exosomes selectively targeted neurons, where they were then internalized, suggesting that exosomes could deliver NGB originating from astrocytes to neurons. It was also observed that in astrocytes, apoptosis is associated with the release of PAR-4/ceramide-containing lipid exosomes [27].

4.2. Exosomes from Cortical Neurons

Exosomes are also secreted from **cortical neurons**, with important consequences. In one study, the biochemical composition of exosomes prepared from the cultured medium of primary cultures of rat cortical neurons at embryonic day 16 was evaluated using mass spectrometry. Proteomic profiling identified an enrichment of integral membrane protein GluR2/3, the α-amino-3-hydroxy-5-methyl-4-isozazolepropionic acid receptors (AMPARs), and the specific cell adhesion molecule L1 [28]. Interestingly, this analysis did not show enrichment of NR1 subunits of the N-methyl-D-Aspartic Acid Receptor 1 (NMDA) glutamate receptor, suggesting that GluR2/3 secretion is specifically facilitated through exosomes. In contrast, these exosomes did not display the plasma membrane protein, NA^+/K^+-ATPase, providing evidence that the exosome fractions were not contaminated with plasma membrane [28].

Further studies showed that mature cortical neurons from the somato-dendritic compartment are capable of releasing exosomes [29]. Here, they showed that the release of exosomes from 15 day cortical and hippocampal neuronal cultures was regulated by calcium influx and glutamatergic synaptic activity. When treated with ibicucullin or pirocotoxin, antagonists of GABA receptors known to enhance glutamatergic spontaneous activity, a mass release of exosomes was detected [29]. As a proof of principle, the subsequent addition of either an AMPAR or NMDA antagonist attenuated the $GABA_A$-induced exosomal secretion. Taken together, these experiments demonstrate that secretion of exosomes is regulated by glutamatergic activity in cortical neurons.

Furthermore, exosomes secreted by cortical neurons upon glutamatergic synapse activation were selectively endocytosed by neurons, whereas the exosomes derived from neuroblastoma cells were taken up by glial and neuronal cells without bias [30]. Thus, the uptake of exosomes is somehow specified by the parental cell, suggesting a novel mechanism of inter-neuronal communication.

4.3. Exosomes from Oligodendrocytes

Oligodendrocytes insulate axons with a multilayered myelin sheath. It has been proposed that exosomes secreted from oligodendrocytes may relay molecular cues that support glia-mediated trophic nutrients to axons [31]. In one study, myelinating oligodendrocytes were found to secrete exosomes in a Ca^{2+}-dependent manner [32]. This observation supports other studies suggesting that exosome release is triggered by neuronal activation [29]. In another study, Frühebeis et al. showed that in contact-independent cocultures of neurons and oligodendrocytes, the neurotransmitter glutamate was able to trigger the secretion of oligodendroglial exosomes [33]. This release was mediated by Ca^{2+} entry through oligodendrogial NBQX (2,3-dihydroxy-6-nitro-7-sulfamoyl-benzo[f]quinoxaline-2,3-dione); NMDA and AMPA receptors [33]. Furthermore, exposure of neurons to oligodendroglial-derived exosomes increased the action potential firing rate, altering both the transcriptome and cellular signal transduction pathways [34]. These exosomes also transferred protective proteins, including catalase and superoxide dismutase (SOD) [34]. Lipid extracts from exosomes isolated from primary cultured oligodendrocytes were analyzed by thin layer chromatography (TLC). These studies identified an enrichment of the canonical myelin lipids galactocerebroside and sulfatide [32]. Proteomic profiling demonstrated that a fraction of these exosomes contained canonical myelin proteins, including myelin proteolipid protein (PLP), 2′3′-cyclic-nucleotide-phosophdiesterase (CNP), myelin oligodendrocyte glycoprotein (MOG), and, to a lesser extent, myelin basic protein (MBP) [32]. Further classification of the proteins identified by mass spectroscopy revealed a spectrum of diverse protein families, including those involved in signal transduction pathways, lipid metabolism, oxidative stress, cellular metabolism, and intriguingly, nuclear proteins [32].

5. Studies of Exosomes in Specific Lysosome Storage Disorders (LSDs)

Lysosomal storage diseases (LSD) include over 70 heritable inborn errors of metabolism characterized by lysosomal dysfunction. Mutations in the genes encoding lysosomal proteins lead to substrate accumulation within the lysosome, which can result in cell dysfunction and cell death [35]. LSDs are individually rare, but as a group have an estimated incidence of around 1 in 5000 [36]. These genetically and clinically heterogeneous disorders affect multiple systems, often manifesting with neurological involvement and neurodegeneration.

LSDs result from defects in lysosomal proteins and enzymes, but also endocytic trafficking proteins, integral membrane proteins, and lipids, as well as regulatory proteins [35,37,38]. Collectively, these disorders can be further divided into subcategories based upon the stored materials, such as mucopolysaccharidoses, glycoproteinoses, and lipidoses [38]. The composition of the accumulated materials is intrinsic to each LSD. It has been proposed that in an effort to alleviate the buildup, these undigested materials are, in part, redirected into the extracellular space by lysosomal exocytosis [39]. In the following section, we will review studies of the release of exosomes/EVs in six specific LSD models (Table 1).

Table 1. Selected Lysosomal Storage Disorders (LSD).

LSD	Metabolite Accumulation	Consequence
Metachromatic leukodystrophy	Sulfatide (spingolipid-3-O-sulfogalactosylceramide)	Increased lysosomal exocytosis
Mucolipidosis type IV	Phospholipids, gangliosides	Increased lysosomal exocytosis
Sialidosis	Sialylated oligosaccharides and glycopeptides	Increased lysosomal exocytosis Identified NEU1 as a negative regulator in lysosomal exocytosis
Cystinosis	Cystine	Microvesicles/exosomes containing wildtype CTNS protein can correct
Niemann-Pick type C	Cholesterol	Increased exosomal-cholesterol secretion in vitro
Gaucher disease	Glucosylceramide, glucosylsphingosine	Increased number of exosomes, aberrant morphology

5.1. Metachromatic Leukodystrophy

Metachromatic leukodystrophy (MLD) is an LSD caused by autosomal recessive mutations in *ARSA*, the gene coding for lysosomal hydrolase arylsulfatase A (ASA) [40]. This enzyme is responsible for the breakdown of the spingolipid-3-O-sulfogalactosylceramide (sulfatide) in oligodendrocytes and distal tubule kidney cells [41]. Patients deficient in this enzyme have increased sulfatides in their urine and cerebrospinal fluid. The buildup of sulfatides damages cells of the CNS, in part by affecting the myelin sheath, as well as the nerve fibers protected by this sheath, resulting in weakness and neurodegeneration. Studies have suggested that the elevated sulfatides present in the urine is a cellular response to dying tubular kidney cells [41]. In an effort to investigate the underlying molecular mechanisms, primary cell cultures of kidney tubule cells from ASA deficient mice were established, demonstrating calcium-induced lysosomal exocytosis [42]. Examination of the content secreted into the cell culture medium showed sulfatides in ASA-deficient cells but not in controls. This study is one of the first to propose that cells are eliminating sulfatides through lysosomal exocytosis. Taken together, this observation provides a potential mechanism for the presence of sulfatides in the biological fluids of patients with MLD.

5.2. Mucolipidosis Type IV

The autosomal recessive LSD Mucolipidosis type IV (MLIV) results in severe neurological and ophthalmologic impairment, motor delay, and gastric dysfunction [43,44]. MLIV is caused by pathologic variants in *MCOLN1*, a member of the transient receptor potential (TRPML1) cation channel gene family [44]. This gene encodes the protein, mucolipin-1 (MLN1), the master Ca^{2+} release channel in the lysosome. However, how the lack of MLIV leads to neurodegeneration is largely unknown. Similar to studies in MLD [42], fibroblasts derived from patients with MLIV also exhibited dramatic impairment in lysosomal exocytosis [45]. This was evaluated by assays measuring the cleavage product of the soluble lysosomal enzyme N-acetyl-β-D-glucosaminidase (NAG). These studies revealed that the amount of NAG released from cultured control fibroblast cell lines was 250-fold higher than the amount released in lines from patients with MLIV [45]. Subcellular localization studies revealed that MLN1 translocates to the plasma membrane and correlates with the percentage of lysosomal organelles available for exocytosis. Transfecting different patient cell lines with wildtype *MLN1* corrected impaired lysosomal exocytosis and restored the channel activity [45]. This work identified the first ion channel, MLN1, found to play a role in lysosomal exocytosis.

Additional studies further examined the role of MLN1 and exosomal release. Depletion of MLN1 from mature adipocytes reduced the exosomal markers CD9, CD81, CD63, and Hsp70 [46]. Notably, isolated plasma membrane from mature adipocytes showed that loss of MLN1 led to a 50% reduction in levels of the lysosomal marker LAMP-1. LAMP-1 is enriched at the plasma membrane when cells are undergoing exocytosis [46]. Taken together, these results indicate that MLN1 plays a role in the trafficking of lysosomes to the plasma membrane, as well as in lysosomal mediated-exosomal secretion.

5.3. Sialidosis

Pathogenic gene variants in *NEU1* disrupt N-acetyl-α-neuraminidase, the lysosomal enzyme that initiates the catabolism of sialyl-glycoconjugates by removing terminal sialic acid residues [47,48]. Perturbations in this pathway cause the LSD sialidosis (also known as ML1) in humans. While there are different types of sialidosis, with differing degrees of clinical severity, they all affect the CNS. Patients with sialidosis have been shown to have diffuse brain atrophy.

Complementary studies, conducted in both murine $neu1^{-/-}$ macrophages and fibroblasts from patients with type II sialidosis [49] showed that cell lines deficient in this lysosomal enzyme had a subcellular redistribution of LAMP-1, a resident lysosomal marker, to the plasma membrane. Supportive experiments using electron microscopy showed that macrophages from a $neu1^{-/-}$ mouse were enriched with "clusters" of lysosomes proximal to the PM, reflecting excessive lysosomal exocytosis. Subsequent studies described the impact of human NEU1 deficiency on exosome release in patient fibroblasts, again showing increased levels of oversialyated LAMP-1 at the PM was accompanied by increased exocytosis.

Functional studies were used to examine the molecular consequences of exosomes released by $neu1^{-/-}$ mice in muscle and connective tissue [50]. Murine $neu1^{-/-}$ fibroblasts exhibited excessive release of exosomes carrying profibrotic signaling molecules, including activated transforming growth factor-β (TGFβ) and wingless-related integration site (WNT)/ β-catenin signaling ligands. These signaling molecules are known to propagate fibrotic signals and trigger myofibroblast transdifferentiation [51,52]. Adding exosomes derived from $neu1^{-/-}$ myofibroblasts into the cultured medium of normal fibroblasts converted them into myofibroblasts [50]. However, when wild-type N-acetyl-α-neuraminidase activity was restored in the *neu1*$^{-/-}$ murine myofibroblasts, exosomes isolated from the rescued cell line no longer converted normal fibroblasts into myofibroblasts, suggesting that restoring N-acetyl-α-neuraminidase activity corrected the excessive release of exosomes carrying profibrotic signaling molecules [50].

5.4. Cystinosis

Cystinosis is a lysosomal storage disease caused by pathogenic variants in the gene *CTNS*, which encodes a lysosomal membrane cystine transporter, cystinosin [53]. This multi-systemic disorder leads to the accumulation of lysosomal cystine and is the main cause of hereditary renal Fanconi syndrome [53]. The addition of microvesicles and/or exosomes derived from both mesenchymal stem cells (MSCs) and transduced insect cells containing wildtype *CTNS* protein to fibroblasts from patients with cystinosis corrected the cystine levels [54,55]. Additional reports have identified **tunneling nanotubules** (TNT) as an alternative endocytic trafficking mechanism that can mediate the cystine clearance. Co-culture assays showed that TNTs produced by wildtype macrophages allowed for the transfer of cystinosin-bearing lysosomes into the cystinosin-deficient fibroblasts [54]. Conversely, cystinotic fibroblasts used the same TNTs to unload aberrant cystine-filled lysosomes into wildtype macrophages. In fact, TNT corrected cystine levels with greater efficiency than secreted exosomes/microvesicles from wildtype MSC or macrophages. Taken together, these observations showed that bidirectional exchange of vesicles and cargo between cell types can occur through TNTs. This work also demonstrated that vesicles released from stem cells are capable of delivering the correct cargo to repair deficits in a neighboring cell.

5.5. Niemann-Pick Type C

Niemann–Pick type C (NPC) disease is caused by bi-allelic variants in two genes, *NPC1* and *NPC2*. Loss of *NPC1* causes abnormal intra-lysosomal accumulation of unesterified cholesterol and sphingolipids in the brain, liver, and spleen [56]. While the age at presentation and the initial manifestations are variable, progressive dementia and neurological signs are almost universal among patients with NPC.

To examine whether *NPC1* impacted exosome secretion, Strauss et al. (2010) showed that both fibroblasts from patients harboring pathogenic *NPC1* variants, as well as siRNA-mediated knockdown of *NPC1* in wild-type oligodendrocytes showed elevated exosomal cholesterol release [57]. Then, oligodendroglial cells were challenged, either by increasing amounts of free cholesterol in the media, or using an inhibitor, U18666A, known to sequester cholesterol into the late endosome/lysosome compartments [57]. In both scenarios, treated cells had a striking increase in exosome secretion. Interestingly, the release of exosomal cholesterol was dependent on the function of the known exosome marker flotillin. Collectively these are the first observations reporting an increase in exosomal cholesterol secretion in cell lines that disrupt *NPC1* function. Taken together, the secretion of exosomal cholesterol in response to lysosomal dysfunction may represent an additional mechanism orchestrating intracellular cholesterol homeostasis. This first study documenting the levels of exosomes in an LSD, requires further validation in in vivo models.

5.6. GaucherDdisease

Gaucher disease (GD), resulting from deficient lysosomal glucocerebrosidase, is caused by bi-allelic variants in *GBA1* and is the most common genetic risk factor for the more common neurodegenerative disorder, Parkinson disease (PD). Deficiencies in this lysosomal enzyme disrupt the conversion of glucosylceramide into glucose and ceramide, resulting in the accumulation of glucosylceramide, as well as its deacylated form glucosylsphingosine, in lysosomes. There are both neuronopathic and non-neuronopathic forms of GD, although the basis for the neuropathology seen is not fully understood.

Recent studies performed using patient plasma indicated that lysosomal dysfunction in patients with GD leads to a striking alteration of plasma exosomal size and morphology [58]. **Dynamic light scattering** (DLS) detected three distinct populations of EVs, finding that the proportion of exosomes around 100 nm in diameter was significantly increased in the GD cohort. Complementary studies using cryo-EM showed an abundance of vesicles with altered morphology in samples from patients with GD. High resolution images of EVs isolated from these patients exhibited multilayered vesicles of larger size, when compared to controls [58]. In contrast to the other LSDs described in this section, the concentration of EVs released did not significantly differ between patients with GD and controls.

5.7. Lysosomal Storage Disorders in General

The focal point of these studies converges on the notion that perturbations in lysosomal function influence lysosomal exocytosis and therefore EV secretion (Table 1). Several studies have demonstrated that lysosomal dysfunction enhances EV secretion by upregulating exocytosis. It has been postulated that elevated EV secretion serves to relieve the accumulation of byproducts in the lysosome. Other studies examining exosome secretion in patients with GD reported an altered morphology when compared to controls, although the total exosome concentration released was similar [58]. As described previously, the accumulation of metabolites and partially undigested cellular materials is specific to each LSD. However, two unifying observations are commonly found in these disorders: 1. increased lysosomal exocytosis, and 2. elevated EV secretion. It is thought that both mechanisms serve as complementary routes to remove the buildup of unwanted waste in the lysosome [39]. Furthermore, it has been suggested that the accumulated byproducts in the lysosome may be shunted to the ILVs found in MVBs. These ILVs, containing unwanted products from the lysosomes, become exosomes when the MVBs fuse with the plasma membrane [39]. These are attractive hypotheses; however crucial unanswered questions remain. The molecular mechanisms detailing the coordinated release of exosomes, whether via the redirection of MVBs and/or lysosomes to the plasma membrane are still unknown. Future work examining the role of exosomes in various LSDs could provide a model system to explore, not only the molecular mechanisms that govern exosome secretion, but also their role in cellular homeostasis.

6. Exosomes as Therapeutic Agents for Treating Lysosomal Storage Disorders

During the past few decades, our ability to treat many of the LSDs has greatly improved. Current treatments include enzyme replacement therapy (ERT) and substrate reduction therapy (SRT), while pharmacological chaperones and gene therapy [59] are emerging options. One challenge in treatment is our current limited ability to deliver therapies across the blood–brain barrier. Extracellular vehicles (EVs) and exosomes could help to address this challenge by serving as drug-delivery vehicles. Since these vesicles can carry cargo between adjacent cells and organs, and efficiently cross the blood–brain barrier [59], they are attractive candidates for drug development. [60].

One LSD for which exosome-based therapy is being explored is Gaucher disease, where preliminary work reported the potential of opto-genetically engineered exosomes for treating GD [61]. A 2019 study described a method of producing enzyme-loaded HEK293-derived exosomes for the targeted delivery of glucocerebrosidase to endocytic compartments of recipient cells [62]. The authors fused glucocerebrosidase to exosomes, targeting the transmembrane protein vesicular stomatitis virus glycoprotein (VSVG), and loaded these fusion proteins onto exosomes. The exosomes were taken up by recipient cells, which showed significantly enhanced gluocerebrosidase activity. They designed exosomes that presented functional enzymes in two different spatial conformations, finding no significant differences [62]. While this approach demonstrated potential, it should be further confirmed using patient-derived or animal models of GD.

The application of EVs for treatment has also been explored for ceroid lipo-fuscinoses 2 (CLN2) or Batten disease. CLN2 is a lysosomal storage disorder that results from dysfunctional lysosomal enzyme tripeptidyl peptidase-1 (TPP1), encoded by *TPP1*. A 2019 study used macrophage-derived EVs to deliver soluble TPP1 protein for the treatment of CLN2 [63]. In one approach, they transfected macrophages with the *TPP1*-encoding plasmid DNA. In another, they loaded naïve EVs with TPP1 therapeutic enzyme ex vitro, using sonication or saponin permeabilization. Both techniques successfully incorporated enzymatically active TPP1 into EVs, which then delivered TPP1 to target cells in an in vitro model of CLN2. Around 70% of the enzyme was delivered to lysosomes, the target organelles. Using a late-infantile neuronal ceroid lipofuscinosis mouse model, they found that the EVs were delivered to the brain, and noted an increased lifespan after intraperitoneal administration of EV-TPP1. This study further supports the potential use of macrophage-derived EVs as drug delivery vehicles for the treatment of LSDs.

Exosome-based strategies are also under investigation for the treatment of NPC. The NPC protein is a large transmembrane cholesterol transporter and these characteristics limit the applicability of an ERT-type or gene therapy approach. Engineered exosomes are currently being developed to carry a functional copy of the NPC protein to neural cells [64].

While exosome therapeutics for LSDs is still an emerging field, recent and ongoing work is promising. As with exosome therapy applied to any other disease, there are still challenges to address before these strategies can be widely implemented. These include determining the exosome's loading capacity and the half-life of the cargo, exploring exosome dosage and biodistribution, and evaluating the kinetics of exosome uptake at the target cells [59]. A better understanding of exosomes, as well as further investigation into their in vivo limitations and any potential immunological response is necessary for the successful development of such therapeutic strategies.

7. Concluding Remarks

This review highlighted the biogenesis and signature of exosomes, their role as intercellular messengers in neuronal circuitry, their fate in a subset of LSDs, and explored the potential applications of exosomes in cell-based therapeutics to treat LSDs. Treatments targeting the nervous system are a crucial unmet need in the LSDs. Further research is also needed to determine both the role and predictability of exosomal cargo as biomarkers for disease states. While the landscape of exosome research continues to evolve, major questions and challenges remain. In particular, in vivo studies capturing the exosomal signature specific to each cell type in the CNS are crucial for interpreting their physiological functions. Such studies will allow us to examine how substrate accumulation or lysosomal dysfunction in the LSDs may influence the spatiotemporal properties of EVs and their impact on the neuronal circuitry in vivo. Further technological advances are required to improve exosomal purification, and improved molecular markers are needed to definitively separate and classify each subpopulation.

A major advantage of the EV transport network over other cellular communication networks (paracrine, autocrine, exocrine) is that EVs can deliver their membrane encapsulated effector cargos across inter-organ distances without becoming diluted or degraded. However, the mechanisms that target a specific subset of EVs to a particular cell type or tissue remain to be explored. While this field is rapidly evolving, further rigorous basic science investigations are needed to better guide the clinical use of exosomes in targeted therapies and diagnostics.

Author Contributions: Their specific contributions are as follows: A.M.G.: Performed literature review and wrote the first draft of the manuscript. E.G.W.: Wrote sections of the manuscript and drafted and prepared the figure. C.M.: Wrote sections of the manuscript and edited the final draft. E.S.: Conceived of and outlined the paper, edited the final versions. All authors have read and agreed to the published version of the manuscript.

Funding: This work was funded by the Intramural Research Programs of the National Human Genome Research Institute, NIGMS PRAT fellowship (AMG) (1FI2GM128643-01) and the National Institutes of Health.

Institutional Review Board Statement: N/A.

Informed Consent Statement: N/A.

Data Availability Statement: N/A.

Acknowledgments: The authors acknowledge Barbara Stubblefield for her help proofreading.

Conflicts of Interest: The authors have no conflicts to disclose.

Appendix A

Vesicles
Enclosed by a lipid bilayer, these tiny spherical sacks are filled with fluid from the parental cell. Depending on their origin, they can carry out a variety of functions including transport and signal transduction.

Extracellular vesicles (EVs)
These lipid bilayer vesicles are naturally released from the cell and range in diameter (50–5000 nm) [65]. Depending on their biogenesis and release pathways, these vesicles include ectosomes, apoptotic bodies, microparticles, microvesicles, and exosomes [66].

Ectosomes
A distinct subtype of EVs that ubiquitously sheds from the plasma membrane. In comparison to exosomes, these vesicles are more variable in size (100–500 nm).

Apoptotic bodies
As another major class of EVs (50–5000 nm) [65], these vesicles are a product of cells undergoing programmed cell death. Increasing evidence suggests that this class of vesicles play a role in immunity surveillance [66].

Exosomes
Nano-sized membrane bound vesicles ranging 70–150 nm in diameter, which begin as intraluminal vesicles found in the multivesicular body (MVB). These released vesicles can be delivered to distant or nearby cells and serve as mediators for intercellular communication.

Exosome cargo
The delivery cargo contained within exosomes includes proteins, lipids, RNAs, DNAs and other cellular components. The molecular contents can be influenced by different physiological and pathological states of the cell. As intercellular communicators, these cargoes can be exchanged, eliminated and illicit cellular response.

Autophagy-lysosomal pathway
An evolutionary conserved process that is activated during stress conditions such as starvation, oxidative stress and other damaging conditions. It involves the bulk degradation of macromolecules or organelles by sending this cargo to the lysosome [67,68].

Lysosome exocytosis
A Ca^{2+} regulated process leading to the extracellular release of lysosomal content. Lysosomes release their contents by migrating from the perinuclear region to the cell surface and fuse with the PM. Exosomes are also present in lysosomes and can be released through this cellular trafficking pathway [46,69].

Autophagosomes
A double membrane compartment that engulfs cytoplasmic substrates destined for degradation. Once the cargo is sequestered, these specialized organelles fuse and deliver their engulfed contents to lysosomes for degradation [67,68].

Messenger RNA (mRNA)
This is a single-stranded RNA molecule that is first transcribed from DNA in the nucleus and then exported to the cytoplasm. This transcript encodes the genetic sequence of a gene which is then translated into protein by ribosome complexes.

MicroRNA (miRNA)
First discovered in *Caenorhabditis elegans* [70,71], these are a subclass of noncoding RNAs, with an average length of 22 nucleotides [72]. They bind to the complimentary sequence of mRNA molecules and turn off gene expression. This post-transcriptional regulation of gene expression can be carried out through a variety of mechanisms. miRNA

has been identified in exosomes, that may be targeted to other cells and modulate gene expression [72].

Endocytosis
A cellular process in which cells internalize materials and nutrients from the outside. This process can be subdivided into four pathways: caveolae, pinocytosis, receptor-mediated endocytosis, and phagocytosis.

Clathrin-coated
Clathrin is a self-polymerizing protein composed of three heavy and light chains that form the triskelion cage. Clathrin coating was first discovered around vesicles invaginating from the plasma membrane and this remains the best characterized transport vesicle.

Early endosome (EE)
As the first compartment of the endocytic pathway, this organelle is found at the periphery of the cell. EEs are noted as tubule-vesicular structures and serve as the principal sorting station.

Endosomal membranes
A collection of intracellular membrane bound organelles that make up the endocytic trafficking network.

Multivesicular bodies (MVB)
A specialized member of the endo-lysosomal compartment that matures from EE by the inward budding into the lumen [7].

Intraluminal vesicles (ILVs)
These vesicles are precursors to exosomes and arise from the inward budding into the lumen of the MVB [7].

Endosomal sorting complex required for transport (ESCRT)
This machinery includes four major complexes ESCRT -0, -I, -II, and -III that form a multicomplex of proteins. Together, these complexes control MVB biogenesis and coordinate the sorting of ubiquitinated membrane proteins to the intraluminal vesicles [73].

Tunneling nanotubules (TnTs)
These long membrane nanotubules protrude from the plasma membrane of one cell and make contacts with another distant cell. This novel route in cell-to-cell communication enables transfer of proteins, cellular organelles, miRNAs and viral pathogens including HIV and prions [74].

Astrocytes
These are specialized glial cells in the CNS. They are the most numerous cell type and harbor a distinct star shaped morphology. This population of cells perform diverse roles such as axon guidance, synaptic support and modulate the blood-brain barrier permeability [75].

Cortical neurons
This class of neurons can be divided into interneurons and projection neurons. Interneurons use GABA as a neurotransmitter while projection neurons utilize glutamate [76].

Oligodendrocytes
This is a specialized glial cell similar to astrocytes whose responsibility is to myelinate the CNS axons [77].

Dynamic Light Scattering
A technique also known as photon correlation spectroscopy, is used to detect the size distribution profile of vesicles by measuring the intensity fluctuations of scattered light when illuminated with a laser beam. This method uses mathematical models derived from Brownian motion and light scattering theory [78].

References

1. Zhang, J.; Li, S.; Li, L.; Li, M.; Guo, C.; Yao, J.; Mi, S. Exosome and exosomal microRNA: Trafficking, sorting, and function. *Genom. Proteom. Bioinform.* **2015**, *13*, 17–24. [CrossRef] [PubMed]
2. Johnstone, R.M.; Adam, M.; Hammond, J.R.; Orr, L.; Turbide, C. Vesicle formation during reticulocyte maturation. Association of plasma membrane activities with released vesicles (exosomes). *J. Biol. Chem.* **1987**, *262*, 9412–9420. [CrossRef]
3. Wolf, P. The nature and significance of platelet products in human plasma. *Br. J. Haematol.* **1967**, *13*, 269–288. [CrossRef] [PubMed]

4. Mulcahy, L.A.; Pink, R.C.; Carter, D.R. Routes and mechanisms of extracellular vesicle uptake. *J. Extracell Vesicles* **2014**, *3*. [CrossRef]
5. Gruenberg, J.; Stenmark, H. The biogenesis of multivesicular endosomes. *Nat. Rev. Mol. Cell Biol.* **2004**, *5*, 317–323. [CrossRef]
6. Kalluri, R.; LeBleu, V.S. The biology, function, and biomedical applications of exosomes. *Science* **2020**, *367*. [CrossRef] [PubMed]
7. Piper, R.C.; Katzmann, D.J. Biogenesis and function of multivesicular bodies. *Annu. Rev. Cell Dev. Biol.* **2007**, *23*, 519–547. [CrossRef]
8. Colombo, M.; Moita, C.; van Niel, G.; Kowal, J.; Vigneron, J.; Benaroch, P.; Manel, N.; Moita, L.F.; Thery, C.; Raposo, G. Analysis of ESCRT functions in exosome biogenesis, composition and secretion highlights the heterogeneity of extracellular vesicles. *J. Cell Sci.* **2013**, *126*, 5553–5565. [CrossRef] [PubMed]
9. Schey, K.L.; Luther, J.M.; Rose, K.L. Proteomics characterization of exosome cargo. *Methods* **2015**, *87*, 75–82. [CrossRef]
10. Chen, S.; Datta-Chaudhuri, A.; Deme, P.; Dickens, A.; Dastgheyb, R.; Bhargava, P.; Bi, H.; Haughey, N.J. Lipidomic characterization of extracellular vesicles in human serum. *J. Circ. Biomark.* **2019**, *8*, 1849454419879848. [CrossRef] [PubMed]
11. Sun, R.; Liu, Y.; Lu, M.; Ding, Q.; Wang, P.; Zhang, H.; Tian, X.; Lu, P.; Meng, D.; Sun, N.; et al. ALIX increases protein content and protective function of iPSC-derived exosomes. *J. Mol. Med. (Berl.)* **2019**, *97*, 829–844. [CrossRef]
12. Yang, F.; Ning, Z.; Ma, L.; Liu, W.; Shao, C.; Shu, Y.; Shen, H. Exosomal miRNAs and miRNA dysregulation in cancer-associated fibroblasts. *Mol. Cancer* **2017**, *16*, 148. [CrossRef]
13. Valadi, H.; Ekstrom, K.; Bossios, A.; Sjostrand, M.; Lee, J.J.; Lotvall, J.O. Exosome-mediated transfer of mRNAs and microRNAs is a novel mechanism of genetic exchange between cells. *Nat. Cell Biol.* **2007**, *9*, 654–659. [CrossRef] [PubMed]
14. Skotland, T.; Hessvik, N.P.; Sandvig, K.; Llorente, A. Exosomal lipid composition and the role of ether lipids and phosphoinositides in exosome biology. *J. Lipid Res.* **2019**, *60*, 9–18. [CrossRef]
15. Trajkovic, K.; Hsu, C.; Chiantia, S.; Rajendran, L.; Wenzel, D.; Wieland, F.; Schwille, P.; Brugger, B.; Simons, M. Ceramide triggers budding of exosome vesicles into multivesicular endosomes. *Science* **2008**, *319*, 1244–1247. [CrossRef] [PubMed]
16. Keerthikumar, S.; Chisanga, D.; Ariyaratne, D.; Al Saffar, H.; Anand, S.; Zhao, K.; Samuel, M.; Pathan, M.; Jois, M.; Chilamkurti, N.; et al. ExoCarta: A Web-Based Compendium of Exosomal Cargo. *J. Mol. Biol.* **2016**, *428*, 688–692. [CrossRef] [PubMed]
17. Maia, J.; Caja, S.; Strano Moraes, M.C.; Couto, N.; Costa-Silva, B. Exosome-Based Cell-Cell Communication in the Tumor Microenvironment. *Front. Cell Dev. Biol.* **2018**, *6*, 18. [CrossRef]
18. Cocucci, E.; Meldolesi, J. Ectosomes and exosomes: Shedding the confusion between extracellular vesicles. *Trends Cell Biol.* **2015**, *25*, 364–372. [CrossRef] [PubMed]
19. Pan, B.T.; Johnstone, R. Selective externalization of the transferrin receptor by sheep reticulocytes in vitro. Response to ligands and inhibitors of endocytosis. *J. Biol. Chem.* **1984**, *259*, 9776–9782. [CrossRef]
20. Kosaka, N.; Iguchi, H.; Hagiwara, K.; Yoshioka, Y.; Takeshita, F.; Ochiya, T. Neutral sphingomyelinase 2 (nSMase2)-dependent exosomal transfer of angiogenic microRNAs regulate cancer cell metastasis. *J. Biol. Chem.* **2013**, *288*, 10849–10859. [CrossRef] [PubMed]
21. Kosaka, N.; Iguchi, H.; Yoshioka, Y.; Takeshita, F.; Matsuki, Y.; Ochiya, T. Secretory mechanisms and intercellular transfer of microRNAs in living cells. *J. Biol. Chem.* **2010**, *285*, 17442–17452. [CrossRef] [PubMed]
22. Baietti, M.F.; Zhang, Z.; Mortier, E.; Melchior, A.; Degeest, G.; Geeraerts, A.; Ivarsson, Y.; Depoortere, F.; Coomans, C.; Vermeiren, E.; et al. Syndecan-syntenin-ALIX regulates the biogenesis of exosomes. *Nat. Cell Biol.* **2012**, *14*, 677–685. [CrossRef] [PubMed]
23. Ostrowski, M.; Carmo, N.B.; Krumeich, S.; Fanget, I.; Raposo, G.; Savina, A.; Moita, C.F.; Schauer, K.; Hume, A.N.; Freitas, R.P.; et al. Rab27a and Rab27b control different steps of the exosome secretion pathway. *Nat. Cell Biol.* **2010**, *12*, 19–30. [CrossRef] [PubMed]
24. Yu, X.; Harris, S.L.; Levine, A.J. The regulation of exosome secretion: A novel function of the p53 protein. *Cancer Res.* **2006**, *66*, 4795–4801. [CrossRef] [PubMed]
25. Santangelo, L.; Giurato, G.; Cicchini, C.; Montaldo, C.; Mancone, C.; Tarallo, R.; Battistelli, C.; Alonzi, T.; Weisz, A.; Tripodi, M. The RNA-Binding Protein SYNCRIP Is a Component of the Hepatocyte Exosomal Machinery Controlling MicroRNA Sorting. *Cell Rep.* **2016**, *17*, 799–808. [CrossRef]
26. You, Y.; Borgmann, K.; Edara, V.V.; Stacy, S.; Ghorpade, A.; Ikezu, T. Activated human astrocyte-derived extracellular vesicles modulate neuronal uptake, differentiation and firing. *J. Extracell Vesicles* **2020**, *9*, 1706801. [CrossRef] [PubMed]
27. Wang, G.; Dinkins, M.; He, Q.; Zhu, G.; Poirier, C.; Campbell, A.; Mayer-Proschel, M.; Bieberich, E. Astrocytes secrete exosomes enriched with proapoptotic ceramide and prostate apoptosis response 4 (PAR-4): Potential mechanism of apoptosis induction in Alzheimer disease (AD). *J. Biol. Chem.* **2012**, *287*, 21384–21395. [CrossRef] [PubMed]
28. Faure, J.; Lachenal, G.; Court, M.; Hirrlinger, J.; Chatellard-Causse, C.; Blot, B.; Grange, J.; Schoehn, G.; Goldberg, Y.; Boyer, V.; et al. Exosomes are released by cultured cortical neurones. *Mol. Cell Neurosci.* **2006**, *31*, 642–648. [CrossRef]
29. Lachenal, G.; Pernet-Gallay, K.; Chivet, M.; Hemming, F.J.; Belly, A.; Bodon, G.; Blot, B.; Haase, G.; Goldberg, Y.; Sadoul, R. Release of exosomes from differentiated neurons and its regulation by synaptic glutamatergic activity. *Mol. Cell Neurosci.* **2011**, *46*, 409–418. [CrossRef] [PubMed]
30. Chivet, M.; Hemming, F.; Pernet-Gallay, K.; Fraboulet, S.; Sadoul, R. Emerging role of neuronal exosomes in the central nervous system. *Front. Physiol.* **2012**, *3*, 145. [CrossRef]
31. Fitzner, D.; Schnaars, M.; van Rossum, D.; Krishnamoorthy, G.; Dibaj, P.; Bakhti, M.; Regen, T.; Hanisch, U.K.; Simons, M. Selective transfer of exosomes from oligodendrocytes to microglia by macropinocytosis. *J. Cell Sci.* **2011**, *124*, 447–458. [CrossRef] [PubMed]

32. Kramer-Albers, E.M.; Bretz, N.; Tenzer, S.; Winterstein, C.; Mobius, W.; Berger, H.; Nave, K.A.; Schild, H.; Trotter, J. Oligodendrocytes secrete exosomes containing major myelin and stress-protective proteins: Trophic support for axons? *Proteom. Clin. Appl.* **2007**, *1*, 1446–1461. [CrossRef] [PubMed]
33. Fruhbeis, C.; Frohlich, D.; Kuo, W.P.; Amphornrat, J.; Thilemann, S.; Saab, A.S.; Kirchhoff, F.; Mobius, W.; Goebbels, S.; Nave, K.A.; et al. Neurotransmitter-triggered transfer of exosomes mediates oligodendrocyte-neuron communication. *PLoS Biol.* **2013**, *11*, e1001604. [CrossRef]
34. Frohlich, D.; Kuo, W.P.; Fruhbeis, C.; Sun, J.J.; Zehendner, C.M.; Luhmann, H.J.; Pinto, S.; Toedling, J.; Trotter, J.; Kramer-Albers, E.M. Multifaceted effects of oligodendroglial exosomes on neurons: Impact on neuronal firing rate, signal transduction and gene regulation. *Philos. Trans. R. Soc. Lond. B Biol. Sci.* **2014**, *369*. [CrossRef]
35. Platt, F.M.; d'Azzo, A.; Davidson, B.L.; Neufeld, E.F.; Tifft, C.J. Lysosomal storage diseases. *Nat. Rev. Dis. Primers* **2018**, *4*, 27. [CrossRef]
36. Meikle, P.J.; Hopwood, J.J.; Clague, A.E.; Carey, W.F. Prevalence of lysosomal storage disorders. *JAMA* **1999**, *281*, 249–254. [CrossRef]
37. Platt, F.M.; Boland, B.; van der Spoel, A.C. The cell biology of disease: Lysosomal storage disorders: The cellular impact of lysosomal dysfunction. *J. Cell Biol.* **2012**, *199*, 723–734. [CrossRef]
38. Kaye, E.M. Lysosomal Storage Diseases. *Curr. Treat. Options Neurol.* **2001**, *3*, 249–256. [CrossRef]
39. Eitan, E.; Suire, C.; Zhang, S.; Mattson, M.P. Impact of lysosome status on extracellular vesicle content and release. *Ageing Res. Rev.* **2016**, *32*, 65–74. [CrossRef] [PubMed]
40. Polten, A.; Fluharty, A.L.; Fluharty, C.B.; Kappler, J.; von Figura, K.; Gieselmann, V. Molecular basis of different forms of metachromatic leukodystrophy. *N. Engl. J. Med.* **1991**, *324*, 18–22. [CrossRef] [PubMed]
41. Gieselmann, V.; Krageloh-Mann, I. Metachromatic leukodystrophy—An update. *Neuropediatrics* **2010**, *41*, 1–6. [CrossRef]
42. Klein, D.; Bussow, H.; Fewou, S.N.; Gieselmann, V. Exocytosis of storage material in a lysosomal disorder. *Biochem. Biophys. Res. Commun.* **2005**, *327*, 663–667. [CrossRef]
43. Bach, G. Mucolipidosis type IV. *Mol. Genet. Metab.* **2001**, *73*, 197–203. [CrossRef]
44. Bargal, R.; Avidan, N.; Olender, T.; Ben Asher, E.; Zeigler, M.; Raas-Rothschild, A.; Frumkin, A.; Ben-Yoseph, O.; Friedlender, Y.; Lancet, D.; et al. Mucolipidosis type IV: Novel MCOLN1 mutations in Jewish and non-Jewish patients and the frequency of the disease in the Ashkenazi Jewish population. *Hum. Mutat.* **2001**, *17*, 397–402. [CrossRef] [PubMed]
45. LaPlante, J.M.; Sun, M.; Falardeau, J.; Dai, D.; Brown, E.M.; Slaugenhaupt, S.A.; Vassilev, P.M. Lysosomal exocytosis is impaired in mucolipidosis type IV. *Mol. Genet. Metab.* **2006**, *89*, 339–348. [CrossRef] [PubMed]
46. Kim, M.S.; Muallem, S.; Kim, S.H.; Kwon, K.B.; Kim, M.S. Exosomal release through TRPML1-mediated lysosomal exocytosis is required for adipogenesis. *Biochem. Biophys. Res. Commun.* **2019**, *510*, 409–415. [CrossRef] [PubMed]
47. Bonten, E.; van der Spoel, A.; Fornerod, M.; Grosveld, G.; d'Azzo, A. Characterization of human lysosomal neuraminidase defines the molecular basis of the metabolic storage disorder sialidosis. *Genes Dev.* **1996**, *10*, 3156–3169. [CrossRef]
48. Rottier, R.J.; Bonten, E.; d'Azzo, A. A point mutation in the neu-1 locus causes the neuraminidase defect in the SM/J mouse. *Hum. Mol. Genet.* **1998**, *7*, 313–321. [CrossRef]
49. Yogalingam, G.; Bonten, E.J.; van de Vlekkert, D.; Hu, H.; Moshiach, S.; Connell, S.A.; d'Azzo, A. Neuraminidase 1 is a negative regulator of lysosomal exocytosis. *Dev. Cell* **2008**, *15*, 74–86. [CrossRef]
50. van de Vlekkert, D.; Demmers, J.; Nguyen, X.X.; Campos, Y.; Machado, E.; Annunziata, I.; Hu, H.; Gomero, E.; Qiu, X.; Bongiovanni, A.; et al. Excessive exosome release is the pathogenic pathway linking a lysosomal deficiency to generalized fibrosis. *Sci. Adv.* **2019**, *5*, eaav3270. [CrossRef]
51. Meng, X.M.; Nikolic-Paterson, D.J.; Lan, H.Y. TGF-beta: The master regulator of fibrosis. *Nat. Rev. Nephrol.* **2016**, *12*, 325–338. [CrossRef] [PubMed]
52. Cao, H.; Wang, C.; Chen, X.; Hou, J.; Xiang, Z.; Shen, Y.; Han, X. Inhibition of Wnt/beta-catenin signaling suppresses myofibroblast differentiation of lung resident mesenchymal stem cells and pulmonary fibrosis. *Sci. Rep.* **2018**, *8*, 13644. [CrossRef] [PubMed]
53. Nesterova, G.; Gahl, W.A. Cystinosis: The evolution of a treatable disease. *Pediatr. Nephrol.* **2013**, *28*, 51–59. [CrossRef] [PubMed]
54. Naphade, S.; Sharma, J.; Gaide Chevronnay, H.P.; Shook, M.A.; Yeagy, B.A.; Rocca, C.J.; Ur, S.N.; Lau, A.J.; Courtoy, P.J.; Cherqui, S. Brief reports: Lysosomal cross-correction by hematopoietic stem cell-derived macrophages via tunneling nanotubes. *Stem Cells* **2015**, *33*, 301–309. [CrossRef] [PubMed]
55. Cherqui, S.; Courtoy, P.J. The renal Fanconi syndrome in cystinosis: Pathogenic insights and therapeutic perspectives. *Nat. Rev. Nephrol.* **2017**, *13*, 115–131. [CrossRef]
56. Chang, T.Y.; Reid, P.C.; Sugii, S.; Ohgami, N.; Cruz, J.C.; Chang, C.C. Niemann-Pick type C disease and intracellular cholesterol trafficking. *J. Biol. Chem.* **2005**, *280*, 20917–20920. [CrossRef]
57. Strauss, K.; Goebel, C.; Runz, H.; Mobius, W.; Weiss, S.; Feussner, I.; Simons, M.; Schneider, A. Exosome secretion ameliorates lysosomal storage of cholesterol in Niemann-Pick type C disease. *J. Biol. Chem.* **2010**, *285*, 26279–26288. [CrossRef]
58. Tatiana, S.; Stanislav, N.; Darya, K.; Luiza, G.; Konstantin, S.; Sergey, L.; Elena, V.; Galina, S.; Nikolai, V.; Arthur, K.; et al. Altered level of plasma exosomes in patients with Gaucher disease. *Eur. J. Med. Genet.* **2020**, *63*, 104038. [CrossRef] [PubMed]
59. Sarko, D.K.; McKinney, C.E. Exosomes: Origins and Therapeutic Potential for Neurodegenerative Disease. *Front. Neurosci.* **2017**, *11*, 82. [CrossRef] [PubMed]

60. Edelmann, M.J.; Maegawa, G.H.B. CNS-Targeting Therapies for Lysosomal Storage Diseases: Current Advances and Challenges. *Front. Mol. Biosci.* **2020**, *7*, 559804. [CrossRef] [PubMed]
61. Choi, K.; Choi, H.; Yim, N.; Ryu, S.-W.; Choi, C. Exosome-based delivery of glucocerebrosidase lysosomal enzyme for treatment of Gaucher disease. *Mol. Genet. Metab.* **2018**, *123*, S31–S32. [CrossRef]
62. Do, M.A.; Levy, D.; Brown, A.; Marriott, G.; Lu, B. Targeted delivery of lysosomal enzymes to the endocytic compartment in human cells using engineered extracellular vesicles. *Sci. Rep.* **2019**, *9*, 17274. [CrossRef] [PubMed]
63. Haney, M.J.; Klyachko, N.L.; Harrison, E.B.; Zhao, Y.; Kabanov, A.V.; Batrakova, E.V. TPP1 Delivery to Lysosomes with Extracellular Vesicles and their Enhanced Brain Distribution in the Animal Model of Batten Disease. *Adv. Healthc. Mater.* **2019**, *8*, e1801271. [CrossRef] [PubMed]
64. Zipkin, M. Exosome redux. *Nat. Biotechnol.* **2019**, *37*, 1395–1400. [CrossRef] [PubMed]
65. Carnino, J.M.; Lee, H.; Jin, Y. Isolation and characterization of extracellular vesicles from Broncho-alveolar lavage fluid: A review and comparison of different methods. *Respir. Res.* **2019**, *20*, 240. [CrossRef] [PubMed]
66. Battistelli, M.; Falcieri, E. Apoptotic Bodies: Particular Extracellular Vesicles Involved in Intercellular Communication. *Biology* **2020**, *9*, 21. [CrossRef] [PubMed]
67. Kenney, D.L.; Benarroch, E.E. The autophagy-lysosomal pathway: General concepts and clinical implications. *Neurology* **2015**, *85*, 634–645. [CrossRef] [PubMed]
68. Eskelinen, E.L.; Saftig, P. Autophagy: A lysosomal degradation pathway with a central role in health and disease. *Biochim. Biophys. Acta* **2009**, *1793*, 664–673. [CrossRef]
69. Machado, E.; White-Gilbertson, S.; van de Vlekkert, D.; Janke, L.; Moshiach, S.; Campos, Y.; Finkelstein, D.; Gomero, E.; Mosca, R.; Qiu, X.; et al. Regulated lysosomal exocytosis mediates cancer progression. *Sci. Adv.* **2015**, *1*, e1500603. [CrossRef] [PubMed]
70. Lee, R.C.; Feinbaum, R.L.; Ambros, V. The C. elegans heterochronic gene lin-4 encodes small RNAs with antisense complementarity to lin-14. *Cell* **1993**, *75*, 843–854. [CrossRef]
71. Wightman, B.; Ha, I.; Ruvkun, G. Posttranscriptional regulation of the heterochronic gene lin-14 by lin-4 mediates temporal pattern formation in C. elegans. *Cell* **1993**, *75*, 855–862. [CrossRef]
72. Chatrchyan, S.; Khachatryan, V.; Sirunyan, A.M.; Tumasyan, A.; Adam, W.; Bergauer, T.; Dragicevic, M.; Ero, J.; Fabjan, C.; Friedl, M.; et al. Search for new physics with a monojet and missing transverse energy in pp collisions at radicals = 7 TeV. *Phys. Rev. Lett.* **2011**, *107*, 201804. [CrossRef] [PubMed]
73. Slagsvold, T.; Pattni, K.; Malerod, L.; Stenmark, H. Endosomal and non-endosomal functions of ESCRT proteins. *Trends Cell Biol.* **2006**, *16*, 317–326. [CrossRef]
74. Kolba, M.D.; Dudka, W.; Zareba-Koziol, M.; Kominek, A.; Ronchi, P.; Turos, L.; Chroscicki, P.; Wlodarczyk, J.; Schwab, Y.; Klejman, A.; et al. Tunneling nanotube-mediated intercellular vesicle and protein transfer in the stroma-provided imatinib resistance in chronic myeloid leukemia cells. *Cell Death Dis.* **2019**, *10*, 817. [CrossRef] [PubMed]
75. Siracusa, R.; Fusco, R.; Cuzzocrea, S. Astrocytes: Role and Functions in Brain Pathologies. *Front. Pharmacol.* **2019**, *10*, 1114. [CrossRef] [PubMed]
76. Campbell, K. Cortical neuron specification: It has its time and place. *Neuron* **2005**, *46*, 373–376. [CrossRef] [PubMed]
77. Bradl, M.; Lassmann, H. Oligodendrocytes: Biology and pathology. *Acta Neuropathol.* **2010**, *119*, 37–53. [CrossRef] [PubMed]
78. van der Pol, E.; Coumans, F.; Varga, Z.; Krumrey, M.; Nieuwland, R. Innovation in detection of microparticles and exosomes. *J. Thromb Haemost* **2013**, *11* (Suppl. 1), 36–45. [CrossRef]

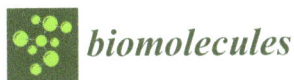

Review

Precision Medicine for Lysosomal Disorders

Filippo Pinto e Vairo [1,2,†], **Diana Rojas Málaga** [3,*,†], **Francyne Kubaski** [4,5,6,7], **Carolina Fischinger Moura de Souza** [4], **Fabiano de Oliveira Poswar** [4], **Guilherme Baldo** [5,8,9,10] and **Roberto Giugliani** [4,5,6,7,8,11]

1. Center for Individualized Medicine, Mayo Clinic, Rochester, MN 55905, USA; vairo.filippo@mayo.edu
2. Department of Clinical Genomics, Mayo Clinic, Rochester, MN 55905, USA
3. Grupo Fleury, São Paulo 04344-070, Brazil
4. Medical Genetics Service, HCPA, Porto Alegre 90035-903, Brazil; fkubaski@udel.edu (F.K.); cfsouza@hcpa.edu.br (C.F.M.d.S.); fposwar@hcpa.edu.br (F.d.O.P.); rgiugliani@hcpa.edu.br (R.G.)
5. Postgraduate Program in Genetics and Molecular Biology, UFRGS, Porto Alegre 91501-970, Brazil; gbaldo@hcpa.edu.br
6. Biodiscovery Laboratory, HCPA, Porto Alegre 90035-903, Brazil
7. INAGEMP, Porto Alegre 90035-004, Brazil
8. Gene Therapy Center, HCPA, Porto Alegre 90035-903, Brazil
9. Department of Physiology and Pharmacology, UFRGS, Porto Alegre 90050-170, Brazil
10. Postgraduate Program in Biological Sciences: Physiology, UFRGS, Porto Alegre 90050-170, Brazil
11. Department of Genetics, UFRGS, Porto Alegre 91501-970, Brazil
* Correspondence: inova.diana@grupofleury.com.br
† These authors contributed equally to this paper.

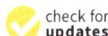

Received: 22 June 2020; Accepted: 23 July 2020; Published: 26 July 2020

Abstract: Precision medicine (PM) is an emerging approach for disease treatment and prevention that accounts for the individual variability in the genes, environment, and lifestyle of each person. Lysosomal diseases (LDs) are a group of genetic metabolic disorders that include approximately 70 monogenic conditions caused by a defect in lysosomal function. LDs may result from primary lysosomal enzyme deficiencies or impairments in membrane-associated proteins, lysosomal enzyme activators, or modifiers that affect lysosomal function. LDs are heterogeneous disorders, and the phenotype of the affected individual depends on the type of substrate and where it accumulates, which may be impacted by the type of genetic change and residual enzymatic activity. LDs are individually rare, with a combined incidence of approximately 1:4000 individuals. Specific therapies are already available for several LDs, and many more are in development. Early identification may enable disease course prediction and a specific intervention, which is very important for clinical outcome. Driven by advances in omics technology, PM aims to provide the most appropriate management for each patient based on the disease susceptibility or treatment response predictions for specific subgroups. In this review, we focused on the emerging diagnostic technologies that may help to optimize the management of each LD patient and the therapeutic options available, as well as in clinical developments that enable customized approaches to be selected for each subject, according to the principles of PM.

Keywords: lysosomal diseases; precision medicine; enzyme replacement therapy; pharmacological chaperones; gene therapy.

1. Introduction

According to the National Institutes of Health (NIH), "precision medicine" (PM) is "an emerging approach for disease treatment and prevention that takes into account individual variability in genes, environment, and lifestyle for each person." The terms "personalized medicine", "individualized medicine", and "precision medicine" have been used interchangeably in recent years; however, precision medicine has been the preferred term since 2015 when the Precision Medicine Initiative (PMI) was launched.

The PMI is a research endeavor funded by the NIH that aims to understand the functional consequences of individual genomic variations and how they interact with the environment to determine the best approach to prevent or treat diseases [1]. PM encompasses the use of advanced diagnostic tools, such as genomic analyses through whole-exome sequencing (WES) or whole-genome sequencing (WGS); other omics, such as metabolomics and epigenomics; advanced imaging; personal and population health information, and big data analytics [2]. Thus, PM refers to the tailoring of the treatment to an individual genetic background, but it does not mean the creation of devices or drugs for only a specific individual. It provides the ability to sort individuals into categories based on their disease susceptibility or predicted response to a treatment. Nonetheless, the term "personalized medicine" may be misleading, suggesting that a unique treatment can be designed for each person, which is not accurate [3].

Lysosomal diseases (LDs) are a group of approximately 70 monogenic disorders caused by a defect in lysosomal function. LDs may result from enzymatic deficiencies (e.g., Gaucher disease (GD)) or impairments in membrane-associated transporters (e.g., cystinosis), enzyme modifiers (e.g., mucolipidosis II and III) or activators (e.g., saposin deficiency) [4]. Although individually rare, the incidence of LDs as a group is estimated to be as high as 1 in 4000 in some countries [5,6]. LDs are heterogeneous disorders, and the phenotype of the affected individual depends on the type of substrate and where it accumulates, as well as the type of genetic change and residual enzymatic activity. Some phenotypes are common to many LDs, such as coarse facies, progressive developmental delay, visceromegaly, and skeletal changes. However, there are disorders that mainly affect the central nervous system (CNS (e.g., neuronal ceroid lipofuscinoses [NCLs])) and others that do not present with primary CNS involvement.

The standard diagnostic work-up for several LDs is based on the clinical presentation; the detection of biomarkers in blood, urine, or cerebrospinal fluid (CSF), and the direct measurement of enzyme activity in leukocytes, plasma, or fibroblasts. Genetic testing is usually performed to confirm or document the biochemical diagnosis but, depending on the disease, might be the only available diagnostic approach.

In the past two decades, pharmaceutical companies have strongly invested in the development of specific therapies for the treatment of LDs, mainly in the form of recombinant enzymes for enzyme replacement therapy (ERT (Table 1)). These medications are usually used intravenously and aim at breaking down the substrates which have accumulated due to an enzymatic deficiency. GD was the first LD to benefit from this approach, with great success. Notably, there is variability in the clinical efficacy due to the severity of the clinical picture, presence of antibodies against the recombinant enzyme, and lack of efficiency in difficult-to-target organs, such as bone, cartilage, and, more importantly, the brain, since the enzyme does not cross the blood–brain barrier (BBB) [7].

Table 1. Market-approved enzyme replacement therapies (ERTs) and hematopoietic stem cell transplantation (HSCT) outcomes.

Disease	Product	Manufacturer	FDA or EMA* Approval	Prescribing Information	Comments on HSCT
Alpha-Mannosidosis	Lamzede®	Chiesi	2018*	https://www.ema.europa.eu/en/documents/product-information/lamzede-epar-product-information_en.pdf	Effective, maybe an alternative to ERT [8]
Fabry disease	Replagal®	Takeda/Shire	2001	https://www.ema.europa.eu/en/documents/product-information/replagal-epar-product-information_en.pdf	Not effective
	Fabrazyme®	Sanofi/Genzyme	2001	www.fabrazyme.com/hcp/pi/fz_us_hc_pi.pdf	
	Fabagal®#	ISU ABXIS	2014#	http://www.abxis.com/eng/product/doc_fabagal.pdf	
Gaucher type I	Cerezyme®*	Sanofi/Genzyme	1994	www.cerezyme.com/-/l/media/files/CerezymeUS/pdf/cerezyme_pi.pdf	Effective, maybe an alternative to ERT [9]
	Velaglucerase alfa	Takeda/Shire	2010	www.accessdata.fda.gov/drugsatfda_docs/label/2010/022575lbl.pdf	
	Elelyso™	Pfizer/Protalix	2012	www.elelyso.com/pdf/ELELYSO_Prescribing_Information.pdf	
	Abcertin®#	ISU ABXIS	2012#	http://www.abxis.com/eng/product/doc_abcertin.pdf	
Lysosomal acid lipase deficiency	Kanuma™	Alexion	2015	https://kanuma.com/hcp	High mortality rate due to transplant related complications, liver failure or sinusoidal obstruction syndrome [10]
Mucopolysaccharidosis I	Aldurazyme®	Sanofi/Genzyme	2003	www.aldurazyme.com/pdf/az_us_hc_pi.pdf	Effective, maybe an alternative to ERT; recommended for patients with the Hurler phenotype if performed early [11]
Mucopolysaccharidosis II	Elaprase®	Takeda/Shire	2006	www.elaprase.com/pdf/Elaprase_US_PI_v6.pdf	Effective if performed in early disease stages before irreversible disease manifestations have occurred [12,13]
	Hunterase®	GC Pharma/Nanolek LLC	2012#	https://www.nanolek.ru/en/product/biotekhnologicheskie/khanteraza/	

Table 1. Cont.

Disease	Product	Manufacturer	FDA or EMA* Approval	Prescribing Information	Comments on HSCT
Mucopolysaccharidosis IVA	Vimizin®	BioMarin	2014	https://vimizim.com/hcp/prescribing-information/	Reported in a few cases, may be an alternative treatment if performed early [14]
Mucopolysaccharidosis VI	Naglazyme™	BioMarin	2005	www.naglazyme.com/en/documents/Naglazyme_Prescribing_Information.pdf	Effective, maybe an alternative to ERT [15]
Mucopolysaccharidosis type VII	Mepsevii™	Ultragenyx	2017	https://www.accessdata.fda.gov/drugsatfda_docs/label/2017/761047s000lbl.pdf	Reported in a few cases, may be an alternative treatment if performed early [16]
Neuronal ceroid lipofuscinosis type 2	Brineura™	BioMarin	2017	https://www.brineura.com/wp-content/themes/jupiter-child/assets/pdfs/resources/Brineura-Dosing-and-Administration-Guide.pdf	Not effective
Pompe disease	Myozyme®	Sanofi/Genzyme	2006	www.accessdata.fda.gov/drugsatfda_docs/label/2008/125141_74lbl.pdf	Not effective
	Lumizyme®	Sanofi/Genzyme	2010	www.accessdata.fda.gov/drugsatfda_docs/label/2010/125291lbl.pdf	

approved in South Korea. * Ceredase was made from placenta and it was the precursor of Cerezyme®.

Before the development of ERT, hematopoietic stem cell transplantation (HSCT) was the only therapy to treat LDs. It has been used successfully to treat GD and neuronopathic forms of mucopolysaccharidosis (MPS) type I, for instance (Table 1).

Another treatment approach is substrate reduction, which aims to decrease the production of the storage material. There are market-approved drugs in this category for GD and Niemann–Pick type C (NPC) and several clinical and preclinical trials for other diseases, such as Fabry disease (FD), Pompe disease (PD), and GM_2 gangliosidosis (GM_2). Regardless of the specific treatment, individuals with LDs usually need a multidisciplinary approach for supportive care to prevent and treat complications, which includes hearing aids, orthoses, speech, respiratory and physical therapies, and psychological support, among others. Importantly, several LDs are targets of researchers and companies interested in gene therapy and genome editing approaches since they are well-characterized monogenic diseases; there are still unmet needs, and even a slight increase in the enzymatic activity could be sufficient to achieve clinical benefits.

The basic concept of PM has been a part of healthcare for many years. Solid organ or bone marrow transplant recipients have always been matched to compatible donors to reduce the risk of complications. For example, in the LD field, ERT dosage has been tailored or even deemed unnecessary. Moreover, hematopoietic stem cell transplantation (HSCT) has been based on the genotype of patients. However, the more comprehensive concept of PM, including novel molecular diagnostic tools and big data analysis, is still relatively limited in medical practice.

In this review, we highlight the advances in the diagnostic approaches and in the development of novel tailored therapies for individuals with LDs.

2. Molecular Diagnosis Advances for Lysosomal Diseases

Among the novel technological drivers of PM, next-generation sequencing (NGS) methods have the greatest effect on the diagnostics of LDs since they are becoming more accessible and affordable [17]. NGS applications include the sequencing of a set of specific genomic regions (targeted NGS panel), WES and WGS. These technologies are powerful approaches to overcome the wide clinical and genetic heterogeneity of LDs, allowing the simultaneous screening of several LD-related genes with shorter turnaround times for the final report [18,19].

In the NGS targeted panel, the genes investigated are known to be related to the patient's phenotype. This approach is heavily dependent on a diagnostic hypothesis that determines which set of genes will be analyzed for each patient, which is disadvantageous when patients with milder or atypical phenotypes are analyzed. In this scenario, a comprehensive gene panel could be helpful, allowing the expansion of the phenotypic spectrum of these disorders. For example, central nervous system involvement is predominant in MPS III, several neuronal ceroid lipofuscinoses, and Tay–Sachs disease, which would justify the inclusion of the associated genes in a neurological-focused panel. Meanwhile, MPS IV-, MPS VI-, or pycnodysostosis-associated genes could be included in a general skeletal dysplasia panel [18]. Whole–exomesequencing (WES) is a standard diagnosisprocedureinmanyplacesandlikewiseisusedtofindnovelgenesassociatedwithrareconditions, such as the newly discovered MPStype (mucopolysaccharidosis–plussyndrome, MPSPS) [20,21], expanding the recognized phenotypic spectrum of known LDs [22,23] and elucidating complex phenotypes [24]. Moreover, several LDs remain undiagnosed after extensive genetic and biochemical investigations due to a wide phenotypic spectrum of nonspecific manifestations or lack of available clinical tests, so WES may be used to identify undiagnosed patients [25]. Although WGS is still not part of a routine clinical diagnosis, it has often been used in a research context to aid in the characterization of complex alterations [26,27]. Notably, ethical aspects are one of the challenges of WES and WGS due to the possibility of identifying variants in genes not related to the main phenotype [28].

Currently, molecular analyses using these three approaches have several roles in LD diagnosis: (1) to confirm the final diagnosis, mainly in milder and atypical cases [29]; (2) to clarify borderline biochemical results in screening and enzymatic assays, as obtained in carriers and pseudodeficiency cases (when enzyme activity is decreased but with no clinical consequences) [30]; (3) to characterize a novel gene associated with a new type of LD, such as the cases of *VPS33A* in MPSPS [21] and *DESG1* in leukodystrophy [31]; (4) for prenatal diagnosis [32,33]; (5) to predict disease severity [34,35]; (6) for the identification of patients with variants amenable to targeted therapy [36,37].

Although next-generation sequencing is revolutionizing LDs diagnosis, the sheer number of distinct conditions, the limited number of patients affected by each rare disease, and the high associated costs represents major challenges for drug development for these diseases.

3. Metabolomics As a New Tool for Diagnosis and Monitoring

The term metabolomics was introduced in 2002 to define the deep analysis of small molecules that are part of metabolic pathways by high-throughput analytical methodologies combined with high-end statistical analyses [38–40]. Due to the complexity of the interactions of metabolites in our complex systems, these molecules should be properly identified and quantified. The main methods employed for these analyses are nuclear magnetic resonance (NMR) spectroscopy and mass spectrometry (MS), which can be additionally coupled to reduced ion suppression with capillary electrophoresis (CE) for polar charged compounds, gas chromatography (GC) for the analysis of volatile compounds or liquid chromatography (LC) for the analysis of polar and nonpolar compounds [40,41].

Metabolomics can be extremely useful for the diagnosis and monitoring of LDs and can also lead to the discovery of novel biomarkers that can be crucial from diagnosis to treatment follow-up. These molecules can even be used for the discovery of novel LDs [40,42,43].

In 2005, the Human Metabolome Project was launched, aiming to identify connections between genes, diseases, and metabolites to aid the investigation of metabolites associated with inborn errors of metabolism that are reported in the human metabolome database (HMDB) [44,45]. The HMDB is currently the largest database of metabolomics, and it can be used to clarify which metabolic pathway is disturbed for each disorder, enabling the identification and study of key metabolites. A classic example of how metabolomics has aided in the diagnosis and monitoring of LDs is the discovery of globotriaosylsphingosine (lyso-Gb3) as a biomarker for FD [46–51].

The two major approaches used in metabolomics studies are based on targeted and untargeted analysis. Targeted metabolomics comprises the analysis of specific metabolites that are usually quantified and compared, leading to the establishment of reference ranges. This panel-based approach can reduce the time of diagnosis for several disorders [51–53]. The untargeted approach consists of analyzing all the detectable metabolites (known and unknown) in any type of sample matrix (tissue or biological fluid) to elucidate whether there are any abnormalities that can be correlated with disorders [53,54]. The matrix-assisted laser desorption/ionization-time of flight mass spectrometry (MALDI-TOF) profiling has been widely used for untargeted metabolomics followed by liquid chromatography tandem mass spectrometry [40,55].

The targeted analysis of metabolites is useful in newborn screening (NBS) of LDs (as a primary target, or in a second-tier analysis), as well as to monitor treatment. However, more recently, an untargeted analysis has also been applied to some LDs. Untargeted metabolomics can deepen the understanding of disease mechanisms, allowing discoveries of better biomarkers, new treatment options and personalized therapies. As an example, a metabolome analysis revealed an abnormal polyamine metabolism in the cerebrospinal fluid (CSF) of patients with neuronopathic forms of mucopolysaccharidosis (MPS). Since treatment options for MPS I vary according to the patient's phenotype, the assessment of these metabolites can help to decide which treatment is more appropriate for each patient [56].

In another study [57] performed in MPS IIIB mice, 231 serum metabolites were altered early in the disease's natural history. The authors treated mice with gene therapy, and almost 90% of these molecules were corrected. Considering the limitations of current biomarkers, these data show that the metabolites can be used as surrogate markers; their normalization could indicate treatment effectiveness and could be potentially used for the adjustment of doses, for example.

4. Next-Generation Treatments

While standard treatments are successful in many instances, there are also certain groups of patients for which these standard approaches are not the best solution. Some alternative therapeutic approaches, such as pharmacological chaperones, gene therapy, and substrate reduction therapy, are in development, with many currently under clinical trials demonstrating great potential (Table 2).

Table 2. Active clinical trials for lysosomal diseases (as of June, 2020).

Disease	Treatment	Product	Expected outcomes	Cons	Status	EudraCT number	NCT Number	Sponsor
Acid Sphingomyelinase Deficiency	Intravenous enzyme replacement therapy	Olipudase alfa	Overall disease improvement	Efficacy to be determined	Terminated	n/a	NCT00410566	Genzyme, a Sanofi Company
Alpha-mannosidosis	Intrathecal administration of cell therapy	Umbilical cord blood-derived oligodendrocyte-like cells	Rapid delivery of donor cells in the CNS; constant enzyme secretion; one-time treatment	Conditioning side-effects; safety and efficacy still to be determined	Recruiting	n/a	NCT02254863	Duke University, Durham, NC
	Intrathecal administration of cell therapy	Umbilical cord blood-derived oligodendrocyte-like cells	Rapid delivery of donor cells in the CNS; constant enzyme secretion; one-time treatment	Conditioning side-effects; safety and efficacy still to be determined	Recruiting	n/a	NCT02254863	Duke University, Durham, NC
Aspartylglucosaminuria	Chaperone therapy	Betaine	Overall disease improvement	Efficacy and safety to be determined	Ongoing	2017-000645-48	n/a	Orphan Europe SARL
Cystinosis	Stop codon read-through	ELX-02	Overall disease improvement	Efficacy and safety to be determined	Terminated	n/a	NCT04069260	Eloxx Pharmaceuticals, Inc.
	ex vivo gene therapy	Lentiviral vector (CTNS-RD-04)	Overall disease improvement	Efficacy and safety to be determined	Recruiting	n/a	NCT03897361	University of California, San Diego
Danon Disease	Gene therapy	AAV9 vector (RP-A501)	Overall disease improvement	Efficacy and safety to be determined	Recruiting	n/a	NCT03882437	Rocket Pharmaceuticals Inc.
Fabry disease	Liver directed gene therapy	AAV Vector (FLT190)	One-time treatment; broad enzyme distribution	Efficacy to be determined	Recruiting	n/a	NCT04040049	Freeline Therapeutics
	Gene therapy	AAV 2/6 vector (ST-920)	One-time treatment; broad enzyme distribution	Efficacy to be determined	Recruiting	n/a	NCT04046224	Sangamo Therapeutics
	Substrate reduction therapy combined with enzyme replacement therapy	Venglustat + agalsidase beta	Overall disease improvement	Efficacy and safety to be determined	Completed	n/a	NCT02228460	Genzyme, a Sanofi Company

Table 2. *Cont.*

Disease	Treatment	Product	Expected outcomes	Cons	Status	EudraCT number	NCT Number	Sponsor
	Enzyme replacement therapy	Pegunigalsidase alfa	Overall disease improvement	Efficacy and safety to be determined	Active, not recruiting	n/a	NCT03018730	Protalix
	Substrate reduction therapy combined with enzyme replacement therapy	Lucerastat+ Fabrazymeor Replagal	Overall disease improvement	Efficacy and safety to be determined	Completed	n/a	NCT02930655	Idorsia Pharmaceuticals Ltd.
	ex vivo gene therapy	Lentiviral vector (AVR-RD-01)	One-time treatment; broad enzyme distribution; less immune response due to the autologous process	Efficacy to be determined	Recruiting	n/a	NCT03454893	AvroBio
Gaucher disease	Chaperone therapy	Ambroxol	Overall disease improvement due to higher enzyme levels	Efficacy and safety to be determined	Recruiting	n/a	NCT03950050	Shaare Zedek Medical Center
	Substrate reduction therapy combined with enzyme replacement therapy	Venglustat + imiglucerase	Overall disease improvement	Efficacy and safety to be determined	Recruiting	n/a	NCT02843035	Genzyme, a Sanofi Company
	ex vivo gene therapy	Lentiviral vector (AVR-RD-02)	Overall disease improvement	Efficacy and safety to be determined	Recruiting	n/a	NCT04145037	AvroBio
Krabbe disease	Intrathecal administration of cell therapy	Umbilical cord blood-derived oligodendrocyte-like cells	Rapid delivery of donor cells in the CNS; constant enzyme secretion; one-time treatment	Conditioning side-effects; safety and efficacy still to be determined	Recruiting	n/a	NCT02254863	Duke University, Durham, NC
	Intracisternal gene therapy	AAV9 vector (LYS-GM101)	Overall disease improvement	Efficacy to be determined	Not yet recruiting	n/a	NCT04273269	Lysogene
GM1 gangliosidosis	Intracisternal gene therapy	AAVhu68 (PBGM01)	Overall disease improvement	Efficacy and safety to be determined	Not yet recruiting	n/a	n/a	PassageBio
	Intravenous gene therapy	AAV9 vector (AAV9-GLB1)	Overall disease improvement	Efficacy to be determined	Recruiting	n/a	NCT03952637	National Human Genome Research Institute

Table 2. Cont.

Disease	Treatment	Product	Expected outcomes	Cons	Status	EudraCT number	NCT Number	Sponsor
GM2 gangliosidosis	Substrate reduction therapy	Miglustat	Overall disease improvement	Efficacy to be determined	Recruiting	n/a	NCT03822013	Tehran University of Medical Sciences
	Substrate reduction therapy	Venglustat			Recruiting	n/a	NCT04221451	Genzyme, a Sanofi Company
	Intrathecal gene therapy	rAAVrh8-HEXA/B	Overall disease improvement	Efficacy and safety to be determined	not yet recruiting	n/a	n/a	Axovant
	Intrathecal administration of cell therapy	Umbilical cord blood-derived oligodendrocyte-like cells	Rapid delivery of donor cells in the CNS; constant enzyme secretion; one-time treatment	Conditioning side-effects; safety and efficacy still to be determined	Recruiting	n/a	NCT02254863	Duke University, Durham, NC
Metachromatic leukodystrophy	Intrathecal enzyme replacement therapy	SHP 611	Overall disease improvement	Efficacy to be determined	Recruiting	2018-003291-12	NCT03771898	Takeda
	Hematopoietic stem cell gene therapy	Lentiviral vector (OTL-200)	Improvement in enzyme levels with sulfatide storage reduction; able to prevent disease if administered in presymptomatic patients; no signs of genotoxicity.	It might not be able to rescue progression in symptomatic patients; long-term follow up is needed to determine possible complications	Active, not recruiting	n/a	NCT01560182	Orchard Therapeutics
	Intrathecal administration of cell therapy	Umbilical cord blood-derived oligodendrocyte-like cells	Rapid delivery of donor cells in the CNS; constant enzyme secretion; one-time treatment	Conditioning side-effects; safety and efficacy still to be determined	Recruiting	n/a	NCT02254863	Duke University, Durham, NC
Mucopolysaccharidosis type I	Enzyme replacement therapy with fusion protein	Valanafusp alfa	Improvement in enzyme levels with reduction in GAG storage in urine, plasma and CSF; drug likely penetrates the BBB	Immune responses that can possibly neutralize the enzyme; efficacy to be determined	Completed	n/a	NCT03053089	ArmaGen, Inc
	Autologous CD34+ HSCT transduced ex vivo gene therapy	Lentiviral vector	Overall disease improvement due to higher enzyme levels	Efficacy and safety to be determined	Recruiting	n/a	NCT03488394	IRCCS San Raffaele

Table 2. Cont.

Disease	Treatment	Product	Expected outcomes	Cons	Status	EudraCT number	NCT Number	Sponsor
	Enzyme replacement therapy with fusion protein	JR-171	Improvement in enzyme levels with reduction in GAG storage in urine, plasma and CSF; drug likely penetrates the BBB	Immune responses that can possibly neutralize the enzyme; efficacy to be determined	Not yet recruiting	n/a	NCT04227600	JCR Pharmaceuticals Co., Ltd.
	Intracisternal gene therapy	AAV9 vector (RGX-111)	Improvement in enzyme levels with reduction in GAG storage; improvement in CNS	Efficacy to be determined	Recruiting	n/a	NCT03580083	Regenxbio Inc.
	Intracisternal gene therapy B32.I38	AAV9 vector (RGX-121)	Improvement in enzyme levels with reduction in GAG storage in urine, plasma and CSF; drug likely penetrates the BBB	Efficacy to be determined	Recruiting	n/a	NCT03566043	Regenxbio Inc.
	Intrathecal enzyme replacement therapy	Idursulfase	Improvement in enzyme levels with reduction in GAG storage in the CSF; improvement in neurological impairment	Efficacy and safety to be determined	Completed	n/a	NCT00920647	Takeda
Mucopolysaccharidosis type II	Intracerebroventricular enzyme replacement therapy	Idursulfase beta	Overall disease improvement	Efficacy and safety to be determined	Completed	n/a	NCT01645189	GC Pharma
	Enzyme replacement therapy with fusion protein	DNL310	Overall disease improvement	Efficacy and safety to be determined	Not yet recruiting	n/a	NCT04251026	Denali Therapeutics Inc.
	Enzyme replacement therapy with fusion protein	JR-141	Improvement in enzyme levels with reduction in GAG storage in urine, plasma and CSF; drug likely penetrates the BBB	Immune responses that can possibly neutralize the enzyme; efficacy to be determined	Enrolling by invitation	n/a	NCT04348136	JCR Pharmaceuticals Co., Ltd.

Table 2. *Cont.*

Disease	Treatment	Product	Expected outcomes	Cons	Status	EudraCT number	NCT Number	Sponsor
	Genome editing	SB-913	One-time treatment; broad enzyme distribution	Immune responses that can possibly neutralize the enzyme; efficacy to be determined	Active, not recruiting	n/a	NCT03041324	Sangamo Therapeutics
	Intrathecal administration of cell therapy**	Umbilical cord blood-derived oligodendrocyte-like cells	Rapid delivery of donor cells in the CNS; constant enzyme secretion; one-time treatment	Conditioning side-effects; safety and efficacy still to be determined	Recruiting	n/a	NCT02254863	Duke University, Durham, NC
	Autologous CD34+ HSCT transduced ex vivo gene therapy	Lentiviral vector	One-time treatment; broad enzyme distribution	Efficacy to be determined	Recruiting	n/a	NCT04201405	University of Manchester
Mucopolysaccharidosis type IIIA	Intravenous gene therapy	AAV09 vector (ABO-102)	Leads to sustained enzyme production in the brain, likely to be one-time treatment, well tolerated	Possible immune response; efficacy still under testing; long-term follow up is needed to determine possible complications	Recruiting	n/a	NCT04088734	Abeona Therapeutics, Inc
	Intracerebral gene therapy	AAV 10 vector (LYS-SAF302)			Recruiting	n/a	NCT03612869	Lysogene
	Intrathecal administration of cell therapy	Umbilical cord blood-derived oligodendrocyte-like cells	Rapid delivery of donor cells in the CNS; constant enzyme secretion; one-time treatment	Conditioning side-effects; safety and efficacy still to be determined	Recruiting	n/a	NCT02254863	Duke University, Durham, NC
	Intracerebroventricular enzyme replacement therapy	AX 250	Overall disease improvement	Efficacy and safety to be determined	enrolling by invitation	n/a	NCT03784287	Allievex Corporation
Mucopolysaccharidosis type IIIB	Intravenous gene therapy with adeno-associated virus (AAV)	AAV9 vector (rAAV9.CMVhNAGLU)	Overall disease improvement	Efficacy to be determined	Recruiting	n/a	NCT03315182	Abeona Therapeutics, Inc

Table 2. Cont.

Disease	Treatment	Product	Expected outcomes	Cons	Status	EudraCT number	NCT Number	Sponsor
	Intracerebral gene therapy	AAV2/5 vector (rAAV2/5-hNaGlu)	Leads to sustained enzyme production in the brain, likely to be one-time treatment, well tolerated	Possible immune response; efficacy still under testing; long-term follow up is needed to determine possible complications	Completed	2012-000856-33	n/a	Institut Pasteur
	Intrathecal administration of cell therapy	Umbilical cord blood-derived oligodendrocyte-like cells	Rapid delivery of donor cells in the CNS; constant enzyme secretion; one-time treatment	Conditioning side-effects; safety and efficacy still to be determined	Recruiting	n/a	NCT02254863	Duke University, Durham, NC
Mucopolysaccharidosis type IVA	Cellular signaling pathway inhibition	Losartan	Improvement on cardiac impairment	Efficacy and safety to be determined	Recruiting	n/a	NCT03632213	Hospital de Clinicas de Porto Alegre
	Substrate reduction therapy	Odiparcil	Overall disease improvement	Efficacy and safety to be determined	Completed	n/a	NCT03370653	Inventiva Pharma
Mucopolysaccharidosis type VI	Cellular signaling pathway inhibition	Losartan	Improvement on cardiac impairment	Efficacy and safety to be determined	Recruiting	n/a	NCT03632213	Hospital de Clinicas de Porto Alegre
	Liver directed gene therapy	AAV2/8 vector (AAV2/8.TBG.hARSB)	Overall disease improvement	Efficacy to be determined	Recruiting	n/a	NCT03173521	Fondazione Telethon
Neuronal Ceroid Lipofuscinosis type 2 (CLN2)	Intracerebral gene therapy	AAV vector (AAVrh.10CUhCLN2)	Overall disease improvement	Efficacy to be determined	Active, not recruiting	n/a	NCT01414985	Weill Medical College of Cornell University
Neuronal Ceroid Lipofuscinosis type 3 (CLN3)	Intrathecal gene therapy	AAV9 vector (AT-GTX-502)	Overall disease improvement	Efficacy to be determined	Active, not recruiting	n/a	NCT03770572	Amicus Therapeutics
Neuronal Ceroid Lipofuscinosis type 6 (CLN6)	Intrathecal gene therapy	AAV9 vector (AT-GTX-501)	Overall disease improvement	Efficacy to be determined	Active, not recruiting	n/a	NCT02725580	Amicus Therapeutics
Niemann-pick type C	Intrathecal administration	2-Hydroxypropyl-Beta-Cyclodextrin	Improvement of liver symptoms	Efficacy and safety to be determined	Recruiting	n/a	NCT03471143	Washington University School of Medicine

Table 2. Cont.

Disease	Treatment	Product	Expected outcomes	Cons	Status	EudraCT number	NCT Number	Sponsor
Pompe disease	Intravenous gene therapy	AAV8 vector (AT845)	Improvement in respiratory function	Efficacy to be determined	Not yet recruiting	n/a	NCT04174105	Audentes Therapeutics
	Intravenous gene therapy	AAV2/8 vector (AAV2/8LSPhGAA)	Improvement in respiratory function	Efficacy to be determined	Recruiting	n/a	NCT03533673	Asklepios Biopharmaceutical, Inc.
	Chaperone + enzyme replacement therapy	AT2221 + ATB200+ alglucosidase alfa	Overall disease improvement	Efficacy to be determined	Ongoing	n/a	NCT03729362	Amicus Therapeutics
	Diaphragm delivery gene therapy	AAV 1 vector (rAAV1-CMV-GAA)	Improvement in respiratory function	Limited results in inspiratory pressure; immune responses; long-term follow up is needed to determine possible complications	Completed	n/a	NCT00976352	University of Florida

5. Small Molecules

Small molecules are low molecular weight synthetic compounds that address the pathophysiological mechanisms of LDs in different manners, such as substrate synthesis inhibition (SSI), the enhancement of enzyme stability, or premature termination codon read-through. These molecules have some advantages over ERT, such as the possibility of being administered orally, the lack of hypersensitive reactions, low manufacturing costs, and more importantly, the ability to cross the BBB [58].

5.1. Pharmacogenomics and Small Molecules

Variants in polymorphic genes that code for some of the cytochrome P450 (CYP) enzymes are known to influence the metabolism of certain drugs. These are called pharmacogenes, and the study of how an individual's genomic profile influences their response to medications is called pharmacogenomics (PGx), which is a core element of PM [59]. Genetic-based drug prescription not only improves the outcome of treatments but also reduces the risk of adverse effects. Individuals with variants that cause less active or inactive alleles are called poor metabolizers. The lack of activity of a pharmacogene may cause an overdose or an increase in the toxicity of a certain medication. On the other hand, ultrarapid metabolizers may experience a lack of efficacy. If the medication is a prodrug (such as clopidogrel), it might not be effective in an individual who is a poor metabolizer or might cause toxicity in someone who is a rapid metabolizer. Notably, over 90% of the population has at least one impactful variant in a pharmacogene, which should prompt a change in dosing or a change in drug prescription [60].

5.2. Substrate Synthesis Inhibition

Miglustat (Zavesca®, Actelion Pharmaceuticals, Allschwil, Switzerland) is a synthetic analog of D-glucose and was the first market-approved SSI drug for the treatment of GD and NPC [61]. Although miglustat has been shown to reduce the accumulation of glycosphingolipids in animal models of other LDs, it has not been approved for the treatment of patients due to a lack of measurable clinical benefits [62]. Interestingly, PM and PGx became more relevant for the LD field after the approval of eliglustat (Cerdelga™, Sanofi-Genzyme, Cambridge, MA, USA) as a treatment option for GD.

Eliglustat is an oral substrate reduction therapeutic that may be used as a first-line therapy for patients with the nonneuropathic form of GD who are not CYP2D6 ultra-rapid metabolizers [63]. However, eliglustat does not cross the BBB, limiting its effects on the neuropathic forms of the disease. Another example is cysteamine, which is the treatment of choice for nephropathic cystinosis since it delays progression of the renal and extrarenal manifestations and has a strong impact on survival rates [64]. Disease progression in NPC patients has been proven to stabilize with intrathecal 2-hydroxypropyl-β-cyclodextrin (HP-β-CD) since it does not cross the BBB [65]. Recently, drug-loaded nanoparticles were tested in NPC mice and were able to reach the CNS at a higher rate than other organs, making them a potential novel approach to treat patients [66]. Based on the preclinical data regarding the reduction of GAG accumulation, genistein has been tested in different types of MPS with conflicting results but an overall lack of clinical benefit. For MPS III, a phase III, randomized, placebo-controlled, clinical trial of high-dose oral genistein (EudraCT number: 2013-001479-18) failed to meet the primary goals, so there is no support for the use of genistein to treat these patients.

5.3. Pharmacological Chaperones

Missense variants may cause protein misfolding, which might lead to premature degradation. Pharmacological chaperones may interact with the mutant enzyme and prevent or delay its degradation. Migalastat (Galafold™, Amicus Therapeutics, Cranbury, NJ, USA) was the first pharmacological chaperone approved for the treatment of adult individuals who have a confirmed diagnosis of FD and a drug-amenable *GLA* missense variant. In addition to migalastat, several compounds have been proven to enhance lysosomal enzyme stability, such as ambroxol [67] and NCG607 [68] for glucocerebrosidase (GCase), progranulin for GCase, cathepsin D, hexosaminidase A [69,70], among others [71]. There are ongoing clinical trials testing chaperones in combination with ERT for PD. Preliminary results show an increase in α-glucosidase activity by two-fold compared with that of ERT alone [72].

5.4. Premature Termination Codon Read-Through

Several LDs are caused by nonsense variants leading to premature termination codons (PTCs), resulting in truncated enzymes. PTCs (or stop codons) are often more deleterious than missense variants because they lead to a loss of allele expression. Therefore, individuals with LDs caused by PTCs usually present severe phenotypes. There are drugs being tested on cell lines and animal models that promote the ribosome to read through PTCs and translate a somewhat functional enzyme. For example, chloramphenicol has been shown to enhance alpha-L-iduronidase (IDUA) activity in cell lines of MPS I patients [73], whereas ataluren has shown effects on the galactocerebrosidase activity in Krabbe disease (KB) mice [74] and on palmitoyl-protein thioesterase 1 activity in NCL mice [75]. Based on these examples, a genetic diagnosis for an individual with LD has become mandatory not only to provide adequate family counseling but also to tailor therapeutic management. To date, there is no market-approved LD-specific drug in this category. However, some aminoglycoside and nonaminoglycoside compounds have shown promising results in cell-based studies for cystinosis [76], neuronal ceroid lipofuscinosis, and others [77].

6. Next-Generation ERT

While alternative therapeutic approaches involving small molecules and gene therapy are being developed, modifications and additions to the ERT field are being explored to improve the range, efficacy and/or convenience of this modality of treatment. Most of these modifications try to address an important unmet need, which relates to the CNS manifestations of LDs, as the standard intravenous ERT is not able to cross the blood–brain barrier (BBB). Other difficulties of standard ERTs are related to the compliance with weekly or biweekly infusions for life and the low efficacy in some tissues/organs. Precision medicine is intrinsically related to these new alternatives, as it is expected that specific patients will better respond to a specific approach, and the choices will be highly related to the genetic background of each affected individual.

6.1. Intrathecal and Intracerebroventricular ERT

To address the neurological manifestations of several LDs, the enzyme should be able to reach the CNS. This does not occur with standard intravenous ERT, as the standard enzyme does not cross the BBB in significant amounts. To physically overcome the BBB, the enzyme may be administered intrathecally (IT) or by intracerebroventricular (ICV) injections. IT-ERT has been attempted for MPS IIIA, but the trial was interrupted due to a lack of efficacy. However, ICV-ERT has already been approved to treat type 2 neuronal ceroid lipofuscinosis–CNL2 (BioMarin Pharmaceuticals). IT-ERT is in clinical development to treat metachromatic leukodystrophy-MLD (Takeda). For severe MPS II, both IT (Takeda) and ICV (Green Cross) ERT administrations are being explored [78].

6.2. Intravenous ERT that Bypasses the BBB

Another approach to address the neurological manifestations of LDs is to use an alternative formulation of the enzyme, which may be provided as a "fusion protein" (also known as a "Trojan horse"). These fusion proteins combine the therapeutic enzyme with an antibody that is able to be recognized by a specific receptor and allowed to cross the BBB. Two examples of this approach are AGT-181, a fusion protein combining IDUA with an antibody that binds to the insulin receptor at the BBB for the treatment of MPS I (Armagen Technologies), and JR-141, a fusion protein combining iduronate sulfatase with an antibody that binds the transferrin receptor in the BBB for the treatment of MPS II (JCR Pharmaceuticals). Improvements in neurodevelopmental tests and neuroimaging biomarkers were reported with the use of AGT-181 in MPS I [79], and a significant decrease in heparan sulfate in the CSF was observed with JR-141 [80]. Other LD targets already disclosed are MPS I, MPS IIIA, MPS IIIB, MPS VII, and PD (JCR Pharmaceuticals), whereas MPS II and MPS IIIA are targeted by an alternative similar approach (Denali Therapeutics).

6.3. Intravenous ERT with Extended Half-Life

Intravenous ERT has a very short half-life in plasma, and infusions should be provided every week or every two weeks, depending on the disease. Some modifications introduced in the recombinant enzyme could extend the half-life and potentially enable longer intervals between infusions, which could represent a significant improvement in the convenience for the patient, as well as a reduction in costs for the health care system. A PEGylated formulation of alfa-galactosidase A is in development (Protalix BioTherapeutics) to treat FD, and the possibility of monthly administration is being explored. The investigators claim that the formulation could potentially have further advantages, in addition to an improved convenience [81].

6.4. ERT Administered via Encapsulated Cells Implanted in the Patient

The lack of convenience of weekly or biweekly infusions for life is also being tentatively addressed by the implantation of capsules containing genetically modified cells. The properties of these capsules prevent patient antibodies from attacking the cells and simultaneously allow the cells to obtain nutrients and produce the enzymes which leave the capsules to reach the tissues and organs [82]. The main advantages of this strategy over standard intravenous ERTs relate to convenience, as the patient will not need to receive regular infusions, and to the continuous release of enzyme (instead of weekly or biweekly pulses of enzyme). The disadvantages are the small surgery needed to implant the encapsulated cells, which will probably need to be repeated from time to time, and the fact that, if the cells produce a standard enzyme, it will not be able to cross the BBB. This strategy, which is being developed for FD and MPS I (Sigilon Therapeutics), could potentially address other LDs.

6.5. Intravenous ERT Combined with Oral Pharmacological Chaperones

A pharmacological chaperone (migalastat) was developed and already approved to treat patients with FD who harbor amenable mutations, as an alternative to ERT. The same product is being clinically tested in combination with ERT in patients with PD (Amicus Therapeutics). In this case, the chaperone would boost the enzyme activity, which is expected to improve outcomes [83].

6.6. Intravenous ERT for Other LDs

The number of LDs that have a specific ERT available is continuously increasing. Acid sphingomyelinase deficiency (ASMD) has acute and chronic forms. Chronic ASMD (formerly known as Niemann–Pick type B disease) has a presentation somewhat similar to that of GD type I with hepatomegaly, splenomegaly, anemia, and thrombocytopenia as well as interstitial lung disease. An intravenous ERT for chronic ASMD (olipudase alfa, Sanofi S.A.) is already in an advanced stage of clinical development [84].

7. Gene Therapy/Genome Editing

Gene therapies for LDs are advancing rapidly. Although not all of them, most LDs present brain involvement, stimulating the development of therapies targeting this organ [85].

There are two gene therapy approaches for brain involvement in LDs. In one case, the vector carrying the therapeutic gene is administered in vivo, either by in situ administration or by an intravenous injection of a vector with a tropism for brain cells [71,86]. The latter can also be used for other LDs without brain involvement by targeting the vector to other organs [87]. One example of a clinical trial using in vivo gene therapy for an LD includes the intraparenchymal injections of a recombinant adeno-associated viral vector serotype 2/5 (rAAV2/5) in children with mucopolysaccharidosis type IIIB [88].

Another possible scenario is hematopoietic stem cell (HSC)-targeted gene therapy. The rationale for this approach is that microglial cells originate from the differentiation of hematopoietic precursor cells. Thus, HSCs can be harvested, corrected ex vivo, and infused back into the patient. Gene-corrected HSCs repopulate the bone marrow and eventually migrate into the brain and differentiate into microglial cells. These cells then secrete the enzyme and cross-correct neurons and other brain cells. Eight out of nine children with metachromatic leukodystrophy who were submitted to an ex vivo gene therapy protocol experienced the prevention of disease onset or a halted disease progression [89], showing the potential of this approach.

Although CRISPR-Cas9 genome editing has been tested in preclinical trials for different LDs [90], so far, only zinc finger-mediated gene editing has been applied in a trial for an LD—Hunter syndrome [91]. The trial is still ongoing, and no efficacy can be inferred at this point, but preliminary results showed no serious adverse effects using this approach.

8. Antisense Oligonucleotide Therapy

Antisense oligonucleotide (ASO) technology has emerged as a powerful therapeutic alternative for the treatment of genetic disorders by targeting cellular RNA and controlling gene expression through several distinct mechanisms. Novel chemical modifications of single-stranded deoxynucleotides allowed the development of next-generation ASOs with enhanced pharmacological properties. This is reflected in the fact that in the past few years, ASO therapies were approved for the treatment of spinal muscular atrophy and Duchenne muscular dystrophy [92].

ASO-based therapies for LDs are focused mainly on restoring the normal splicing of mutated transcripts. At least 600 mutations that affect precursor mRNA (pre-mRNA) splicing have been described in patients with LDs. Most are private variants, but a common splicing variant accounts for up to 70% of the pathogenic alleles for PD, FD, mucolipidosis type II/III, and Tay–Sachs disease, representing excellent candidates for this type of approach [93].

The first attempt to develop an ASO therapy for an LD was performed in a cellular model of NPC disease carrying a variant that creates a cryptic donor splice site, resulting in the incorporation of 194 bp of intron nine as a new exon (pseudoexon) [94]. The strategy was able to restore normal splicing. Since then, several other studies have reported this approach in the treatment of late-onset PD caused by the c.-32-13T>G variant present in 40–70% of the alleles [95] and for MPS type II [96].

Recently, an unprecedented example of precision medicine for LD was published. Kim et al. [26] reported the discovery, development, and administration of milasen, a splice-modulating antisense oligonucleotide drug tailored to a single patient. Mila was a six-year-old girl with CLN7 neuronal ceroid lipofuscinosis, which is a fatal neurodegenerative condition. After a WGS analysis, a known pathogenic variant was found in trans with a novel insertion of an SVA (SINE-VNTR-Alu) retrotransposon in *MFSD8*. The SVA causes misplicing of the MFSD8 mRNA and leads to premature translational termination. The researchers customized an ASO that blocked the cryptic splice-acceptor site, increased the ratio of normal to mutant mRNA and restored the *MFSD8* expression. Moreover, there was a decrease in intracellular vacuolization in the patient's fibroblasts. Due to clinical urgency and promising in vitro results, the Food and Drug Administration (FDA)-approved milasen to be administered by intrathecal injection to this single patient in ascending doses. As a result, seizures decreased from 30 episodes per day lasting 1 to 2 min to just a few episodes lasting a few seconds. Remarkably, the path from the identification of the variants to the development of the tailored drug and clinical deployment occurred in less than 12 months [26].

9. Combination of Therapies

When the first therapies for LDs were announced, they were focused on correcting the primary enzymatic defect and some of the most striking symptoms. However, LDs are multisystem diseases with difficult-to-treat affected organs, so monotherapies frequently do not improve all symptoms. Similar to multifactorial diseases, a combination of therapies may be necessary to achieve the best therapeutic response. For example, ERT has limited success in treating bone, cartilage, and the heart in MPS I, II, and VI. In patients with PD in advanced stages of the disease, skeletal muscle impairment remains refractory to ERT [97].

Although CNS administration of ERT, HSCT, or gene therapy circumvents the BBB, the widespread involvement of multiple brain regions in LDs and the inability of treatments to diffuse freely throughout the parenchyma result in only partial correction of CNS pathology [98].

There are combined strategies in clinical and preclinical trials for LDs. The most common combination therapy for a LDs leverages the success of ERT by coupling it with chaperones, SSIs, gene therapy, or HSCT. (i) ERT and HSCT are therapeutic options to halt the disease progression but are not curative. HSCT is the standard of care for children with severe MPS I, and ERT is typically initiated prior to transplantation to improve somatic symptoms and the ability to tolerate conditioning and transplants. Despite HSCT, growth failure with short stature along with musculoskeletal complications remains a prominent manifestation of MPS IH. ERT in combination with HSCT also enhances cognitive outcomes. The real benefit of ERT post-HSCT is still under evaluation [99,100]. (ii) For SSI + ERT, the oral selective glucosylceramide synthase inhibitor (venglustat) is under investigation for the treatment of GD type 3. Combined with ERT (imiglucerase), it is being assessed in the phase 2 LEAP trial in 11 patients aged ≥18 years to evaluate neurological outcomes since venglustat has been shown to cross the BBB [101]. (iii) For gene therapy and HSCT, HSCT synergized with CNS-directed AAV-mediated ERT reduced storage, decreased neuroinflammation, improved motor deficits, and dramatically improved the lifespan of an NCL animal model [102]. (iv) For CNS-directed gene therapy, systemic SSI, and HSCT, this combination modality has been studied in a preclinical mouse model of KD. Simultaneously, treating multiple pathogenic targets resulted in an unprecedented increase in life span with improved motor function, persistent GALC expression, nearly normal psychosine levels, and decreased neuroinflammation [103].

Although combinations of therapies that involve gene therapy or genome editing are still not available for patients, the data from preclinical trials are very promising. Understanding the pathophysiology of LDs and identifying the secondary mechanisms involved in the pathogenesis, such as ER stress, altered lipid trafficking, autophagy impairment, inflammation, and altered calcium homeostasis, will aid in the development of personalized therapies for the diverse symptoms of LDs [13].

10. Concluding Remarks

The goal of PM is to use biological knowledge and health information to predict disease risk, understand disease pathophysiology, identify disease subcategories, improve diagnoses, and provide tailored treatment strategies to achieve the best possible outcomes. In the LD field, Mila´s case mentioned above perfectly illustrates how recently developed technologies, such as whole-genome sequencing and antisense approaches, allowed the delineation of pathways for ultrapersonalized medicine.

Although PM has the potential to profoundly improve LD management, the required advances will take some time to become routine. For example, the collection and analysis of patients' data will be invaluable for PM to reach its potential in this field. Clinical and research laboratories often create biorepositories, whose power depends on the number and types of samples. It is a great challenge to develop biorepositories for LDs since there are limited numbers of individuals reported due to rarity or underdiagnoses. However, this challenge might be overcome by national and international collaborative efforts and multicenter data sharing, data collection standardization, and patient education on the benefits of sharing experiences and samples.

Recent advances in omics are already being used and have been instrumental in directing clinical decision making. The integration of multiomics data has the potential to drive real changes in PM and will be crucial to understanding the biological and cellular mechanisms of LD-causing variants and developing novel approaches for LD treatment in an individualized manner. However, the analysis and interpretation of omics data is challenging, especially because they are highly complex and voluminous; for this purpose, the development of novel bioinformatics methods and databases will be necessary.

Finally, this article intended to highlight the novel diagnosis and treatment modalities for LDs based on a PM approach. Even though novel therapies such as antisense oligonucleotides and genome editing are still in their early stages, they have already shown promising results in the clinical setting, suggesting that they are real possibility for several LDs in the near future.

Author Contributions: F.P.e.V., D.R.M., and R.G. designed the study, performed the research, analyzed the data, and wrote and reviewed the paper. F.K., F.d.O.P., C.F.M.d.S., and G.B. performed the research and wrote and reviewed the paper. All authors were involved in the reviewing and editing of the manuscript. All authors approved the final version. All authors have read and agreed to the published version of the manuscript.

Funding: FK and FOP conducted this review during scholarship financed by CAPES. GB and RG are recipients of CNPq research scholarships. The work received support from CNPq grants 303219/19-0 and 465549/2014-4, CAPES (grant 88887.136366/2017-00), FAPERGS (grant 17/2551-0000521-0) and FIPE/HCPA (2017-0664 and 2017-0685).

Conflicts of Interest: RG has served as a speaker, a consultant or an advisory board member for Amicus, Abeona, BioMarin, Inventiva, Janssen, JCR Pharmaceuticals, Lysogene, PTC, Regenxbio, Sanofi, Sobi, Takeda and Ultragenyx; has received research grants from Allevex, Amicus, Armagen, BioMarin, GC Pharma, JCR Pharmaceuticals, Lysogene, Regenxbio, Sanofi, and Takeda, and has received travel expenses to attend scientific meetings from Amicus, BioMarin, JCR Pharmaceuticals, Sanofi, Takeda, and Ultragenyx. The other authors have no conflicts of interest to disclose.

References

1. Pinto, E.V.F.; Lazaridis, K.N. Individualized medicine comes to the liver clinic. *J. Hepatol.* **2019**, *70*, 1057–1059. [CrossRef] [PubMed]
2. Hou, Y.C.; Yu, H.C.; Martin, R.; Cirulli, E.T.; Schenker-Ahmed, N.M.; Hicks, M.; Cohen, I.V.; Jönsson, T.J.; Heister, R.; Napier, L.; et al. Precision medicine integrating whole-genome sequencing, comprehensive metabolomics, and advanced imaging. *Proc. Natl. Acad. Sci. USA* **2020**, *117*, 3053–3062. [CrossRef] [PubMed]
3. *Toward Precision Medicine: Building a Knowledge Network for Biomedical Research and a New Taxonomy of Disease*; National Academies Press: Washington, DC, USA, 2011. [CrossRef]
4. Platt, F.M.; d'Azzo, A.; Davidson, B.L.; Neufeld, E.F.; Tifft, C.J. Lysosomal storage diseases. *Nat. Rev. Dis. Primers* **2018**, *4*, 27. [CrossRef] [PubMed]
5. Fuller, M.; Meikle, P.J.; Hopwood, J.J. Epidemiology of lysosomal storage diseases: An overview. In *Fabry Disease: Perspectives from 5 Years of FOS*; Mehta, A., Beck, M., Sunder-Plassmann, G., Eds.; Oxford PharmaGenesis Ltd.: Oxford, UK, 2006.
6. Giugliani, R.; Federhen, A.; Michelin-Tirelli, K.; Riegel, M.; Burin, M. Relative frequency and estimated minimal frequency of Lysosomal Storage Diseases in Brazil: Report from a Reference Laboratory. *Genet. Mol. Biol.* **2017**, *40*, 31–39. [CrossRef] [PubMed]
7. Beck, M. Treatment strategies for lysosomal storage disorders. *Dev. Med. Child Neurol.* **2018**, *60*, 13–18. [CrossRef] [PubMed]
8. Mynarek, M.; Tolar, J.; Albert, M.H.; Escolar, M.L.; Boelens, J.J.; Cowan, M.J.; Finnegan, N.; Glomstein, A.; Jacobsohn, D.A.; Kühl, J.S.; et al. Allogeneic Hematopoietic SCT for Alpha-Mannosidosis: An Analysis of 17 Patients. *Bone Marrow Transplant.* **2012**, *47*, 352–359. [CrossRef]
9. Somaraju, U.R.; Tadepalli, K. 'Cochrane Database of Systematic Reviews Hematopoietic Stem Cell Transplantation for Gaucher Disease (Review) Hematopoietic Stem Cell Transplantation for Gaucher Disease. *Hematop. Stem Cell Transplant. Gauch. Dis.* **2017**, *10*. [CrossRef]
10. Gramatges, M.M.; Dvorak, C.C.; Regula, D.P.; Enns, G.M.; Weinberg, K.; Agarwal, R. Pathological Evidence of Wolman's Disease Following Hematopoietic Stem Cell Transplantation despite Correction of Lysosomal Acid Lipase Activity. *Bone Marrow Transplant.* **2009**, 449–450. [CrossRef]
11. Aldenhoven, M.; Van Den Broek, B.T.A.; Wynn, R.F.; O'Meara, A.; Veys, P.; Rovelli, A.; Jones, S.A.; Parini, R.; Van Hasselt, P.M.; Renard, M.; et al. Quality of Life of Hurler Syndrome Patients after Successful Hematopoietic Stem Cell Transplantation. *Blood Adv.* **2017**, *1*, 2236–2242. [CrossRef]
12. Barth, A.L.; Horovitz, D.D.G. Hematopoietic Stem Cell Transplantation in Mucopolysaccharidosis Type II. *J. Inborn Errors Metab. Screen.* **2018**, *6*, e180008. [CrossRef]

13. Barth, L.; de Magalhães, T.S.P.C.; Reis, A.B.R.; de Oliveira, M.L.; Scalco, F.B.; Cavalcanti, N.C.; Silva, D.S.E.; Torres, D.A.; Costa, A.A.P.; Bonfim, C.; et al. Early Hematopoietic Stem Cell Transplantation in a Patient with Severe Mucopolysaccharidosis II: A 7 Years Follow-Up. *Mol. Genet. Metab. Rep.* **2017**, *12*, 62–68. [CrossRef] [PubMed]
14. Yabe, H.; Tanaka, A.; Chinen, Y.; Kato, S.; Sawamoto, K.; Yasuda, E.; Shintaku, H.; Suzuki, Y.; Orii, T.; Tomatsu, S. Hematopoietic Stem Cell Transplantation for Morquio A Syndrome. *Mol. Genet. Metab.* **2016**, *117*, 84–94. [CrossRef] [PubMed]
15. Turbeville, S.; Nicely, H.; Douglas Rizzo, J.; Pedersen, T.L.; Orchard, P.J.; Horwitz, M.E.; Horwitz, E.M.; Veys, P.; Bonfim, C.; Al-Seraihy, A. Clinical Outcomes Following Hematopoietic Stem Cell Transplantation for the Treatment of Mucopolysaccharidosis VI. *Mol. Genet. Metab.* **2011**, *102*, 111–115. [CrossRef] [PubMed]
16. Orii, K.; Suzuki, Y.; Tomatsu, S.; Orii, T.; Fukao, T. Long-Term Follow-up Posthematopoietic Stem Cell Transplantation in a Japanese Patient with Type-VII Mucopolysaccharidosis. *Diagnostics* **2020**, *10*, 105. [CrossRef]
17. Jameson, J.L.; Longo, D.L. Precision medicine–personalized, problematic, and promising. *N. Engl. J. Med.* **2015**, *372*, 2229–2234. [CrossRef]
18. Brusius-Facchin, A.C.; Rojas Malaga, D.; Leistner-Segal, S.; Giugliani, R. Recent advances in molecular testing to improve early diagnosis in children with mucopolysaccharidoses. *Expert Rev. Mol. Diagn.* **2018**, *18*, 855–866. [CrossRef]
19. Nashabat, M.; Al-Khenaizan, S.; Alfadhel, M. Report of a Case that Expands the Phenotype of Infantile Krabbe Disease. *Am. J. Case Rep.* **2019**, *20*, 643–646. [CrossRef]
20. Kondo, H.; Maksimova, N.; Otomo, T.; Kato, H.; Imai, A.; Asano, Y.; Kobayashi, K.; Nojima, S.; Nakaya, A.; Hamada, Y.; et al. Mutation in VPS33A affects metabolism of glycosaminoglycans: A new type of mucopolysaccharidosis with severe systemic symptoms. *Hum. Mol. Genet.* **2017**, *26*, 173–183. [CrossRef]
21. Dursun, A.; Yalnizoglu, D.; Gerdan, O.F.; Yucel-Yilmaz, D.; Sagiroglu, M.S.; Yuksel, B.; Gucer, S.; Sivri, S.; Ozgul, R.K. A probable new syndrome with the storage disease phenotype caused by the VPS33A gene mutation. *Clin. Dysmorphol.* **2017**, *26*, 1–12. [CrossRef]
22. Nikkel, S.M.; Huang, L.; Lachman, R.; Beaulieu, C.L.; Schwartzentruber, J.; Majewski, J.; Geraghty, M.T.; Boycott, K.M.; Consortium, F.C. Whole-exome sequencing expands the phenotype of Hunter syndrome. *Clin. Genet.* **2014**, *86*, 172–176. [CrossRef]
23. Zeng, Q.; Fan, Y.; Wang, L.; Huang, Z.; Gu, X.; Yu, Y. Molecular defects identified by whole exome sequencing in a child with atypical mucopolysaccharidosis IIIB. *J. Pediatr. Endocrinol. Metab.* **2017**, *30*, 463–469. [CrossRef]
24. Kaissi, A.A.; Hofstaetter, J.; Weigel, G.; Grill, F.; Ganger, R.; Kircher, S.G. The constellation of skeletal deformities in a family with mixed types of mucopolysaccharidoses: Case report. *Medicine* **2016**, *95*, e4561. [CrossRef] [PubMed]
25. Vairo, F.P.; Boczek, N.J.; Cousin, M.A.; Kaiwar, C.; Blackburn, P.R.; Conboy, E.; Lanpher, B.C.; Gavrilova, R.H.; Pichurin, P.N.; Lazaridis, K.N.; et al. The prevalence of diseases caused by lysosome-related genes in a cohort of undiagnosed patients. *Mol. Genet. Metab. Rep.* **2017**, *13*, 46–51. [CrossRef] [PubMed]
26. Kim, J.; Hu, C.; Moufawad El Achkar, C.; Black, L.E.; Douville, J.; Larson, A.; Pendergast, M.K.; Goldkind, S.F.; Lee, E.A.; Kuniholm, A.; et al. Patient-Customized Oligonucleotide Therapy for a Rare Genetic Disease. *N. Engl. J. Med.* **2019**, *381*, 1644–1652. [CrossRef] [PubMed]
27. Blomqvist, M.; Smeland, M.F.; Lindgren, J.; Sikora, P.; Riise Stensland, H.M.F.; Asin-Cayuela, J. beta-Mannosidosis caused by a novel homozygous intragenic inverted duplication in MANBA. *Cold Spring Harb. Mol. Case Stud.* **2019**, *5*. [CrossRef]
28. Ashton-Prolla, P.; Goldim, J.R.; Vairo, F.P.; da Silveira Matte, U.; Sequeiros, J. Genomic analysis in the clinic: Benefits and challenges for health care professionals and patients in Brazil. *J. Community Genet.* **2015**, *6*, 275–283. [CrossRef]
29. Pinto, E.V.F.; Conboy, E.; de Souza, C.F.M.; Jones, A.; Barnett, S.S.; Klee, E.W.; Lanpher, B.C. Diagnosis of Attenuated Mucopolysaccharidosis VI: Clinical, Biochemical, and Genetic Pitfalls. *Pediatrics* **2018**, *142*. [CrossRef]
30. Bravo, H.; Neto, E.C.; Schulte, J.; Pereira, J.; Filho, C.S.; Bittencourt, F.; Sebastiao, F.; Bender, F.; de Magalhaes, A.P.S.; Guidobono, R.; et al. Investigation of newborns with abnormal results in a newborn screening program for four lysosomal storage diseases in Brazil. *Mol. Genet. Metab. Rep.* **2017**, *12*, 92–97. [CrossRef]

31. Pant, D.C.; Dorboz, I.; Schluter, A.; Fourcade, S.; Launay, N.; Joya, J.; Aguilera-Albesa, S.; Yoldi, M.E.; Casasnovas, C.; Willis, M.J.; et al. Loss of the sphingolipid desaturase DEGS1 causes hypomyelinating leukodystrophy. *J. Clin. Investig.* **2019**, *129*, 1240–1256. [CrossRef]
32. Li, D.; Lin, Y.; Huang, Y.; Zhang, W.; Jiang, M.; Li, X.; Zhao, X.; Sheng, H.; Yin, X.; Su, X.; et al. Early prenatal diagnosis of lysosomal storage disorders by enzymatic and molecular analysis. *Prenat. Diagn.* **2018**, *38*, 779–787. [CrossRef]
33. Zhang, J.; Chen, H.; Kornreich, R.; Yu, C. Prenatal Diagnosis of Tay-Sachs Disease. *Methods Mol. Biol.* **2019**, *1885*, 233–250. [CrossRef] [PubMed]
34. Ou, L.; Przybilla, M.J.; Whitley, C.B. SAAMP 2.0: An algorithm to predict genotype-phenotype correlation of lysosomal storage diseases. *Clin. Genet.* **2018**, *93*, 1008–1014. [CrossRef]
35. Scott, H.S.; Litjens, T.; Nelson, P.V.; Brooks, D.A.; Hopwood, J.J.; Morris, C.P. alpha-L-iduronidase mutations (Q70X and P533R) associate with a severe Hurler phenotype. *Hum. Mutat.* **1992**, *1*, 333–339. [CrossRef] [PubMed]
36. Hein, L.K.; Bawden, M.; Muller, V.J.; Sillence, D.; Hopwood, J.J.; Brooks, D.A. alpha-L-iduronidase premature stop codons and potential read-through in mucopolysaccharidosis type I patients. *J. Mol. Biol.* **2004**, *338*, 453–462. [CrossRef]
37. Nowak, A.; Huynh-Do, U.; Krayenbuehl, P.A.; Beuschlein, F.; Schiffmann, R.; Barbey, F. Fabry disease genotype, phenotype, and migalastat amenability: Insights from a national cohort. *J. Inherit. Metab. Dis.* **2020**, *43*, 326–333. [CrossRef] [PubMed]
38. Fiehn, O. Metabolomics—The link between genotypes and phenotypes. *Plant Mol. Biol.* **2002**, *48*, 155–171. [CrossRef] [PubMed]
39. Nicholson, J.K.; Holmes, E.; Kinross, J.M.; Darzi, A.W.; Takats, Z.; Lindon, J.C. Metabolic phenotyping in clinical and surgical environments. *Nature* **2012**, *491*, 384–392. [CrossRef] [PubMed]
40. Mussap, M.; Zaffanello, M.; Fanos, V. Metabolomics: A challenge for detecting and monitoring inborn errors of metabolism. *Ann. Transl. Med.* **2018**, *6*, 338. [CrossRef]
41. Gonzalez-Dominguez, A.; Duran-Guerrero, E.; Fernandez-Recamales, A.; Lechuga-Sancho, A.M.; Sayago, A.; Schwarz, M.; Segundo, C.; Gonzalez-Dominguez, R. An Overview on the Importance of Combining Complementary Analytical Platforms in Metabolomic Research. *Curr. Top. Med. Chem.* **2017**, *17*, 3289–3295. [CrossRef]
42. Tebani, A.; Abily-Donval, L.; Afonso, C.; Marret, S.; Bekri, S. Clinical Metabolomics: The New Metabolic Window for Inborn Errors of Metabolism Investigations in the Post-Genomic Era. *Int. J. Mol. Sci.* **2016**, *17*, 1167. [CrossRef]
43. Sandlers, Y. The future perspective: Metabolomics in laboratory medicine for inborn errors of metabolism. *Transl. Res.* **2017**, *189*, 65–75. [CrossRef] [PubMed]
44. Wishart, D.S.; Feunang, Y.D.; Marcu, A.; Guo, A.C.; Liang, K.; Vazquez-Fresno, R.; Sajed, T.; Johnson, D.; Li, C.; Karu, N.; et al. HMDB 4.0: The human metabolome database for 2018. *Nucleic Acids Res.* **2018**, *46*, D608–D617. [CrossRef] [PubMed]
45. Mandal, R.; Chamot, D.; Wishart, D.S. The role of the Human Metabolome Database in inborn errors of metabolism. *J. Inherit. Metab. Dis.* **2018**, *41*, 329–336. [CrossRef] [PubMed]
46. Auray-Blais, C.; Boutin, M.; Gagnon, R.; Dupont, F.O.; Lavoie, P.; Clarke, J.T. Urinary globotriaosylsphingosine-related biomarkers for Fabry disease targeted by metabolomics. *Anal. Chem.* **2012**, *84*, 2745–2753. [CrossRef]
47. Auray-Blais, C.; Boutin, M. Novel gb(3) isoforms detected in urine of fabry disease patients: A metabolomic study. *Curr. Med. Chem.* **2012**, *19*, 3241–3252. [CrossRef]
48. Manwaring, V.; Boutin, M.; Auray-Blais, C. A metabolomic study to identify new globotriaosylceramide-related biomarkers in the plasma of Fabry disease patients. *Anal. Chem.* **2013**, *85*, 9039–9048. [CrossRef]
49. Dupont, F.O.; Gagnon, R.; Boutin, M.; Auray-Blais, C. A metabolomic study reveals novel plasma lyso-Gb3 analogs as Fabry disease biomarkers. *Curr. Med. Chem.* **2013**, *20*, 280–288. [CrossRef]
50. Mashima, R.; Okuyama, T.; Ohira, M. Biomarkers for Lysosomal Storage Disorders with an Emphasis on Mass Spectrometry. *Int. J. Mol. Sci.* **2020**, *21*, 2704. [CrossRef]

51. Janeckova, H.; Hron, K.; Wojtowicz, P.; Hlidkova, E.; Baresova, A.; Friedecky, D.; Zidkova, L.; Hornik, P.; Behulova, D.; Prochazkova, D.; et al. Targeted metabolomic analysis of plasma samples for the diagnosis of inherited metabolic disorders. *J. Chromatogr. A* **2012**, *1226*, 11–17. [CrossRef]
52. Jacob, M.; Malkawi, A.; Albast, N.; Al Bougha, S.; Lopata, A.; Dasouki, M.; Abdel Rahman, A.M. A targeted metabolomics approach for clinical diagnosis of inborn errors of metabolism. *Anal. Chim. Acta* **2018**, *1025*, 141–153. [CrossRef]
53. Coene, K.L.M.; Kluijtmans, L.A.J.; van der Heeft, E.; Engelke, U.F.H.; de Boer, S.; Hoegen, B.; Kwast, H.J.T.; van de Vorst, M.; Huigen, M.; Keularts, I.; et al. Next-generation metabolic screening: Targeted and untargeted metabolomics for the diagnosis of inborn errors of metabolism in individual patients. *J. Inherit. Metab. Dis.* **2018**, *41*, 337–353. [CrossRef] [PubMed]
54. Gertsman, I.; Barshop, B.A. Promises and pitfalls of untargeted metabolomics. *J. Inherit. Metab. Dis.* **2018**, *41*, 355–366. [CrossRef] [PubMed]
55. Hajduk, J.; Matysiak, J.; Kokot, Z.J. Challenges in biomarker discovery with MALDI-TOF MS. *Clin. Chim. Acta* **2016**, *458*, 84–98. [CrossRef] [PubMed]
56. Hinderer, C.; Katz, N.; Louboutin, J.P.; Bell, P.; Tolar, J.; Orchard, P.J.; Lund, T.C.; Nayal, M.; Weng, L.; Mesaros, C.; et al. Abnormal polyamine metabolism is unique to the neuropathic forms of MPS: Potential for biomarker development and insight into pathogenesis. *Hum. Mol. Genet.* **2017**, *26*, 3837–3849. [CrossRef]
57. Fu, H.; Meadows, A.S.; Ware, T.; Mohney, R.P.; McCarty, D.M. Near-Complete Correction of Profound Metabolomic Impairments Corresponding to Functional Benefit in MPS IIIB Mice after IV rAAV9-hNAGLU Gene Delivery. *Mol. Ther.* **2017**, *25*, 792–802. [CrossRef]
58. Poswar, F.O.; Vairo, F.; Burin, M.; Michelin-Tirelli, K.; Brusius-Facchin, A.C.; Kubaski, F.; Souza, C.F.M.; Baldo, G.; Giugliani, R. Lysosomal diseases: Overview on current diagnosis and treatment. *Genet. Mol. Biol.* **2019**, *42*, 165–177. [CrossRef]
59. Weinshilboum, R. Inheritance and drug response. *N. Engl. J. Med.* **2003**, *348*, 529–537. [CrossRef]
60. Van Driest, S.L.; Shi, Y.; Bowton, E.A.; Schildcrout, J.S.; Peterson, J.F.; Pulley, J.; Denny, J.C.; Roden, D.M. Clinically actionable genotypes among 10,000 patients with preemptive pharmacogenomic testing. *Clin. Pharmacol. Ther.* **2014**, *95*, 423–431. [CrossRef]
61. Cox, T.M.; Aerts, J.M.; Andria, G.; Beck, M.; Belmatoug, N.; Bembi, B.; Chertkoff, R.; Vom Dahl, S.; Elstein, D.; Erikson, A.; et al. The role of the iminosugar N-butyldeoxynojirimycin (miglustat) in the management of type I (non-neuronopathic) Gaucher disease: A position statement. *J. Inherit. Metab. Dis.* **2003**, *26*, 513–526. [CrossRef]
62. Shapiro, B.E.; Pastores, G.M.; Gianutsos, J.; Luzy, C.; Kolodny, E.H. Miglustat in late-onset Tay-Sachs disease: A 12-month, randomized, controlled clinical study with 24 months of extended treatment. *Genet. Med.* **2009**, *11*, 425–433. [CrossRef]
63. Peterschmitt, M.J.; Cox, G.F.; Ibrahim, J.; MacDougall, J.; Underhill, L.H.; Patel, P.; Gaemers, S.J.M. A pooled analysis of adverse events in 393 adults with Gaucher disease type 1 from four clinical trials of oral eliglustat: Evaluation of frequency, timing, and duration. *Blood Cells Mol. Dis.* **2018**, *68*, 185–191. [CrossRef] [PubMed]
64. Ariceta, G.; Giordano, V.; Santos, F. Effects of long-term cysteamine treatment in patients with cystinosis. *Pediatr. Nephrol.* **2019**, *34*, 571–578. [CrossRef] [PubMed]
65. Megias-Vericat, J.E.; Garcia-Robles, A.; Company-Albir, M.J.; Fernandez-Megia, M.J.; Perez-Miralles, F.C.; Lopez-Briz, E.; Casanova, B.; Poveda, J.L. Early experience with compassionate use of 2 hydroxypropyl-beta-cyclodextrin for Niemann-Pick type C disease: Review of initial published cases. *Neurol. Sci.* **2017**, *38*, 727–743. [CrossRef] [PubMed]
66. Donida, B.; Raabe, M.; Tauffner, B.; de Farias, M.A.; Machado, A.Z.; Timm, F.; Kessler, R.G.; Hammerschmidt, T.G.; Reinhardt, L.S.; Brito, V.B.; et al. Nanoparticles containing beta-cyclodextrin potentially useful for the treatment of Niemann-Pick C. *J. Inherit. Metab. Dis.* **2020**, *43*, 586–601. [CrossRef] [PubMed]
67. Kim, Y.M.; Yum, M.S.; Heo, S.H.; Kim, T.; Jin, H.K.; Bae, J.S.; Seo, G.H.; Oh, A.; Yoon, H.M.; Lim, H.T.; et al. Pharmacologic properties of high-dose ambroxol in four patients with Gaucher disease and myoclonic epilepsy. *J. Med. Genet.* **2020**, *57*, 124–131. [CrossRef]

68. Aflaki, E.; Borger, D.K.; Moaven, N.; Stubblefield, B.K.; Rogers, S.A.; Patnaik, S.; Schoenen, F.J.; Westbroek, W.; Zheng, W.; Sullivan, P.; et al. A New Glucocerebrosidase Chaperone Reduces alpha-Synuclein and Glycolipid Levels in iPSC-Derived Dopaminergic Neurons from Patients with Gaucher Disease and Parkinsonism. *J. Neurosci.* **2016**, *36*, 7441–7452. [CrossRef]
69. Chen, Y.; Jian, J.; Hettinghouse, A.; Zhao, X.; Setchell, K.D.R.; Sun, Y.; Liu, C.J. Progranulin associates with hexosaminidase A and ameliorates GM2 ganglioside accumulation and lysosomal storage in Tay-Sachs disease. *J. Mol. Med.* **2018**, *96*, 1359–1373. [CrossRef]
70. Jian, J.; Hettinghouse, A.; Liu, C.J. Progranulin acts as a shared chaperone and regulates multiple lysosomal enzymes. *Genes Dis.* **2017**, *4*, 125–126. [CrossRef]
71. Giugliani, R.; Vairo, F.; Kubaski, F.; Poswar, F.; Riegel, M.; Baldo, G.; Saute, J.A. Neurological manifestations of lysosomal disorders and emerging therapies targeting the CNS. *Lancet Child Adolesc. Health* **2018**, *2*, 56–68. [CrossRef]
72. Kishnani, P.; Tarnopolsky, M.; Roberts, M.; Sivakumar, K.; Dasouki, M.; Dimachkie, M.M.; Finanger, E.; Goker-Alpan, O.; Guter, K.A.; Mozaffar, T.; et al. Duvoglustat HCl Increases Systemic and Tissue Exposure of Active Acid alpha-Glucosidase in Pompe Patients Co-administered with Alglucosidase alpha. *Mol. Ther.* **2017**, *25*, 1199–1208. [CrossRef]
73. Mayer, F.Q.; Artigalas, O.A.; Lagranha, V.L.; Baldo, G.; Schwartz, I.V.; Matte, U.; Giugliani, R. Chloramphenicol enhances IDUA activity on fibroblasts from mucopolysaccharidosis I patients. *Curr. Pharm. Biotechnol.* **2013**, *14*, 194–198. [CrossRef] [PubMed]
74. Luddi, A.; Crifasi, L.; Capaldo, A.; Piomboni, P.; Costantino-Ceccarini, E. Suppression of galactocerebrosidase premature termination codon and rescue of galactocerebrosidase activity in twitcher cells. *J. Neurosci. Res.* **2016**, *94*, 1273–1283. [CrossRef] [PubMed]
75. Thada, V.; Miller, J.N.; Kovacs, A.D.; Pearce, D.A. Tissue-specific variation in nonsense mutant transcript level and drug-induced read-through efficiency in the Cln1(R151X) mouse model of INCL. *J. Cell. Mol. Med.* **2016**, *20*, 381–385. [CrossRef] [PubMed]
76. Brasell, E.J.; Chu, L.; El Kares, R.; Seo, J.H.; Loesch, R.; Iglesias, D.M.; Goodyer, P. The aminoglycoside geneticin permits translational readthrough of the CTNS W138X nonsense mutation in fibroblasts from patients with nephropathic cystinosis. *Pediatr. Nephrol.* **2019**, *34*, 873–881. [CrossRef] [PubMed]
77. Baradaran-Heravi, A.; Balgi, A.D.; Zimmerman, C.; Choi, K.; Shidmoossavee, F.S.; Tan, J.S.; Bergeaud, C.; Krause, A.; Flibotte, S.; Shimizu, Y.; et al. Novel small molecules potentiate premature termination codon readthrough by aminoglycosides. *Nucleic Acids Res.* **2016**, *44*, 6583–6598. [CrossRef] [PubMed]
78. Giugliani, R.; Dalla Corte, A.; Poswar, F.; Vancella, C.; Horovitz, D.; Riegel, M.; Baldo, G.; Vairo, F. Intrathecal/Intracerebroventricular enzyme replacement therapy for the mucopolysaccharidoses: Efficacy, safety, and prospects. *Exp. Opin. Orphan Drugs* **2018**, *6*, 403–411. [CrossRef]
79. Giugliani, R.; Giugliani, L.; de Oliveira Poswar, F.; Donis, K.C.; Corte, A.D.; Schmidt, M.; Boado, R.J.; Nestrasil, I.; Nguyen, C.; Chen, S.; et al. Neurocognitive and somatic stabilization in pediatric patients with severe Mucopolysaccharidosis Type I after 52 weeks of intravenous brain-penetrating insulin receptor antibody-iduronidase fusion protein (valanafusp alpha): An open label phase 1-2 trial. *Orphanet J. Rare Dis.* **2018**, *13*, 110. [CrossRef]
80. Okuyama, T.; Eto, Y.; Sakai, N.; Minami, K.; Yamamoto, T.; Sonoda, H.; Yamaoka, M.; Tachibana, K.; Hirato, T.; Sato, Y. Iduronate-2-Sulfatase with Anti-human Transferrin Receptor Antibody for Neuropathic Mucopolysaccharidosis II: A Phase 1/2 Trial. *Mol. Ther.* **2019**, *27*, 456–464. [CrossRef]
81. Schiffmann, R.; Goker-Alpan, O.; Holida, M.; Giraldo, P.; Barisoni, L.; Colvin, R.B.; Jennette, C.J.; Maegawa, G.; Boyadjiev, S.A.; Gonzalez, D.; et al. Pegunigalsidase alfa, a novel PEGylated enzyme replacement therapy for Fabry disease, provides sustained plasma concentrations and favorable pharmacodynamics: A 1-year Phase 1/2 clinical trial. *J. Inherit. Metab. Dis.* **2019**, *42*, 534–544. [CrossRef]
82. Baldo, G.; Mayer, F.Q.; Martinelli, B.; Meyer, F.S.; Burin, M.; Meurer, L.; Tavares, A.M.; Giugliani, R.; Matte, U. Intraperitoneal implant of recombinant encapsulated cells overexpressing alpha-L-iduronidase partially corrects visceral pathology in mucopolysaccharidosis type I mice. *Cytotherapy* **2012**, *14*, 860–867. [CrossRef]
83. Xu, S.; Lun, Y.; Frascella, M.; Garcia, A.; Soska, R.; Nair, A.; Ponery, A.S.; Schilling, A.; Feng, J.; Tuske, S.; et al. Improved efficacy of a next-generation ERT in murine Pompe disease. *JCI Insight* **2019**, *4*. [CrossRef] [PubMed]

84. Wasserstein, M.P.; Diaz, G.A.; Lachmann, R.H.; Jouvin, M.H.; Nandy, I.; Ji, A.J.; Puga, A.C. Olipudase alfa for treatment of acid sphingomyelinase deficiency (ASMD): Safety and efficacy in adults treated for 30 months. *J. Inherit Metab. Dis.* **2018**, *41*, 829–838. [CrossRef] [PubMed]
85. Ohashi, T. Gene therapy for lysosomal storage diseases and peroxisomal diseases. *J. Hum. Genet.* **2019**, *64*, 139–143. [CrossRef] [PubMed]
86. Gonzalez E, B.G. Gene Therapy for Lysosomal Storage Disorders: Recent Advances and Limitations. *J. Inborn Errors Metab. Screen.* **2017**, *5*, 1–6. [CrossRef]
87. Corti, M.; Liberati, C.; Smith, B.K.; Lawson, L.A.; Tuna, I.S.; Conlon, T.J.; Coleman, K.E.; Islam, S.; Herzog, R.W.; Fuller, D.D.; et al. Safety of Intradiaphragmatic Delivery of Adeno-Associated Virus-Mediated Alpha-Glucosidase (rAAV1-CMV-hGAA) Gene Therapy in Children Affected by Pompe Disease. *Hum. Gene Ther. Clin. Dev.* **2017**, *28*, 208–218. [CrossRef]
88. Tardieu, M.; Zerah, M.; Gougeon, M.L.; Ausseil, J.; de Bournonville, S.; Husson, B.; Zafeiriou, D.; Parenti, G.; Bourget, P.; Poirier, B.; et al. Intracerebral gene therapy in children with mucopolysaccharidosis type IIIB syndrome: An uncontrolled phase 1/2 clinical trial. *Lancet Neurol.* **2017**, *16*, 712–720. [CrossRef]
89. Sessa, M.; Lorioli, L.; Fumagalli, F.; Acquati, S.; Redaelli, D.; Baldoli, C.; Canale, S.; Lopez, I.D.; Morena, F.; Calabria, A.; et al. Lentiviral haemopoietic stem-cell gene therapy in early-onset metachromatic leukodystrophy: An ad-hoc analysis of a non-randomised, open-label, phase 1/2 trial. *Lancet* **2016**, *388*, 476–487. [CrossRef]
90. Poletto, E.; Baldo, G.; Gomez-Ospina, N. Genome Editing for Mucopolysaccharidoses. *Int. J. Mol. Sci.* **2020**, *21*, 500. [CrossRef]
91. Sheridan, C. Sangamo's landmark genome editing trial gets mixed reception. *Nat. Biotechnol.* **2018**, *36*, 907–908. [CrossRef]
92. Rinaldi, C.; Wood, M.J.A. Antisense oligonucleotides: The next frontier for treatment of neurological disorders. *Nat. Rev. Neurol.* **2018**, *14*, 9–21. [CrossRef]
93. Dardis, A.; Buratti, E. Impact, Characterization, and Rescue of Pre-mRNA Splicing Mutations in Lysosomal Storage Disorders. *Genes* **2018**, *9*, 73. [CrossRef]
94. Rodriguez-Pascau, L.; Coll, M.J.; Vilageliu, L.; Grinberg, D. Antisense oligonucleotide treatment for a pseudoexon-generating mutation in the NPC1 gene causing Niemann-Pick type C disease. *Hum. Mutat.* **2009**, *30*, E993–E1001. [CrossRef] [PubMed]
95. van der Wal, E.; Bergsma, A.J.; Pijnenburg, J.M.; van der Ploeg, A.T.; Pijnappel, W. Antisense Oligonucleotides Promote Exon Inclusion and Correct the Common c.-32-13T>G GAA Splicing Variant in Pompe Disease. *Mol. Ther. Nucleic Acids* **2017**, *7*, 90–100. [CrossRef] [PubMed]
96. Matos, L.; Goncalves, V.; Pinto, E.; Laranjeira, F.; Prata, M.J.; Jordan, P.; Desviat, L.R.; Perez, B.; Alves, S. Functional analysis of splicing mutations in the IDS gene and the use of antisense oligonucleotides to exploit an alternative therapy for MPS II. *Biochim. Biophys. Acta* **2015**, *1852*, 2712–2721. [CrossRef] [PubMed]
97. Parenti, G.; Andria, G.; Ballabio, A. Lysosomal storage diseases: From pathophysiology to therapy. *Annu. Rev. Med.* **2015**, *66*, 471–486. [CrossRef] [PubMed]
98. Macauley, S.L. Combination Therapies for Lysosomal Storage Diseases: A Complex Answer to a Simple Problem. *Pediatr. Endocrinol. Rev.* **2016**, *13* (Suppl. 1), 639–648. [PubMed]
99. Eisengart, J.B.; Jarnes, J.; Ahmed, A.; Nestrasil, I.; Ziegler, R.; Delaney, K.; Shapiro, E.; Whitley, C. Long-term cognitive and somatic outcomes of enzyme replacement therapy in untransplanted Hurler syndrome. *Mol. Genet. Metab. Rep.* **2017**, *13*, 64–68. [CrossRef]
100. Ng, M.; Gupta, A.; Lund, T.; Orchard, P. Impact of extended post-HSCT enzyme replacement therapy (ERT) on linear growth in mucopolysaccharidosis type IH (MPS IH). *Mol. Genet. Metab.* **2020**, *129*, S115–S116. [CrossRef]
101. Schiffmann, R.; Cox, T.M.; Ida, H.; Mengel Mistry, P.; Crawford, N.; Gaemers, S.; Jih, A.; Peterschmitt, M.J.; Sharma, J.; Zhang, Q.; et al. Venglustat combined with imiglucerase positively affects neurological features and brain connectivity in adults with Gaucher disease type 3. *Mol. Genet. Metab.* **2020**, *129*, S144–S145. [CrossRef]

102. Roberts, M.S.; Macauley, S.L.; Wong, A.M.; Yilmas, D.; Hohm, S.; Cooper, J.D.; Sands, M.S. Combination small molecule PPT1 mimetic and CNS-directed gene therapy as a treatment for infantile neuronal ceroid lipofuscinosis. *J. Inherit. Metab. Dis.* **2012**, *35*, 847–857. [CrossRef]
103. Hawkins-Salsbury, J.A.; Shea, L.; Jiang, X.; Hunter, D.A.; Guzman, A.M.; Reddy, A.S.; Qin, E.Y.; Li, Y.; Gray, S.J.; Ory, D.S.; et al. Mechanism-based combination treatment dramatically increases therapeutic efficacy in murine globoid cell leukodystrophy. *J. Neurosci.* **2015**, *35*, 6495–6505. [CrossRef] [PubMed]

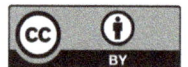

© 2020 by the authors. Licensee MDPI, Basel, Switzerland. This article is an open access article distributed under the terms and conditions of the Creative Commons Attribution (CC BY) license (http://creativecommons.org/licenses/by/4.0/).

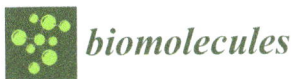

Review

Pompe Disease: New Developments in an Old Lysosomal Storage Disorder

Naresh K. Meena and Nina Raben *

Cell and Developmental Biology Center, National Heart, Lung, and Blood Institute, NIH, Bethesda, MD 20892, USA; nareshkumar.meena@nih.gov
* Correspondence: rabenn@mail.nih.gov

Received: 27 August 2020; Accepted: 15 September 2020; Published: 18 September 2020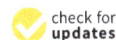

Abstract: Pompe disease, also known as glycogen storage disease type II, is caused by the lack or deficiency of a single enzyme, lysosomal acid alpha-glucosidase, leading to severe cardiac and skeletal muscle myopathy due to progressive accumulation of glycogen. The discovery that acid alpha-glucosidase resides in the lysosome gave rise to the concept of lysosomal storage diseases, and Pompe disease became the first among many monogenic diseases caused by loss of lysosomal enzyme activities. The only disease-specific treatment available for Pompe disease patients is enzyme replacement therapy (ERT) which aims to halt the natural course of the illness. Both the success and limitations of ERT provided novel insights in the pathophysiology of the disease and motivated the scientific community to develop the next generation of therapies that have already progressed to the clinic.

Keywords: Pompe disease; lysosome; lysosomal targeting; autophagy; enzyme replacement therapy; gene therapy; muscle; satellite cells

1. Introduction

Pompe disease, also known as Type II glycogen storage disease (GSDII), is a rare autosomal recessive neuromuscular disorder that affects people of all ages. This severe, often fatal illness gained a well-deserved reputation for being the first recognized lysosomal storage disorder, a group which now includes more than 50 entities [1]. In the 1960s, some thirty years after the first description of the illness by Joannes Cassianus Pompe [2], the mystery behind massive accumulation of glycogen in multiple tissues in autopsy reports from the affected individuals was solved: the patients were missing the enzyme, acid alpha-glucosidase (GAA), which had an acidic pH optimum, and glycogen was stored in a membrane-bound organelle, suggesting its lysosomal origin [3]. This enzyme is uniquely responsible for total hydrolysis of glycogen to glucose in the lysosome, and its deficiency manifests as a multisystem disorder with predominant involvement of skeletal and cardiac muscles.

The estimated frequency of the disease is often cited as 1 in 40,000 live births [4], but recent implementation of newborn screening (NBS) for Pompe disease revealed a much higher frequency [5,6]. The first such a program was enacted in Taiwan in 2005 [7], followed by several other countries including the US, where the recommendation by the Advisory Committee on Heritable Disorders in Newborns and Children to add Pompe disease to the Recommended Uniform Screening Panel was finally approved in 2015.

The enzyme is synthesized as a 110-kD precursor, which is glycosylated in the endoplasmic reticulum (ER) and phosphorylated on mannose residues in Golgi apparatus on its way to the late endosome/lysosomes, where the enzyme undergoes extensive proteolytic processing yielding, through a 95-kD endosomal intermediate, fully processed 76- and 70-kD mature lysosomal forms with higher affinity for the natural substrate, glycogen [8,9]. These posttranslational modifications, common to many lysosomal hydrolases [10], ensure their transport to the lysosomal system through the mannose-6-phosphate (M6P) receptor-mediated pathway [11]. Importantly, a portion of the precursor protein can be secreted, taken up by ubiquitous cell surface M6P receptors, and delivered to the lysosome through the endocytic pathway, thus providing the basis for enzyme replacement therapy for Pompe and other lysosomal storage disorders. The structure of recombinant human GAA has been solved by X-ray crystallography [12].

The severity of the disease largely corresponds to the nature of the genetic defect and the degree of residual enzyme activity, giving rise to a wide range of phenotypes that differ in the age of onset and the rate of progression [13,14]. Although this condition represents a single disease continuum, two discrete phenotypes are broadly accepted: the most severe and rapidly fatal infantile onset form and a milder late onset form with or without cardiac involvement respectively.

More than 500 mutations have been reported, including insertions, deletions, splice site, nonsense, and missense mutations (pompevariantdatabase.nl). Most are unique to families, but some are common in particular ethnic groups, such as the Dutch, Chinese from Taiwan, African-Americans, etc., (reviewed in [15]). The most common defect in Caucasians with late-onset disease is the leaky intronic mutation (c.-32-13T>G IVS1) [16] which allows for the generation of low levels of normal enzyme [17–19]. A recent study demonstrated that in a subset of patients, the IVS1 mutant allele contains a genetic modifier (c510C>T; a synonymous mutation) which further reduces the amount of active enzyme [20]. The advances in new molecular techniques, such as a generic-splicing assay, minigene analysis, SNP array analysis, and targeted Sanger sequencing, significantly expanded the scope of genetic diagnostic analysis in Pompe disease patients [21].

Following years of drug development, preclinical studies in a mouse model [22,23], and two pivotal clinical trials [24,25], recombinant human GAA-a drug called alglucosidase alfa (rhGAA; Myozyme© (ex-US) and Lumizyme© (US); Genzyme, Cambridge, Massachusetts)-received broad-label marketing approval for the treatment of Pompe disease in 2006. Enzyme replacement therapy (ERT) became the first disease-specific treatment and remains the only approved therapy for Pompe disease. In this review we will explore how the therapy changed the disease landscape by altering clinical picture, stimulating efforts to better understand the pathogenesis, and motivating industry and academia to develop next-generation treatments.

2. An Expanded Set of Clinical Characteristics

Pompe disease presents with a wide range of clinical characteristics and different life expectancy depending on the age at onset. Two major distinctive clinical phenotypes are recognized based on the age at which the symptoms appear and the presence or absence of cardiomyopathy: the most severe classic infantile onset type (IOPD) includes patients with less than 1% of GAA activity who develop symptoms within the first year of life and, if left untreated, rarely survive beyond 18 months; the milder late-onset type (LOPD) with higher enzyme activity may become apparent in childhood, adolescence, or adulthood.

Patients with IOPD present with rapidly progressive hypertrophic cardiomyopathy, left ventricular outflow obstruction, elevated creatine kinase, generalized muscle weakness, hypotonia, macroglossia, failure to thrive, respiratory distress and loss of independent ventilation. Major motor milestones, such as the ability to roll over, sit, or stand, are not achieved; the majority of patients die from a combination of heart and respiratory failure. Although this most devastating type is clinically homogeneous, there is an important distinction among the patients in that some produce non-functional enzyme (cross-reactive immunological material (CRIM)-positive), whereas others produce no enzyme at all (CRIM-negative). Additionally, a subset of patients with similar age of onset and clinical presentations but without/or less severe cardiomyopathy and absence of left ventricular outflow obstruction are classified as non-classic IOPD; delayed motor skills and severe progressive muscle weakness leading to respiratory failure by early childhood are main characteristics of the disease in this subgroup [26,27].

The introduction of ERT has been a major breakthrough in the field, and the treatment proved to be most beneficial for patients with IOPD who survive significantly longer due to a remarkable effect of the drug on cardiac size and function. The reversal of hypertrophic cardiomyopathy and the improvement of cardiac function were observed in most patients within the first months on ERT. This effect of the drug was already evident in the first clinical trials [24,25], and the expectation was that the treatment would convert the most severe infantile form to a milder late-onset type. However, in more than a decade since the regulatory approval of the drug, it became clear that this is not the case. The survivors, in particular long-term survivors develop a new phenotype that reflects multisystem involvement with some of the symptoms that have not been previously ascribed to Pompe disease [28]. Almost all long-term survivors are plagued with muscle weakness despite ERT, leading to a characteristic gait pattern, lumbar hyperlordosis, and progressive scoliosis. Respiratory dysfunction that results from both muscular and neural deficits [29] is a common problem necessitating non-invasive or invasive assisted ventilation. Hearing loss, ptosis, a motor speech disorder, and much reduced speech intelligibility are all manifestations of a new emerging phenotype [28] (reviewed in [30]). Additional symptoms include swallowing difficulties, gastro-esophageal reflux, and aspiration leading to increased risk of upper respiratory tract infections and pneumonia. Accumulation of excess glycogen in the brain of patient with IOPD [31] may lead to neurocognitive impairment in a number of patients [32]. A recent study [33] reported progressive white matter lesions which affect cognitive and neuropsychological development in ERT-treated patients with IOPD who reached adulthood. These changes were not seen previously because of early fatality in untreated IOPD patients.

Several basic conclusions can be drawn: A number of patients still die within the first years of life despite ERT; the response to ERT in CRIM-negative patients is confounded by an immune response against the enzyme [34] and is less effective even with immunomodulation; the best results are achieved when the patients are afforded very early treatment-within the first few days of life-which became feasible with the initiation of newborn screening [35]. However, even under the best-case scenario, when ERT was initiated within the first 10 days of life in CRIM-positive IOPD patients, airway abnormalities and speech disorders were still observed over the course of 8 years in a retrospective study [36]. Finally, a new phenotype with clinical manifestations of the CNS lesions requires additional intervention since the neurological manifestations are not amenable to ERT and raises new questions about how treatment will be shaped in the future.

The symptoms of limb-girdle muscle weakness, respiratory dysfunction, and hyperCKemia at any time beyond 12 months of age are the main characteristics of the late-onset form Pompe disease. Initial signs, such as exercise intolerance, muscle pain, and fatigue, are often overlooked or ignored leading to a delayed diagnosis [37,38]. Later on, slowly progressive deterioration of axial, limb-girdle, and respiratory muscle, particularly the diaphragm, eventually leads to wheelchair-dependency and assisted ventilation. The lower airway smooth muscles involvement (well documented in a mouse model [39]) contributes to respiratory problems, and respiratory failure is the main cause of death in LOPD even in patients on ERT.

The view of LOPD has shifted away from its original definition as primarily a muscle disorder. As in IOPD, the expanded spectrum of clinical manifestations reflects the involvement of multiple tissues and organs, thus establishing the multisystem nature of this illness. The emerging new features of the disease include vascular and cerebrovascular defects, for example, intracranial aneurysm or dilative arteriopathy, hearing loss, central and peripheral nervous system abnormalities, scoliosis, progressive loss of bone mass, as well as gastrointestinal and urinary tract symptoms [40] (reviewed in [41]). A small subset of LOPD patients develop cardiomyopathy which improves on ERT [42].

The majority of LOPD patients benefit from ERT in that the therapy improves or stabilizes motor and respiratory function but skeletal muscle weakness persists, and many show signs of disease progression [43,44]. Inefficient glycogen clearance in smooth muscle of vascular, ocular, gastrointestinal, and respiratory systems has been reported in ERT-treated patients (reviewed in [45]). A number of patients still require ventilation and become wheelchair dependent despite several years on ERT [46]. A recent long-term (10 years) prospective study reported that the initial positive response to therapy in the first 3–5 years was followed by a secondary decline in walking ability, muscle strength, and pulmonary function [47].

Overall, there is a great deal of variability in LOPD patients' response to therapy, ranging from those who continue to respond well up to 8–10 years to those who do not respond at all. Although the reasons of this variability are not exactly understood, the extent of underlying muscle pathology is, no doubt, an important factor. Not surprisingly, a detailed analysis of muscle biopsies from a large cohort of LOPD patients before the ERT initiation demonstrated a correlation between the severity of muscle damage and response to therapy. However, no correlation between the duration of the disease and more severe muscle damage was observed, and there was no meaningful genotype–phenotype correlation in this group [48].

The lack of any clinical stabilization or improvement in the first 2 years of treatment or deterioration of clinical condition despite therapy constitute the reasons to consider the discontinuation of ERT; these criteria are included in the guidelines developed by a multidisciplinary expert committee of the European Pompe consortium (EPOC). Interestingly, no acceleration in decline was observed in several patients who discontinued ERT in accordance with the established criteria [49,50], suggesting that at least in some cases ERT is of dubious benefit. As for the timing to start ERT, the European consensus states that only symptomatic patients with confirmed diagnosis should be treated. However, this practice may not last long because LOPD patients, diagnosed through new-born screening and carefully followed up, were shown to have overt or subtle symptoms much earlier than expected [51]. The search for reliable biomarkers to aid in diagnosis, progression, and response to ERT has remained elusive over the past decades. In this regard, of particular interest is the recent identification of circulating microRNAs as potential biomarkers of Pompe disease [52,53] (reviewed in [54]). These new biomarkers, in particular miR-133a, can help monitor the efficacy of the current and emerging therapies by serial sampling through liquid biopsies.

3. Beyond the Lysosome: Pathogenic Cascade and Muscle Regeneration

Our understanding of the mechanisms driving the pathogenesis of muscle damage in Pompe disease is rapidly evolving. Not long ago, the pathogenesis was viewed as a process that occurs in stages, including gradual glycogen buildup in the lysosomal lumen, lysosomal membrane rupture due to the mechanical pressure, a discharge of glycogen and potentially toxic materials into the cytoplasm, and finally the destruction of muscle architecture [55]. These somewhat loosely defined morphological stages as well as normal looking myofibers next to the affected ones, can indeed be recognized in a biopsy from the same LOPD patient. This heterogeneity in the degree of myofibers damage within a single muscle bundle is one of the mysteries in Pompe disease. In contrast, muscle morphology in IOPD patients is more homogeneous, normal fibers are commonly absent, and muscle architecture is lost in most cells.

The first "blow" to this simplistic view of the pathogenesis came from the experiments in GAA KO mice (KO) [56]. Ultrastructural and morphological observations revealed the presence of large areas of autophagic accumulation in muscle samples from KO [22]. Following this initial finding, we began to unravel the contribution of autophagy to the pathophysiology of Pompe disease.

Macroautophagy (often referred to as autophagy) is a major degradative pathway that delivers cytoplasmic cargo to the lysosome where the final breakdown occurs. Various types of cargo including a portion of the cytoplasm, misfolded protein aggregates, glycogen, and in the case of eukaryotes, malfunctioning organelles, are transported to the lysosome in newly formed double membrane-bound vesicles, called autophagosomes, that fuse with lysosomes. This process requires the recruitment and assembly of multiple components of the autophagy machinery. Basal autophagic activity maintains tissue homeostasis and serves as quality control mechanism by promoting the degradation of toxic protein aggregates and aberrant organelles [57]. Aside from its basal role, autophagic activity can be induced in response to a variety of stress conditions, providing an adaptive mechanism to ensure the cell's survival [58,59].

Skeletal muscles rely heavily on autophagy because muscle fibers are terminally differentiated cells unable to divide and dilute aberrant proteins and organelles through cell division [60]. It is now well-established that too much or too little autophagic activity can negatively affect muscle function and result in muscle wasting [61,62]. Accumulation of autophagic debris is a prominent feature of a group of muscle disorders, including Pompe disease, called autophagic vacuolar myopathies [63].

The sheer size of the areas occupied by the piles of autophagic debris in muscle fibers in KO mice is quite remarkable. Long stretches of autophagic accumulation, often extending the whole length of the fibers and located in their cores, can be visualized by confocal microscopy of single muscle fibers immunostained with lysosomal (LAMP1) and autophagosomal (LC3) markers. Ultrastructural studies revealed the contents of the autophagic areas: classical double-membrane autophagosomes with undigested materials or glycogen particles, glycogen-laden lysosomes with broken borders, multivesicular bodies, and multimembrane concentric membranous structures. These areas are completely devoid of sarcomere structure and, therefore, are unable to contract. Indeed, there is a significant reduction in muscle force ex vivo in KO compared to WT [64].

The molecular mechanism underlying the defective autophagy in the diseased muscle involves both increased formation of autophagosomes (induction of autophagy) and their inefficient fusion with lysosomes (autophagic block). Elevated levels of proteins required for the initial steps of autophagy (autophagosome nucleation and maturation), such as VPS15 protein kinase, the lipid kinase catalytic subunit VPS34, and the regulatory protein Beclin1, in muscle biopsies from KO and Pompe patients [65,66] argue for autophagy induction. The mechanism of this surge in autophagy is not exactly clear. Likewise, the mechanism of impaired autophagosomal-lysosomal fusion, which can be directly observed by time-lapse microscopy of live fibers co-stained with LC3/LAMP1 [67], is not fully understood. Our recent finding of increased levels of galectin 3, a sensitive marker of endosomal/lysosomal damage, in KO muscle offers a possible explanation for the defective fusion [66].

Defective autophagy, a major secondary abnormality in the affected muscles, can have dire consequences: oxidative stress, accumulation of aberrant mitochondria and autophagic substrates, such as p62/SQSTM1 and potentially toxic high molecular weight K63-linked ubiquitinated protein aggregates. Furthermore, autophagic buildup negatively affects trafficking and lysosomal delivery of the therapeutic enzyme [67–69] and contributes to poor skeletal muscle response to ERT [70,71]. Importantly, autophagic accumulation and elevated levels of galectin 3 can be detected as early as in 6-week-old KO mice, well before the disease becomes clinically apparent [66].

Yet another layer in the pathogenic cascade of muscle damage in Pompe disease involves dysregulation of lysosome-based signaling pathways. Gone is the view of the lysosome as a low-key cellular recycling center. New research over the past decade positions this organelle at the center of metabolic signaling pathways. The lysosome integrates multiple environmental signals to maintain cellular homeostasis by regulating the switch between anabolic and catabolic state. Two major kinases that have broadly opposing effects-the nutrient-sensitive mammalian target of rapamycin complex 1 (mTORC1) and the energy-sensing AMP-activated protein kinase alpha 1 (AMPK)-play principal roles in controlling metabolic programs. Much is now understood about the role of the lysosome as a platform for the activation of these kinases, and how these two signaling pathways cross-talk directly and indirectly at multiple levels to balance ATP-consuming biosynthetic and ATP-producing catabolic pathways and to send feedback signals for lysosomal biogenesis and autophagy [72]. The communication and coordination between the mTORC1 and AMPK pathways involve an ever-growing number of signaling intermediates, but this field is beyond the scope of this review. Here, we will name only those few that have been analyzed in Pompe disease.

The recruitment of mTORC1 to the lysosomal membrane under nutrient-rich condition brings the kinase to close proximity to its activator, Ras homologue enriched in brain (RHEB), which resides on lysosomes. RHEB is negatively regulated by the tuberous sclerosis complex (TSC2) leading to the inhibition of mTORC1 activity. In its turn, TSC integrates a range of inputs including AMPK pathway [73,74] (reviewed in [75–78]). Activation of AMPK by upstream liver kinase B1 (LKB1) [79] occurs on the surface of late endosome/lysosome, where AMPK phosphorylates and activate the TSC complex, thereby inactivating RHEB and mTORC1 signaling [76]. When nutrients are plenty, mTORC1 phosphorylates and inactivates a key initiator of autophagy, ULK1, on Ser758 to inhibit autophagy and prevent its interaction with AMPK [80]. On the other hand, AMPK phosphorylates ULK1 on multiple different sites (e.g., Ser317 and Ser777) to activate ULK1 and induce autophagy [80,81].

The dysregulation of AMPK and mTORC1 signaling pathways and defective autophagy have been linked to changes in muscle function and disease [61,82,83] (reviewed in [84]). Extensive analysis of the upstream inputs and downstream targets of AMPK and mTORC1 in cultured GAA-deficient myotubes and in muscle samples from KO mice, performed in our lab, demonstrated a dysregulation of these two pathways in the diseased muscle cells. Increased levels of LKB1 and an increase in the amount of LKB1-mediated Thr^{172} AMPK phosphorylation indicated activation of AMPK, suggesting that the affected muscles are energy deficient. Increased phosphorylation of two downstream AMPK targets-acetyl CoA carboxylase (ACC Ser^{79}) and TBC1D1 (Ser^{660})-confirmed the activation of the LKB1/AMPK pathway. In line with this notion, AMPK-mediated phosphorylation of $TSC2^{S1387}$ and $ULK-1^{S317}$ were markedly increased in KO muscle, whereas mTORC1 activity was decreased as measured by the phosphorylation levels of its downstream targets, EIF4EBP1 and the p70 ribosomal protein S6 kinase [85,86]. What is intriguing about the mTORC1 status in the affected muscle is that this kinase is able to properly move to the lysosome under nutrient-rich condition but unable to move away from the lysosomal surface under starvation, as shown by immunostaining of GAA-deficient myotubes with LAMP1/mTORC1 [85]. The disturbance of mTORC1 signaling was also reported in GAA-deficient C2C12 myoblasts, and in human fibroblasts and induced pluripotent stem cells (iPSCs) from infantile Pompe disease patients [87,88]. Thus, it appears that activation of the LKB1-AMPK pathway and excessive accumulation of TSC2 at the lysosomal surface are responsible for the diminished mTORC1 activity and activation of autophagy in Pompe muscle.

In developing and growing muscle, mTORC1 is viewed as a key regulator of skeletal muscle mass [89]. Indeed, reactivation of mTORC1 in vivo in muscle of KO mice by AAV-mediated TSC knockdown or arginine supplementation resulted in the reversal of muscle atrophy and a striking removal of autophagic buildup [85]. A similar effect was observed in a model of another muscle disorder: activation of mTOR ameliorated muscle atrophy in valosin-containing protein associated inclusion body myopathy (VCP-IBM) [90].

Finally, our recent studies demonstrated a metabolic re-programming in muscle samples derived from KO mice. The metabolome profile of the diseased muscle reflected the state of limited glucose availability and revealed a decrease in glycolysis and a shift from carbohydrate to lipids as the main energy source. Lower than normal glycolysis was also observed in human primary myoblasts from Pompe disease patients [91]. It is worth mentioning that metabolic pathways are highly conserved through evolution, and metabolic similarities between rodents and humans are very comparable despite the commonly observed differences in the phenotype of many mouse models of human diseases, including Pompe disease. In addition, a consistent increase in glycogen synthesis precursors in KO muscle-galactose 1-phosphate and UDP-glucose, the immediate glucose donor for glycogen synthesis-suggests inhibition of cytosolic glycogen synthesis [92]. Thus, progressive lysosomal glycogen accumulation in the diseased muscle sets off a cascade of events, such as altered autophagy and muscle proteostasis, oxidative stress, and dysregulation of major signaling and metabolic pathways (Figure 1). Despite a significant progress in our understanding of the molecular mechanisms of muscle damage in Pompe disease, we are still far from having the whole picture [93].

A somewhat disappointing result of ERT in reversing skeletal muscle pathology became a driving force behind yet another new direction in the field, namely exploring the regenerative capacity of skeletal muscle in Pompe disease. Muscle wasting and atrophy are not only the result of increased breakdown of damaged muscle cells, but also a decreased ability of satellite cells to replace lost myofibers (reviewed in [94]). Activation of Pax7-positive multipotent satellite cells is a prerequisite for muscle regenerative response [95] (reviewed in [96]). These cells, located between the sarcolemma and basal lamina of myofibers, typically exist in adult muscle in mitotically quiescent state, but when activated begin to proliferate and differentiate, leading to the replenishment of the quiescent satellite cell reserve and the formation of new myofibers for muscle repair.

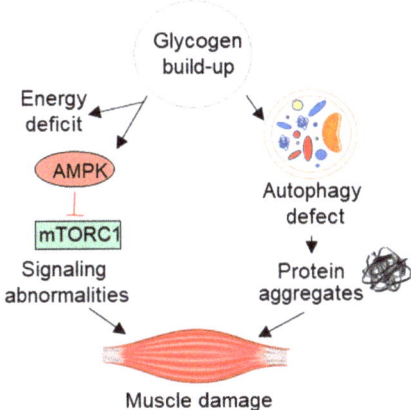

Figure 1. Pathogenic cascade of muscle damage in Pompe disease.

Importantly, analysis of muscle biopsies from both IOPD and LOPD patients indicated that the pool of Pax7-positive satellite cells was well preserved in each group independent of the disease severity, but the regenerative activity of muscle was absent; mild regenerative response was detected only in some classic infantile patients [97]. These data provided indirect evidence of a failure of satellite cell activation in Pompe disease. In the follow-up studies in murine models of Pompe disease, two independent groups [98,99] demonstrated that despite extensive muscle damage, the number of regenerating fibers in adult animals is essentially negligible. Remarkably, the satellite cells were fully functional and were able to robustly respond to acute and repeated muscle injury induced by cardiotoxin or barium chloride leading to efficient muscle regeneration comparable to that in WT controls. Thus, muscle from GAA-KO mice regenerated efficiently in response to exogenous insult but failed to do so to counteract relentless damage during the course of the disease. Resolving the apparent conundrum of why muscle SCs remain inactive in Pompe disease, while still retaining their potential to become activated, may open up new therapeutic venues. Given the role of autophagy in providing nutrients needed to meet the bioenergetic demands during transition of satellite cells from quiescence into an activated state [100], defective autophagy in the diseased muscle may be responsible for the missing activation signal.

4. Evolution of Therapy

There is no doubt that Pompe disease patients have benefited from alglucosidase alfa treatment. Although it is clear that the current drug is no panacea, the therapy has added years and quality of life to the lives of people with the disease. It is also equally clear that a more efficient therapy is much needed. The number of studies designed to improve the therapy, both in vitro and in vivo in mouse models, has skyrocketed in past years. Multiple approaches, such as substrate reduction therapy, inhibition of autophagy and modulation of mTORC1 signaling, chaperone therapy, stimulation of lysosomal exocytosis, antisense oligonucleotides, etc., have been explored as a potential alternative or adjunct therapies. We refer the reader to several recent reviews on these subjects [101–103]. Instead, we will cover the strategies that have already moved to the clinic and focus on the completed, ongoing, or enrolling clinical trials evaluating the effects of new recombinant enzymes and gene therapy.

A major shortcoming of the current standard of care is the inability of alglucosidase alfa to reach skeletal muscle efficiently; in fact, less than 1% of i.v. bolus administered enzyme ends up in muscle [104]. As mentioned above, the cation-independent mannose 6-phosphate receptor (CI-M6PR) has been exploited to deliver the exogenous recombinant enzymes for the treatment of lysosomal storage disorders. The receptor binds its ligands, the M6P bearing proteins, at the cell surface and transports the cargo to acidic late endosomal compartment, where the proteins and the receptor part ways, so that the proteins move to the lysosome whereas the receptor is recycled for the next round of ligand transport. A major reason for the suboptimal efficacy of alglucosidase alfa in skeletal muscle is that M6P-enzyme represents only a small fraction of the drug since its overall content of M6P glycan is low [23]. The problem is further compounded by the relatively low abundance of CI-MPR in muscle tissue [105,106].

4.1. Next-Generation ERT

Notably, the less than optimal intrinsic quality of alglucosidase alfa was understood years ago, as indicated by the efforts in the early 2000s to enhance the delivery of the therapeutic enzyme to the affected muscle by carbohydrate remodeling of the original enzyme to increase the amount of M6P [107]. This early work and an extended follow-up study [108] led to the development of a modified glycoengineered enzyme with a synthetic oligosaccharide harboring mannose 6-phosphate (M6P) residues. This new recombinant human GAA, called neo-GAA, with much improved affinity for the CI-MPR and uptake by muscle cells, showed more efficient glycogen clearance in immunotolerized KO mice compared to the unmodified enzyme, particularly in younger mice. Muscle glycogen reduction was also achieved in older symptomatic KO mice, but the improvement in motor function was only marginal [108].

Neo-GAA (Avalglucosidase alfa; Sanofi Genzyme, Cambridge, MA, USA), a second-generation glycoengineered recombinant GAA with increased bis-M6P levels, was first evaluated for safety and tolerability in a now completed clinical trial (NCT01898364). The results of this Phase 1/2 open-labeled, ascending-dose (5, 10, and 20 mg/kg biweekly over the course of 24 weeks) study in previously ERT-treated (switch group) and -untreated (naïve group) LOPD patients was recently published [109]. Neo-GAA was overall well-tolerated and safe; only two of the 24 enrolled patients discontinued because of the drug-related serious adverse events. Based on the glycogen levels in baseline quadriceps biopsies (~6% of tissue area), patients from both groups were considered to be mildly affected. Although the assessment of efficacy was not a part of the protocol, exploratory efficacy parameters showed a slight improvement in pulmonary function in ERT-naïve and no decline in ERT-switch patients. A Phase 3 study to compare the safety and efficacy of neo-GAA and alglucosidase alfa in previously untreated LOPD was initiated in 2016 and is ongoing (COMET; NCT02782741). In the randomized, double-blind portion of the study, patients received either neo-GAA or alglucosidase alfa (standard of care) for 49 weeks; thereafter, all patients participated in ongoing open-label treatment with neo-GAA. In addition, the company's clinical development program includes several other exploratory efficacy studies with neo-GAA in LOPD and IOPD patients.

Another new investigational drug, AT-GAA (Amicus Therapeutics, Cranbury, NJ, USA) is the combination of a novel non-modified rhGAA bearing high bis-M6P (Amicus proprietary cell line) with a pharmacological chaperone (AT2221; N-butyldeoxynojirimycin; NB-DNJ, miglustat) for stabilizing the enzyme in the circulation (reviewed in [104]). Both preclinical and clinical studies in Pompe disease patients demonstrated that small molecules chaperones increased the stability and bioavailability of the therapeutic enzyme [103,110–112].

In a large preclinical study in KO mice, AT-GAA was shown to significantly outperform alglucosidase alfa in all measured outcomes: GAA uptake and activity, muscle strength, reduction in lysosomal size and glycogen levels, and mitigation of autophagic defect [92]. Furthermore, long-term treatment of KO with AT-GAA completely reversed muscle lysosomal glycogen accumulation, eliminated autophagic buildup in >80% of muscle fibers, and to a large degree restored AMPK/mTORC1 signaling, muscle proteostasis, and metabolic abnormalities [66]. This outcome is in striking contrast with the limited effect of a long-term treatment of KO mice with alglucosidase alfa at a similar dose of 20 mg/kg [22].

AT-GAA was evaluated in Phase 1/2 clinical trial in ERT-switch and naïve non-ambulatory LOPD patients; the drug was well-tolerated with a low number of infusion-associated reactions and showed promising results, as evidenced by improvement in muscle function, increase in upper-body muscle strength, and patient-reported outcomes (reviewed in [104]). Two Phase 3 studies, one comparing AT-GAA with alglucosidase alfa/placebo (PROPEL Study; NCT03729362; active, not recruiting), and the second one (ZIP Study: NCT03911505; recruiting) evaluating the pharmacokinetics, safety, efficacy, and pharmacodynamic of AT-GAA in LOPD patients were initiated in 2018 and 2019 respectively.

An attempt was made to target both lysosomal and extra-lysosomal glycogen accumulation in the affected muscle. VAL-1221 (Valerion Therapeutics, Concord, MA, USA) is a CHO-produced fusion protein containing the 110 kDa human GAA precursor and the Fab fragment of a murine lupus anti-DNA antibody, 3E10. This monoclonal anti-DNA antibody were shown to penetrate living cells and move to the nucleus through the equilibrative nucleoside transporter 2 (ENT2) [113–115]. Experiments in cultured L6 myoblasts and fibroblasts derived from Pompe disease patients as well as in vivo studies in KO mice suggested a potential benefit of this fusion protein [116]. However, in our experience, VAL-1221 in KO mice did not show any improvement in muscle glycogen content (unpublished data). A Phase 1/2 dose-escalation clinical trial (NCT02898753) of VAL-1221 in previously treated LOPD patients was initiated in 2017 [117], but the results of this study were not validated by peer review. As of June 2020, the company terminated this trial in the US and UK.

Finally, a combination of alglucosidase alfa with β2 agonists, clenbuterol, or albuterol, was shown to enhance the efficacy of the therapeutic enzyme owing to the increased expression of CI-MPR in skeletal muscle [118,119]. A pilot study of albuterol plus ERT in LOPD patients who were not improving further following more than two years on ERT alone showed the benefit of this approach [120]. A phase 1/2 double-blind, randomized, placebo-controlled 52-week study (NCT01942590) of clenbuterol in LOPD patients treated with ERT provided evidence for safety and showed a modest improvement in motor function [121]. This study (initiated in 2013) is now completed. Table 1 summarizes the above-mentioned clinical trials.

4.2. Gene Therapy

There is a dramatic surge in the number of drug candidates for gene therapy to combat human diseases, and Pompe disease is no exception. The limitations of the currently available ERT, along with the requirement for frequent life-long i.v. infusions, and the inability of the therapeutic enzyme to cross BBB, make the development of gene therapy for Pompe disease an attractive option. Over the past years, the field has witnessed the explosion of gene therapy studies testing different types of vectors, various promoters, numerous elements of the transgene expression cassette, and routes of delivery in preclinical setting. These studies are discussed in several recent reviews [102,122–125]. Here, we focused on already initiated and planned gene-therapy-based clinical trials using nonpathogenic adeno-associated virus (AAV) as a vector (Table 1). Unlike the wild type virus, the recombinant AAV genome largely remains in an episomal form in the nucleus and has a low frequency of integration in the host cell genome (reviewed in [126]). AAV quickly became the vectors of choice for Pompe disease gene therapy.

Based on the results of the early preclinical studies evaluating the effect of systemic or intramuscular administration of AAV vectors in KO mice [127–129], the first-in-human trial of gene therapy for Pompe disease began in 2006, thus marking a milestone in the field. This was an open label, Phase 1/2 trial (NCT00976352) using direct injection of rAAV2/1-CMV-hGAA into the diaphragm of a small group of children who required assisted ventilation despite ERT. The study confirmed safety and showed a tendency to improve respiratory function in some patients [130–132].

Phase 1/2 clinical trial evaluating the feasibility of two successive intramuscular (into tibialis anterior muscle) administration of an AAV9 vector expressing GAA is ongoing and is recruiting patients with LOPD (NCT02240407). The recombinant AAV carries the codon-optimized acid alpha-glucosidase under the control of human desmin enhancer/promoter (rAAV9-DES-hGAA). The immune modulation strategy using Rituximab and Sirolimus prior and after the first administration of the vector is designed to prevent the immune response against the AAV capsid and the transgene, thus allowing for the second vector administration. The same group of researchers from University of Florida are planning to initiate a new Phase 1/2 clinical trial of systemic injection of rAAV9-DES-GAA in 3–5-year-old IOPD patients.

Another approach-hepatic gene transfer-relies on a remarkable ability of hepatocytes to produce and secrete the expressed protein into the bloodstream, thus providing a steady supply of the therapeutic enzyme for the uptake by other tissues. Early studies on KO mice demonstrated that a single i.v. administration of a modified adenovirus (AV) vector encoding human GAA resulted in efficient liver transduction, secretion of the GAA precursor, and clearance of lysosomal glycogen accumulation in skeletal and cardiac muscles [133]. These results along with the follow-up studies [134,135] provided a solid foundation for using what is now called "liver depot gene therapy" in Pompe disease. However, the use of AAV vectors is now highly preferred for achieving a long-term persistent therapeutic gene transfer.

The unique immunologic properties of the liver allow for the induction of immune tolerance to foreign antigens through a regulatory T-cell mediated mechanism (reviewed in [136]). Indeed, AAV-mediated liver-specific expression of human GAA in KO mice was shown to prevent the formation of anti-GAA antibody when the vector was administered prior to the start of ERT, thus improving ERT efficacy [137–139]. The concept of induction of tolerance to the therapeutic enzyme delivered during ERT by low-dose AAV vector administration is termed "immunomodulatory gene therapy" [140]. Multiple preclinical studies have explored the impact of different AAV serotypes and promoters, vector dosages, and modifications of the GAA sequence, such as the signal peptide and codon optimization, to enhance GAA secretion into the bloodstream and to better control humoral immune responses (reviewed in [123,124,141]). These studies have culminated in the first liver gene therapy clinical trials for Pompe disease.

Table 1. Next generation therapies for Pompe disease.

Intervention/Treatment	Characteristics/Delivery Method	Company/Institution	Clinical Trial Phase/Identifier	References
ERT				
neo-GAA	Glycoengineered recombinant GAA with increased bis-M6P levels (avalglucosidase alfa)	Genzyme, a Sanofi Company	Completed/NCT01898364 Phase 3/NCT02782741	Zhu et al. [108] Pena et al. [109]
AT-GAA (ATB200/AT2221)	rhGAA bearing high bis-M6P with a pharmacological chaperone (miglustat)	Amicus Therapeutics	Phase 3/NCT03729362 Phase 3/NCT03911505	Khanna et al. [111] Xu et al. [92] Meena et al. [66]
VAL-1221	Fusion protein containing antibody 3E10 and rhGAA	Valerion Therapeutics	Terminated/NCT02898753	Weisbart et al. [114,115] Yi et al. [116] Kishnani et al. [117]
ERT + Clenbuterol	Alglucosidase alfa with β2-adrenergic agonist clenbuterol	Duke University	Completed/NCT01942590	Koeberl et al. [118–121]
Gene Therapy				
rAAV2/1-CMV-hGAA	Intramuscular injection into the diaphragm	University of Florida	Completed/NCT00976352	Smith et al. [130] Byrne et al. [131] Corti et al. [132]
rAAV9-DES-hGAA	Intramuscular re-administration	Lacerta Therapeutics/University of Florida	Phase 1/2/NCT02240407	Salabarria et al. [125]
AAV2/8-LSPhGAA	Screening for eligibility Ascending dose intravenous administration	Duke University Asklepios Biopharmaceutical/Duke University	Completed/NCT03285126 Phase 1/2/ NCT03533673	Kishnani et al. [141] Han et al. [142]
SPK-3006 (AAV liver directed secretable GAA)	Intravenous administration	Spark Therapeutics	Phase 1/2/ NCT04093349	Puzzo et al. [143] Cagin et al. [144]

ERT: enzyme replacement therapy; M6P: mannose-6-phosphate; clinical trials listed in this table are registered as of August 2020.

A Phase 1 clinical trial (NCT03533673) of liver depot gene therapy in adult patients is designed to evaluate an rAAV serotype 8 vector carrying the human GAA under the control of liver-specific promoter (AAV2/8-LSPhGAA). This is an ongoing open label, randomized study (currently recruiting). A careful consideration of the vector dosage for this trial was based on the preclinical data showing effective biochemical correction of skeletal muscle at a dose of 2×10^{12} vg/kg, and induction of immune tolerance to the ERT delivered rhGAA (with only partial correction of the muscle defect) at a minimum effective dose of 2×10^{11} vg/kg [142]. These data justified a starting dose of 1.6×10^{12} vg/kg for Phase 1 clinical trial [141]. This clinical trial was preceded by a Pompe gene therapy trial (NCT03285126; completed), designed to determine eligibility for the forthcoming trial in adults with LOPD.

Another Phase 1/2 liver transfer gene therapy clinical trial (NCT04093349; RESOLUTE), initiated by Spark Therapeutics is recruiting patients with LOPD receiving ERT. The study is designed to evaluate the safety, tolerability, and efficacy of investigational liver-directed AAV gene therapy of the secretable GAA (SPK-3006) in adults, treated in sequential dose-level cohorts. Preclinical studies using this AAV8-mediated liver gene transfer of an engineered secretable GAA (secGAA) resulted in high and stable levels of GAA in the circulation and rescued muscle and CNS pathology in adult and severely affected older KO mice without development of humoral immune responses to the enzyme [143,144].

An inherent limitation of hepatic gene transfer is that AAV episomal vectors will be diluted over time in the developing and growing liver, eventually leading to the loss of vector genomes and transgene expression. This creates a major problem for treatment of pediatric patients with the disease, who are likely to require a second round of vector administration and immunosuppression to prevent the formation of neutralizing antibodies. In general, the success of liver-directed gene therapy for Pompe disease relies on both secretion of large amount of precursor GAA and its efficient CI-MPR-mediated uptake and lysosomal trafficking in distant organs. As with traditional ERT, the same requirement for high M6P content and affinity for the CI-MPR applies to the liver-produced secreted GAA to achieve efficient targeting and correction of muscle defect. This raises a possibility of generating an "ideal" transgene expression cassette to allow for the maximally reduced dose of vector. Although challenging, the era of gene therapy for Pompe disease has arrived, and the therapy has the potential to one day become a lifelong cure.

Author Contributions: N.K.M. performed many of the experiments described in Section 3, collected and reviewed materials, and participated in preparation of the manuscript; N.R. collected and analyzed the literature and wrote the paper. All authors have read and agreed to the published version of the manuscript.

Funding: This work was supported by the Intramural Research Program of the NHLBI of the National Institutes of Health. Meena was supported in part by a CRADA between NIH and Amicus Therapeutics.

Conflicts of Interest: The authors declare no conflict of interest.

References

1. Martina, J.A.; Raben, N.; Puertollano, R. SnapShot: Lysosomal Storage Diseases. *Cell* **2020**, *180*, 602. [CrossRef]
2. Pompe, J.C. Over idiopatische hypertrophie van het hart. *Ned. Tijdschr. Geneeskd.* **1932**, *76*, 304.
3. Hers, H.G. Alpha-glucosidase deficiency in generalize glycogen storage disease (Pompe's disease). *Biochem. J.* **1963**, *86*, 11. [CrossRef] [PubMed]
4. Martiniuk, F.; Chen, A.; Mack, A.; Arvanitopoulos, E.; Chen, Y.; Rom, W.N.; Codd, W.J.; Hanna, B.; Alcabes, P.; Raben, N.; et al. Carrier frequency for glycogen storage disease type II in New York and estimates of affected individuals born with the disease. *Am. J. Med Genet.* **1998**, *79*, 69–72. [CrossRef]
5. Bodamer, O.; Scott, C.R.; Giugliani, R.; Pompe Disease Newborn Screening Working Group; on behalf of the Pompe Disease Newborn Screening Working Group. Newborn Screening for Pompe Disease. *Pediatrics* **2017**, *140*, S4–S13. [CrossRef] [PubMed]
6. Tang, H.; Feuchtbaum, L.; Sciortino, S.; Matteson, J.; Mathur, D.; Bishop, T.; Olney, R.S. The First Year Experience of Newborn Screening for Pompe Disease in California. *Int. J. Neonatal Screen* **2020**, *6*, 9. [CrossRef]

7. Chien, Y.H.; Chiang, S.-C.; Zhang, X.K.; Keutzer, J.; Lee, N.-C.; Huang, A.-C.; Chen, C.-A.; Wu, M.-H.; Huang, P.-H.; Tsai, F.-J.; et al. Early Detection of Pompe Disease by Newborn Screening Is Feasible: Results From the Taiwan Screening Program. *Pediatrics* **2008**, *122*, e39–e45. [CrossRef]
8. Wisselaar, H.A.; Kroos, M.A.; Hermans, M.M.; Van Beeumen, J.; Reuser, A.J. Structural and functional changes of lysosomal acid alpha-glucosidase during intracellular transport and maturation. *J. Boil. Chem.* **1993**, *268*, 2223–2231.
9. Moreland, R.J.; Jin, X.; Zhang, X.K.; Decker, R.W.; Albee, K.L.; Lee, K.L.; Cauthron, R.D.; Brewer, K.; Edmunds, T.; Canfield, W.M. Lysosomal Acid α-Glucosidase Consists of Four Different Peptides Processed from a Single Chain Precursor. *J. Boil. Chem.* **2004**, *280*, 6780–6791. [CrossRef]
10. Dahms, N.M.; Lobel, P.; Kornfeld, S. Mannose 6-phosphate receptors and lysosomal enzyme targeting. *J. Boil. Chem.* **1989**, *264*.
11. Ghosh, P.; Dahms, N.M.; Kornfeld, S. Mannose 6-phosphate receptors: New twists in the tale. *Nat. Rev. Mol. Cell Boil.* **2003**, *4*, 202–213. [CrossRef]
12. Roig-Zamboni, V.; Cobucci-Ponzano, B.; Iacono, R.; Ferrara, M.C.; Germany, S.; Bourne, Y.; Parenti, G.; Moracci, M.; Sulzenbacher, G. Structure of human lysosomal acid α-glucosidase–a guide for the treatment of Pompe disease. *Nat. Commun.* **2017**, *8*, 1111. [CrossRef]
13. Hirschhorn, R.; Reuser, A.J. *Glycogen Storage Disease Type II: Acid Alphaglucosidase (Acid Maltase) Deficiency. The Metabolic and Molecular Basis of Inherited Disease*; McGraw-Hill: New York, NY, USA, 2001.
14. Güngör, D.; Reuser, A.J. How to describe the clinical spectrum in Pompe disease? *Am. J. Med Genet. Part A* **2013**, *161*, 399–400. [CrossRef] [PubMed]
15. Peruzzo, P.; Pavan, E.; Dardis, A. Molecular genetics of Pompe disease: A comprehensive overview. *Ann. Transl. Med.* **2019**, *7*, 278. [CrossRef] [PubMed]
16. Huie, M.L.; Chen, A.S.; Tsujino, S.; Shanske, S.; DiMauro, S.; Engel, A.G.; Hirschhorn, R. Aberrant splicing in adult onset glycogen storage disease type II (GSDII): Molecular identification of an IVS1 (-13T–>G) mutation in a majority of patients and a novel IVS10 (+1GT–>CT) mutation. *Hum. Mol. Genet.* **1994**, *3*, 1.
17. Boerkoel, C.F.; Exelbert, R.; Nicastri, C.; Nichols, R.C.; Miller, F.W.; Plotz, P.H.; Raben, N. Leaky splicing mutation in the acid maltase gene is associated with delayed onset of glycogenosis type II. *Am. J. Hum. Genet.* **1995**, *56*, 887–897. [PubMed]
18. Raben, N.; Nichols, R.C.; Martiniuk, F.; Plotz, P.H. A model of mRNA splicing in adult lysosomal storage disease (glycogenosis type II). *Hum. Mol. Genet.* **1996**, *5*, 995–1000. [CrossRef] [PubMed]
19. Dardis, A.; Zanin, I.; Zampieri, S.; Stuani, C.; Pianta, A.; Romanello, M.; Baralle, F.E.; Bembi, B.; Buratti, E. Functional characterization of the common c.-32-13T>G mutation of GAA gene: Identification of potential therapeutic agents. *Nucleic Acids Res.* **2013**, *42*, 1291–1302. [CrossRef] [PubMed]
20. Bergsma, A.J.; In't Groen, S.L.; van den Dorpel, J.J.; van den Hout, H.J.; van der Beek, N.A.; Schoser, B.; Toscano, A.; Musumeci, O.; Bembi, B.; Dardis, A.; et al. A genetic modifier of symptom onset in Pompe disease. *EBioMedicine* **2019**, *43*, 553–561. [CrossRef]
21. In't Groen, S.L.; de Faria, D.O.; Iuliano, A.; van den Hout, J.M.; Douben, H.; Dijkhuizen, T.; Cassiman, D.; Witters, P.; Romero, M.Á.B.; de Klein, A.; et al. Novel GAA Variants and Mosaicism in Pompe Disease Identified by Extended Analyses of Patients with an Incomplete DNA Diagnosis. *Mol. Ther. Methods Clin. Dev.* **2020**, *17*, 337–348. [CrossRef]
22. Raben, N.; Danon, M.; Gilbert, A.; Dwivedi, S.; Collins, B.; Thurberg, B.; Mattaliano, R.; Nagaraju, K.; Plotz, P. Enzyme replacement therapy in the mouse model of Pompe disease. *Mol. Genet. Metab.* **2003**, *80*, 159–169. [CrossRef] [PubMed]
23. McVie-Wylie, A.; Lee, K.; Qiu, H.; Jin, X.; Do, H.; Gotschall, R.; Thurberg, B.; Rogers, C.; Raben, N.; O'Callaghan, M.; et al. Biochemical and pharmacological characterization of different recombinant acid α-glucosidase preparations evaluated for the treatment of Pompe disease. *Mol. Genet. Metab.* **2008**, *94*, 448–455. [CrossRef] [PubMed]
24. Kishnani, P.S.; Corzo, D.; Nicolino, M.; Byrne, B.; Mandel, H.; Hwu, W.L.; Leslie, N.; Levine, J.; Spenser, C.; McDonald, M.; et al. Recombinant human acid [alpha]-glucosidase: Major clinical benefits in infantile-onset Pompe disease. *Neurology* **2007**, *68*, 99–109. [CrossRef] [PubMed]
25. Nicolino, M.; Byrne, B.; Wraith, J.E.; Leslie, N.; Mandel, H.; Freyer, D.R.; Arnold, G.L.; Pivnick, E.K.; Ottinger, C.J.; Robinson, P.H.; et al. Clinical outcomes after long-term treatment with alglucosidase alfa in infants and children with advanced Pompe disease. *Genet. Med.* **2009**, *11*, 210–219. [CrossRef]

26. Slonim, A.E.; Bulone, L.; Ritz, S.; Goldberg, T.; Chen, A.; Martiniuk, F. Identification of two subtypes of infantile acid maltase deficiency. *J. Pediatr.* **2000**, *137*, 283–285. [CrossRef]
27. Kishnani, P.S.; Hwu, W.-L.; Mandel, H.; Nicolino, M.; Yong, F.; Corzo, D. A retrospective, multinational, multicenter study on the natural history of infantile-onset Pompe disease. *J. Pediatr.* **2006**, *148*, 671–676. [CrossRef]
28. Prater, S.N.; Banugaria, S.G.; DeArmey, S.M.; Botha, E.G.; Stege, E.M.; E Case, L.; Jones, H.N.; Phornphutkul, C.; Wang, R.Y.; Young, S.P.; et al. The emerging phenotype of long-term survivors with infantile Pompe disease. *Genet. Med.* **2012**, *14*, 800–810. [CrossRef]
29. DeRuisseau, L.R.; Fuller, D.D.; Qiu, K.; DeRuisseau, K.C.; Donnelly, W.H.; Mah, C.; Reier, P.J.; Byrne, B.J. Neural deficits contribute to respiratory insufficiency in Pompe disease. *Proc. Natl. Acad. Sci. USA* **2009**, *106*, 9419–9424. [CrossRef]
30. Hahn, A.; Schänzer, A. Long-term outcome and unmet needs in infantile-onset Pompe disease. *Ann. Transl. Med.* **2019**, *7*, 283. [CrossRef]
31. Pena, L.D.M.; Proia, A.D.; Kishnani, P.S.; Zschocke, J. Postmortem Findings and Clinical Correlates in Individuals with Infantile-Onset Pompe Disease. *JIMD Rep.* **2015**, *23*, 45–54. [CrossRef]
32. McIntosh, P.T.; Hobson-Webb, L.D.; Kazi, Z.B.; Prater, S.N.; Banugaria, S.G.; Austin, S.; Wang, R.; Enterline, D.S.; Frush, D.P.; Kishnani, P.S. Neuroimaging findings in infantile Pompe patients treated with enzyme replacement therapy. *Mol. Genet. Metab.* **2018**, *123*, 85–91. [CrossRef] [PubMed]
33. Ebbink, B.J.; Poelman, E.; Aarsen, F.K.; Hoogenboom-Plug, I.; Régal, L.; Muentjes, C.; Beek, N.A.M.E.V.D.; Lequin, M.H.; Van Der Ploeg, A.T.; Hout, J.M. Classic infantile Pompe patients approaching adulthood: A cohort study on consequences for the brain. *Dev. Med. Child Neurol.* **2018**, *60*, 579–586. [CrossRef]
34. Kishnani, P.S.; Goldenberg, P.C.; DeArmey, S.L.; Heller, J.; Benjamin, D.; Young, S.; Bali, D.; Smith, S.A.; Li, J.S.; Mandel, H.; et al. Cross-reactive immunologic material status affects treatment outcomes in Pompe disease infants. *Mol. Genet. Metab.* **2010**, *99*, 26–33. [CrossRef]
35. Chien, Y.H.; Hwu, W.-L.; Lee, N.-C. Pompe Disease: Early Diagnosis and Early Treatment Make a Difference. *Pediatr. Neonatol.* **2013**, *54*, 219–227. [CrossRef] [PubMed]
36. Yang, C.; Niu, D.; Tai, S.; Wang, T.; Su, H.; Huang, L.; Soong, W. Airway abnormalities in very early treated infantile-onset Pompe disease: A large-scale survey by flexible bronchoscopy. *Am. J. Med Genet. Part A* **2020**, *182*, 721–729. [CrossRef] [PubMed]
37. Güngör, D.; de Vries, J.M.; Brusse, E.; Kruijshaar, M.E.; Hop, W.C.; Murawska, M.; van den Berg, L.E.; Reuser, A.J.; van Doorn, P.A.; Hagemans, M.L.; et al. Enzyme replacement therapy and fatigue in adults with Pompe disease. *Mol. Genet. Metab.* **2013**, *109*, 174–178. [CrossRef] [PubMed]
38. Güngör, D.; Schober, A.; Kruijshaar, M.; Plug, I.; Karabul, N.; Deschauer, M.; Van Doorn, P.; Van Der Ploeg, A.; Schoser, B.; Hanisch, F. Pain in adult patients with Pompe disease. *Mol. Genet. Metab.* **2013**, *109*, 371–376. [CrossRef]
39. Keeler, A.M.; Liu, D.; Zieger, M.; Xiong, L.; Salemi, J.; Bellvé, K.; Byrne, B.J.; Fuller, D.D.; ZhuGe, R.; ElMallah, M.K. Airway smooth muscle dysfunction in Pompe (GAA-/-) mice. *Am. J. Physiol. Lung Cell. Mol. Physiol.* **2017**, *312*, L873–L881. [CrossRef]
40. Chan, J.; Desai, A.K.; Kazi, Z.B.; Corey, K.; Austin, S.; Webb, L.D.H.; E Case, L.; Jones, H.N.; Kishnani, P.S. The emerging phenotype of late-onset Pompe disease: A systematic literature review. *Mol. Genet. Metab.* **2017**, *120*, 163–172. [CrossRef]
41. Toscano, A.; Rodolico, C.; Musumeci, O. Multisystem late onset Pompe disease (LOPD): An update on clinical aspects. *Ann. Transl. Med.* **2019**, *7*, 284. [CrossRef]
42. Alandy-Dy, J.; Wencel, M.; Hall, K.; Simon, J.; Chen, Y.; Valenti, E.; Yang, J.; Bali, D.; Lakatos, A.; Goyal, N.; et al. Variable clinical features and genotype-phenotype correlations in 18 patients with late-onset Pompe disease. *Ann. Transl. Med.* **2019**, *7*, 276. [CrossRef] [PubMed]
43. Anderson, L.J.; Henley, W.; Wyatt, K.M.; Nikolaou, V.; Waldek, S.; Hughes, D.; Lachmann, R.H.; Logan, S. Effectiveness of enzyme replacement therapy in adults with late-onset Pompe disease: Results from the NCS-LSD cohort study. *J. Inherit. Metab. Dis.* **2014**, *37*, 945–952. [CrossRef]
44. Schoser, B.; Stewart, A.; Kanters, S.; Hamed, A.; Jansen, J.; Chan, K.; Karamouzian, M.; Toscano, A. Survival and long-term outcomes in late-onset Pompe disease following alglucosidase alfa treatment: A systematic review and meta-analysis. *J. Neurol.* **2016**, *264*, 621–630. [CrossRef]

45. McCall, A.L.; Salemi, J.; Bhanap, P.; Strickland, L.M.; Elmallah, M.K. The impact of Pompe disease on smooth muscle: A review. *J. Smooth Muscle Res.* **2018**, *54*, 100–118. [CrossRef] [PubMed]
46. Stepien, K.M.; Hendriksz, C.J.; Roberts, M.; Sharma, R. Observational clinical study of 22 adult-onset Pompe disease patients undergoing enzyme replacement therapy over 5years. *Mol. Genet. Metab.* **2016**, *117*, 413–418. [CrossRef] [PubMed]
47. Harlaar, L.; Hogrel, J.-Y.; Perniconi, B.; Kruijshaar, M.E.; Rizopoulos, D.; Taouagh, N.; Canal, A.; Brusse, E.; Van Doorn, P.A.; Van Der Ploeg, A.T.; et al. Large variation in effects during 10 years of enzyme therapy in adults with Pompe disease. *Neurology* **2019**, *93*, e1756–e1767. [CrossRef]
48. Kulessa, M.; Weyer-Menkhoff, I.; Viergutz, L.; Kornblum, C.; Claeys, K.G.; Schneider, I.; Plöckinger, U.; Young, P.; Boentert, M.; Vielhaber, S.; et al. An integrative correlation of myopathology, phenotype and genotype in late onset Pompe disease. *Neuropathol. Appl. Neurobiol.* **2019**, *46*, 359–374. [CrossRef]
49. Van Der Ploeg, A.T.; Kruijshaar, M.E.; Toscano, A.; Laforet, P.; Angelini, C.; Lachmann, R.H.; Pascual, S.I.P.; Roberts, M.; Rösler, K.; Stulnig, T.M.; et al. European consensus for starting and stopping enzyme replacement therapy in adult patients with Pompe disease: A 10-year experience. *Eur. J. Neurol.* **2017**, *24*, 768-e31. [CrossRef]
50. Van Kooten, H.; Harlaar, L.; Van Der Beek, N.; Van Doorn, P.; Van Der Ploeg, A.; Brusse, E.; Chair, W.V.D.P.; Ditters, I.; Hoogendijk-Boon, M.; Huidekoper, H.; et al. Discontinuation of enzyme replacement therapy in adults with Pompe disease: Evaluating the European POmpe Consortium stop criteria. *Neuromuscul. Disord.* **2020**, *30*, 59–66. [CrossRef]
51. Rairikar, M.V.; Case, L.E.; Bailey, L.A.; Kazi, Z.B.; Desai, A.K.; Berrier, K.L.; Coats, J.; Gandy, R.; Quinones, R.; Kishnani, P.S. Insight into the phenotype of infants with Pompe disease identified by newborn screening with the common c.-32-13T>G "late-onset" GAA variant. *Mol. Genet. Metab.* **2017**, *122*, 99–107. [CrossRef]
52. Tarallo, A.; Carissimo, A.; Gatto, F.; Nusco, E.; Toscano, A.; Musumeci, O.; Coletta, M.; Karali, M.; Acampora, E.; Damiano, C.; et al. microRNAs as biomarkers in Pompe disease. *Genet. Med.* **2018**, *21*, 591–600. [CrossRef] [PubMed]
53. Carrasco-Rozas, A.; Fernández-Simón, E.; Lleixà, M.C.; Belmonte, I.; Pedrosa-Hernandez, I.; Montiel-Morillo, E.; Nuñez-Peralta, C.; Llauger Rossello, J.; Segovia, S.; De Luna, N.; et al. Identification of serum microRNAs as potential biomarkers in Pompe disease. *Ann. Clin. Transl. Neurol.* **2019**, *6*, 1214–1224. [CrossRef]
54. Taverna, S.; Cammarata, G.; Colomba, P.; Sciarrino, S.; Zizzo, C.; Francofonte, D.; Zora, M.; Scalia, S.; Brando, C.; Curto, A.L.; et al. Pompe disease: Pathogenesis, molecular genetics and diagnosis. *Aging* **2020**, *12*. [CrossRef] [PubMed]
55. Thurberg, B.; Maloney, C.L.; Vaccaro, C.; Afonso, K.; Tsai, A.C.-H.; Bossen, E.; Kishnani, P.S.; O'Callaghan, M. Characterization of pre- and post-treatment pathology after enzyme replacement therapy for pompe disease. *Lab. Investig.* **2006**, *86*, 1208–1220. [CrossRef]
56. Raben, N.; Nagaraju, K.; Lee, E.; Kessler, P.; Byrne, B.; Lee, L.; Lamarca, M.; King, C.; Ward, J.; Sauer, B.; et al. Targeted Disruption of the Acid α-Glucosidase Gene in Mice Causes an Illness with Critical Features of Both Infantile and Adult Human Glycogen Storage Disease Type II. *J. Boil. Chem.* **1998**, *273*, 19086–19092. [CrossRef] [PubMed]
57. Mizushima, N.; Levine, B.; Cuervo, A.M.; Klionsky, D.J. Autophagy fights disease through cellular self-digestion. *Nature* **2008**, *451*, 1069–1075. [CrossRef] [PubMed]
58. Mizushima, N.; Yamamoto, A.; Matsui, M.; Yoshimori, T.; Ohsumi, Y. In Vivo Analysis of Autophagy in Response to Nutrient Starvation Using Transgenic Mice Expressing a Fluorescent Autophagosome Marker. *Mol. Boil. Cell* **2004**, *15*, 1101–1111. [CrossRef] [PubMed]
59. Onodera, J.; Ohsumi, Y. Autophagy Is Required for Maintenance of Amino Acid Levels and Protein Synthesis under Nitrogen Starvation. *J. Boil. Chem.* **2005**, *280*, 31582–31586. [CrossRef]
60. Gundersen, K. Muscle memory and a new cellular model for muscle atrophy and hypertrophy. *J. Exp. Boil.* **2016**, *219*, 235–242. [CrossRef]
61. Masiero, E.; Agatea, L.; Mammucari, C.; Blaauw, B.; Loro, E.; Komatsu, M.; Metzger, D.; Reggiani, C.; Schiaffino, S.; Sandri, M. Autophagy Is Required to Maintain Muscle Mass. *Cell Metab.* **2009**, *10*, 507–515. [CrossRef]
62. Masiero, E.; Sandri, M. Autophagy inhibition induces atrophy and myopathy in adult skeletal muscles. *Autophagy* **2010**, *6*, 307–309. [CrossRef]

63. Nishino, I. Autophagic Vacuolar Myopathy. *Semin. Pediatr. Neurol.* **2006**, *13*, 90–95. [CrossRef] [PubMed]
64. Xu, S.; Galperin, M.; Melvin, G.; Horowits, R.; Raben, N.; Plotz, P.; Yu, L. Impaired organization and function of myofilaments in single muscle fibers from a mouse model of Pompe disease. *J. Appl. Physiol.* **2010**, *108*, 1383–1388. [CrossRef] [PubMed]
65. Nascimbeni, A.C.; Fanin, M.; Angelini, C.; Sandri, M. Autophagy dysregulation in Danon disease. *Cell Death Dis.* **2017**, *8*, e2565. [CrossRef] [PubMed]
66. Meena, N.K.; Ralston, E.; Raben, N.; Puertollano, R. Enzyme Replacement Therapy Can Reverse Pathogenic Cascade in Pompe Disease. *Mol. Ther. Methods Clin. Dev.* **2020**, *18*, 199–214. [CrossRef]
67. Spampanato, C.; Feeney, E.; Li, L.; Cardone, M.; Lim, J.-A.; Annunziata, F.; Zare, H.; Polishchuk, R.; Puertollano, R.; Parenti, G.; et al. Transcription factor EB (TFEB) is a new therapeutic target for Pompe disease. *EMBO Mol. Med.* **2013**, *5*, 691–706. [CrossRef]
68. Fukuda, T.; Ewan, L.; Bauer, M.; Mattaliano, R.J.; Zaal, K.; Ralston, E.; Plotz, P.H.; Raben, N. Dysfunction of endocytic and autophagic pathways in a lysosomal storage disease. *Ann. Neurol.* **2006**, *59*, 700–708. [CrossRef]
69. Nascimbeni, A.C.; Fanin, M.; Tasca, E.; Angelini, C.; Sandri, M. Impaired autophagy affects acid α-glucosidase processing and enzyme replacement therapy efficacy in late-onset glycogen storage disease type II. *Neuropathol. Appl. Neurobiol.* **2015**, *41*, 672–675. [CrossRef]
70. Shea, L.; Raben, N. Autophagy in skeletal muscle: Implications for Pompe disease. *Int. J. Clin. Pharmacol. Ther.* **2009**, *47*, S42–S47. [CrossRef]
71. Fukuda, T.; Ahearn, M.; Roberts, A.; Mattaliano, R.J.; Zaal, K.; Ralston, E.; Plotz, P.H.; Raben, N. Autophagy and Mistargeting of Therapeutic Enzyme in Skeletal Muscle in Pompe Disease. *Mol. Ther.* **2006**, *14*, 831–839. [CrossRef]
72. Inoki, K.; Kim, J.; Guan, K.-L. AMPK and mTOR in Cellular Energy Homeostasis and Drug Targets. *Annu. Rev. Pharmacol. Toxicol.* **2012**, *52*, 381–400. [CrossRef] [PubMed]
73. Sancak, Y.; Bar-Peled, L.; Zoncu, R.; Markhard, A.L.; Nada, S.; Sabatini, D.M. Ragulator-Rag Complex Targets mTORC1 to the Lysosomal Surface and Is Necessary for Its Activation by Amino Acids. *Cell* **2010**, *141*, 290–303. [CrossRef] [PubMed]
74. Zoncu, R.; Bar-Peled, L.; Efeyan, A.; Wang, S.; Sancak, Y.; Sabatini, D.M. mTORC1 Senses Lysosomal Amino Acids Through an Inside-Out Mechanism That Requires the Vacuolar H+-ATPase. *Science* **2011**, *334*, 678–683. [CrossRef]
75. Bar-Peled, L.; Sabatini, D.M. Regulation of mTORC1 by amino acids. *Trends Cell Boil.* **2014**, *24*, 400–406. [CrossRef] [PubMed]
76. Inoki, K.; Li, Y.; Xu, T.; Guan, K.-L. Rheb GTPase is a direct target of TSC2 GAP activity and regulates mTOR signaling. *Genes Dev.* **2003**, *17*, 1829–1834. [CrossRef]
77. Demetriades, C.; Plescher, M.; Teleman, A.A. Lysosomal recruitment of TSC2 is a universal response to cellular stress. *Nat. Commun.* **2016**, *7*, 10662. [CrossRef]
78. Menon, S.; Dibble, C.C.; Talbott, G.; Hoxhaj, G.; Valvezan, A.J.; Takahashi, H.; Cantley, L.C.; Manning, B.D. Spatial control of the TSC complex integrates insulin and nutrient regulation of mTORC1 at the lysosome. *Cell* **2014**, *156*, 771–785. [CrossRef]
79. Sakamoto, K.; Zarrinpashneh, E.; Budas, G.R.; Pouleur, A.-C.; Dutta, A.; Prescott, A.R.; Vanoverschelde, J.-L.J.; Ashworth, A.; Jovanović, A.; Alessi, D.R.; et al. Deficiency of LKB1 in heart prevents ischemia-mediated activation of AMPKalpha2 but not AMPKalpha1. *Am. J. Physiol. Metab.* **2005**, *290*, E780–E788. [CrossRef]
80. Kim, J.; Kundu, M.; Viollet, B.; Guan, K.-L. AMPK and mTOR regulate autophagy through direct phosphorylation of Ulk1. *Nat. Cell Biol.* **2011**, *13*, 132–141. [CrossRef]
81. Egan, D.F.; Kim, J.; Shaw, R.J.; Guan, K.-L. The autophagy initiating kinase ULK1 is regulated via opposing phosphorylation by AMPK and mTOR. *Autophagy* **2011**, *7*, 645–646. [CrossRef]
82. Bentzinger, C.F.; Lin, S.; Romanino, K.; Castets, P.; Guridi, M.; Summermatter, S.; Handschin, C.; Tintignac, L.; Hall, M.N.; Rüegg, M.A. Differential response of skeletal muscles to mTORC1 signaling during atrophy and hypertrophy. *Skelet. Muscle* **2013**, *3*, 6. [CrossRef] [PubMed]
83. Grumati, P.; Coletto, L.; Sabatelli, P.; Cescon, M.; Angelin, A.; Bertaggia, E.; Blaauw, B.; Urciuolo, A.; Tiepolo, T.; Merlini, L.; et al. Autophagy is defective in collagen VI muscular dystrophies, and its reactivation rescues myofiber degeneration. *Nat. Med.* **2010**, *16*, 1313–1320. [CrossRef]

84. Sandri, M.; Coletto, L.; Grumati, P.; Bonaldo, P. Misregulation of autophagy and protein degradation systems in myopathies and muscular dystrophies. *J. Cell Sci.* **2013**, *126*, 5325–5333. [CrossRef] [PubMed]
85. Lim, J.; Li, L.; Shirihai, O.S.; Trudeau, K.M.; Puertollano, R.; Raben, N. Modulation of mTOR signaling as a strategy for the treatment of Pompe disease. *EMBO Mol. Med.* **2017**, *9*, 353–370. [CrossRef]
86. Lim, J.-A.; Sun, B.; Puertollano, R.; Raben, N. Therapeutic Benefit of Autophagy Modulation in Pompe Disease. *Mol. Ther.* **2018**, *26*, 1783–1796. [CrossRef]
87. Shemesh, A.; Wang, Y.; Yang, Y.; Yang, G.S.; Johnson, D.E.; Backer, J.M.; Pessin, J.E.; Zong, H. Suppression of mTOR1 Activation in Acid- alpha -Glucosidase Deficient Cells and Mice is Ameliorated by Leucine Supplementation. *Am. J. Physiol. Regul. Integr. Comp. Physiol.* **2014**. [CrossRef]
88. Yoshida, T.; Awaya, T.; Jonouchi, T.; Kimura, R.; Kimura, S.; Era, T.; Heike, T.; Sakurai, H. A Skeletal Muscle Model of Infantile-onset Pompe Disease with Patient-specific iPS Cells. *Sci. Rep.* **2017**, *7*, 13473. [CrossRef] [PubMed]
89. Yoon, M.-S. mTOR as a Key Regulator in Maintaining Skeletal Muscle Mass. *Front. Physiol.* **2017**, *8*. [CrossRef]
90. Ching, J.K.; Elizabeth, S.V.; Ju, J.-S.; Lusk, C.; Pittman, S.K.; Weihl, C.C. mTOR dysfunction contributes to vacuolar pathology and weakness in valosin-containing protein associated inclusion body myopathy. *Hum. Mol. Genet.* **2012**, *22*, 1167–1179. [CrossRef]
91. Hintze, S.; Limmer, S.; Dabrowska-Schlepp, P.; Berg, B.; Krieghoff, N.; Busch, A.; Schaaf, A.; Meinke, P.; Schoser, B. Moss-Derived Human Recombinant GAA Provides an Optimized Enzyme Uptake in Differentiated Human Muscle Cells of Pompe Disease. *Int. J. Mol. Sci.* **2020**, *21*, 2642. [CrossRef]
92. Xu, S.; Lun, Y.; Frascella, M.; Garcia, A.; Soska, R.; Nair, A.; Ponery, A.S.; Schilling, A.; Feng, J.; Tuske, S.; et al. Improved efficacy of a next-generation ERT in murine Pompe disease. *JCI Insight* **2019**, *4*, 125358. [CrossRef]
93. Schoser, B. Pompe disease: What are we missing? *Ann. Transl. Med.* **2019**, *7*, 292. [CrossRef]
94. Yin, H.; Price, F.; Rudnicki, M.A. Satellite Cells and the Muscle Stem Cell Niche. *Physiol. Rev.* **2013**, *93*, 23–67. [CrossRef]
95. Lepper, C.; Partridge, T.A.; Fan, C.-M. An absolute requirement for Pax7-positive satellite cells in acute injury-induced skeletal muscle regeneration. *Development* **2011**, *138*, 3639–3646. [CrossRef] [PubMed]
96. Rudnicki, M.A.; Le Grand, F.; McKinnell, I.; Kuang, S. The Molecular Regulation of Muscle Stem Cell Function. *Cold Spring Harb. Symp. Quant. Boil.* **2008**, *73*, 323–331. [CrossRef] [PubMed]
97. Schaaf, G.; Van Gestel, T.J.M.; Brusse, E.; Verdijk, R.M.; De Coo, I.F.M.; Van Doorn, P.A.; Van Der Ploeg, A.T.; Pijnappel, W.P. Lack of robust satellite cell activation and muscle regeneration during the progression of Pompe disease. *Acta Neuropathol. Commun.* **2015**, *3*, 65. [CrossRef] [PubMed]
98. Schaaf, G.; Van Gestel, T.J.M.; In't Groen, S.L.; De Jong, B.; Boomaars, B.; Tarallo, A.; Cardone, M.; Parenti, G.; Van Der Ploeg, A.T.; Pijnappel, W.P. Satellite cells maintain regenerative capacity but fail to repair disease-associated muscle damage in mice with Pompe disease. *Acta Neuropathol. Commun.* **2018**, *6*, 119. [CrossRef] [PubMed]
99. Lagalice, L.; Pichon, J.; Gougeon, E.; Soussi, S.; Deniaud, J.; Ledevin, M.; Maurier, V.; Leroux, I.; Durand, S.; Ciron, C.; et al. Satellite cells fail to contribute to muscle repair but are functional in Pompe disease (glycogenosis type II). *Acta Neuropathol. Commun.* **2018**, *6*, 116. [CrossRef] [PubMed]
100. Tang, A.H.; Rando, T.A. Induction of autophagy supports the bioenergetic demands of quiescent muscle stem cell activation. *EMBO J.* **2014**, *33*, 2782–2797. [CrossRef]
101. Lim, J.-A.; Li, L.; Raben, N. Pompe disease: From pathophysiology to therapy and back again. *Front. Aging Neurosci.* **2014**, *6*. [CrossRef]
102. Kohler, L.; Puertollano, R.; Raben, N. Pompe Disease: From Basic Science to Therapy. *Neurotherapeutics* **2018**, *15*, 928–942. [CrossRef]
103. Parenti, G.; Andria, G.; Valenzano, K.J. Pharmacological Chaperone Therapy: Preclinical Development, Clinical Translation, and Prospects for the Treatment of Lysosomal Storage Disorders. *Mol. Ther.* **2015**, *23*, 1138–1148. [CrossRef] [PubMed]
104. Do, H.V.; Khanna, R.; Gotschall, R. Challenges in treating Pompe disease: An industry perspective. *Ann. Transl. Med.* **2019**, *7*, 291. [CrossRef] [PubMed]
105. Wenk, J.; Hille, A.; Von Figura, K. Quantitation of Mr 46000 and Mr 300000 mannose 6-phosphate receptors in human cells and tissues. *Biochem. Int.* **1991**, *23*.

106. Funk, B.; Kessler, U.; Eisenmenger, W.; Hansmann, A.; Kolb, H.J.; Kiess, W. Expression of the insulin-like growth factor-II/mannose-6-phosphate receptor in multiple human tissues during fetal life and early infancy. *J. Clin. Endocrinol. Metab.* **1992**, *75*, 424–431.
107. Zhu, Y.; Li, X.; McVie-Wylie, A.; Jiang, C.; Thurberg, B.L.; Raben, N.; Mattaliano, R.J.; Cheng, S.H. Carbohydrate-remodelled acid α-glucosidase with higher affinity for the cation-independent mannose 6-phosphate receptor demonstrates improved delivery to muscles of Pompe mice. *Biochem. J.* **2005**, *389*, 619–628. [CrossRef]
108. Zhu, Y.; Jiang, J.-L.; Gumlaw, N.K.; Zhang, J.; Bercury, S.D.; Ziegler, R.J.; Lee, K.; Kudo, M.; Canfield, W.M.; Edmunds, T.; et al. Glycoengineered Acid α-Glucosidase with Improved Efficacy at Correcting the Metabolic Aberrations and Motor Function Deficits in a Mouse Model of Pompe Disease. *Mol. Ther.* **2009**, *17*, 954–963. [CrossRef]
109. Pena, L.D.M.; Barohn, R.J.; Byrne, B.J.; Desnuelle, C.; Goker-Alpan, O.; Ladha, S.; Laforêt, P.; Mengel, K.E.; Pestronk, A.; Pouget, J.; et al. Safety, tolerability, pharmacokinetics, pharmacodynamics, and exploratory efficacy of the novel enzyme replacement therapy avalglucosidase alfa (neoGAA) in treatment-naïve and alglucosidase alfa-treated patients with late-onset Pompe disease: A phase 1, open-label, multicenter, multinational, ascending dose study. *Neuromuscul. Disord.* **2019**, *29*, 167–186. [CrossRef]
110. Porto, C.; Cardone, M.; Fontana, F.; Rossi, B.; Tuzzi, M.R.; Tarallo, A.; Barone, M.V.; Andria, G.; Parenti, G. The Pharmacological Chaperone N-butyldeoxynojirimycin Enhances Enzyme Replacement Therapy in Pompe Disease Fibroblasts. *Mol. Ther.* **2009**, *17*, 964–971. [CrossRef]
111. Khanna, R.; Flanagan, J.J.; Feng, J.; Soska, R.; Frascella, M.; Pellegrino, L.J.; Lun, Y.; Guillen, D.; Lockhart, D.J.; Valenzano, K.J. The Pharmacological Chaperone AT2220 Increases Recombinant Human Acid α-Glucosidase Uptake and Glycogen Reduction in a Mouse Model of Pompe Disease. *PLoS ONE* **2012**, *7*, e40776. [CrossRef]
112. Parenti, G.; Fecarotta, S.; La Marca, G.; Rossi, B.; Ascione, S.; Donati, M.A.; Morandi, L.O.; Ravaglia, S.; Pichiecchio, A.; Ombrone, D.; et al. A Chaperone Enhances Blood α-Glucosidase Activity in Pompe Disease Patients Treated with Enzyme Replacement Therapy. *Mol. Ther.* **2014**, *22*, 2004–2012. [CrossRef] [PubMed]
113. Hansen, J.E.; Tse, C.-M.; Chan, G.; Heinze, E.R.; Nishimura, R.N.; Weisbart, R.H. Intranuclear Protein Transduction through a Nucleoside Salvage Pathway. *J. Boil. Chem.* **2007**, *282*, 20790–20793. [CrossRef] [PubMed]
114. Weisbart, R.H.; Gera, J.; Chan, G.; Hansen, J.E.; Li, E.; Cloninger, C.; Levine, A.J.; Nishimura, R.N. A Cell-Penetrating Bispecific Antibody for Therapeutic Regulation of Intracellular Targets. *Mol. Cancer Ther.* **2012**, *11*, 2169–2173. [CrossRef] [PubMed]
115. Weisbart, R.H.; Chan, G.; Jordaan, G.; Noble, P.W.; Liu, Y.; Glazer, P.M.; Nishimura, R.N.; Hansen, J.E. DNA-dependent targeting of cell nuclei by a lupus autoantibody. *Sci. Rep.* **2015**, *5*, 12022. [CrossRef]
116. Yi, H.; Sun, T.; Armstrong, D.; Borneman, S.; Yang, C.; Austin, S.; Kishnani, P.S.; Sun, B. Antibody-mediated enzyme replacement therapy targeting both lysosomal and cytoplasmic glycogen in Pompe disease. *J. Mol. Med.* **2017**, *95*, 513–521. [CrossRef]
117. Kishnani, P.; Lachmann, R.; Mozaffar, T.; Walters, C.; Case, L.; Appleby, M.; Libri, V.; Kak, M.; Wencel, M.; Landy, H. Safety and efficacy of VAL-1221, a novel fusion protein targeting cytoplasmic glycogen, in patients with late-onset Pompe disease. *Mol. Genet. Metab.* **2019**, *126*, S85–S86. [CrossRef]
118. Koeberl, D.; Luo, X.; Sun, B.; McVie-Wylie, A.; Dai, J.; Li, S.; Banugaria, S.G.; Chen, Y.-T.; Bali, D.S. Enhanced efficacy of enzyme replacement therapy in Pompe disease through mannose-6-phosphate receptor expression in skeletal muscle. *Mol. Genet. Metab.* **2011**, *103*, 107–112. [CrossRef]
119. Koeberl, D.D.; Li, S.; Dai, J.; Thurberg, B.L.; Bali, D.; Kishnani, P.S. Beta2 Agonists enhance the efficacy of simultaneous enzyme replacement therapy in murine Pompe disease. *Mol. Genet. Metab.* **2012**, *105*, 221–227. [CrossRef]
120. Koeberl, D.; Austin, S.; E Case, L.; Smith, E.C.; Buckley, A.F.; Young, S.P.; Bali, D.; Kishnani, P.S. Adjunctive albuterol enhances the response to enzyme replacement therapy in late-onset Pompe disease. *FASEB J.* **2014**, *28*, 2171–2176. [CrossRef]
121. Koeberl, D.; E Case, L.; Smith, E.C.; Walters, C.; Han, S.-O.; Li, Y.; Chen, W.; Hornik, C.P.; Huffman, K.M.; Kraus, W.E.; et al. Correction of Biochemical Abnormalities and Improved Muscle Function in a Phase I/II Clinical Trial of Clenbuterol in Pompe Disease. *Mol. Ther.* **2018**, *26*, 2304–2314. [CrossRef]
122. Doerfler, P.A.; Nayak, S.; Corti, M.; Morel, L.; Herzog, R.W.; Byrne, B.J. Targeted approaches to induce immune tolerance for Pompe disease therapy. *Mol. Ther. Methods Clin. Dev.* **2016**, *3*, 15053. [CrossRef]

123. Ronzitti, G.; Collaud, F.; Laforet, P.; Mingozzi, F. Progress and challenges of gene therapy for Pompe disease. *Ann. Transl. Med.* **2019**, *7*, 287. [CrossRef]
124. Byrne, B.J.; Fuller, D.D.; Smith, B.K.; Clement, N.; Coleman, K.; Cleaver, B.; Vaught, L.; Falk, D.J.; McCall, A.; Corti, M. Pompe disease gene therapy: Neural manifestations require consideration of CNS directed therapy. *Ann. Transl. Med.* **2019**, *7*, 290. [CrossRef]
125. Salabarria, S.; Nair, J.; Clement, N.; Smith, B.; Raben, N.; Fuller, D.; Byrne, B.J.; Corti, M. Advancements in AAV-mediated Gene Therapy for Pompe Disease. *J. Neuromuscul. Dis.* **2020**, *7*, 15–31. [CrossRef] [PubMed]
126. Mingozzi, F.; High, K.A. Overcoming the Host Immune Response to Adeno-Associated Virus Gene Delivery Vectors: The Race Between Clearance, Tolerance, Neutralization, and Escape. *Annu. Rev. Virol.* **2017**, *4*, 511–534. [CrossRef] [PubMed]
127. Mah, C.S.; Pacak, C.A.; Cresawn, K.O.; DeRuisseau, L.R.; Germain, S.; Lewis, M.A.; Cloutier, D.A.; Fuller, D.D.; Byrne, B.J. Physiological Correction of Pompe Disease by Systemic Delivery of Adeno-associated Virus Serotype 1 Vectors. *Mol. Ther.* **2007**, *15*, 501–507. [CrossRef] [PubMed]
128. Mah, C.S.; Falk, D.J.; Germain, S.A.; Kelley, J.S.; Lewis, M.A.; A Cloutier, D.; DeRuisseau, L.R.; Conlon, T.J.; Cresawn, K.O.; Fraites, T.J., Jr.; et al. Gel-mediated Delivery of AAV1 Vectors Corrects Ventilatory Function in Pompe Mice with Established Disease. *Mol. Ther.* **2010**, *18*, 502–510. [CrossRef] [PubMed]
129. Elmallah, M.K.; Falk, D.J.; Nayak, S.; Federico, R.A.; Sandhu, M.S.; Poirier, A.; Byrne, B.J.; Fuller, D.D. Sustained Correction of Motoneuron Histopathology Following Intramuscular Delivery of AAV in Pompe Mice. *Mol. Ther.* **2014**, *22*, 702–712. [CrossRef] [PubMed]
130. Smith, B.K.; Collins, S.W.; Conlon, T.J.; Mah, C.S.; Lawson, L.A.; Martin, A.D.; Fuller, D.D.; Cleaver, B.D.; Clement, N.; Phillips, D.; et al. Phase I/II Trial of Adeno-Associated Virus–Mediated Alpha-Glucosidase Gene Therapy to the Diaphragm for Chronic Respiratory Failure in Pompe Disease: Initial Safety and Ventilatory Outcomes. *Hum. Gene Ther.* **2013**, *24*, 630–640. [CrossRef] [PubMed]
131. Byrne, P.I.; Collins, S.; Mah, C.C.; Smith, B.; Conlon, T.; Martin, S.D. Phase I/II trial of diaphragm delivery of recombinant adeno-associated virus acid alpha-glucosidase (rAAaV1-CMV-GAA) gene vector in patients with Pompe disease. *Hum. Gene Ther. Clin. Dev.* **2014**, *25*, 134–163. [CrossRef]
132. Corti, M.; Liberati, C.; Smith, B.K.; Lawson, L.A.; Tuna, I.S.; Conlon, T.J.; Coleman, K.E.; Islam, S.; Herzog, R.W.; Fuller, D.D.; et al. Safety of Intradiaphragmatic Delivery of Adeno-Associated Virus-Mediated Alpha-Glucosidase (rAAV1-CMV-hGAA) Gene Therapy in Children Affected by Pompe Disease. *Hum. Gene Ther. Clin. Dev.* **2017**, *28*, 208–218. [CrossRef] [PubMed]
133. Amalfitano, A.; McVie-Wylie, A.J.; Hu, H.; Dawson, T.L.; Raben, N.; Plotz, P.; Chen, Y.T. Systemic correction of the muscle disorder glycogen storage disease type II after hepatic targeting of a modified adenovirus vector encoding human acid-α-glucosidase. *Proc. Natl. Acad. Sci. USA* **1999**, *96*, 8861–8866. [CrossRef]
134. Kiang, A.; Hartman, Z.C.; Liao, S.; Xu, F.; Serra, D.; Palmer, D.J.; Ng, P.; Amalfitano, A.; Kiang, Z.C.H.A. Fully Deleted Adenovirus Persistently Expressing GAA Accomplishes Long-Term Skeletal Muscle Glycogen Correction in Tolerant and Nontolerant GSD-II Mice. *Mol. Ther.* **2006**, *13*, 127–134. [CrossRef] [PubMed]
135. Rastall, D.P.W.; Seregin, S.S.; Aldhamen, Y.A.; Kaiser, L.; Mullins, C.; Liou, A.; Ing, F.; Pereria-Hicks, C.; Godbehere-Roosa, S.; Palmer, D.; et al. Long-term, high-level hepatic secretion of acid α-glucosidase for Pompe disease achieved in non-human primates using helper-dependent adenovirus. *Gene Ther.* **2016**, *23*, 743–752. [CrossRef] [PubMed]
136. Mingozzi, F.; High, K.A. Therapeutic in vivo gene transfer for genetic disease using AAV: Progress and challenges. *Nat. Rev. Genet.* **2011**, *12*, 341–355. [CrossRef] [PubMed]
137. Franco, L.M.; Sun, B.; Yang, X.; Bird, A.; Zhang, H.; Schneider, A.; Brown, T.; Young, S.P.; Clay, T.M.; Amalfitano, A.; et al. Evasion of Immune Responses to Introduced Human Acid α-Glucosidase by Liver-Restricted Expression in Glycogen Storage Disease Type II. *Mol. Ther.* **2005**, *12*, 876–884. [CrossRef] [PubMed]
138. Sun, B.; Bird, A.; Young, S.P.; Kishnani, P.S.; Chen, Y.-T.; Koeberl, D. Enhanced Response to Enzyme Replacement Therapy in Pompe Disease after the Induction of Immune Tolerance. *Am. J. Hum. Genet.* **2007**, *81*, 1042–1049. [CrossRef] [PubMed]
139. Sun, B.; Kulis, M.D.; Young, S.P.; Hobeika, A.C.; Li, S.; Bird, A.; Zhang, H.; Li, Y.; Clay, T.M.; Burks, W.; et al. Immunomodulatory Gene Therapy Prevents Antibody Formation and Lethal Hypersensitivity Reactions in Murine Pompe Disease. *Mol. Ther.* **2010**, *18*, 353–360. [CrossRef]

140. Bond, J.; Kishnani, P.; Koeberl, D. Immunomodulatory, liver depot gene therapy for Pompe disease. *Cell. Immunol.* **2019**, *342*, 103737. [CrossRef]
141. Kishnani, P.S.; Koeberl, D. Liver depot gene therapy for Pompe disease. *Ann. Transl. Med.* **2019**, *7*, 288. [CrossRef]
142. Han, S.-O.; Ronzitti, G.; Arnson, B.; Leborgne, C.; Li, S.; Mingozzi, F.; Koeberl, D. Low-Dose Liver-Targeted Gene Therapy for Pompe Disease Enhances Therapeutic Efficacy of ERT via Immune Tolerance Induction. *Mol. Ther. Methods Clin. Dev.* **2017**, *4*, 126–136. [CrossRef] [PubMed]
143. Puzzo, F.; Colella, P.; Biferi, M.G.; Bali, D.; Paulk, N.K.; Vidal, P.; Collaud, F.; Simon-Sola, M.; Charles, S.; Hardet, R.; et al. Rescue of Pompe disease in mice by AAV-mediated liver delivery of secretable acid α-glucosidase. *Sci. Transl. Med.* **2017**, *9*, eaam6375. [CrossRef] [PubMed]
144. Cagin, U.; Puzzo, F.; Gomez, M.J.; Moya-Nilges, M.; Sellier, P.; Abad, C.; Van Wittenberghe, L.; Daniele, N.; Guerchet, N.; Gjata, B.; et al. Rescue of Advanced Pompe Disease in Mice with Hepatic Expression of Secretable Acid α-Glucosidase. *Mol. Ther.* **2020**, *28*. [CrossRef] [PubMed]

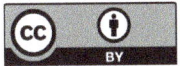

© 2020 by the authors. Licensee MDPI, Basel, Switzerland. This article is an open access article distributed under the terms and conditions of the Creative Commons Attribution (CC BY) license (http://creativecommons.org/licenses/by/4.0/).

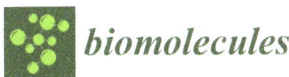

Article

The Release of a Soluble Glycosylated Protein from Glycogen by Recombinant Lysosomal α-Glucosidase (rhGAA) In Vitro and Its Presence in Serum In Vivo

Allen K. Murray [1,2]

1. HIBM Research Group, Inc., Chatsworth, CA 21053, USA; amurray1@glycantechnologies.com or allen@hibm.org; Tel.: +1-949-689-9664
2. Glycan Technologies, Inc., P.O. Box 17993, Irvine, CA 92623, USA

Received: 31 October 2020; Accepted: 23 November 2020; Published: 29 November 2020

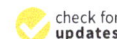

Abstract: In studies on the degradation of glycogen by rhGAA, a glycosylated protein core material was found which consists of about 5–6% of the total starting glycogen. There was an additional 25% of the glycogen unaccounted for based on glucose released. After incubation of glycogen with rhGAA until no more glucose was released, no other carbohydrate was detected on HPAEC-PAD. Several oligosaccharides are then detectable if the medium is first boiled in 0.1 N HCl or incubated with trypsin. It is present in serum either in an HCl extract or in a trypsin digest. The characteristics of the in vivo serum material are identical to the material in the in vitro incubation medium. One oligosaccharide cannot be further degraded by rhGAA, from the incubation medium as well as from serum co-elute on HPAEC-PAD. Several masked oligosaccharides in serum contain m-inositol, e-inositol, and sorbitol as the major carbohydrates. The presence of this glycosylated protein in serum is a fraction of glycogen that is degraded outside the lysosome and the cell. The glycosylated protein in the serum is not present in the serum of Pompe mice not on ERT, but it is present in the serum of Pompe disease patients who are on ERT, so it is a biomarker of GAA degradation of lysosomal glycogen.

Keywords: rhGAA; Pompe disease; glycogen; lysosomal α-glucosidase; GAA biomarker

1. Introduction

The deficiency of the lysosomal of α-glucosidase (GAA) in Pompe disease tissue, also known as type II glycogenosis and acid maltase deficiency, was identified in 1963 [1]. The initial publication did report the ability to release glucose from glycogen but did not specifically report α-1,6-glucosidase activity. The specificity of the lysosomal α-glucosidase to hydrolyze α-1,6 linkages was reported for the dog liver enzyme in 1964 [2] and its absence was reported in human Pompe disease tissues in 1970 [3]. The enzyme has multiple activities including α-1,4-glucosidase, α-1,6-glucosidase, transglucanase, transglucosylation, maltase and glucamylase. It is subject to substrate inhibition by maltooligosaccharides above a concentration of 5 mM [4–8]. However, the substrate concentration is not known in vivo or in vitro since the molecular weight or the concentration of the soluble fraction of glycogen is not known. The ability of the enzyme to degrade glycogen was reported as 91%, however, the inability to completely degrade Pompe glycogen when it was 80% degraded by the lysosomal α-glucosidase followed by phosphorylase and debrancher was reported in 1970 [5]. In another publication, the α-glucosidase was reported as able to convert 95% of the glycogen to glucose [6]. However, this is likely the comparison of glucose released by the enzyme compared to glucose released by acid hydrolysis as was previously published from the same laboratory. The ability to detect very small amounts of other carbohydrates was not available at that time. A problem with these two studies is that it appears that they used commercially isolated glycogen which I have found to be partially degraded by harsh isolation procedures. It is assumed that only glucose is released in vivo, but from earlier work with glycogen as a substrate, it appears that oligosaccharides are also released in vitro and are then degraded to glucose [9].

Enzyme replacement therapy using recombinant human GAA [rhGAA] for Pompe disease has been facilitated by the development of the knockout mouse model which is deficient in the lysosomal α-glucosidase [10]. There are reports of residual carbohydrate in the muscle tissue of the Pompe mouse following a course of enzyme replacement therapy (ERT) [10] as well as in biopsy muscle tissue from patients following ERT has also been reported [11,12]. The initial interest to begin this work was the presence of what was called residual glycogen in the cytoplasm of Pompe mouse tissue following ERT. At that time, I knew that glycogen was not a homopolymer of glucose, so the broader question was, could rhGAA completely degrade glycogen? It seems surprising that the question was not addressed before ERT began. This residual carbohydrate has been called glycogen in publications but it has not been isolated and identified. All that has been published is that it stains with PAS, indicating it contains carbohydrate.

The initial goal of this work was to determine if rhGAA could completely degrade glycogen. A core glycosylated protein, which is glycosylated primarily with inositol and sorbitol, iditol and has minor constituents of glucose, galactose, and mannose, as well as galactosamine and glucosamine, was identified. The mass of which consists of about 5–6% of the initial glycogen in the incubation tube [9]. It is likely that the residual carbohydrate material in tissue consists of the non-glucan portion of glycogen that cannot be degraded by rhGAA or possibly glycogen that has been modified by some pathophysiological process during storage. This present work is the result of an unexpected observation of that earlier work. The mass of glucose released by rhGAA and the residual glycosylated protein do not equal the mass of starting glycogen so about another 25% of the glycogen was unaccounted for. It is this unaccounted for glucan and a glycosylated protein containing primarily inositol and sorbitol which are the subjects of this report. About 70–75% of the mass of glycogen is released as glucose by the action of rhGAA in vitro. After approximately four days of in vitro incubation of glycogen with rhGAA, the glucose released reaches a plateau and no more glucose is released. No carbohydrate was detected in the medium that eluted after glucose by HPAEC-PAD on a CarboPac PA1 column. If the medium was first boiled in 0.1 N HCl for 30 min, a number of oligosaccharides were detected. Incubation with trypsin also exposed oligosaccharides for detection. It appears that this is a case of a protein masking carbohydrate which is unusual but some cases have been reported [13,14]. The soluble glycosylated protein in the medium is bound by Dowex 50W, which is evidence of binding as a charged entity such as a protein but it is not bound by concanavalin A which binds carbohydrates containing glucose or mannose, including glycogen [15]. Based on these characteristics and the possibility of the involvement of lysosomal exocytosis, serum was investigated and this soluble glycosylated protein was found to be present in serum.

2. Materials and Methods

2.1. Glycogen Substrates

Sigma, Type IX bovine liver glycogen, SigmaAldrich, St. Louis, MO, USA, is extracted by the method of Bell and Young, [16] which involves boiling and TCA precipitation of proteins at elevated temperature. This method is quite harsh compared to the method of isolation of the human glycogen in this report. All chemicals were of Reagent Grade or higher. Concanavalin A, monosaccharide and oligosaccharide standards and TFA were purchased from Sigma Aldrich, St. Louis, MO, USA. Dowex 50W was obtained from Bio-Rad, Hercules, CA, USA.

2.2. Human Glycogen Samples

Human glycogen samples were extracted by the method of Mordoh, Krisman, and Leloir [17] with the addition of five freeze-thaw steps to ensure the rupture of lysosomes. This method was chosen because it was reported that the isolated glycogen appeared to be identical to native glycogen isolated from liver as judged by its rate of sedimentation and its appearance under the electron microscope. Glycogen isolated by this method has been shown to be paracrystalline [18]. The glycogens were characterized for a number of parameters including average chain length, protein content, amino acid composition, RNA content, phosphate content, β-amolysis, iodine absorbance, interior chain length, and external chain length [19,20]. The protein content was less than one per cent for two of the three samples. All glycogens were hydrated for at least 18 h before incubations. Glycogen solutions were never frozen.

2.3. Source

Autopsy liver tissue from an 18-month-old female with Pompe disease (type II glycogenosis) and liver tissue from two adult male accident victims. The Pompe liver and the Control 1 liver were obtained at autopsy. In the case of Control 2, the patient was an organ donor on life support so the liver tissue was obtained immediately on termination of life support. All liver tissue was stored at −76 °C until the glycogen isolation. The case of the Pompe disease patient and an enzyme replacement trial with lysosomal α-glucosidase linked to low density lipoprotein has been previously reported [21].

The IRB approval was UC Irvine, UCI/ 2008-6631, and the genomic analysis of patients was reported [22].

2.4. Enzyme Assays

Recombinant human GAA (rhGAA) was provided by Sanofi Genzyme, Framingham, MA, USA, which is the 110 kDa precursor which is converted to the mature form in the tissue in ERT. Assay mixtures consisted of 1 mL volume containing 500 μg or more of glycogen as indicated, 50 mM sodium acetate buffer, pH 4.6, and 10 μL or 25 μL of rhGAA (5 μg/μL) as indicated. The reactions were incubated at 37 °C under toluene to prevent microbial growth. At various time points, as indicated in the figures, the reaction mixture was mixed on a vortex mixer, then centrifuged at 16,000× g for 5 min to precipitate any insoluble material. Then, a 100 μL or 200 μL aliquot was extracted and boiled for 5 min. The sample was then centrifuged at 16,000× g for 5 min to precipitate any insoluble material and the supernatant was analyzed for carbohydrates by HPAEC-PAD on a PA1 column. The remaining incubation mixture was mixed on a vortex mixer and returned to the water bath.

2.5. Carbohydrate Analysis

HPAEC-PAD was performed on a Dionex DX-600 ion chromatograph using a CarboPac PA1 column. (Thermo Fisher Scientific, Dionex, Thermo Elecdtron North America, LLC, Madison, WI, USA) The eluent was 150 mM sodium hydroxide, isocratic from 0 to 5 min, then a linear sodium acetate gradient from 5 to 25 min going from 0 to 57% 500 mM NaOAc in 150 mM NaOH at a flow rate of 1 mL/min. Fractions of 0.25 mL were collected using a Gilson 201 fraction collector. Fractions were partially reduced in volume on a Speed Vac to a volume less than 1.0 mL and then dialyzed overnight against 18.3 megohm water in 1.0 mL chambers against a 500 MWCO membrane. Fractions were taken to dryness in a Speed-Vac. The fractions were then hydrolyzed with 2 N TFA at 100 °C for two hours after which they were taken to dryness in a Speed-Vac. If it was determined that hydrolysis was incomplete, as evidenced by changes on passage through a Dowex column, samples were hydrolyzed again with 4 N TFA at 120 °C for 1 to 4 h. Monosaccharides and sugar alcohols were determined using a CarboPac MA1 column with isocratic elution with 480 mM NaOH at a flow rate of 0.4 mL/min. The waveform for carbohydrate analysis had a potential of +0.1 V from 0 to 0.40 s, −2.0 V from 0.41 to 0.42 s, +0.6 V from 0.43 to 0.44 s, and −0.1 V from 0.44 to 0.50 s with integration from 0.20 to 0.40 s. Data analysis was performed using Dionex Chromeleon 6.60 software.

2.6. Protein Determination

Protein determination was by a modification of the method of Lowry et al. [23]. A control experiment of protein determination on BSA showed no significant difference between samples of before and after hydrolysis for comparison.

3. Results

3.1. Incubation Medium Analysis

Demonstration of the oligomers in glycogen and their relationship to degradation by rhGAA is shown in Figure 1A–C. Figure 1A shows the incubation medium from rhGAA degradation of Control 2 glycogen at 4 and 6 days of incubation, which only shows glucose released in the lower two plots, after four days no more glucose was released for up to 14 days. However, when the medium was extracted with 0.1 N HCl at 100 °C for 30 min, oligosaccharides were detected as shown in the middle two plots. Then, when the medium was treated with 2 N TFA for 2 h at 100 °C to degrade oligosaccharides to monosaccharides, the result was the surprising appearance of more oligosaccharides particularly with Control 2 glycogen in the 6 day medium as shown in the top two plots. It should be pointed out that at day 4, additional medium and enzyme were added. This particular glycogen sample, Control 2, appears to have a higher degree of complexity as shown in Murray [9]. This result was not as apparent in other glycogen samples. This particular glycogen sample was obtained from an organ donor who was maintained on life support until the organs could be harvested so this liver tissue was then frozen immediately. Some suggest that degradation of glycogen is apparent at 15 min after death. These results, and others, suggest that changes begin to take place very soon after death which may be why this glycogen may be somewhat different than other glycogens from tissue obtained at autopsy. Figure 1B,C demonstrates that the oligomers in TFA extracts can be degraded by rhGAA, however this is most apparent in the day 4 samples, which is due to the fact that the day 4 samples contains incubation medium from the beginning of the experiment. There are shifts in the retention times of residual peaks which appear to correspond to the residual material originally obtained from rhGAA degradation. The identification of the fraction which is released by the 0.1 N HCl contains about 18% of the mass of the initial glycogen sample. The characteristic which results in the appearance of the oligosaccharides on HCl extraction of the medium is of interest since this was totally unexpected. The residual material fractions all contain protein.

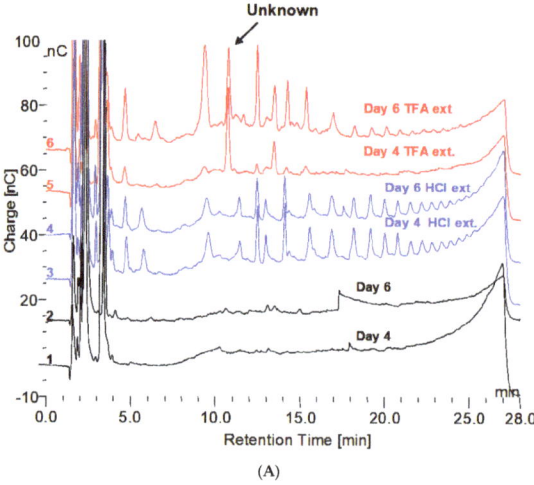

(A)

Figure 1. *Cont.*

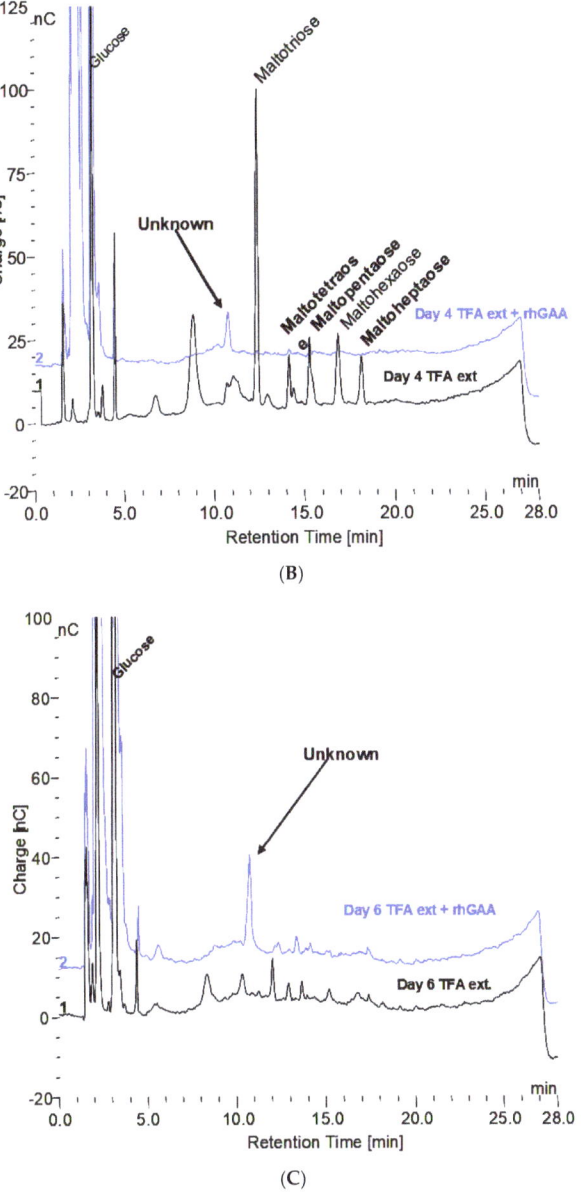

Figure 1. (**A**) Incubation medium of Control 2 with rhGAA after 4 and 6 days, HCl extract of the same and 2N TFA hydrolyzate of same. (**B**) Incubation medium of Control 2 glycogen with rhGAA after 4 days: 2N TFA hydrolyzate and same incubated with rhGAA. (**C**) Incubation medium of Control 2 glycogen with rhGAA after 6 days: 2N TFA hydrolyzate and same incubated with rhGAA.

Reaction mixture from rhGAA degradation of Control 2 glycogen was subjected to the scheme shown in Figure 2A. At each of the six steps, the sample was analyzed and the results are shown in Figure 2B.

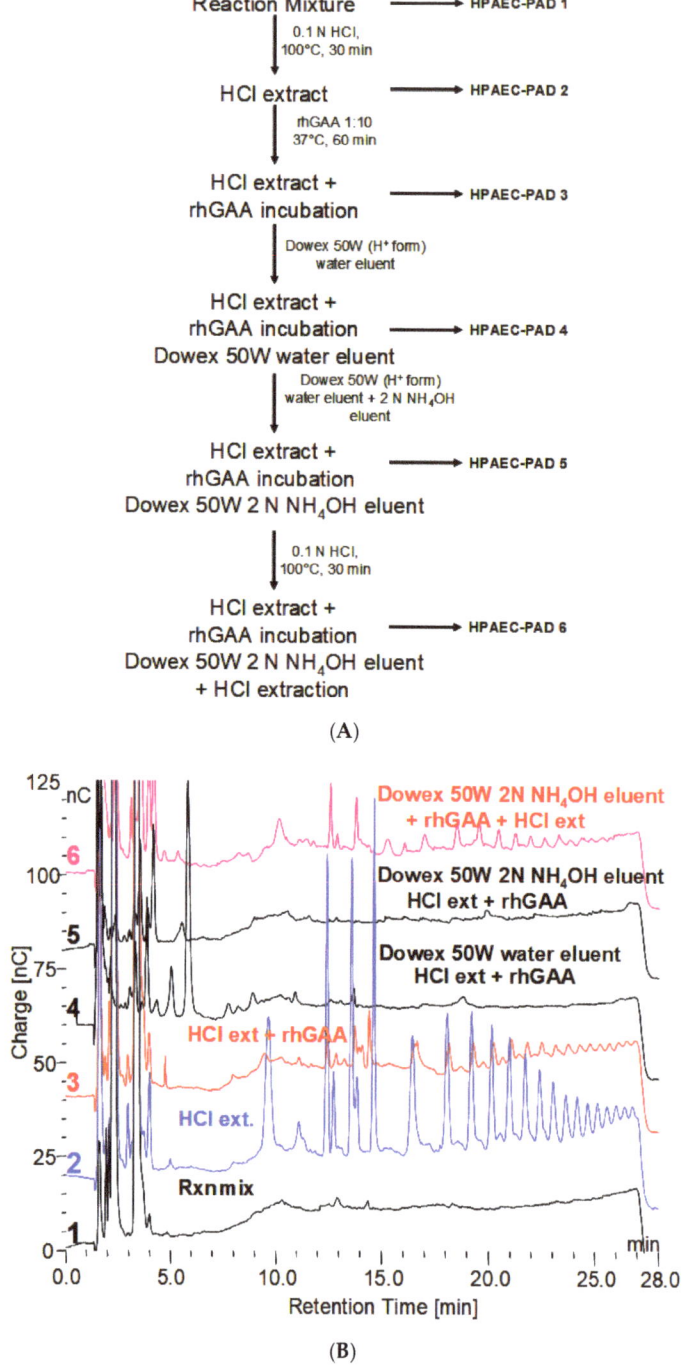

Figure 2. (**A**) Extraction procedures for incubation medium from rhGAA degradation of Control 2 glycogen after no more glucose is released. HPAEC-PAD numbers 1–6 refer to chromatograms 1–6 in 2B. (**B**) Results of samples analysis at each of sic steps in 2A.

3.2. Characteristics of the Glycogen Fraction that is not Degraded by rhGAA

1. HPAEC-PAD does not reveal any significant peaks that elute after monosaccharides. Which indicates no carbohydrates with ionizable hydroxyl groups are present?
2. Extraction with 0.1 N HCl at 100 °C for 30 min reveals maltooligosaccharides from DP 2 to about 18 on HPAEC-PAD.
3. The material in the incubation medium binds to a Dowex 50W ion exchange column and elutes in 2.0 N NH_4OH. This is indicative of binding by a charged species such as protein or amino acids. After taken to dryness, it can be extracted with 0.1 N HCl at 100 °C to reveal the maltooligosaccharides.
4. Incubation with amyloglucosidase does not do anything to the samples.
5. Incubation with trypsin reveals some smaller oligosaccharides that elute in the region of up to about DP 4 and one at about DP 7 or 8. Additionally, trypsin treatment before HCl extraction appears to facilitate the appearance of more larger oligosaccharides. This is indicative of oligosaccharides being released or their appearance facilitated by the removal of protein.
6. Incubation with concanavalin A does not appear to bind the material. This indicates the absence of exposed glucose or mannose residues, including glycogen, which would be bound by the concanavalin A protein [14].

3.3. Summary of Characteristics

- Lack of chemical detection of ionizable hydroxyls of carbohydrate.
- Lack of biological recognition of carbohydrate by rhGAA, concanavalin A, or amyloglucosidase.
- Binding to Dowex 50W indicative of a charged species.
- Exposure of carbohydrate by incubation with a protease (trypsin).

These characteristics led to the conclusion that the material contains carbohydrate material which is masked by protein. There are reports in the literature of carbohydrate masked by protein. Since the material was not detected to be carbohydrate chemically, or by glycosidases and concanavalin A, it is possible that it is not recognized by the biological system. It was considered to be possible that it could be released outside the cell by the lysosomal exocytosis mechanism in which the lysosomal membrane fuses with the cell membrane and the lysosomal contents are expelled from the cell [24,25]. This has been shown for the export of stored glycogen from Pompe mouse cells in culture [26,27] and for the release of lysosomal enzymes in urine [28]. If that were the case, then it seemed reasonable that this material might be found in blood or urine. Normal human serum was investigated and the material was found to be present, indicating that this may be part of the normal mechanism of degradation for lysosomal glycogen.

3.4. Serum Investigation

About 200 µL of blood was obtained from a fingertip needle stick of a normal individual and added to 300 µL of 0.9% NaCl in a conical 1.5 mL tube and immediately centrifuged for 10 min at 10,000× g and allowed to clot. The serum was then diluted 1:10 and 1:20 and analyzed by HPAEC-PAD directly as well as after extraction with 0.1 N HCl for 30 min at 100 °C. The serum, HCl extract, and HCl extract following in vitro incubation of glycogen with rhGAA are shown in Figure 3A. The peak labeled "Unknown" is present in all of the serum samples analyzed. However, there was significant variability in the oligosaccharide content of the HCl extracts between different serum samples from the same source from day to day. The oligosaccharides varied but the unknown peak was consistently the same. The clot at the bottom of the serum but above the red blood cells was extracted. The HCl extract of the clot is characterized by abundant oligosaccharides. Since the clot contains fibrin and as a protein its function is to bind proteins or other components of blood, it is not surprising that the clot bound oligosaccharides, which appear to be conjugated to protein. Following HCl extraction, the oligosaccharides are readily degraded in vitro by rhGAA but the rhGAA does not degrade the unknown. The degradation of the oligosaccharides results in an increase in the size of the unknown peak.

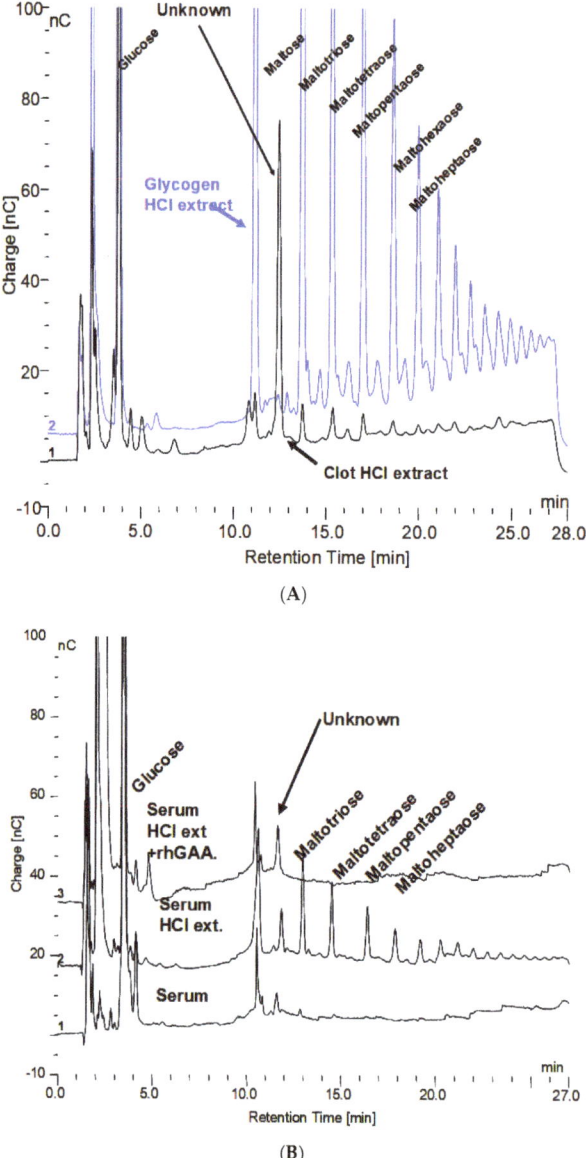

Figure 3. (**A**) Glycogen HCl extract showing maltooligosaccharides DP2-16 and clot HCl extract with array of maltooligosaccharides and the Unknown. (**B**) Serum, serum HCl extract, and serum HCl extract after rhGAA incubation.

The HCl extract of the clot shown in Figure 3A contains almost the full array of malto-oligosaccharides from DP2-16. The small peaks between the oligosaccharide peaks in Figure 3A are the glycosylated protein peaks associated with the oligosaccharides [20], as well as the unknown.

The rhGAA degradation of the oligosaccharides in the clot extract exposes the unknown and leaves the small peaks as well as some of the oligosaccharide peaks, which is shown in Figure 3B. The oligosaccharide peaks would likely not be there if a longer incubation was used. The chromatograms for the clot HCl extract before and after rhGAA degradation are shown in Figure 4A. The retention times for components can vary in different solutions as is the case with the HCl extract of incubation medium and the HCl extract of serum or the clot. This can be due to salt concentrations and other components of the solution. Therefore, to establish the identity of the material from the two different sources, equal volumes of both solutions containing the same amount of the unknown were combined and the mixture was chromatographed. In this case, the result was only one peak, which was symmetrical with no leading or trailing shoulders indicative of identity of the material from both sources as shown in Figure 4B. In this case, the Control 2 glycogen HCl extract was from day 8 of a rhGAA degradation of glycogen where the unknown was the only oligosaccharide remaining. It should be pointed out that there may be slight differences in absolute retention times of components but not in relative retention times. This is due to the fact that some chromatograms were obtained with only the electrochemical detector in use and other times with the addition of the photodiode array detector, which is in line ahead of the electrochemical detector, resulting in a slight delay in elution of peaks detected by the electrochemical detector.

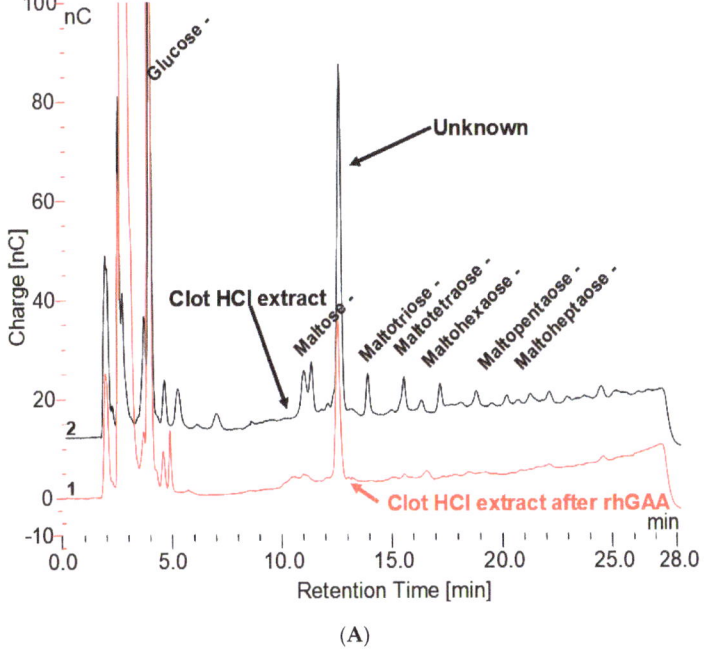

(A)

Figure 4. Cont.

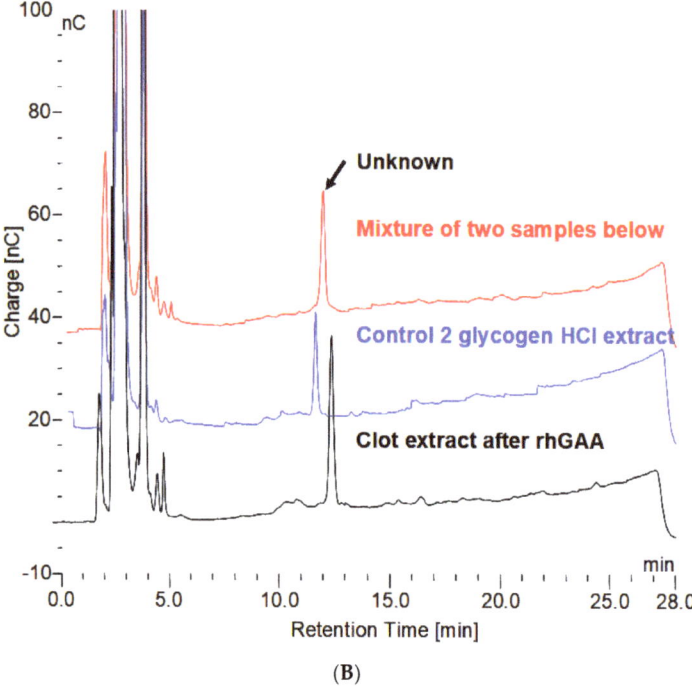

(B)

Figure 4. (**A**) Clot HCl extract before and after degradation with rhGAA demonstrating the Unknown is not degraded. (**B**) HCl extract of Control 2 glycogen, HCl extract of clot following rhGAA degradation, and a mixture of equal parts of both extracts demonstrating one symmetrical peak.

3.5. Masking of Carbohydrate by Protein

From the initial observation of the in vitro degradation of glycogen, that the apparent absence of oligosaccharides in the incubation medium could be overcome by boiling in 0.1 N HCl for 30 min or by trypsin, the concern became one of the comparison of the methods. An overnight or 24 h incubation with trypsin did not reveal as much of the terminal oligosaccharide, which is not degraded by GAA as was released by the HCl treatment. However, longer trypsin incubation releases much more of the material as shown in Figure 5A. It is also apparent that the HCl treatment results in a shift to a slightly longer retention time as well as variable release of the other oligosaccharides. The chymotrypsin treatment appears to release more oligosaccharide material, although it takes longer, as shown in Figure 5B. The products released are reproducible. The first two peaks with retention times of about 9 and 11 min as well as the last oligosaccharide with a retention time of 26 min are the major ones and as a result the ones of major interest. They all still have peptide material attached as shown in plots which show both the electrochemical detector and the absorbance at 280 nm. The retention times do shift slightly when other proteases are used due to the different specificity of which amino acids the proteases cleave.

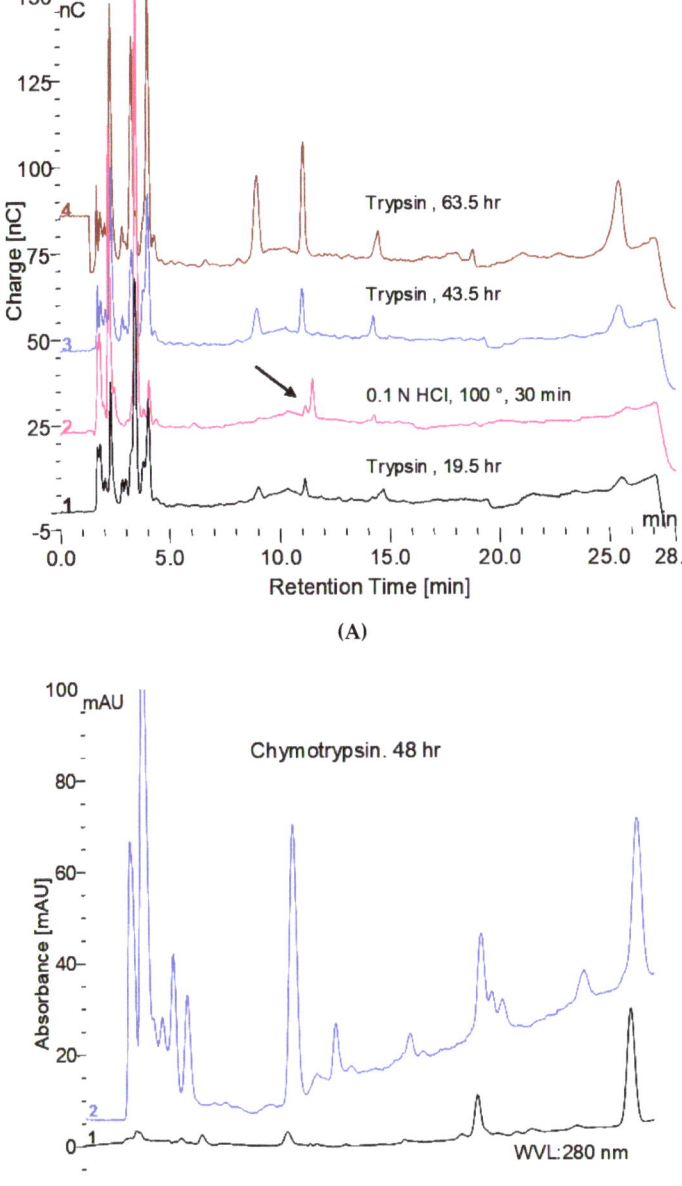

Figure 5. (**A**) Release of peptide bound oligosaccharides by trypsin and 0.1 N HCl. The HCl treatment was at the beginning. The trypsin treatment was for the indicated time at 37 °C under toluene. (**B**) Release of peptide bound oligosaccharides by chymotrypsin showing carbohydrate in blue and protein in black.

3.6. Fraction Collection and Evidence of Protein Masking by Carbohydrate in Serum

The effect of doubling the concentration of trypsin used as well as chymotrypsin was tried. In 48 h incubation, doubling the trypsin concentration did not have a noticeable effect on the result. Chymotrypsin was more effective at the same concentration as trypsin. Proteinase K was also tried but there is a problem with proteinase K since it contains a number of oligosaccharides in the enzyme preparation which makes it problematic for collection of fractions.

Six fractions were collected from a trypsin incubation mixture which are labeled 1–6 in the top panel of Figure 6. As mentioned earlier fractions 1, 2, and 6 are quantitatively the major ones of interest. These fractions were collected from multiple chromatographic runs into the same tubes. Below the top chromatograms, the parallel treatments of fractions 1 and 2 are shown. The fractions were partially concentrated on a Speed-Vac and then dialyzed against water at room temperature overnight using a 500 MWCO membrane in 1 mL dialyzers. Following dialysis, no oligosaccharides were detected as shown in the top chromatogram for each sample. There were a few small peaks at about 2–3 min retention time which represent sugar alcohols and a small peak at about 3.5 min which represents glucose galactose and mannose are not separated from glucose under these conditions. Next, the fractions were hydrolyzed in 2 N trifluoroacetic acid at 100 °C for two hours and then taken to dryness in the Speed-Vac. The fractions were then made up to 1.0 mL in water. Chromatography again on the PA1 column revealed increased monosaccharides but no oligosaccharides as shown in the second chromatogram for each fraction. The fractions were then analyzed by chromatography on an MA1 column which revealed inositol, sorbitol, hexoses, and xylose in 2-2 (Shown in Figures 7 and 8). The samples were then passed over a Dowex 50W column to remove amino acids. The material which passed through was then analyzed by chromatography on the MA1 column which indicated increased inositol and sorbitol (shown in Figures 7 and 8). This was likely due to additional hydrolysis on the resin which is not uncommon. Since it was apparent that everything had not been hydrolyzed the samples were then hydrolyzed in 4 N TFA at 120 °C for two hours, dried on a Speed-Vac and made up to 1.0 mL in water. Subsequent chromatography on an MA1 column revealed significantly more *m*-inositol, *e*-inositol, sorbitol, and xylitol (tentative) as well as hexoses and less xylose in 2-2 as shown in the bottom chromatogram for each fraction. During acid hydrolysis to release carbohydrates, although some carbohydrates are released with increasing time, others may be degraded. In this case, during the 4 N TFA hydrolysis, some glucose and a significant amount of xylose are degraded with increased time. This final TFA hydrolyzate is shown for both fractions in the bottom panel of Figure 6.

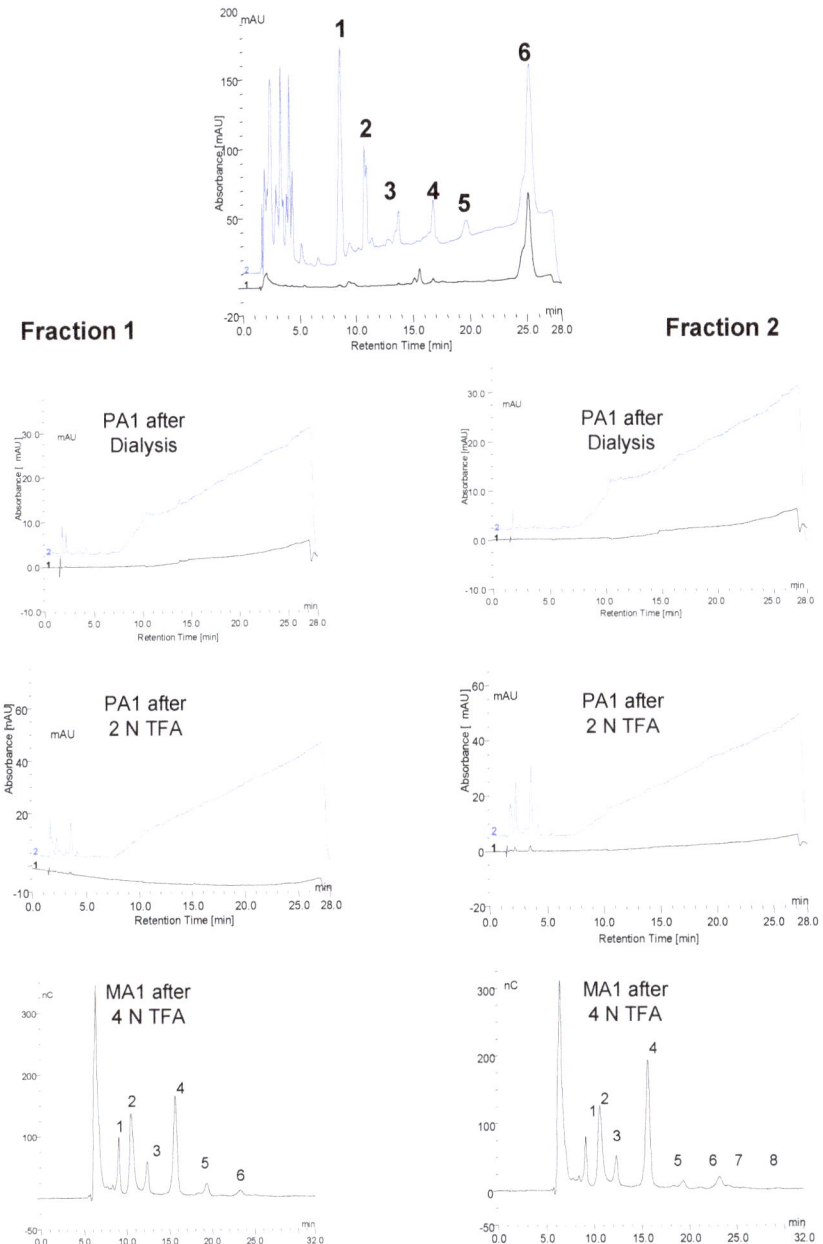

Figure 6. The top chromatogram shows the fractions collected. The three chromatograms on the left show fraction 1 after dialysis, after hydrolysis with 2 N TFA and after hydrolysis with 4 N TFA from top to bottom. The three chromatograms on the right show the same three treatments of Fraction 2. Carbohydrates: 1, *myo*-inositol:2, *epi*-inositol: 3, Xylitol: 4, Sorbitol: 5, Manitol: 6, Glucose: 7, Xylose: 8, Galactose.

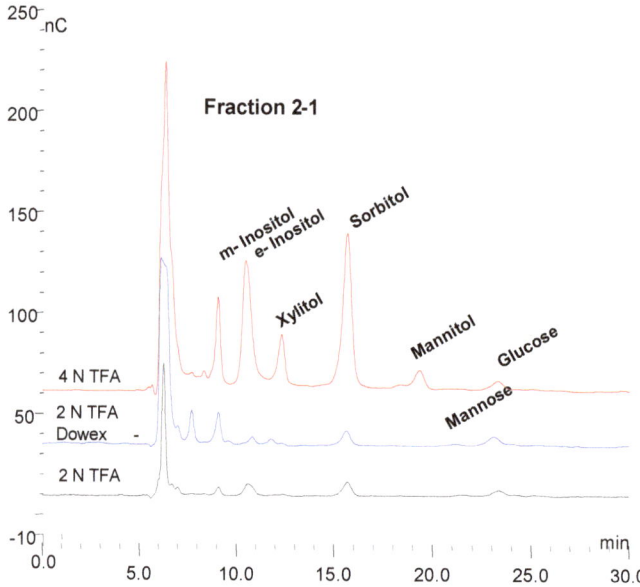

Figure 7. The monosaccharide chromatograms for Fraction 1 (2-1) are shown from bottom to top for 2 N TFA hydrolyzate, Dowex 50W column, and 4 N TFA hydrolyzate.

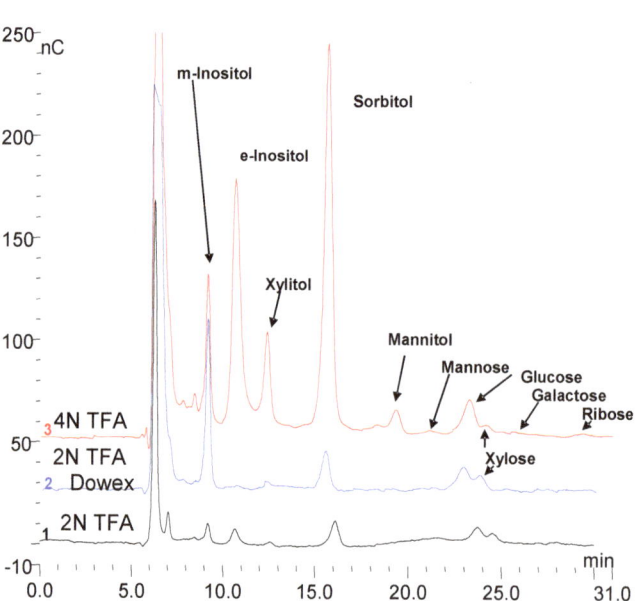

Figure 8. The monosaccharide chromatograms for Fraction 2 (2-2) are shown from bottom to top for 2 N TFA hydrolyzate, Dowex 50 column, and 4 N TFA hydrolyzate.

It is apparent from this sequence that the initial fractions from the collection in the 150 mM NaOH/NaOAc elution medium are altered by the dialysis to remove the salt. Those peaks are then not apparent when the dialyzed sample is chromatographed. However, TFA hydrolysis of the fractions demonstrates that the material was present but that it was masked. Therefore, it appears that the initial in vivo material from serum or the incubation medium from in vitro rhGAA degradation is masked by protein. After proteolysis with enzymes, there apparently is still enough peptide material attached to mask the carbohydrate after dialysis. It may be possible to remove more peptide material by using proteases with different specificities. It appears that after initial hydrolysis with 0.1 N HCl at 100 °C for 30 min to expose the carbohydrate, the removal of salt by dialysis then permits a configuration change to again mask the carbohydrate. This is the case for both the material from the in vitro rhGAA incubations and the in vivo material isolated from serum.

3.7. Monosaccharide Composition of Fractions

The three monosaccharide chromatograms for Fraction 1(2-1) after hydrolysis in 2 N TFA, followed by passage through a Dowex 50W column and hydrolysis in 4 N TFA are shown in Figure 7. After each step, the dried sample was made up to 1.0 mL. Since 25 µL samples were injected on the column in each case, the losses between steps were minimal. The increasingly broad injection peak is indicative of samples containing protein since proteins and amino acids are not retarded on the column.

The three monosaccharide chromatograms for Fraction 2(2-2) after hydrolysis in 2 N TFA, followed by passage through a Dowex 50W column and hydrolysis in 4 N TFA are shown in Figure 8. The monosaccharide composition of the six fractions is shown in Figure 9.

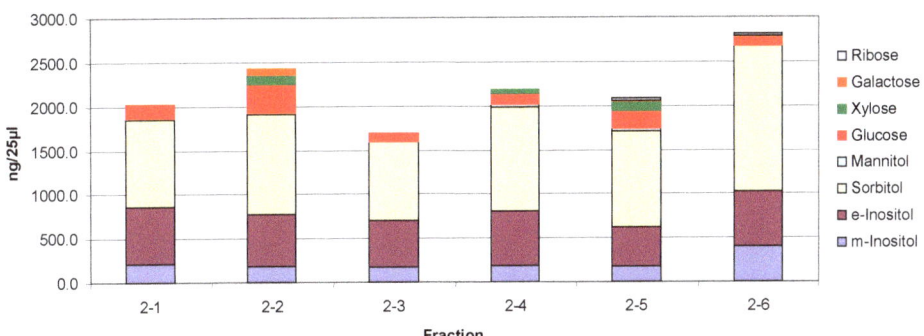

Figure 9. Monosaccharide composition of fractions.

From the carbohydrate composition of the fractions it appears that the major components are the two inositols, sorbitol, xylitol, and mannitol are relatively similar and that the variability occurs in the monosaccharides. However, it is important to keep in mind that these are the monosaccharide compositions of oligosaccharides that still have some peptide attached. On incubation with rhGAA, all of them except 2-2 are degraded with an increase in 2-2 and free glucose, which indicates that although glucose is only a minor constituent, it likely is in a critical position. This is suggestive that at least a portion of the other glycopeptides are being converted to 2-2. There is still peptide attached but it is not known if the peptide is the same for all of them so it is not yet possible to determine with absolute specificity the quantitative interrelationships. It is very likely that there are multiple glycosylation sites, each having a different monosaccharide composition as will be discussed later.

The question of whether these in vivo fractions are intact components of glycogen or whether they have undergone some modification by GAA, or any other enzymes, is an open question since GAA does have glucanase, glucantransferase, and glucosyltransferase activities under the same conditions in which it has glucosyl hydrolase activity [4–9]. There is a commonly held belief that GAA only breaks glycogen down to glucose but it breaks down glycogen to some oligosaccharides which then are later degraded to glucose [9].

The carbohydrate composition of these soluble glycosylated proteins is unique by consisting mainly of inositols and sorbitol with some iditol. Inositol and sorbitol are not known to be found on any other protein. Literature searches do not reveal any glycosylated proteins published with these as the major carbohydrate. In fact, a search does not reveal any publication of a glycosylated protein with sorbitol

Figure 10 shows the HPAEC-PAD chromatograms of the 0.1 N HCl extracts from the serum of two Pompe mice that did not receiver ERT and the serum of three Pompe disease patients that are on ERT. These results are what would be expected if the unknown peak of interest (2-2 in Figure 6) is really a terminal degradation product of GAA degradation of glycogen. The unexpected result in Figure 10 is the large peak at about 18 min retention time in the serum of the Pompe mice. The retention time is what would be expected for maltoheptaose. The peak was collected and incubated with trypsin, which resulted in several peaks with shorter retention times. Each of those peaks was collected, hydrolyzed, and monosaccharide composition determined. Each had a different composition, but combined, they consisted of the inositols, iditol, and sorbitol with lesser amounts of glucose, galactose, and mannose. So, they appear to be related to the other glycosylated proteins from glycogen. The fact that this peak is present in the serum of Pompe mice not on ERT and absent from the serum of Pompe patients on ERT also implies that it is related. The serum of Pompe mice on ERT will be investigated as soon as it is available. It is unclear how this peak may be related to glycogen but based on its presence in the serum of Pompe mice not on ERT, its absence from normal serum or serum of Pompe patients on ERT and the similarity of its carbohydrate composition to the other soluble glycosylated proteins, it appears that it is related.

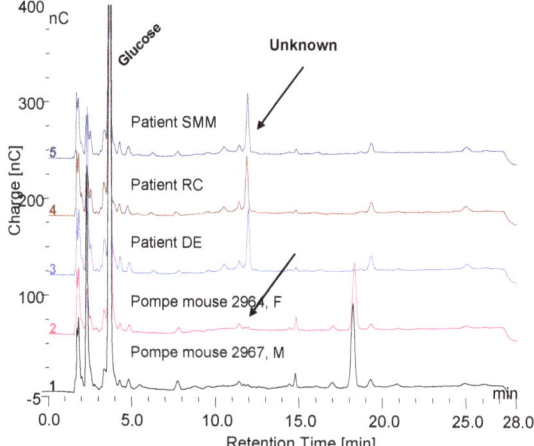

Figure 10. The 0.1 N HCl extracts of serum, 1:10 from two Pompe mice, age 8.7 months and three Pompe patients. The peak at about 18 min in the Pompe mouse serum is a glycosylated protein containing *m*-inositol, sorbitol and glucose as major components as well as galactose and mannose.

A summary of the various fractions isolated following in vitro degradation of glycogen by rhGAA as well as the fractions isolated from normal serum, in vivo, is shown in Figure 11.

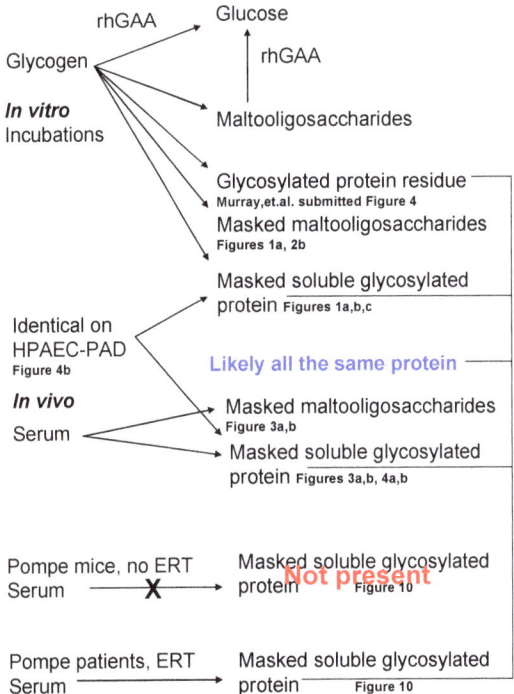

Figure 11. Summary of the metabolites discussed and reference to the figures showing them. The top portion shows metabolites from the in vitro incubations and the bottom portion shows in vivo metabolites isolated from serum.

4. Discussion

A soluble fraction of glycogen that is not completely degraded in vitro by rhGAA contains at least 20% of the initial glycogen. The fact that the carbohydrate cannot be detected unless the incubation medium is boiled in 0.1 N HCl for 30 min or incubated with a protease such as trypsin or chymotrypsin for up to 48 h indicates that the carbohydrate is masked by protein. If the carbohydrate was exposed on the surface of the protein, it would be detected. Following protease incubation, all but one of the oligosaccharides can be degraded or modified in vitro by rhGAA. The one major oligosaccharide in serum that cannot be degraded in vitro by rhGAA following the HCl or protease treatment persists as a terminal metabolite of in vivo GAA degradation of glycogen which is peak 2-2 in Figure 9. As the peaks from serum that can be degraded in vitro by rhGAA disappear, peak 2-2 that is not be degraded increases in magnitude as the other peaks are degraded. As mentioned earlier, this has not been determined to be a quantitative conversion. This metabolite has an identical chromatographic retention time to an unknown previously detected from in vitro glycogen degradation by rhGAA and it has a similar monosaccharide composition as well.

Perhaps if calibrated with the proportion of glycogen degraded, this terminal metabolite could possibly be useful to quantitatively assess lysosomal glycogen degradation in vivo. However, since glycogen is not homogeneous, such a determination may be difficult to achieve without a better understanding of the structure of glycogen. It should be kept in mind that such experiments would not account for ongoing replenishment of lysosomal glycogen by phagocytosis which is assumed to be the case for turnover in lysosomal function in tissues and has been demonstrated in fibroblast culture [29]. One would assume that the lysosomal population would reflect a steady state appearance of glycogen uptake and degradation but the real time case may be more complex than that. Once more is known about the protein masking the carbohydrate, much more will be understood. It is possible an antibody could be raised against the protein or glycopeptides for analysis to determine the localization of complete lysosomal glycogen degradation.

It will be important to investigate the site of degradation of this glycosylated protein as it may be useful in the study of normal lysosomal glycogen in muscle. Liver or kidneys are likely sites of degradation. There is a neutral α-glucosidase in liver which is known to degrade maltooligosaccharides but it can not degrade glycogen [30]. The endogenous substrate for this enzyme is not known, yet there are other α-glucosidases present including some involved in glycosylation of glycoproteins. There is also a reported maltase in kidney for which there is no known substrate, but glucose is not a major component of this glycoprotein. It should be pointed out that glycogenin and the glycosylated protein appear to occupy different points of attachment to the polysaccharide.

Glycogenin is a self glucosylating protein which acquires 10–20 glucose residues, which then serve as the primer for the glucosyl residues of glycogen [31]. The glycosylated protein in this work is found associated with each oligosaccharide derived from the polysaccharide whether released by weak acid or enzymatic hydrolysis. Each one must differ in carbohydrate composition to account for their chromatographic separation; however, they could differ by a repeating unit. This implies that it likely is associated along the length of the polymer, while glycogenin is attached at the nonreducing end. It has been shown that glycogenin can attach xylose in the first position of glucosylation [32].

Comparison of the carbohydrate portions of unknowns 2-1 to 2-6 indicate that all have protein, inositols, sorbitol, mannose, glucose, and galactose and three appear to have xylose. The identification of xylitol is tentative.

During this work, the reasoning was that if the carbohydrate could not be detected by either chemical or biological means, then perhaps the cell could not recognize it as carbohydrate either. As mentioned earlier, there are precedents for the lysosomal exocytosis following degradation of a substance up to a point at which the lysosomal membrane fuses with the cell membrane and expels the material from the cell [24–28]. Although the terminal glycogen degradation product was found in serum, only a very small peak which was unresolved was found in urine that could possibly be attributed to this unknown metabolite. Based on co-chromatography, the soluble glycosylated protein found in serum in vivo which cannot be degraded by rhGAA in vitro appears to be the same as that in the incubation medium from rhGAA degradation of glycogen in vitro. Further degradation with proteases demonstrated that 6 oligosaccharide bound peptides were found, which could be expected since the HCl would not be a specific cleavage agent. On occasion, only four oligosaccharide-peptides were found. However, in all cases, there are quantitatively three major ones. All but one of the oligosaccharides can be degraded or at least significantly modified with rhGAA in vitro even though glucose is not a major constituent. Given the unknown effects of sometimes different conditions or different proteases used, it is reasonable to suspect differences in the appearance of the minor oligosaccharide-peptide species. It should be pointed out that the extraction of the incubation medium of rhGAA degradation of glycogen in vitro also contains a series of masked maltooligosaccharides, which were not apparent before the HCl extraction, which then can be degraded by rhGAA as shown in Figure 1A,B, but they have to first be treated with HCl or protease to be detected. The same is true for the HCl extract from serum as shown in Figures 3B and 4A. So, it is apparent that a significant portion of glycogen contains carbohydrate masked by protein which is degraded outside of the lysosome and subsequently the cell. Some of it is the typical maltooligosaccharide array which can be degraded in vitro by a further exposure to rhGAA and then there is the group of peptide bound oligosaccharides which contain inositol and sorbitol as their major carbohydrate components. It appears that the typical maltooligosaccharides, which are also masked, are peptide bound. However, based on other work, it would appear that all of the maltooligosaccharides contain the protein which is conjugated to inositol and sorbitol based on the chromatograms in which they appear to have the small peaks of the glycosylated protein [20]. The site(s) of degradation of the maltooligosaccharides masked by protein is also an important question because, although they can be degraded in vitro by rhGAA, they would not be exposed to GAA in vivo. If the protein were removed it, could be that they are degraded by one or more of the other α-glucosidases mentioned. It may be that the protein component of these protein bound maltooligosaccharides is the same as the soluble glycosylated protein unknown, fraction 2-2 in Figure 9 as suggested in Figure 11.

These results contribute to the observations of degradation of lysosomal glycogen. The question of where this soluble glycosylated protein is ultimately degraded is added to the list of unknowns as well as the site of degradation of the masked maltooligosaccharides. The fact that this soluble glycosylated protein has protein masking carbohydrate is significant. Such masking is known in biochemistry but I have not found any report for glycogen or for serum components [13,14]. To work out the details of this soluble glycosylated protein, sufficient quantities will be required which will require the collection of many fractions of the glycosylated protein associated with each oligosaccharide. The serum from 100–200 μL of blood contains as much soluble glycosylated protein as several 1 mL incubation tubes with 500 μg of glycogen in each. In comparison, the rat lysosomal fraction from about 140 g of muscle tissue was found to contain about 900 μg of glycogen in 10 mL. The original intent of this work was to isolate the lysosomal fraction from rat muscle and then monitor the degradation of the endogenous glycogen by the GAA in the fraction. However, if this work had begun with animals, the soluble glycosylated protein likely would not have been found or at least it would not have been found for a very long time. This now adds incentive to isolate the lysosomal glycogen and compare it to cytoplasmic glycogen as well as to do a comparison of proglycogen and macroglycogen from both the lysosomal fraction and the cytoplasmic fraction of tissue as well as to compare muscle and liver glycogen.

It is important to understand the masking mechanism to be able to quantify the soluble glycosylated protein as well as to understand the role of lysosomal glycogen in normal metabolism. Does this masking affect our methods of glycogen determination using amyloglucosidase? Should a proteolytic step be used before the amyloglucosidase degradation? These are now questions to be considered and experiments to be performed.

It is likely that the glycosylated protein residue from degradation of glycogen by rhGAA in vitro, the glycosylated protein associated with the masked oligosaccharides, as well as the glycosylated protein terminal glycogen degradation product are all the same protein based on their carbohydrate composition and possible location of their association with glycogen as indicated in Figure 11. It might be that degradation of the glucan then leaves protein attached and depending on ionic conditions, the protein may cover the carbohydrate to mask it.

One of the most interesting points of these results is that the glucose and sorbitol content of these polymers is greater than the quantity of free glucose in the same volume of blood. It is likely that one reason this has not been reported is due to the masking. There also appears to be some self-assembly of protein/carbohydrate when isolated fractions are dialyzed which also complicates things. This self-assembly is not unknown in polysaccharides. A TFA hydrolyzate of serum indicates that one of the most abundant carbohydrates is sorbitol, which is more abundant than glucose.

A similar glycosylated protein has been found in cellulose and corn starch, which also contains mannose, glucose, and galactose, with the major components being inositols, iditol, and sorbitol [20]. Sorbitol, also known as glucitol, is the intermediate between glucose and fructose. The inositol content is more difficult to determine since significantly more inositol is liberated by hydrolysis in 4 N TFA at 120 °C than is liberated in 2 N TFA at 100 °C, indicating that it is more difficult to extract. In fact, as shown in Figure 8, significantly more *m*-inositol was liberated by the passage of the sample over the Dowex 50W column of the 2 N TFA hydrolyzate and then much more by hydrolysis with 4 N TFA of the material passed over the Dowex 50W column. This is also true of *myo*-inositol in glycosylphosphotidyl inositol [GPI] anchor proteins. One reason that inositol and sorbitol may not have been reported as components of polysaccharides such as cellulose, starch, and glycogen may be that much of the earlier work was done using GLC where, for volatility, monosaccharides were converted to alditol acetates and *m*-inositol was added as an internal standard [33].

This terminal metabolite from the degradation of glycogen by GAA and its masking by protein will provide a mechanism as a biomarker by which to gain direct information on the function of lysosomal glycogen and perhaps its role in muscle physiology. Up to this point, our understanding of lysosomal glycogen has been limited to its accumulation in Pompe disease. Perhaps now we can begin to understand the role of lysosomal glycogen and if the impairment if its degradation pathway contributes to the pathophysiology of Pompe disease in a manner different than that attributed to the accumulation of glycogen. This information will permit a better basic understanding of Pompe disease and a better understanding of ERT and how it mimics the normal lysosomal glycogen pathway as well as how it may differ from that pathway if, in fact, it does differ.

This biomarker will enable an assessment of the effectiveness of ERT in Pompe patients in a relatively short time period of days. It could be monitored easily since only a pinprick is required for the small amount of blood needed. It will be possible to determine the most effective frequency of enzyme administration, particularly if it is found to vary among patients. The current two week interval may not be optimal for all patients so this will enable an assessment of GAA activity during the interval between administrations to assess the enzyme activity over the time period.

5. Conclusions

The breakdown of glycogen by rhGAA in vitro only releases enough glucose to account for about 75% of the mass of starting glycogen. About 5–6% is attributed to a glycosylated protein core which has inositols, sorbitol as the major carbohydrates, as well as glucosamine, galactosamine, glucose, and galactose. About another 18% is released as maltooligosaccharides masked by protein and the remainder is a soluble glycosylated protein also masked. The masked carbohydrate and the soluble glycosylated protein are found in normal serum, which is evidence that degradation of about 25% of the lysosomal glycogen occurs outside of the lysosome and outside of the cell. This appears to be facilitated by lysosomal exocytosis. The soluble glycosylated protein is a terminal degradation product of GAA degradation of lysosomal glycogen. This soluble glycosylated protein is not present in the serum of Pompe mice which are not on ERT but it is present in the serum of Pompe patients on ERT and normal individuals. This soluble glycosylated protein is a biomarker for degradation of glycogen by GAA and should be useful to assess ERT in patients. Since the glycosylated protein appears to be a terminal degradation product of GAA degradation of glycogen, it has potential to be very useful to monitor such degradation in relatively short time periods. As such, it should be possible to monitor the degradation of lysosomal glycogen essentially on a daily basis, if desired, to monitor such activity in the interval between administrations of rhGAA. This should enable a better understanding of the whole ERT process and may lead to improved treatment practices.

Funding: This work was supported by a grant from Sanofi Genzyme GZ-2017-11675.

Acknowledgments: I would like to thank Virginia Kimonis, M.D. for serum samples from Pompe mice and human Pompe patients on ERT.

Conflicts of Interest: Author declares no conflicts of interest.

Abbreviations

BSA	bovine serum albumin
ERT	enzyme replacement therapy
GAA	Lysosomal α-glucosidase
rhGAA	recombinant human lysosomal α-glucosidase
HPAEC-PAD	high performance anion exchange chromatography-pulsed amperometric detection
HPLC	high performance liquid chromatography
GLC	gas liquid chromatography
TFA	trifluoroacetic acid
PAS	periodic acid Schiff stain.

References

1. Hers, H.G. α-Glucosidase deficiency in generalized glycogen-storage disease (Pompe's disease). *Biochem. J.* **1963**, *86*, 11–16. [CrossRef] [PubMed]
2. Torres, H.N.; Olavarria, J.M. Liver α-Glucosidases. *J. Biol. Chem.* **1964**, *239*, 2427–2434. [PubMed]
3. Brown, B.I.; Brown, D.H.; Jeffrey, P.L. Simultaneous Absence of α-1,4-Glucosidase and α-1,6-Glucosidase Activities (pH4) in Tissues of Children with Type II Glycogen Storage Disease. *Biochemistry* **1970**, *9*, 1423–1428. [CrossRef] [PubMed]
4. Jeffrey, P.L.; Brown, D.H.; Brown, B.I. Lysosomal α-glucosidase. I. Purification and properties of the rat liver enzyme. *Biochemistry* **1970**, *9*, 1403–1415. [CrossRef] [PubMed]
5. Jeffrey, P.L.; Brown, D.H.; Brown, B.I. Lysosomal α-glucosidase. II. Kinetics of action of the rat liver enzyme. *Biochemistry* **1970**, *9*, 1416–1422. [CrossRef] [PubMed]
6. Palmer, T.N. The substrate specificity of acid α-glucosidase from rabbit Mu muscle. *Biochem. J.* **1971**, *124*, 701–711. [CrossRef] [PubMed]
7. Palmer, T.N. The Maltase, Glucoamylase and Transglucosylase Activities of Acid α-Glucosidase from Rabbit Muscle. *Biochem. J.* **1971**, *124*, 713–724. [CrossRef]
8. Hers, H.; Van Hoof, F. Enzymes of glycogen degradation in biopsy material. *Methods Enzymol.* **1966**, *8*, 525–532. [CrossRef]
9. Murray, A.K. The action of recombinant lysosomal α-glucosidase [rhGAA] and amyloglucosidase on bovine and human liver glycogen. submitted.
10. Raben, N.; NFukuda, O.; Gilbert, A.L.; de Jong, D.; Thurberg, B.L.; Mattaliano, R.J.; Meikle, P.; Hopwood, J.J.; Nagashima, K.; Nagaraju, K.; et al. Replacing Acid α-Glucosidase in Pompe Disease: Recombinant and Transgenic Enzymes are Equipotent, but Neither Completely Clears Glycogen from Type II Muscle Fibers. *Mol. Ther.* **2005**, *11*, 48–56. [CrossRef]
11. Del Rizzo, M.; Fanin, M.; Cerutti, A.; Cazzorla, C.; Milanesi, O.; Nascimbeni, A.C.; Angelini, C.; Giordano, L.; Bordugo, A.; Burlina, A. Long-term follow-up results in enzyme replacement therapy for Pompe disease: A case report. *J. Inherit. Metab. Dis.* **2010**, *33*, 389–393. [CrossRef]
12. Van Der Ploeg, A.; Carlier, P.G.; Carlier, R.-Y.; Kissel, J.; Schoser, B.; Wenninger, S.; Pestronk, A.; Barohn, R.J.; Dimachkie, M.M.; Goker-Alpan, O.; et al. Prospective exploratory muscle biopsy, imaging, and functional assessment in patients with late-onset Pompe disease treated with alglucosidase alfa: The EMBASSY Study. *Mol. Genet. Metab.* **2016**, *119*, 115–123. [CrossRef] [PubMed]
13. Dapson, R.W. Histochemistry of mucus in the skin of the frog, Rana pipiens. *Anat. Rec. Adv. Integr. Anat. Evol. Biol.* **1970**, *166*, 615–625. [CrossRef] [PubMed]
14. Leger, R.S.; Cooper, R.; Charnley, A. Cuticle-degrading enzymes of entomopathogenic fungi: Cuticle degradation in vitro by enzymes from entomopathogens. *J. Invertebr. Pathol.* **1986**, *47*, 167–177. [CrossRef]
15. Montgomery, R. Determination of glycogen. *Arch. Biochem. Biophys.* **1957**, *67*, 378–386. [CrossRef]
16. Bell, D.J.; Young, F.G. Observations on the Chemistry of Liver Glycogen. *Biochem. J.* **1934**, *28*, 882–889. [CrossRef] [PubMed]
17. Mordoh, J.; Krisman, C.R.; Leloir, L.F. Further studies on high molecular weight liver glycogen. *Arch. Biochem. Biophys.* **1966**, *113*, 265–272. [CrossRef]
18. De Wulf, H.; Hers, H.G. Paracrystalline Glycogen. In *Biochemistry of the Glycosidic Linkage*; PAABS Symposium Vol. 2; Piras, R., Pontis, H.G., Eds.; Academic Press: New York, NY, USA, 1972; pp. 399–402.
19. Metzenberg, A.B. Structural Feathers of Stored Glycogen in a Case of Pompe's Disease [Glycogenosis Type II]. Master's Thesis, University of California, Irvine, CA, USA, 1980.
20. Murray, A.K.; Metzenberg, A.B.; Nichols, R.L. Polysaccharide similarities: Glycosylated protein cores of glycogen, starch and cellulose. submitted.
21. Williams, J.C.; Murray, A.K. Enzyme replacement in Pompe disease with an alpha-glucosidase-low density lipoprotein complex. *Birth defects Orig. Artic. Ser.* **1980**, *16*, 415–423.
22. Alandy-Dy, J.; Wencel, M.; Hall, K.; Simon, J.; Chen, Y.; Valenti, E.; Yang, J.; Bali, D.; Lakatos, A.; Goyal, N.; et al. Variable clinical features and genotype-phenotype correlations in 18 patients with late-onset Pompe disease. *Ann. Transl. Med.* **2019**, *7*, 276. [CrossRef]
23. Lowry, O.H.; Rosebrough, N.J.; Farr, A.L.; Randall, R.J. Protein measurement with the Folin phenol reagent. *J. Biol. Chem.* **1951**, *193*, 265–275.

24. Medina, D.L.; Fraldi, A.; Bouche, V.; Annunziata, F.; Mansueto, G.; Spampanato, C.; Puri, C.; Pignata, A.; Martina, J.A.; Sardiello, M.; et al. Transcriptional Activation of Lysosomal Exocytosis Promotes Cellular Clearance. *Dev. Cell* **2011**, *21*, 421–430. [CrossRef]
25. Rao, S.K.; Huynh, C.; Proux-Gillardeaux, V.; Galli, T.; Andrews, N.W. Identification of SNAREs Involved in Synaptotagmin VII-regulated Lysosomal Exocytosis. *J. Biol. Chem.* **2004**, *279*, 20471–20479. [CrossRef] [PubMed]
26. Spampanato, C.; Feeney, E.; Li, L.; Cardone, M.; Lim, J.-A.; Zare, F.A.H.; Polishchuk, R.; Puertollano, R.; Parenti, G.; Ballabio, A.; et al. Transcription factor EB [TFEB] is a new.therapeutic target for Pompe disease. *EMBO Mol. Med.* **2013**, *5*, 691–706. [CrossRef] [PubMed]
27. Li, H.M.; Feeney, E.; Li, L.; Zare, H.; Puertollano, R.; Raben, N. WITHDRAWN: Clearance of lysosomal glycogen accumulation by Transcription factor EB (TFEB) in muscle cells from lysosomal alpha-glucosidase deficient mice. *Biochem. Biophys. Res. Commun.* **2013**. [CrossRef]
28. Paigen, K.; Peterson, J. Coordinacy of lysosomal enzyme excretion in human urine. *J. Clin. Investig.* **1978**, *61*, 751–762. [CrossRef] [PubMed]
29. Brown, D.H.; Waindle, L.M.; Brown, B.I. The apparent activity in vivo of the lysosomal pathway of glycogen catabolism in cultured human skin fibroblasts from patients with type III glycogen storage disease. *J. Biol. Chem.* **1978**, *253*, 5005–5011. [PubMed]
30. Brown, B.I.; Brown, D.H. The subcellular distribution of enzymes in type II glycogenosis and the occurrence of an oligo-α-1,4-glucan glucohydrolase in human tissues. *Biochim. Biophys. Acta* **1965**, *110*, 124–133. [CrossRef]
31. Roach, P.J.; DePaoli-Roach, A.A.; Hurley, T.D.; Tagliabracci, V.S. Glycogen and its metabolism: Some new developments and old themes. *Biochem. J.* **2012**, *441*, 763–787. [CrossRef]
32. Rodén, L.; Ananth, S.; Campbell, P.; Manzella, S.; Meezan, E. Xylosyl transfer to an endogenous renal acceptor. Purification of the transferase and the acceptor and their identification as glycogenin. *J. Biol. Chem.* **1994**, *269*, 11509–11513.
33. Bukovac, M.J.; Olien, W.C. Ethephon-Induced Gummosis in Sour Cherry (*Prunus cerasus* L.): 1. Effect on xylem function and shoot water status. *Plant Physiol.* **1982**, *70*, 547–555.

Publisher's Note: MDPI stays neutral with regard to jurisdictional claims in published maps and institutional affiliations.

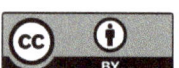

© 2020 by the author. Licensee MDPI, Basel, Switzerland. This article is an open access article distributed under the terms and conditions of the Creative Commons Attribution (CC BY) license (http://creativecommons.org/licenses/by/4.0/).

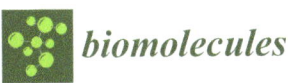

Review

Fabry Disease: Molecular Basis, Pathophysiology, Diagnostics and Potential Therapeutic Directions

Ken Kok [1], Kimberley C. Zwiers [1], Rolf G. Boot [1], Hermen S. Overkleeft [2], Johannes M. F. G. Aerts [1,*] and Marta Artola [1,*]

1 Department of Medical Biochemistry, Leiden Institute of Chemistry, Leiden University, P.O. Box 9502, 2300 RA Leiden, The Netherlands; k.kok@lic.leidenuniv.nl (K.K.); k.c.zwiers@lic.leidenuniv.nl (K.C.Z.); r.g.boot@LIC.leidenuniv.nl (R.G.B.)
2 Department of Bio-organic Synthesis, Leiden Institute of Chemistry, Leiden University, P.O. Box 9502, 2300 RA Leiden, The Netherlands; h.s.overkleeft@chem.leidenuniv.nl
* Correspondence: j.m.f.g.aerts@lic.leidenuniv.nl (J.M.F.G.A.); m.e.artola@lic.leidenuniv.nl (M.A.)

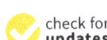

Abstract: Fabry disease (FD) is a lysosomal storage disorder (LSD) characterized by the deficiency of α-galactosidase A (α-GalA) and the consequent accumulation of toxic metabolites such as globotriaosylceramide (Gb3) and globotriaosylsphingosine (lysoGb3). Early diagnosis and appropriate timely treatment of FD patients are crucial to prevent tissue damage and organ failure which no treatment can reverse. LSDs might profit from four main therapeutic strategies, but hitherto there is no cure. Among the therapeutic possibilities are intravenous administered enzyme replacement therapy (ERT), oral pharmacological chaperone therapy (PCT) or enzyme stabilizers, substrate reduction therapy (SRT) and the more recent gene/RNA therapy. Unfortunately, FD patients can only benefit from ERT and, since 2016, PCT, both always combined with supportive adjunctive and preventive therapies to clinically manage FD-related chronic renal, cardiac and neurological complications. Gene therapy for FD is currently studied and further strategies such as substrate reduction therapy (SRT) and novel PCTs are under investigation. In this review, we discuss the molecular basis of FD, the pathophysiology and diagnostic procedures, together with the current treatments and potential therapeutic avenues that FD patients could benefit from in the future.

Keywords: lysosomal storage disorders; Fabry disease; α-galactosidase A; A4GALT; globotriaosylceramide (Gb3); globotriaosyl-sphingosine (lysoGb3); enzyme replacement therapy; pharmacological chaperone therapy; substrate reduction therapy

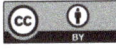

1. Introduction

In 1898, two dermatologists, Johannes Fabry in Dortmund and William Anderson in London, reported similar patients with characteristic skin lesions, so-called angiokeratoma corporis diffusum [1,2]. The inherited disorder became known as Anderson–Fabry disease, nowadays generally referred to as Fabry disease (FD). A striking feature of FD (OMIM 301500) is the characteristic lipid deposits, named zebrabodies, prominently encountered in endothelial cells but lesser also in other cell types [3]. The main component of the storage material was identified by Sweeley and Klionsky as the globoside globotriaosylceramide (Gb3), initially named ceramidetrihexoside (CTH) [4]. Additional accumulating glycosphingolipids in FD patients such as galabiosylceramide (Gb2) and blood group B, B1 and P[1] antigens can be observed, all sharing a terminal α-galactosyl moiety [3]. The molecular basis for lipid abnormalities was firstly elucidated by Brady and coworkers, demonstrating the deficiency of lysosomal acid α-galactosidase activity converting Gb3 to lactosylceramide (LacCer) [5]. A convenient enzyme assay for diagnosis of FD was next developed by Kint, employing an artificial chromogenic α-galactoside substrate [6]. Subsequent research revealed that the reduced α-galactosidase activity in FD patients stems from the lysosomal enzyme α-galactosidase A (α-GalA) that is encoded by the *GLA* gene located at chromosome Xq22 [3]. Of note, an ancient gene duplication has led to two relatively homologous genes: *GLA* and *NAGA*. *NAGA* (also known as α-Galactosidase B (α-GalB)), locus 22q13.2, evolved into an *N*-acetylgalactosaminidase cleaving α-*N*-acetylgalactosamine from glycoconjugates [7,8]. Mutations in *NAGA* cause Schindler disease and Kanzaki disease [9]. α-GalA and α-GalB are both inhibited in enzymatic activity by galactose but only α-GalB is inhibited by *N*-acetylgalactosamine [10]. The globoside Gb3 is degraded by α-GalA, although a minor α-GalB activity towards this metabolite has been reported [11]. The α-GalA enzyme is synthesized as a 429 aa precursor that is processed to a 398 aa glycoprotein functioning as a homodimer [11,12]. The three N-linked glycans of α-GalA acquire mannose-6-phosphate moieties that assist the enzyme's sorting to lysosomes by mannose-6-phosphate receptors. The activity of α-GalA towards the lipid substrate is enhanced by the activator protein saposin B and negatively charged lipids [3]. Close to 1000 mutations have meanwhile been identified in the *GLA* gene, of which most are missense mutations. Thanks to the work of many, particularly by Sakuraba and colleagues, the consequences at the enzyme level of several α-GalA mutations are known [13]. However, the impact of a large number of the presently reported α-GalA mutations remains unclear [14]. So-called α-GalA mutations of unknown significance are often not associated with clearly reduced α-galactosidase activity, promoting the debate as to whether they truly are causing FD [15].

2. Clinical Manifestation of FD

The classic disease manifestation of FD has been extensively described for males [3,16]. Generally, these FD hemizygotes show α-GalA mutations with no or very little residual α-galactosidase activity. Besides the characteristic angiokeratoma, the patients develop corneal opacity (cornea verticillata), neuropathic pain (acroparasthesias), intolerance to heat, inability to sweat, micro-albuminuria and increased intima media thickness. Later in life, the patients develop progressive kidney disease, cardiac symptoms and cerebrovascular disease (stroke). These late-onset symptoms are indistinguishable from similar complications of other origin commonly occurring in the general population. The renal disease usually involves progressive proteinuria following a decline in the glomerular filtration rate (GFR). The final outcome is end-stage renal disease requiring dialysis and kidney transplantation. The heterogeneous cardiac complications may include progressive hypertrophic cardiomyopathy, conduction defects and arrhythmia, atrial fibrillation, valvular disease and coronary artery stenosis. Regarding cerebrovascular complications, ischemic stroke and transient attacks occur relatively commonly. Brain MRI often reveals asymptomatic lesions in the white matter [3].

It has only more recently been appreciated that a significant portion of female FD heterozygotes develop complications, although usually in an attenuated form compared to male FD hemizygotes [17]. Due to X chromosome inactivation (Lyonization), wherein there is (random) transcriptional silencing of one of the X chromosomes in each cell, FD females are mosaic for the expression of α-GalA. Skewed X-inactivation favoring the mutant α-galactosidase A allele in female FD heterozygotes is associated with more severe disease manifestation [18]. In FD females, chronic renal insufficiency is rare. The manifestation of symptoms in FD females is remarkable given the known mosaic of α-GalA-containing and α-GalA-deficient cells in their tissues and the considerable levels of active α-GalA in the circulation [3]. Of note, heterozygous carriers of another X-linked lysosomal storage disorder (LSD) caused by iduronate 2-sulphatase deficiency, Hunter disease (HD), lack symptoms [19]. Apparently, in the case of HD, but not FD, sufficient complementation occurs in deficient cells of female heterozygotes owing to the uptake of secreted enzymes by normal cells [20]. Importantly, atypical variants of FD have been recognized. In these individuals, the disease is restricted to a single organ, particularly the heart and kidneys [21]. FD is now considered to be the most common LSD [16,22]. An accurate estimation of the prevalence is complicated by the great phenotypic heterogeneity. The estimated birth prevalence of classic FD is 0.42 per 100,000 male births in the Netherlands. The actual total prevalence of FD is higher because of under diagnosis of female patients and atypical disease manifestations. Newborn screening studies based on identification of abnormalities in the *GLA* gene or deficiency in α-GalA activity suggest a birth prevalence of at least 1 in 4000 in European populations [23], and higher frequencies have even been noted in Taiwan [24].

3. Storage Cells and Secondary Storage Lipids

The clinical symptoms and signs of FD differ fundamentally from other sphingolipidoses such as Gaucher disease (GD), in which lipid-laden macrophages are prominent and thought to contribute to characteristic symptoms such as hepatosplenomegaly and pancytopenia [25]. In sharp contrast, multiple cell types accumulate lipids in classic FD patients [26]. In the kidney, for example, lipid deposits are detected by electron microscopy in podocytes, endothelial glomerular cells and distal tubular cells [27]. Another peculiarity of FD is the relative mild outcome of complete α-GalA deficiency encountered in most classic FD males. There are no infantile and severe juvenile FD phenotypes as observed for other sphingolipidoses. Moreover, in FD, there is a remarkable discrepancy between the onset of lipid storage and that of symptoms. Gb3 storage in classic FD males already occurs in utero in endothelial cells and macrophages [28]. However, clinical symptoms develop only late in life. The same discrepancy is noted in α-GalA-deficient FD mice and rats [29,30]. Lipid-laden macrophages have been observed in the liver of classic FD males. Consistent with this, chitotriosidase, an established plasma biomarker of sphingolipid-accumulating macrophages in GD patients, is also elevated in the plasma of classic FD males [31,32]. This is not the case in FD females, suggesting that their macrophages are complemented by enzymes released from surrounding cells in contrast to other cell types [33].

A hallmark of FD is the marked elevation of water-soluble deacylated Gb3, also known as globotriaosyl-sphingosine (lysoGb3) [34]. The sphingoid base lysoGb3 is formed by the enzyme acid ceramidase from accumulating Gb3 in lysosomes [35]. LysoGb3 can leave cells and reach the circulation, resulting in over a hundred-fold elevated plasma levels in classic FD males. LysoGb3 is even clearly raised in the plasma of many female FD heterozygotes. Increases in lysoGb3 were also observed in the urine of FD patients. A similar lysoGb3 abnormality was detected in FD mice [36]. Several investigators have meanwhile confirmed the value of elevated plasma lysoGb3 as a biomarker of classic FD, including demonstration of abnormal lysoGb3 in urine [37–40]. Prominent sources of plasma lysoGb3 are likely the endothelium and liver, and the increased plasma lipid appears not to reflect one particular symptom [25,41].

4. Pathophysiology

It is well established that accumulation of Gb3 during α-GalA deficiency takes place in lysosomes, but the subsequent mechanisms causing cellular dysfunction, and ultimately symptoms, are still poorly understood [25,42]. As with other inherited glycosphingolipidoses, lipid-laden lysosomes can be envisioned to cause impaired autophagic flux, including mitophagy, contributing to the observed mitochondrial dysfunction in fibroblasts of FD patients [43–45]. Likewise, dysfunction of the endoplasmic reticulum may occur as suggested by the observed induction of the unfolded protein response in cells of some FD patients [46]. Fibrosis, inflammation and oxidative stress seem to play key roles in pathogenesis [47–50]. It has been hypothesized that lysoGb3 may also act as a pathogenic factor in FD [25,51]. A significant correlation of lysoGb3 lifetime exposure with overall disease severity was noted for classic male and female FD patients [41]. Indeed, lysoGb3 promotes smooth muscle cell proliferation, which fits with the increased intima media thickness and arterial stiffness in FD [29]. Furthermore, evidence has been provided that lysoGb3 at concentrations occurring in FD males damages nociceptive neurons, consistent with the reported pain in the extremities of classic FD males [52]. Lifetime exposure to lysoGb3 was found to correlate very significantly with the cold detection threshold and thermal sensory limen of the upper limb [53]. Next, lysoGb3 is thought to contribute to podocyte loss and glomerulus fibrosis, important aspects of the renal disease in FD patients [54,55]. Finally, lysoGb3, at concentrations as in FD patients, is found to inhibit endothelial nitric oxide synthase (eNOS) and thus may contribute to the vasculopathy in FD [56,57].

There appear to be other cellular consequences of α-GalA deficiency beyond the lysosome. The autophagy–lysosome pathway (ALP) is an important recycling pathway that mediates cell survival [58]. Disruption of the ALP is a common hallmark of lysosomal storage disorders, including Fabry disorders [59–61]. Likewise, in sphingolipid disorders such as Gaucher disease and Fabry disease, disturbed mitochondrial function and energy balance have been noted (for an excellent review on this topic, see Ivanova et al. 2020) [45]. Moreover, infiltration of lymphocytes and macrophages in tissues of FD, including the heart, has been observed, suggesting a role for inflammation in tissue damage. Possibly, chronic inflammation in FD, and associated oxidative stress, promotes organ damage (for a review, see Rozenfeld et al. [48]).

5. Diagnosis

Monitoring of disease manifestations and therapeutic efficacy of FD treatment is essential for the clinical management of FD patients. Disease onset and progression can be determined by clinical, radiological and laboratory analysis. However, the efficacy of a clinical treatment is sometimes challenging to assess due to high variability among patients. In addition, some pathological consequences of FD such as advanced renal failure are irreversible. Nevertheless, biomarkers play a very important role in disease and treatment monitorization [62].

The diagnosis of classic FD males is straightforward: identification of *GLA* gene mutations encoding an absent or evidently dysfunctional α-GalA protein. Extremely low α-GalA activity in leukocytes, fibroblasts and dried blood spots can be conveniently demonstrated using artificial water-soluble substrates, such as 4-methylumbelliferyl-α-galactoside [25]. Detection of elevated concentrations of plasma and urinary Gb3 and lysoGb3 can be used to further confirm diagnosis [29,37,62]. Sensitive LC-MS methods for this have been developed [63–66]. Enzyme activity assays are not always informative for FD females, particularly those with unfavorably skewed X-inactivation. Detection of elevated lysoGb3 is very helpful then to confirm FD diagnosis in females. Problematic is the diagnosis of atypical FD patients presenting with an uncharacteristic symptom (e.g., albuminuria, left ventricular hypertrophy or white matter lesions) in combination with an abnormality in the *GLA* gene with unknown consequences. This is often accompanied by a relatively high residual enzyme activity in cells and no clear abnormality in plasma or urinary Gb3 and lysoGb3 concentrations. Analysis of biopsies and demonstration of deposits of Gb3 are considered, in problematic cases, as helpful to support diagnosis [67,68]. Biochemical monitoring of disease in FD patients increasingly relies on the measurement of plasma lysoGb3; however, it should be kept in mind that the lipid levels do not reflect a particular symptom [69].

6. α-GalA: Reaction Mechanism and Activity-Based Probes (ABPs)

Glycosidases are hydrolytic enzymes that ensure the cleavage of glycosidic linkages in (oligo) saccharides and glycoconjugates, and they have been essential for the breakdown of various glyco(sphingo)lipids such as globotriaosylceramide (Gb3), which together with lysoGb3 is the predominant glycosphingolipid that accumulates in FD patients. α-GalA, an exo-retaining galactosidase member of the GH27 family (cazypedia.org), is responsible for the breakdown of Gb3 into lactosylceramide (LacCer) and galactose [70]. α-GalA cleaves the terminal α-linked galactose units from polysaccharides, glycolipids and glycoproteins [5]. α-GalA and its related lysosomal counterpart α-N-acetylgalactosaminidase (NAGA), also known as α-galactosidase B (α-GalB), which cleaves terminal α-linked N-acetylgalactosamine (α-GalNAc) moieties, are the only human retaining α-galactosidases known [71]. Their active sites only differ in two amino acid residues, which accommodate the C-2 substituent of the enzymatic substrate [12,71]. α-GalB can accommodate larger C-2 substituents (Figure 1A) in contrast to α-GalA (Figure 1B) which only allows a secondary hydroxyl at the C-2 position. Interestingly, by changing these two active site residues in either enzyme, the substrate specificity can be interchanged [71]. In addition to the C-2 position, the substituent and conformation at the C-6 position also play an important role in determining the reactivity of carbohydrates and the selectivity of chemical glycosylation reactions by influencing the stability of the oxocarbenium ion [72]. Most side chains of unbound "free" sugar molecules populate either a *gauche,gauche* (*gg*), *gauche,trans* (*gt*) or *trans,gauche* (*tg*) conformation, in which these abbreviations refer to the stereochemical relation between the O6-C6, O5-C5 and C4-C5 bonds. This results in the *gg* conformation being the most favorable for the formation of oxocarbenium ions [72]. However, this is highly influenced by the stereochemistry of the substituent at the C4 position which is reflected by the fact that the C6 side chains of galactose-configured molecules tend to adopt the *gt* conformation since the *gg* conformation results in an energy penalty due to both C6 and C4 substituents having an axial orientation. Interestingly, these stereochemical preferences are also reflected in the way glycosidases bind their substrates. In the case of α-galactosidases, they have a preference for binding their substrates in the *gt* conformation, thereby avoiding additional energy penalties but still maintaining the highly stabilizing effect on the oxocarbenium ion transition state that the substrate adopts during hydrolysis [72].

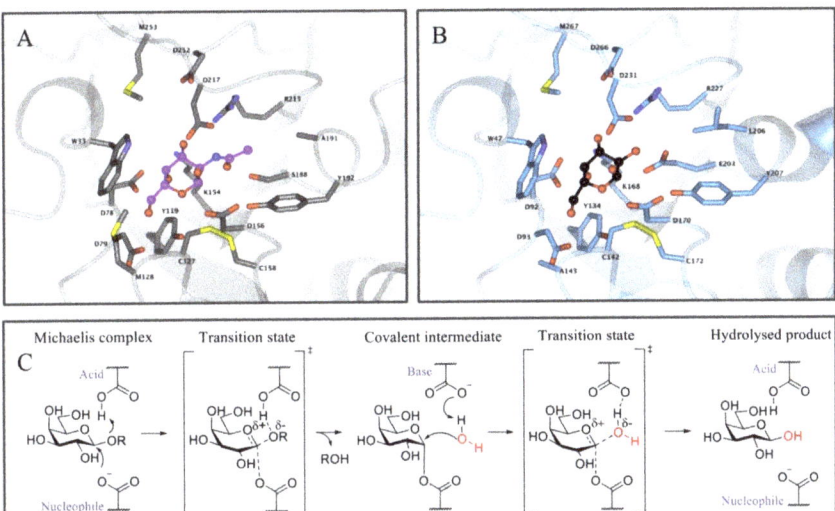

Figure 1. Enzyme structure and reaction mechanism of α-N-acetylgalactosaminidase (α-GalB) and α-galactosidase A (α-GalA). (**A**) Active site of α-GalB (gray) with GalNAc (blue) bound in the pocket. (**B**) Active site of α-GalA (blue) with galactose (black). Larger C-2 substituents cannot be accommodated in α-GalA due to the presence of residues L206 and E203. Structures were obtained from the Protein Data Bank (PDB) IDs 3H55, 3H54 or 3GXP and visualized using CCP4MG. (**C**) Koshland double displacement mechanism of retaining α-GalA.

Apart from the structural similarities between α-GalA and α-GalB, both enzymes retain galactosidases, which means that cleavage of the glycosidic linkage in the enzymatic substrate results in retention of the stereochemistry at the anomeric position of the terminal galactose moiety [73]. This retention of stereochemistry at the anomeric position is driven by a Koshland double displacement mechanism (Figure 1C) [74,75]. In the first step of this mechanism, the nucleophilic residue attacks at the anomeric center of the substrate, while the acid/base residue protonates the leaving group (LacCer in the case of α-GalA). This first step results in the formation of a covalent intermediate via an oxocarbenium ion-like transition state [75]. For the second step, the acid/base amino acid deprotonates a water molecule which concomitantly performs a nucleophilic attack at the anomeric center of the covalently bound substrate. This second step also follows a second oxocarbenium ion-like transition state which results in hydrolysis of the substrate with net retention of the stereochemistry at the anomeric position. X-ray crystal structures revealed that the roles of the nucleophile and the catalytic acid/base in α-GalA were performed by aspartic acid residues D170 and D231, respectively [12]. In addition, the crystal structure showed that α-GalA is a homodimeric glycoprotein and each of the monomers contains two domains, one active site domain and one C-terminal domain containing eight antiparallel β-strands and two sheets. Furthermore, it was found that each monomer contains three N-glycosylation sites that are important for the transport of the enzyme towards the lysosome mediated by the mannose-6-phosphate receptor [12].

Due to their medical implications, multiple inhibitors have been developed over the years that affect both α-galactosidases and more specifically α-GalA. These inhibitors can generally be divided into reversible or irreversible inhibitors. Irreversible inhibitors bind covalently to the enzyme, thereby capitalizing on the Koshland double displacement mechanism. Thus, these inhibitors often utilize an electrophilic trap to capture the nucleophilic residue in the enzyme active site. Some of the oldest irreversible glycosidase inhibitors, which were also designed for α-galactosidases, are fluorinated sugars such as **1** [76] (Figure 2). The fluorine atom causes an inductive effect, which makes it more difficult for the substrate to enter the positively charged oxocarbenium ion transition state and impairs its hydrolysis. Unfortunately, these fluorinated sugars showed modest to no inhibition of α-galactosidases from green coffee bean and *Aspergillus niger*. Epoxides are commonly used electrophilic traps and they were first used as α-galactosidase inhibitors in the form of conduritol C **2** [77]. This epoxide-based inhibitor was further developed into the synthetic form of the cyclophellitol epoxide **3** [78,79]. Unfortunately, epoxide **3** is not a selective α-GalA inhibitor since it also inhibits β-galactosidases GLB1 and GALC [79]. In addition to the epoxides, their nitrogen-based counterpart α-galactose-configured aziridine **4** [78] has shown to be a potent inhibitor of α-GalA (apparent IC_{50} = 40 nM) [79]. However, similar to epoxide **3**, the aziridine is not selective for α-GalA and displays a decent inhibition of GLB1 (apparent IC_{50} = 0.93 μM) and GALC (apparent IC_{50} = 1.1 μM). Both epoxide- and aziridine-based inhibitors make use of the $^4C_1 \rightarrow {^4H_3} \rightarrow {^1S_3}$ conformational itineraries of retaining α-galactosidases [75], mimicking the $^4H_3$ transition state which is also adopted by β-galactosidases [80]. Recently, α-Gal-cyclosulfate **5** has been synthesized as a potential α-GalA inhibitor which mimics the initial $^4C_1$ Michaelis complex [79]. Its chair conformation may render this inhibitor selective towards α-GalA (apparent IC_{50} = 25 μM) and binds covalently to the enzyme adopting a $^1S_3$ bound conformation [79].

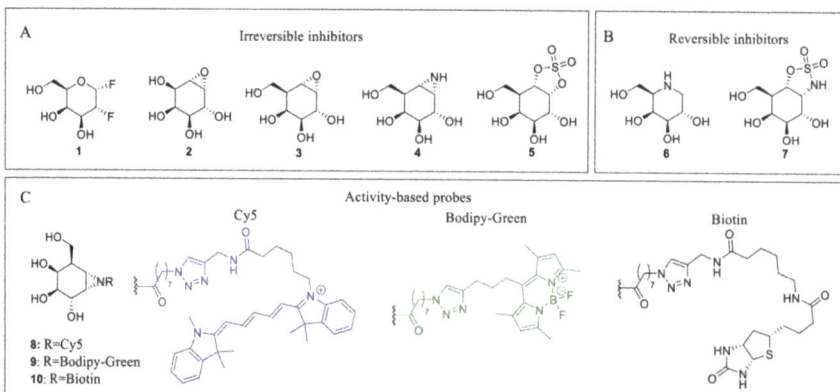

Figure 2. α-GalA inhibitors and activity-based probes (ABPs). (**A**) Irreversible inhibitors: 2-deoxy-2-fluoro-D-galactosyl fluoride **1**, conduritol C **2**, cyclophellitol epoxide **3**, cyclophellitol aziridine **4** and cyclosulfate **5**. (**B**) Reversible inhibitors: Gal-DNJ **6**; cyclosulfamidate **7**. (**C**) ABPs: Cy5 probe **8** (blue), Bodipy-green probe **9** (green) and biotinylated probe **10** (black).

Next to these covalent compounds, one of the first α-GalA inhibitors that is currently used in the clinic is the reversible inhibitor 1-deoxy-galactonojirimycin (DGJ, **6**) [81] which exploits non-covalent interactions. The endocyclic nitrogen of **6** can become protonated, forming an ion pair with a negatively charged amino acid residue in the α-GalA active site. Iminosugar **6** is a potent α-GalA inhibitor (IC$_{50}$ = 79 nM) but lacks selectivity since it also inhibits both GLB1 and β-glucosidase GBA [79]. As a potential alternative for **7**, selective cyclosulfamidate **7** was designed [79]. The cyclosulfamidate is a reversible inhibitor that results from the replacement of one of the endocyclic oxygens of the cyclosulfate **5** by a nitrogen atom. This replacement severely decreases its leaving group capacity, turning cyclosulfamidate **7** into a reversible inhibitor mimicking the Michaelis complex conformation. Although cyclosulfamidate **7** is a more selective inhibitor, it presents a lower inhibitory potency than iminosugar **6**.

Apart from their application as irreversible inhibitors, epoxide- and aziridine-based inhibitors have also been functionalized into activity-based probes (ABPs) for the labeling of various glycosidases in biochemical assays [80]. Modification of aziridine **4** with acyl-based fluorophores (**8** and **9**) and biotin (**10**) tags results in valuable biochemical tools to study α-GalA [82]. These ABPs have shown great selectivity towards α-GalA and α-GalB and can be used in competitive activity-based protein profiling (cABPP) assays to screen new inhibitors or to profile enzyme activity in cell extracts. In particular, ABPs **8** and **10** have been used to study the activity of α-GalA and α-GalB from plant extracts to study the potential enzyme production from *Nicotiana Benthamiana* (*N. Benthamiana*) [10]. In addition, these probes have also been used to identify a novel α-galactosidase from *N. Benthamiana* named α-galactosidase A1.1 [83]. This plant-derived enzyme presents significant structural similarities with α-GalA, an improved stability over a broad pH range and a similar ability to hydrolyze both Gb3 and LysoGb3, representing a potential therapeutic alternative for ERT-based FD management.

7. Present α-GalA-Centered Therapy Approaches

Until a few decades ago, there was no effective treatment available for inherited lysosomal storage diseases (LSDs). The management of most LSDs consisted only of supportive care. For some of the disorders, particularly mucopolysaccharidosis I-H (MPS I-H) and globoid cell leukodystrophy, bone marrow transplantation was performed [84,85]. A breakthrough regarding treatment of LSDs was accomplished by Roscoe Brady, who pioneered, with colleagues at the National Institutes of Health (NIH) in Bethesda, the development of an effective enzyme supplementation for non-neuronopathic type 1 Gaucher disease patients [86,87]. Currently, LSDs treatment capitalizes on four main therapeutic strategies (Figure 3). Intravenous supplementation of administered enzyme replacement therapy (ERT) increases the enzyme levels in the body, while oral pharmacological chaperones (PCT) have shown to promote the correct folding of amenable mutated glycosidases and retrieve residual activity levels. Substrate reduction therapy (SRT) aims to inhibit the biosynthesis of the accumulated metabolites. More recently, gene/RNA therapy allows the insertion of the gene encoding the deficient enzyme in patient cells. Unfortunately, FD patients can presently benefit only from ERT and, since 2016, PCT, both always combined with supportive adjunctive and preventive care.

Enzyme replacement therapy (ERT) is based on chronic two-weekly infusion of (now recombinant) glucocerebrosidase targeted to macrophages by the presence of terminal mannose residues in its N-linked glycans (Figure 3A). The success of the intervention prompted the development of similar ERT approaches for other LSDs, including FD. For this purpose, two different recombinant α-GalA preparations were independently developed in academic centers and subsequently pharmaceutical companies [88,89]. On 3 August 2001, both enzymes for ERT of FD were approved as the first orphan drugs in Europe: agalsidase alfa (Replagal®, Shire HGT [90]) and agalsidase beta (Fabrazyme®, Sanofi Genzyme [90]). The production of the two enzymes is fundamentally different: agalsidase alfa is produced by gene promotor activation in fibroblasts and agalsidase beta by conventional cDNA technology in CHO cells. This difference seemed highly relevant since mRNA editing had been reported for α-GalA. Theoretically, mRNA editing of agalsidase alfa, but not of agalsidase beta, would cause an amino acid difference at position 396 of both enzymes. Detailed analysis of the amino acid composition of both enzymes revealed that α-GalA mRNA is not edited [91]. Both recombinant enzymes, differing slightly in glycan composition, were found to be comparable when tested on in vitro specific activity and uptake by cultured fibroblasts [91,92]. Recent studies with different cultured cells revealed that uptake of recombinant α-GalA (clathrin- and caveolae-dependent endocytosis) might be cell type-specific [93]. Of note, in a human podocyte cell line, three endocytic receptors, IGF2R/M6P, megalin and sortilin, were reported to be involved in α-Gal A uptake [94]. Attention has been focused on improving the tissue distribution of therapeutic enzymes by the generation of α-GalA glycoforms. Elegant chemoenzymatic synthesis was employed by Fairbanks and colleagues to replace the glycans of recombinant α-GalA by synthetized mannose-6-phosphate-rich structures [95]. More recently, engineered CHO cell lines were used to generate specific α-GalA glycoforms [96]. Bolus injection in FD mice revealed the impact of glycan composition on the biodistribution of α-GalA. Unexpectedly, an α-2-3 sialylated (SA) glycoform of α-GalA was found to exhibit improved circulation and biodistribution [96]. It should, however, be kept in mind that translating the outcome of a bolus injection administered via the tail vein in mice to the biodistribution in FD patients is tricky.

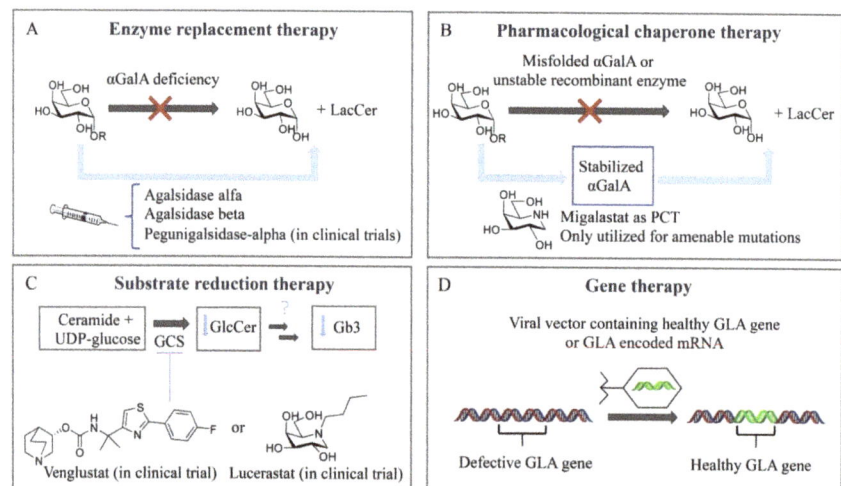

Figure 3. Therapeutic strategies for treatment of Fabry disease. (**A**) Enzyme replacement therapy (ERT). (**B**) Pharmacological chaperone therapy (PCT). (**C**) Substrate reduction therapy (SRT). (**D**) Gene therapy.

Both agalsidases alfa and beta are now approved in many countries throughout the world, but agalsidase alfa is still not approved by the US Food and Drug Administration (FDA). A recombinant α-GalA named Pegunigalsidase-alfa (PRX-102, prh-α-GalA from Protalix) that is produced in tobacco cells and has been chemically modified with polyethyleneglycol (PEG) is currently being investigated in clinical trials [97]. Such chemical modification offers protein stabilization, increased half-life and an improved biodistribution profile [98]. The registered ERTs (agalsidase beta at a standard dose of 1 mg/kg bw/2 wks and agalsidase alfa at a standard dose of 0.2 mg/kg bw/2 wks, similar in costs) were both found to result in clearance of storage material in heart and kidney biopsies. Based on this, ERT was hoped to protect kidney and cardiac function, but more recent data indicate that new clinical events (such as development of end-stage renal failure, myocardial infarction, ventricular fibrillation or cerebrovascular events) may occur in FD patients during ERT. Male sex, classical phenotype and increasing age at treatment initiation are risk factors for progression of disease while on ERT. Other risk factors are reduced renal function, proteinuria, cardiac hypertrophy and fibrosis, hypertension and occurrence of events before the start of ERT. An earlier start of ERT, especially in male patients with classic FD, is thought to improve the treatment outcome [68,99].

The impact of ERT on plasma lysoGb3 levels in FD patients has been, and still is, widely monitored [25]. Plasma lysoGb3 in classic FD patients was found to decrease rapidly after the start of ERT with several regimens in an enzyme dose-dependent manner [100]. After 3 months of treatment, plasma lysoGb3 levels tended to become stable but complete corrections were rare. On the other hand, a reduction in ERT was found to lead to increases in Gb3/lysoGb3 levels in most FD patients investigated [101]. Some classic FD males showed, after a few months of ERT at a similar enzyme dose, a relapse in plasma lysoGb3 levels, which prompted the analysis of a possible antibody response to the therapeutic enzyme. Indeed, the occurrence of antibodies is observed in about 70% of classic FD males receiving ERT [102,103]. Most classic FD males completely lack the α-GalA protein and an immunological response to the infused foreign therapeutic protein is not surprising. The antibodies formed in classic FD male patients receiving agalsidase alfa or beta comparably bind to both recombinant enzymes in vitro and neutralize enzyme activity in vitro [103]. The correction of plasma lysoGb3 during ERT is much less prominent in FD males with antibodies than those without [103]. Similarly, urinary Gb3 levels also hardly correct in FD males with antibodies [103]. The clinical consequences of neutralizing antibodies were unclear for many years. Bénichou et al. observed significantly impaired Gb3 clearance in skin biopsies of patients treated with ERT showing high antibody titers [104]. A five-year study with 68 male FD patients treated with ERT showed that 40% presented serum-mediated antibody inhibition of enzyme, which was associated with increased lyso-Gb3, higher risks for FD-associated symptoms and impaired cardiac and renal function [25]. The cause(s) for the limited response to ERT is (are) not known. Likely, the induction of (neutralizing) antibodies against a therapeutic protein in classic FD males contributes to this. Inadequate ERT biodistribution has also been highlighted, with few enzymes reaching podocytes and cardiac myocytes [28,29].

A seminal work by Ishii and colleagues revealed that specific mutant forms of α-GalA that misfold in the endoplasmic reticulum and are subsequently prematurely degraded can be partly rescued by galactose and more potently by 1-deoxygalactonojirimycin [105–107]. These findings prompted the development of 1-deoxygalactonojirimycin as a pharmacological chaperone named Migalastat (Galafold®, Amicus Therapeutics), which was approved in 2016 in Europe and Canada (USA approval was delayed to 2018) as an alternative therapeutic approach, representing the only oral treatment for FD (Figure 3B) [108]. This small iminosugar reversibly binds to the enzymatic active site in the endoplasmic reticulum (ER) and stabilizes, at low concentrations, particular mutant forms of α-GalA (known as amenable mutant forms), promoting the proper folding of the enzyme, maturation and its trafficking to lysosomes [106,109]. The more acidic lysosomal pH (compared with a neutral pH in the ER) and the high concentration of the Gb3 metabolite in the lysosome displace the reversible small chaperone from the active site and the active enzyme is then able to hydrolyze the accumulated substrates at the lysosomal interface. However, this therapeutic strategy is limited to a specific number of mutations. It is estimated that only 35–50% of FD patients present a migalastat-amenable mutation [110,111]. Interestingly, several recent studies on FD patients with amenable mutations suggest that switching from ERT with agalsidase alfa or beta to migalastat can be a valid, safe and well-tolerated strategy [111–113]. A more recent strategy involves the joint administration of a recombinant enzyme and a pharmacological chaperone [112–115], aiming to stabilize the recombinant enzyme in circulation with the final goal of increasing the concentration of the enzyme that may reach the affected tissues, and allowing the use of lower enzyme doses and prolonged intervals between IV administrations, which should ultimately decrease the side effects and treatment cost and, more importantly, improve the quality of life of FD patients [116]. In particular, migalastat presents a synergetic effect in cultured fibroblasts from FD patients and increases the tissue uptake of recombinant human α-GalA in FD mice [113,115]. A conceptually new class of enzyme stabilizers, cyclophellitol cyclosulfamidates, have recently been described to stabilize algasidase beta and increase α-GalA activity in FD fibroblasts, assisting the functional correction of lysoGb3 metabolite accumulation [79]. Positive allosteric modulators are also under investigation which could afford safer daily dose regimens by avoiding the use of active site binders with a potential inhibitory effect. In particular, in silico docking leads to the identification of 2,6-dithiopurine, an allosteric ligand that stabilizes lysosomal α-GalA in vitro and rescues a particular mutant form, A230T, which is a non-amenable mutation for PCT 1-deoxygalactonojirimycin [117].

Extensive research efforts have been made towards a better FD therapy over the past twenty years, and clinical trials have resulted in FDA- and/or EMA-approved ERT and PCT. Importantly, new research in the field moves towards SRT and gene/RNA therapy to fill the gap of this yet not curable disease. Substrate reduction therapy (SRT) relies on small molecules capable of inhibiting the biosynthesis of the metabolites that accumulate in the lysosome (Figure 3C). SRT using GlcCer synthase (GCS) inhibitors such as miglustat and eliglustat is already on the market for the treatment of Gaucher disease type I, and miglustat is approved for Niemann–Pick Type C, a rare progressive genetic disorder characterized by the deficient transport of cholesterol and lipids inside cells. Both drugs inhibit GCS, which blocks the first step in glycosphingolipid biosynthesis [118]. In particular, venglustat/ibiglustat [119] and lucerastat [120] are currently under evaluation as oral GCS inhibitors for FD (NCT02228460 and NCT02930655 are the respective clinical trials). Efforts and directions towards SRT for FD with specific inhibition of A4GALT, the responsible glycosyltransferase for the synthesis of Gb3, will be further discussed in this review.

Gene therapy is based on the insertion of a correcting gene, encoding the deficient enzyme, in patient cells (Figure 3D). The correcting gene is usually delivered through a vector such as adeno-associated virus (AAV), lentivirus, retrovirus or a non-viral-based system that can then alter the DNA or RNA transcript used for the synthesis of the enzyme of interest. By inserting the nonmutant *GLA* gene, gene therapy aims to correct the enzyme deficiency and reduce the accumulation of Gb3 and lysoGb3 and eventually prevent organ damage in FD patients. A first-in-human clinical study for the treatment with autologous stem cell transplantation using CD34+ cells transduced with the lentiviral vector containing the human *GLA* gene started in Canada in 2016 (NCT02800070). Avobrio is also currently running a phase II clinical trial (NCT03454893) to study the efficacy and safety of a gene therapy (AVR-RD-01) for the treatment of classic FD patients. Recently, two new gene therapies (ST-920 and FLT190) making use of an AAV vector encoding human α-GalA cDNA with specific liver expression cassettes have been described to increase plasma and tissue α-GalA activities in an FD mouse model and are in phase I/II clinical trials (NCT04046224 and NCT04040049) [121–123]. Messenger RNA (mRNA) is also emerging as a new class of therapy for the treatment of rare monogenic disorders. In particular, the efficacy of a messenger mRNA encoding the α-GalA enzyme has been reported in FD α-GalA knockout mice through an IV bolus administration of α-GalA mRNA encapsulated in lipid nanoparticles (0.05–0.5 mg/kg) [124]. Of note, gene therapeutic correction has to be accomplished in the CNS for most LSDs, but not necessarily in FD. Cerebrovascular dysfunction in FD patients resulting in neurological deficits stems largely from stenosis of small vessels and enlargement of large vessels may result in neurological deficits [125].

8. A4GALT: Reaction Mechanism and Enzymatic Products

α-1,4-Galactosyltransferase (A4GALT, Gb3 synthase) is the enzyme responsible for the synthesis of Gb3 from LacCer and UDP-galactose catalyzing the formation of an α-glycosidic 1,4 linkage between the anomeric center of the UDP-Gal donor and the LacCer acceptor. This retaining galactosyltransferase is a member of the GT32 family of glycosyltransferases (EC 2.4.1.228, www.cazy.org, accessed on 08-02-2021). In line with many glycosyltransferases, structural and mechanistic information regarding A4GALT is scarce and the exact mechanism is still a matter of debate, making the rational design of inhibitors a very a challenging process. While no crystal structure of A4GALT has been obtained hitherto, the bacterial homologue LgtC (~20% homology) from *Neisseria meningitidis* has shown the presence of a critical carboxylate residue (Asp190) in its active site, potentially situated on the beta face of UDP-Gal and in the vicinity of the lactosylceramide acceptor [126,127]. This carboxylate pointed to the hypothesis of a double displacement mechanism similar to the one employed by retaining glycosidases (Figures 4 and 5A). However, this amino acid is 8.9 Å away from the donor UDP-Gal and a conformational change would be necessary during catalysis to allow an appropriate positioning. The alternative hypothesis invokes an S_Ni-like mechanism (Figure 5B) in which both the incoming nucleophile and leaving UDP group find occupancy in the enzyme active site at the same time [128,129]. Structural studies also showed the presence of a Mn^{2+} cation within the active site of the enzyme. This metal ion interacts with an Asp-X-Asp (DXD) motif and with the diphosphate leaving group of the UDP-Gal donor. Coordination of Mn^{2+} to the diphosphate leaving group assists the departure of the leaving group (UDP) by stabilizing the negative charge [127]. Unveiling the A4GALT mechanism is of great interest for FD, for which clinical targeting is hampered by a complete lack of effective inhibitors.

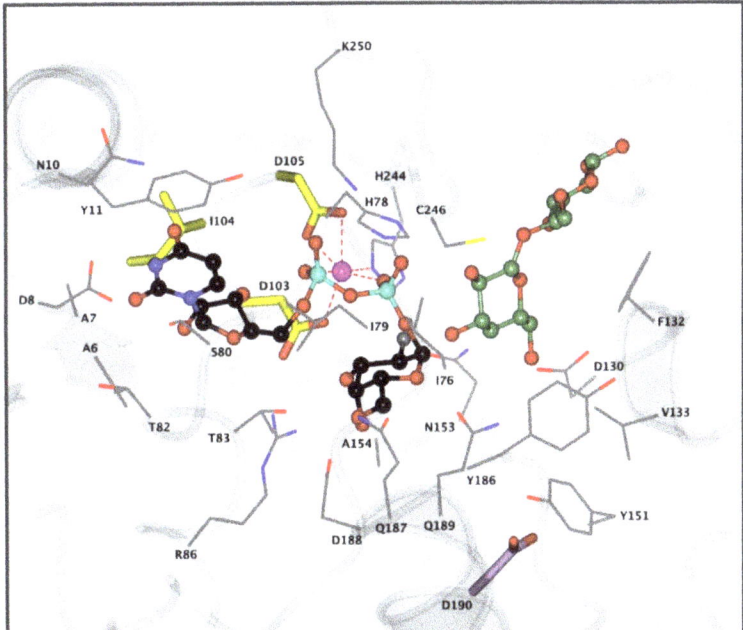

Figure 4. Active site of bacterial A4GALT homologue LgtC. Enzyme active site containing donor analogue UDP-2FGal (black) and acceptor analogue 4′-deoxylactose (green) bound in the pocket. The Mn^{2+} cation (pink) coordinates with the diphosphate group of UDP-Gal and the DXD motif (yellow) to assist in catalysis. Residue D190 (purple) is positioned 8.9 Å away from the UDP-Gal donor and is visualized for clarity. Structure was obtained from the Protein Data Bank (PDB) ID 1GA8 and visualized using CCP4MG.

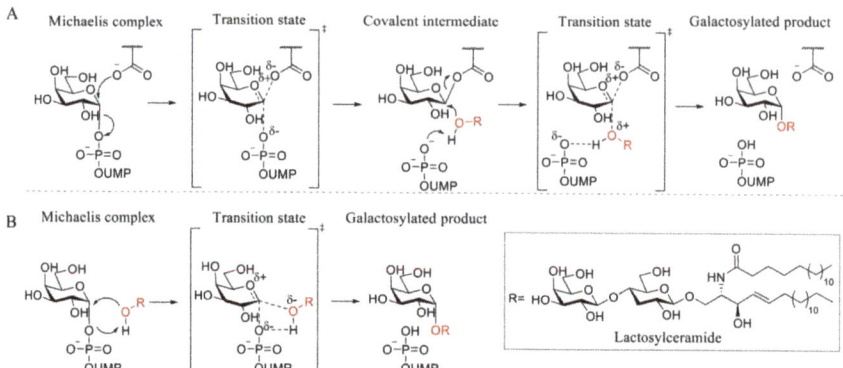

Figure 5. Proposed A4GALT mechanisms. (**A**) Koshland double displacement mechanism of retaining glycosyltransferases (GTs). (**B**) Front-face (S_Ni-like) mechanism of retaining GTs.

Current treatment of FD focused on restoring α-GalA activity through ERT or PCT has shown, as previously discussed, limited clinical efficacy. An attractive therapeutic alternative would be the use of SRT which, for instance, has predominantly been successful for the treatment of Gaucher disease [130]. FDA-approved miglustat and eliglustat inhibit GCS, thereby reducing glucosylceramide levels. Of note, the reduction in GlcCer levels would also indirectly reduce the amount of Gb3 formed by A4GALT. However, when compared to GBA activity in Gaucher patients, male patients suffering from FD have extremely low to non-existent activity of α-GalA [131], meaning that full inhibition of GCS would be required. Complete inactivation of GCS could bring serious health risks since glucosylceramide is a key intermediate for the synthesis of other glycosphingolipids (GSLs) essential for various cellular processes such as cell signaling, membrane stability and immunogenicity [132].

Selective inhibition of A4GALT would, in principle, not interfere with the synthesis of other related GSLs. A4GALT is responsible for the synthesis of Gb3, also known as CD77 or the P^k antigen, and the P1 antigen [133,134]. Both glycosphingolipids, P^k and P1, are blood group antigens belonging to the P1PK system. While P^k is a highly frequent antigen on red blood cells (over 99.9% of humans), P1 is present only in a small fraction of the population. The P1 antigen is formed through the coupling between neolactotetraosylceramide (paragloboside) and the UDP-gal donor [135]. P^k and P1 are both expressed on the surface of human red blood cells. Recently, it has been shown that the p.Q211E variant of A4GALT is also able to synthesize NOR antigens, which are rare glycosphingolipids with a terminal Gal(α1–4)GalNAc moiety present in erythrocytes of patients with NOR polyagglutination syndrome [135,136] (Figure 6A). Importantly, the existence of some individuals with a genetic deficiency in A4GALT without obvious clinical consequences suggests that selective inhibition of this enzyme could be well tolerated by FD patients [137,138].

Gb3 is the main receptor for Shiga toxins which are released by shigella species and Shiga-like toxins produced by certain strains of *Escherichia coli* (*E. coli*) called Shiga-like toxin-producing *E. coli* (STEC), also referred to as verocytotoxin (VT)-producing *E. coli* (VTEC) [139]. The bacteria usually enter the body via contaminated food or water and can cause serious health problems such as hemorrhagic colitis, which can eventually progress towards hemolytic–uremic syndrome (HUS) [140]. The most common toxins are Shiga toxin 1 (stx1) and Shiga toxin 2 (stx2) and both utilize Gb3 as their cell surface receptor with a similar intracellular mechanism of action [141]. Interestingly, similar to A4GALT knockout mice that are insensitive towards Shiga toxins, increased levels of Gb3 in FD mice also protect the mice against Shiga toxins. However, after administration of recombinant human α-GalA and restoring normal Gb3 levels, FD mice became susceptible to the bacterial toxin [142].

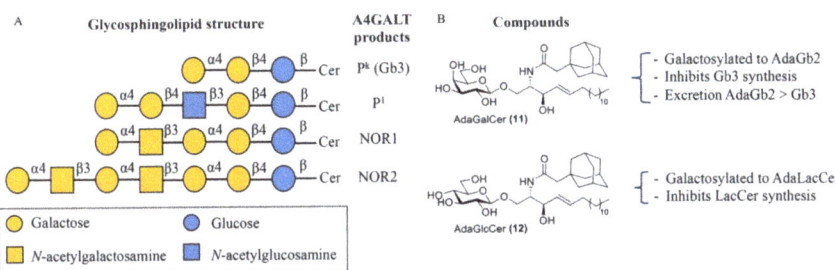

Figure 6. A4GALT glycosphingolipid (GSL) products and Gb3 modulators. (**A**) Structures of glycosphingolipids produced by A4GALT. (**B**) AdaGalCer **11** and AdaGlcCer **12** and their effect on GSL production.

Recently, genome-wide CRISPR-Cas9 knockout screens in Shiga toxins revealed that the lysosomal-associated protein transmembrane 4 alpha (LAPTM4A) is a key player in the biosynthesis of Gb3 [143,144], and LAPTM4A knockout cells showed to be resistant towards Shiga toxins by impairing the binding of the toxins to the cell surface due to the lack of Gb3 [143]. However, the absence of LAPTM4A did not affect A4GALT levels or its proper localization with A4GALT in the Golgi complex. Further analysis showed that the second luminal domain of LAPTM4A plays a key role in the interaction with A4GALT and the eventual synthesis of Gb3 [144]. Moreover, it was shown that replacing only the second luminal domain of LAPTM4A in the homologous LAPTM4B also restores Gb3 synthesis [144]. The fact that A4GALT activity in vitro, with an artificial lipid substrate (NBD-LacCer), is not dependent on the presence of LAPTM4A suggests that this protein could be involved in the presentation of the lipid substrate (LacCer) from membranes to the enzyme [144]. However, additional studies towards the structure and function of LAPTM4A are necessary to fully understand its exact role in Gb3 metabolism. Importantly, due to the relation between LAPTM4A and A4GALT and the resulting influence on cellular Gb3 levels, LAPTM4A or their protein–protein interaction could also be a potential therapeutic target for the treatment of FD.

9. A4GALT Inhibitors and Future Directions

Lowering Gb3 levels remains an important, though challenging, therapeutic strategy for FD. Despite the important role of GTs in various biochemical processes, these enzymes have been relatively unexplored compared to GHs and their respective inhibitors. In general, GT inhibitors are predominantly developed via a rational design approach based on donor or acceptor analogues or by high-throughput screening (HTS) [145]. The first and most logical therapeutic target for SRT in FD is A4GALT. However, no inhibitors have seen the light and only adamantyl-functionalized galactosylceramide (adaGalCer) has shown competition with the LacCer substrate and inhibits Gb3 synthesis in cells [146]. One main reason for the slower development of A4GALT inhibitors may be the lack of structural and mechanistic information concerning the enzyme.

Adamantyl galactosylceramide (adaGalCer) and glucosylceramide (adaGlcCer) are A4GALT acceptor analogues with a modified ceramide fatty acid tail functionalized with an adamantane (Figure 6B). These compounds alter GSL metabolism. In particular, adaGalCer acts as a substrate for A4GALT and is able to lower Gb3 levels at an IC_{50} concentration of 40 μM in FD cells [146]. Of note, enzymatic galactosylation of the inhibitor results in the formation of the adaGb2 product with unknown physiological consequences. However, this artificial more apolar metabolite was 10-fold more effectively excreted to the medium than Gb3 in cells, suggesting a better elimination and a potential solution to Gb3 accumulation. On the other hand, adaGlcCer is converted to adaLacCer and inhibits LacCer synthesis.

A second rational strategy for development of A4GALT inhibitors could be the synthesis of UDP-Gal mimics. Following the success of GH inhibitors, fluorinated donors with a fluorine at their C2 or C5 position functionalized with a UDP group at the anomeric position have been developed as slow inhibitors of retaining glycosyltransferases [147–149]. UDP-carba-Gal analogues, in which the pyranose oxygen atom is replaced by a carbon atom, have also been developed as GT inhibitors and, in general, are very stable competitive inhibitors [150]. In addition, iminosugar donors have been described as GT inhibitors and show electronic and structural similarity by mimicking the positive charge in the oxocarbenium ion transition state [151]. C-glycosides, in which the exocyclic oxygen is replaced by a carbon, also function as donor mimics without being prone to hydrolysis by GHs [152], and a C1-C2 alkene-based analogue conformationally mimicking the oxocarbenium ion transition state resulted in a low-affinity β-galactosyltransferase inhibitor [153]. Different modifications at the nucleotide base have been exploited as well [154]. For instance, attachment of a 5-formylthien-2-yl group to the 5′ position of the base resulted in a nanomolar inhibitor of several different GalTs by blocking the movement of a key mobile loop in the enzyme structure [155]. Of note, the selectivity of UDP-based inhibitors is questionable since a particular UDP-sugar donor functions as a substrate for multiple GTs.

Importantly, the identification of new A4GALT inhibitors could provide important structural and mechanistic insights. Proteomics combined with crystallographic studies using mechanism-based inhibitors could shed some light on the presence or absence of a covalent enzyme inhibitor intermediate and determine if the enzyme actually catalyzes the glycosylation via a double displacement mechanism or a S_Ni-like concerted front-face mechanism. For these inhibitors to become a reality, future research towards effective A4GALT biochemical assays and new HTS methodologies to potentiate the discovery of new binders, together with A4GALT crystallographic studies, appears essential.

10. Concluding Remarks

The detailed knowledge on the molecular basis of FD has not yet resulted in a very effective treatment. Ongoing research on modified enzymes without immunological responses and the design of new treatment modalities, such as gene therapy, enzyme stabilizers or SRT targeting A4GALT in a selective and controlled manner, hold promise to reach major improvements in this direction.

Funding: This research received no external funding.

Institutional Review Board Statement: Not applicable.

Informed Consent Statement: Not applicable.

Data Availability Statement: Not applicable.

Conflicts of Interest: The authors declare no conflict of interest.

References

1. Anderson, W. A Case of Angeo-Keratoma. *Br. J. Dermatol.* **1898**, *10*, 113–117. [CrossRef]
2. Fabry, J. Ein Beitrag zur Kenntniss der Purpura haemorrhagica nodularis (Purpura papulosa haemorrhagica Hebrae). *Arch. Dermatol. Res.* **1898**, *43*, 187–200. [CrossRef]
3. Desnick, R.J.; Ioannou, Y.A. α-Galactosidase a Deficiency. Fabry Disease. The Metabolic and Molecular Bases of Inherited Disease, 8th ed.; Scriver, C.R., Beaudet, A.L., Sly, W.S., Valle, D., Eds.; McGraw-Hill: New York, NY, USA, 2001.
4. Sweeley, C.C.; Klionsky, B. Fabry's Disease: Classification as a sphingolipidosis and partial char-acterization of a novel glycolipid. *J. Biol. Chem.* **1963**, *238*, 3148–3150. [CrossRef]
5. Brady, R.O.; Gal, A.E.; Bradley, R.M.; Martensson, E.; Warshaw, A.L.; Laster, L. Enzymatic Defect in Fabry's Disease. *N. Engl. J. Med.* **1967**, *276*, 1163–1167. [CrossRef]
6. Kint, J.A. Fabry's Disease: Alpha-Galactosidase Deficiency. *Science* **1970**, *167*, 1268–1269. [CrossRef]
7. Hamers, M.N.; Westerveld, A.; Khan, M.; Tager, J.M. Characterization of α-galactosidase isoen-zymes in normal and fabry human-Chinese hamster somatic cell hybrids. *Hum. Genet.* **1977**, *36*, 289–297. [CrossRef] [PubMed]
8. De Groot, P.G.; Westerveld, A.; Khan, P.M.; Tager, J.M. Localization of a gene for human α-galactosidase B (=N-Acetyl-α-D-Galactosaminidase) on chromosome 22. *Qual. Life Res.* **1978**, *44*, 305–312. [CrossRef]

9. Sakuraba, H.; Matsuzawa, F.; Aikawa, S.-I.; Doi, H.; Kotani, M.; Nakada, H.; Fukushige, T.; Kanzaki, T. Structural and immunocytochemical studies on α-N-acetylgalactosaminidase deficiency (Schindler/Kanzaki disease). *J. Hum. Genet.* **2003**, *49*, 1–8. [CrossRef]
10. Kytidou, K.; Beenakker, T.J.M.; Westerhof, L.B.; Hokke, C.H.; Moolenaar, G.F.; Goosen, N.; Mirzaian, M.; Ferraz, M.J.; de Geus, M.A.R.; Kallemeijn, W.W.; et al. Human Alpha Galactosidases Transiently Produced in Nicotiana benthamiana Leaves: New Insights in Substrate Specificities with Relevance for Fabry Disease. *Front. Plant. Sci.* **2017**, *8*, 1026. [CrossRef]
11. Dean, K.J.; Sweeley, C.C. Studies on human liver α-galactosidases. II. Purification and enzymatic properties of α-galactosidase B (α-N-acetylgalactosaminidase). *J. Biol. Chem.* **1979**, *254*, 10001–10005. [CrossRef]
12. Garman, S.C.; Garboczi, D.N. The Molecular Defect Leading to Fabry Disease: Structure of Human α-Galactosidase. *J. Mol. Biol.* **2004**, *337*, 319–335. [CrossRef]
13. Sakuraba, H. Fabry disease in a Japanese population-molecular and biochemical characteris-tics. *Mol. Genet. Metab. Rep.* **2018**, *17*, 73–79. [CrossRef]
14. Smid, B.E.; Hollak, C.E.M.; Poorthuis, B.J.H.M.; Weerman, M.A.V.D.B.; Florquin, S.; Kok, W.E.M.; Deprez, R.H.L.; Timmermans, J.; Linthorst, G.E. Diagnostic dilemmas in Fabry disease: A case series study on GLA mutations of unknown clinical significance. *Clin. Genet.* **2015**, *88*, 161–166. [CrossRef] [PubMed]
15. Schiffmann, R.; Fuller, M.; Clarke, L.A.; Aerts, J.M.F.G. Is it Fabry disease? *Genet. Med.* **2016**, *18*, 1181–1185. [CrossRef]
16. Germain, D.P. Fabry disease. *Orphanet J. Rare Dis.* **2010**, *5*, 30. [CrossRef] [PubMed]
17. MacDermot, K.D.; Holmes, A.; Miners, A.H. Natural history of Fabry disease in affected males and obligate carrier females. *J. Inherit. Metab. Dis.* **2001**, *24*, 13–14. [CrossRef] [PubMed]
18. Elstein, D.; Schachamorov, E.; Beeri, R.; Altarescu, G. X-inactivation in Fabry disease. *Gene* **2012**, *505*, 266–268. [CrossRef] [PubMed]
19. D'Avanzo, F.; Rigon, L.; Zanetti, A.; Tomanin, R. Mucopolysaccharidosis Type II: One Hundred Years of Research, Diagnosis, and Treatment. *Int. J. Mol. Sci.* **2020**, *21*, 1258. [CrossRef]
20. Hickman, S.; Neufeld, E.F. A hypothesis for I-cell disease: Defective hydrolases that do not enter lysosomes. *Biochem. Biophys. Res. Commun.* **1972**, *49*, 992–999. [CrossRef]
21. Schiffmann, R. Fabry disease. *Pharmacol. Ther.* **2009**, *122*, 65–77. [CrossRef]
22. Van der Tol, L.; Smid, B.E.; Poorthuis, B.J.H.M.; Biegstraaten, M.; Deprez, R.H.L.; Linthorst, G.E.; Hollak, C.E.M. A systematic review on screening for Fabry disease: Prevalence of individuals with genetic variants of unknown significance. *J. Med. Genet.* **2013**, *51*, 1–9. [CrossRef]
23. Spada, M.; Pagliardini, S.; Yasuda, M.; Tukel, T.; Thiagarajan, G.; Sakuraba, H.; Ponzone, A.; Desnick, R.J. High Incidence of Later-Onset Fabry Disease Revealed by Newborn Screening. *Am. J. Hum. Genet.* **2006**, *79*, 31–40. [CrossRef] [PubMed]
24. Lin, H.-Y. High incidence of the cardiac variant of Fabry disease revealed by newborn screen-ing in the Taiwan Chinese population. *Circ. Cardiovasc. Genet.* **2009**, *2*, 450–456. [CrossRef]
25. Ferraz, M.J.; Kallemeijn, W.W.; Mirzaian, M.; Moro, D.H.; Marques, A.R.A.; Wisse, P.; Boot, R.G.; Willems, L.I.; Overkleeft, H.; Aerts, J. Gaucher disease and Fabry disease: New markers and insights in pathophysiology for two distinct glycosphingolipidoses. *Biochim. Biophys. Acta Mol. Cell Biol. Lipids* **2014**, *1841*, 811–825. [CrossRef] [PubMed]
26. Yogasundaram, H.; Kim, D.; Oudit, O.; Thompson, R.B.; Weidemann, F.; Oudit, G.Y. Clinical Features, Diagnosis, and Management of Patients With Anderson-Fabry Cardiomyopathy. *Can. J. Cardiol.* **2017**, *33*, 883–897. [CrossRef]
27. Thurberg, B.L. Globotriaosylceramide accumulation in the Fabry kidney is cleared from mul-tiple cell types after enzyme replacement therapy. *Kidney Int.* **2002**, *62*, 1933–1946. [CrossRef] [PubMed]
28. Vedder, A.C.; Strijland, A.; Weerman, M.A.V.B.; Florquin, S.; Aerts, J.M.F.G.; Hollak, C.E.M. Manifestations of Fabry disease in placental tissue. *J. Inherit. Metab. Dis.* **2006**, *29*, 106–111. [CrossRef]
29. Ohshima, T.; Murray, G.J.; Swaim, W.D.; Longenecker, G.; Quirk, J.M.; Cardarelli, C.O.; Sugimoto, Y.; Pastan, I.; Gottesman, M.M.; Brady, R.O.; et al. α-Galactosidase A deficient mice: A model of Fabry disease. *Proc. Natl. Acad. Sci. USA* **1997**, *94*, 2540–2544. [CrossRef]
30. Miller, J.J. α-Galactosidase A-deficient rats accumulate glycosphingolipids and develop car-diorenal phenotypes of Fabry disease. *FASEB J. Off. Publ. Fed. Am. Soc. Exp. Biol.* **2019**, *33*, 418–429.
31. Bussink, A.P.; van Eijk, M.; Renkema, G.H.; Aerts, J.M.; Boot, R.G. The Biology of the Gaucher Cell: The Cradle of Human Chitinases. *Virus Entry* **2006**, *252*, 71–128. [CrossRef]
32. Vedder, A.; Cox-Brinkman, J.; Hollak, C.; Linthorst, G.; Groener, J.; Helmond, M.; Scheij, S.; Aerts, J.M. Plasma chitotriosidase in male Fabry patients: A marker for monitoring lipid-laden macrophages and their correction by enzyme replacement therapy. *Mol. Genet. Metab.* **2006**, *89*, 239–244. [CrossRef] [PubMed]
33. Fuller, M.; Mellett, N.; Hein, L.K.; Brooks, D.A.; Meikle, P.J. Absence of α-galactosidase cross-correction in Fabry heterozygote cultured skin fibroblasts. *Mol. Genet. Metab.* **2015**, *114*, 268–273. [CrossRef]
34. Aerts, J.M.; Groener, J.E.; Kuiper, S.; Donker-Koopman, W.E.; Strijland, A.; Ottenhoff, R.; van Roomen, C.; Mirzaian, M.; Wijburg, F.A.; Linthorst, G.E.; et al. Elevated globotriaosylsphingosine is a hallmark of Fabry disease. *Proc. Natl. Acad. Sci. USA* **2008**, *105*, 2812–2817. [CrossRef]

35. Ferraz, M.J.; Marques, A.R.; Appelman, M.D.; Verhoek, M.; Strijland, A.; Mirzaian, M.; Aerts, J.M. Lysosomal glycosphingolipid catabolism by acid ceramidase: Formation of gly-cosphingoid bases during deficiency of glycosidases. *FEBS Lett.* **2016**, *590*, 716–725. [CrossRef]
36. Ferraz, M.J.; Marques, A.R.A.; Gaspar, P.; Mirzaian, M.; van Roomen, C.; Ottenhoff, R.; Alfonso, P.; Irún, P.; Giraldo, P.; Wisse, P.; et al. Lyso-glycosphingolipid abnormalities in different murine models of lysosomal storage disorders. *Mol. Genet. Metab.* **2016**, *117*, 186–193. [CrossRef]
37. Togawa, T.; Kodama, T.; Suzuki, T.; Sugawara, K.; Tsukimura, T.; Ohashi, T.; Ishige, N.; Suzuki, K.; Kitagawa, T.; Sakuraba, H. Plasma globotriaosylsphingosine as a biomarker of Fabry disease. *Mol. Genet. Metab.* **2010**, *100*, 257–261. [CrossRef]
38. Krüger, R.; Tholey, A.; Jakoby, T.; Vogelsberger, R.; Mönnikes, R.; Rossmann, H.; Beck, M.; Lackner, K.J. Quantification of the Fabry marker lysoGb3 in human plasma by tandem mass spectrometry. *J. Chromatogr. B* **2012**, *883–884*, 128–135. [CrossRef] [PubMed]
39. Boutin, M.; Auray-Blais, C. Multiplex tandem mass spectrometry analysis of novel plasma lyso-Gb3-related analogues in Fabry disease. *Anal. Chem.* **2014**, *86*, 3476–3483. [CrossRef]
40. Talbot, A.; Nicholls, K.; Fletcher, J.M.; Fuller, M. A simple method for quantification of plasma globotriaosylsphingosine: Utility for Fabry disease. *Mol. Genet. Metab.* **2017**, *122*, 121–125. [CrossRef]
41. Rombach, S.; Dekker, N.; Bouwman, M.; Linthorst, G.; Zwinderman, A.; Wijburg, F.; Kuiper, S.; Weerman, M.V.B.; Groener, J.; Poorthuis, B.; et al. Plasma globotriaosylsphingosine: Diagnostic value and relation to clinical manifestations of Fabry disease. *Biochim. Biophys. Acta Mol. Basis Dis.* **2010**, *1802*, 741–748. [CrossRef] [PubMed]
42. Miller, J.J.; Kanack, A.J.; Dahms, N.M. Progress in the understanding and treatment of Fabry disease. *Biochim. Biophys. Acta Gen. Subj.* **2020**, *1864*, 129437. [CrossRef]
43. Lücke, T.; Höppner, W.; Schmidt, E.; Illsinger, S.; Das, A.M. Fabry disease: Reduced activities of respiratory chain enzymes with decreased levels of energy-rich phosphates in fibroblasts. *Mol. Genet. Metab.* **2004**, *82*, 93–97. [CrossRef]
44. Stepien, K.M.; Roncaroli, F.; Turton, N.; Hendriksz, C.J.; Roberts, M.; Heaton, R.A.; Hargreaves, I.P. Mechanisms of Mitochondrial Dysfunction in Lysosomal Storage Disorders: A Review. *J. Clin. Med.* **2020**, *9*, 2596. [CrossRef] [PubMed]
45. Ivanova, M. Altered Sphingolipids Metabolism Damaged Mitochondrial Functions: Lessons Learned From Gaucher and Fabry Diseases. *J. Clin. Med.* **2020**, *9*, 1116. [CrossRef]
46. Ishii, S.; Chang, H.-H.; Kawasaki, K.; Yasuda, K.; Wu, H.-L.; Garman, S.C.; Fan, J.-Q. Mutant α-galactosidase A enzymes identified in Fabry disease patients with residual enzyme activity: Biochemical characterization and restoration of normal intracellular processing by 1-deoxygalactonojirimycin. *Biochem. J.* **2007**, *406*, 285–295. [CrossRef]
47. Rozenfeld, P.; Feriozzi, S. Contribution of inflammatory pathways to Fabry disease pathogenesis. *Mol. Genet. Metab.* **2017**, *122*, 19–27. [CrossRef] [PubMed]
48. Weidemann, F. Fibrosis: A key feature of Fabry disease with potential therapeutic implica-tions. *Orphanet J. Rare Dis.* **2013**, *8*, 116. [CrossRef] [PubMed]
49. Shen, J.-S.; Meng, X.-L.; Moore, D.F.; Quirk, J.M.; Shayman, J.A.; Schiffmann, R.; Kaneski, C.R. Globotriaosylceramide induces oxidative stress and up-regulates cell adhesion molecule expression in Fabry disease endothelial cells. *Mol. Genet. Metab.* **2008**, *95*, 163–168. [CrossRef]
50. Shu, L.; Vivekanandan-Giri, A.; Pennathur, S.; Smid, B.E.; Aerts, J.M.; Hollak, C.E.; Shayman, J.A. Establishing 3-nitrotyrosine as a biomarker for the vasculopathy of Fabry disease. *Kidney Int.* **2014**, *86*, 58–66. [CrossRef]
51. Van Eijk, M.; Ferraz, M.J.; Boot, R.G.; Aerts, J.M. Lyso-glycosphingolipids: Presence and consequences. *Essays Biochem.* **2020**, *64*, 565–578. [CrossRef]
52. Choi, L.; Vernon, J.; Kopach, O.; Minett, M.; Mills, K.; Clayton, P.; Meert, T.; Wood, J.N. The Fabry disease-associated lipid Lyso-Gb3 enhances voltage-gated calcium currents in sensory neurons and causes pain. *Neurosci. Lett.* **2015**, *594*, 163–168. [CrossRef]
53. Biegstraaten, M.; Hollak, C.E.M.; Bakkers, M.; Faber, C.G.; Aerts, J.M.F.G.; van Schaik, I.N. Small fiber neuropathy in Fabry disease. *Mol. Genet. Metab.* **2012**, *106*, 135–141. [CrossRef]
54. Sanchez-Niño, M.D. Globotriaosylsphingosine actions on human glomerular podocytes: Im-plications for Fabry nephropathy. *Nephrol. Dial. Transplant. Off. Publ. Eur. Dial. Transpl. Assoc. Eur. Ren. Assoc.* **2011**, *26*, 1797–1802.
55. Sanchez-Niño, M.D.; Carpio, D.; Sanz, A.B.; Ruiz-Ortega, M.; Mezzano, S.; Ortiz, A. Lyso-Gb3 activates Notch1 in human podocytes. *Hum. Mol. Genet.* **2015**, *24*, 5720–5732. [CrossRef] [PubMed]
56. Kaissarian, N.; Kang, J.; Shu, L.; Ferraz, M.J.; Aerts, J.M.; Shayman, J.A. Dissociation of globotriaosylceramide and impaired endothelial function in α-galactosidase-A deficient EA.hy926 cells. *Mol. Genet. Metab.* **2018**, *125*, 338–344. [CrossRef] [PubMed]
57. Rombach, S.M.; Twickler, T.B.; Aerts, J.M.F.G.; Linthorst, G.E.; Wijburg, F.A.; Hollak, C.E. MVasculopathy in patients with Fabry disease: Current controversies and re-search directions. *Mol. Genet. Metab.* **2010**, *99*, 99–108. [CrossRef]
58. Loos, B.; Engelbrecht, A.-M.; Lockshin, R.A.; Klionsky, D.J.; Zakeri, Z. The variability of au-tophagy and cell death susceptibility: Unanswered questions. *Autophagy* **2013**, *9*, 1270–1285. [CrossRef] [PubMed]
59. Nelson, M.P. Autophagy-lysosome pathway associated neuropathology and axonal degenera-tion in the brains of alpha-galactosidase A-deficient mice. *Acta Neuropathol. Commun.* **2014**, *2*, 20. [CrossRef] [PubMed]
60. Chévrier, M.; Brakch, N.; Céline, L.; Genty, D.; Ramdani, Y.; Moll, S.; Djavaheri-Mergny, M.; Brasse-Lagnel, C.; Laquerrière, A.L.A.; Barbey, F.; et al. Autophagosome maturation is impaired in Fabry disease. *Autophagy* **2010**, *6*, 589–599. [CrossRef] [PubMed]

61. Uchino, M. A histochemical and electron microscopic study of skeletal and cardiac muscle from a Fabry disease patient and carrier. *Acta Neuropathol.* **1995**, *90*, 334–338. [CrossRef]
62. Aerts, J.M.; Kallemeijn, W.W.; Wegdam, W.; Ferraz, M.J.; van Breemen, M.J.; Dekker, N.; Kramer, G.; Poorthuis, B.J.; Groener, J.E.M.; Cox-Brinkman, J.; et al. Biomarkers in the diagnosis of lysosomal storage disorders: Proteins, lipids, and inhibodies. *J. Inherit. Metab. Dis.* **2011**, *34*, 605–619. [CrossRef]
63. Gold, H.; Mirzaian, M.; Dekker, N.; Ferraz, M.J.; Lugtenburg, J.; Codée, J.D.C.; van der Marel, G.A.; Overkleeft, H.S.; Linthorst, G.E.; Groener, J.E.M.; et al. Quantification of Globotriaosylsphingosine in Plasma and Urine of Fabry Patients by Stable Isotope Ultraperformance Liquid Chromatography–Tandem Mass Spectrometry. *Clin. Chem.* **2013**, *59*, 547–556. [CrossRef]
64. Mirzaian, M. Simultaneous quantitation of sphingoid bases by UPLC-ESI-MS/MS with identi-cal 13 C-encoded internal standards. *Clin. Chim. Acta* **2017**, *466*, 178–184. [CrossRef]
65. Boutin, M.; Lavoie, P.; Abaoui, M.; Auray-Blais, C. Tandem Mass Spectrometry Quantitation of Lyso-Gb 3 and Six Related Analogs in Plasma for Fabry Disease Patients. *Curr. Protoc. Hum. Genet.* **2016**, *90*, 17.23.1–17.23.9. [CrossRef] [PubMed]
66. Polo, G.; Burlina, A.P.; Ranieri, E.; Colucci, F.; Rubert, L.; Pascarella, A.; Burlina, A.B. Plasma and dried blood spot lysosphingolipids for the diagnosis of different sphin-golipidoses: A comparative study. *Clin. Chem. Lab. Med.* **2019**, *57*, 1863–1874. [CrossRef] [PubMed]
67. Houge, G. Fabry or not Fabry-a question of ascertainment. *Eur. J. Hum. Genet. EJHG* **2011**, *19*, 1111. [CrossRef] [PubMed]
68. Svarstad, E.; Marti, H.P. The Changing Landscape of Fabry Disease. *Clin. J. Am. Soc. Nephrol.* **2020**, *15*, 569–576. [CrossRef]
69. Bichet, D.G.; Aerts, J.M.; Llm, C.A.-B.; Maruyama, H.; Mehta, A.B.; Skuban, N.; Krusinska, E.; Schiffmann, R. Correction: Assessment of plasma lyso-Gb3 for clinical monitoring of treatment response in migalastat-treated patients with Fabry disease. *Genet. Med.* **2021**, *23*, 238. [CrossRef]
70. Lombard, V.; Ramulu, H.G.; Drula, E.; Coutinho, P.M.; Henrissat, B. The carbohydrate-active enzymes database (CAZy) in 2013. *Nucleic Acids Res.* **2014**, *42*, D490–D495. [CrossRef]
71. Tomasic, I.B.; Metcalf, M.C.; Guce, A.I.; Clark, N.E.; Garman, S.C. Interconversion of the spec-ificities of human lysosomal enzymes associated with Fabry and Schindler diseases. *J. Biol. Chem.* **2010**, *285*, 21560–21566. [CrossRef]
72. Crich, D.; Quirke, J.C.K. Glycoside hydrolases restrict the side chain conformation of their sub-strates to gain additional transition state stabilization. *J. Am. Chem. Soc.* **2020**, *142*, 16965–16973.
73. Guce, A.I.; Clark, N.E.; Salgado, E.N.; Ivanen, D.R.; Kulminskaya, A.A.; Brumer, H.; Garman, S.C. Catalytic Mechanism of Human α-Galactosidase. *J. Biol. Chem.* **2010**, *285*, 3625–3632. [CrossRef]
74. Koshland, D.E. Stereochemistry and the mechanism of enzymatic reactions. *Biol. Rev.* **1953**, *28*, 416–436. [CrossRef]
75. Speciale, G.; Thompson, A.J.; Davies, G.J.; Williams, S.J. Dissecting conformational contribu-tions to glycosidase catalysis and inhibition. *Curr. Opin. Struct. Biol.* **2014**, *28*, 1–13. [CrossRef]
76. Withers, S.G.; Rupitz, K.; Street, I.P. 2-Deoxy-2-fluoro-D-glycosyl fluorides. A new class of specific mechanism-based glycosidase inhibitors. *J. Biol. Chem.* **1988**, *263*, 17–20. [CrossRef]
77. November, F.L. Active site-directed inhibition of galactosidases by conduritol C epoxides (1,2-anhydro-EPI-NEO-inositol). *Febs Lett.* **1981**, *135*, 139–144.
78. Willems, L.I.; Beenakker, T.J.M.; Murray, B.; Gagestein, B.; Elst, H.V.D.; van Rijssel, E.R.; Codee, J.D.C.; Kallemeijn, W.W.; Aerts, J.M.; van der Marel, G.A.; et al. Synthesis of α- and β-Galactopyranose-Configured Isomers of Cyclophellitol and Cyclophellitol Aziridine. *Eur. J. Org. Chem.* **2014**, *2014*, 6044–6056. [CrossRef]
79. Artola, M. α-d-Gal-cyclophellitol cyclosulfamidate is a Michaelis complex analog that stabi-lizes therapeutic lysosomal α-galactosidase A in Fabry disease. *Chem. Sci.* **2019**, *10*, 9233–9243. [CrossRef]
80. Wu, L.; Armstrong, Z.; Schröder, S.P.; de Boer, C.; Artola, M.; Aerts, J.M.; Overkleeft, H.S.; Davies, G.J. An overview of activity-based probes for glycosidases. *Curr. Opin. Chem. Biol.* **2019**, *53*, 25–36. [CrossRef] [PubMed]
81. Legler, G.; Pohl, S. Synthesis of 5-amino-5-deoxy-d-galactopyranose and 1,5-dideoxy-1,5-imino-d-galactitol, and their inhibition of α- and β-d-galactosidases. *Carbohydr. Res.* **1986**, *155*, 119–129. [CrossRef]
82. Willems, L.I.; Beenakker, T.J.M.; Murray, B.; Scheij, S.; Kallemeijn, W.W.; Boot, R.G.; Verhoek, M.; Donker-Koopman, W.E.; Ferraz, M.J.; van Rijssel, E.R.; et al. Potent and Selective Activity-Based Probes for GH27 Human Retaining α-Galactosidases. *J. Am. Chem. Soc.* **2014**, *136*, 11622–11625. [CrossRef] [PubMed]
83. Kytidou, K.; Beekwilder, J.; Artola, M.; van Meel, E.; Wilbers, R.H.; Moolenaar, G.F.; Aerts, J.M. Nicotiana benthamianaα-galactosidase A1.1 can functionally complement human α-galactosidase A deficiency associated with Fabry disease. *J. Biol. Chem.* **2018**, *293*, 10042–10058. [CrossRef] [PubMed]
84. Hoogerbrugge, P.; Brouwer, O.; Bordigoni, P.; Cornu, G.; Kapaun, P.; Ortega, J.; O'Meara, A.; Souillet, G.; Frappaz, D.; Blanche, S.; et al. Allogeneic bone marrow transplantation for lysosomal storage diseases. *Lancet* **1995**, *345*, 1398–1402. [CrossRef]
85. Rovelli, A.M. The controversial and changing role of haematopoietic cell transplantation for lyso-somal storage disorders: An update. *Bone Marrow Transplant.* **2008**, *41* (Suppl. 2), S87–S89. [CrossRef]
86. Brady, R.O. Enzyme replacement therapy: Conception, chaos and culmination. *Philos. Trans. R. Soc. B Biol. Sci.* **2003**, *358*, 915–919. [CrossRef]
87. Aerts, J.M.; Cox, T.M. Roscoe O. Brady: Physician whose pioneering discoveries in lipid bio-chemistry revolutionized treatment and understanding of lysosomal diseases. *Blood Cells. Mol. Dis.* **2018**, *68*, 4–8. [CrossRef] [PubMed]

88. Eng, C.M.; Guffon, N.; Wilcox, W.R.; Germain, D.P.; Lee, P.; Waldek, S.; Caplan, L.; Linthorst, G.E.; Desnick, R.J. Safety and Efficacy of Recombinant Human α-Galactosidase A Replacement Therapy in Fabry's Disease. *N. Engl. J. Med.* **2001**, *345*, 9–16. [CrossRef] [PubMed]
89. Schiffmann, R. Enzyme replacement therapy in fabry disease a randomized controlled trial. *J. Am. Med. Assoc.* **2001**, *285*, 2743–2749. [CrossRef]
90. European Medicines Agency Replagal. European Medicines Agency. Available online: https://www.ema.europa.eu/en/documents/product-information/replagal-epar-product-information_en.pdf (accessed on 8 February 2021).
91. Blom, D.; Speijer, D.; Linthorst, G.E.; Donker-Koopman, W.G.; Strijland, A.; Aerts, J.M. Recombinant Enzyme Therapy for Fabry Disease: Absence of Editing of Human α-Galactosidase A mRNA. *Am. J. Hum. Genet.* **2003**, *72*, 23–31. [CrossRef]
92. Sakuraba, H. Comparison of the effects of agalsidase alfa and agalsidase beta on cultured hu-man Fabry fibroblasts and Fabry mice. *J. Hum. Genet.* **2006**, *51*, 180–188. [CrossRef]
93. Ivanova, M.M. Rapid Clathrin-Mediated Uptake of Recombinant α-Gal-A to Lysosome Acti-vates Autophagy. *Biomolecules* **2020**, *10*, 837. [CrossRef]
94. Prabakaran, T.; Nielsen, R.; Larsen, J.V.; Sørensen, S.S.; Rasmussen, U.F.-; Saleem, M.A.; Petersen, C.M.; Verroust, P.J.; Christensen, E.I. Receptor-Mediated Endocytosis of α-Galactosidase A in Human Podocytes in Fabry Disease. *PLoS ONE* **2011**, *6*, e25065. [CrossRef]
95. Priyanka, P.; Parsons, T.B.; Miller, A.; Platt, F.M.; Fairbanks, A.J. Chemoenzymatic Synthesis of a Phosphorylated Glycoprotein. *Angew. Chem. Int. Ed.* **2016**, *55*, 5058–5061. [CrossRef]
96. Tian, W.; Ye, Z.; Wang, S.; Schulz, M.A.; van Coillie, J.; Sun, L.; Chen, Y.-H.; Narimatsu, Y.; Hansen, L.; Kristensen, C.; et al. The glycosylation design space for recombinant lysosomal replacement enzymes produced in CHO cells. *Nat. Commun.* **2019**, *10*, 1–13. [CrossRef] [PubMed]
97. Ruderfer, I.; Shulman, A.; Kizhner, T.; Azulay, Y.; Nataf, Y.; Tekoah, Y.; Shaaltiel, Y. Development and Analytical Characterization of Pegunigalsidase Alfa, a Chemi-cally Cross-Linked Plant Recombinant Human α-Galactosidase-A for Treatment of Fabry Disease. *Bioconjug. Chem.* **2018**, *29*, 1630–1639. [CrossRef] [PubMed]
98. Schiffmann, R. Pegunigalsidase alfa, a novel PEGylated enzyme replacement therapy for Fab-ry disease, provides sustained plasma concentrations and favorable pharmacodynamics: A 1-year Phase 1/2 clinical trial. *J. Inherit. Metab. Dis.* **2019**, *42*, 534–544.
99. Van der Veen, S.J.; Hollak, C.E.M.; van Kuilenburg, A.B.P.; Langeveld, M. Developments in the treatment of Fabry disease. *J. Inherit. Metab. Dis.* **2020**, *43*, 908–921. [CrossRef]
100. Smid, B.E.; Rombach, S.M.; Aerts, J.M.; Kuiper, S.; Mirzaian, M.; Overkleeft, H.S.; Poorthuis, B.J.H.M.; Hollak, C.E.M.; Groener, J.E.M.; Linthorst, G.E. Consequences of a global enzyme shortage of agalsidase beta in adult Dutch Fabry patients. *Orphanet J. Rare Dis.* **2011**, *6*, 69. [CrossRef]
101. Linthorst, G.E.; Hollak, C.E.M.; Donker-Koopman, W.E.; Strijland, A.; Aerts, J.M.F.G. En-zyme therapy for Fabry disease: Neutralizing antibodies toward agalsidase alpha and beta. *Kidney Int.* **2004**, *66*, 1589–1595. [CrossRef]
102. Sakuraba, H.; Togawa, T.; Tsukimura, T.; Kato, H. Plasma lyso-Gb3: A biomarker for monitoring fabry patients during enzyme replacement therapy. *Clin. Exp. Nephrol.* **2018**, *22*, 843–849. [CrossRef] [PubMed]
103. Rombach, S.M.; Aerts, J.M.F.G.; Poorthuis, B.J.H.M.; Groener, J.E.M.; Donker-Koopman, W.; Hendriks, E.; Mirzaian, M.; Kuiper, S.; Wijburg, F.A.; Hollak, C.E.M.; et al. Long-Term Effect of Antibodies against Infused Alpha-Galactosidase A in Fabry Disease on Plasma and Urinary (lyso)Gb3 Reduction and Treatment Outcome. *PLoS ONE* **2012**, *7*, e47805. [CrossRef] [PubMed]
104. Bénichou, B.; Goyal, S.; Sung, C.; Norfleet, A.M.; O'Brien, F. A retrospective analysis of the po-tential impact of IgG antibodies to agalsidase beta on efficacy during enzyme replacement therapy for Fabry disease. *Mol. Genet. Metab.* **2009**, *96*, 4–12. [CrossRef]
105. Ishii, S.; Kase, R.; Sakuraba, H.; Suzuki, Y. Characterization of a Mutant α-Galactosidase Gene Product for the Late-Onset Cardiac Form of Fabry Disease. *Biochem. Biophys. Res. Commun.* **1993**, *197*, 1585–1589. [CrossRef]
106. Fan, J.-Q.; Ishii, S.; Asano, N.; Suzuki, Y. Accelerated transport and maturation of lysosomal α–galactosidase A in Fabry lymphoblasts by an enzyme inhibitor. *Nat. Med.* **1999**, *5*, 112–115. [CrossRef] [PubMed]
107. Asano, N.; Ishii, S.; Kizu, H.; Ikeda, K.; Yasuda, K.; Kato, A.; Martin, O.R.; Fan, J.-Q. In vitro inhibition and intracellular enhancement of lysosomal α-galactosidase A activity in Fabry lymphoblasts by 1-deoxygalactonojirimycin and its derivatives. *JBIC J. Biol. Inorg. Chem.* **2000**, *267*, 4179–4186. [CrossRef] [PubMed]
108. Markham, A. Migalastat: First Global Approval. *Drugs* **2016**, *76*, 1147–1152. [CrossRef]
109. Germain, D.P.; Hughes, D.A.; Nicholls, K.; Bichet, D.G.; Giugliani, R.; Wilcox, W.R.; Feliciani, C.; Shankar, S.P.; Ezgu, F.; Amartino, H.; et al. Treatment of Fabry's Disease with the Pharmacologic Chaperone Migalastat. *N. Engl. J. Med.* **2016**, *375*, 545–555. [CrossRef] [PubMed]
110. Hughes, D.A.; Nicholls, K.; Shankar, S.P.; Sunder-Plassmann, G.; Koeller, D.; Nedd, K.; Vockley, G.; Hamazaki, T.; Lachmann, R.; Ohashi, T.; et al. Oral pharmacological chaperone migalastat compared with enzyme replacement therapy in Fabry disease: 18-month results from the randomised phase III ATTRACT study. *J. Med. Genet.* **2017**, *54*, 288–296. [CrossRef]
111. Benjamin, E.R.; Della-Valle, M.C.; Wu, X.; Katz, E.; Pruthi, F.; Bond, S.; Bronfin, B.; Williams, H.; Yu, J.; Bichet, D.G.; et al. The validation of pharmacogenetics for the identification of Fabry patients to be treated with migalastat. *Genet. Med.* **2017**, *19*, 430–438. [CrossRef] [PubMed]

112. Porto, C.; Cardone, M.; Fontana, F.; Rossi, B.; Tuzzi, M.R.; Tarallo, A.; Parenti, G. The pharmacological chaperone N-butyldeoxynojirimycin enhances enzyme re-placement therapy in pompe disease fibroblasts. *Mol. Ther.* **2009**, *17*, 964–971. [CrossRef]
113. Pisani, A.; Porto, C.; Andria, G.; Parenti, G. Synergy between the pharmacological chaperone 1-deoxygalactonojirimycin and agalsidase alpha in cultured fibroblasts from patients with Fabry dis-ease. *J. Inherit. Metab. Dis.* **2014**, *37*, 145–146. [CrossRef]
114. Porto, C.; Pisani, A.; Rosa, M.; Acampora, E.; Avolio, V.; Tuzzi, M.R.; Visciano, B.; Gagliardo, C.; Materazzi, S.; la Marca, G.; et al. Synergy between the pharmacological chaperone 1-deoxygalactonojirimycin and the human recombinant alpha-galactosidase A in cultured fibroblasts from patients with Fabry disease. *J. Inherit. Metab. Dis.* **2011**, *35*, 513–520. [CrossRef]
115. Benjamin, E.R.; Khanna, R.; Schilling, A.; Flanagan, J.J.; Pellegrino, L.J.; Brignol, N.; Lun, Y.; Guillen, D.; E Ranes, B.; Frascella, M.; et al. Co-administration With the Pharmacological Chaperone AT1001 Increases Recombinant Human α-Galactosidase A Tissue Uptake and Improves Substrate Reduction in Fabry Mice. *Mol. Ther.* **2012**, *20*, 717–726. [CrossRef] [PubMed]
116. Warnock, D.G.; Bichet, D.G.; Holida, M.; Goker-Alpan, O.; Nicholls, K.; Thomas, M.; Eyskens, F.; Shankar, S.; Adera, M.; Sitaraman, S.; et al. Oral Migalastat HCl Leads to Greater Systemic Exposure and Tissue Levels of Active α-Galactosidase A in Fabry Patients when Co-Administered with Infused Agalsidase. *PLoS ONE* **2015**, *10*, e0134341. [CrossRef]
117. Citro, V.; Peña-García, J.; Den-Haan, H.; Pérez-Sánchez, H.; del Prete, R.; Liguori, L.; Cimmaruta, C.; Lukas, J.; Cubellis, M.V.; Andreotti, G. Identification of an Allosteric Binding Site on Human Lysosomal Alpha-Galactosidase Opens the Way to New Pharmacological Chaperones for Fabry Disease. *PLoS ONE* **2016**, *11*, e0165463. [CrossRef]
118. Smid, B.E.; Ferraz, M.J.; Verhoek, M.; Mirzaian, M.; Wisse, P.; Overkleeft, H.S.; Hollak, C.E.; Aerts, J.M. Biochemical response to substrate reduction therapy versus enzyme replacement therapy in Gaucher disease type 1 patients. *Orphanet J. Rare Dis.* **2016**, *11*, 1–12. [CrossRef] [PubMed]
119. Peterschmitt, M.J.; Crawford, N.P.S.; Gaemers, S.J.M.; Ji, A.J.; Sharma, J.; Pham, T.T. Pharmacokinetics, Pharmacodynamics, Safety, and Tolerability of Oral Venglustat in Healthy Volunteers. *Clin. Pharmacol. Drug Dev.* **2021**, *10*, 86–98. [CrossRef]
120. Guérard, N.; Morand, O.; Dingemanse, J. Lucerastat, an iminosugar with potential as substrate reduction therapy for glycolipid storage disorders: Safety, tolerability, and pharmacokinetics in healthy subjects. *Orphanet J. Rare Dis.* **2017**, *12*, 1–10. [CrossRef]
121. Yasuda, M.; Huston, M.W.; Pagant, S.; Gan, L.; St. Martin, S.; Sproul, S.; Richards, D.; Ballaron, S.; Hettini, K.; Ledeboer, A.; et al. AAV2/6 Gene Therapy in a Murine Model of Fabry Disease Results in Supraphysiological Enzyme Activity and Effective Substrate Reduction. *Mol. Ther. Methods Clin. Dev.* **2020**, *18*, 607–619. [CrossRef] [PubMed]
122. Huston, M.W.; Yasuda, M.; Pagant, S.; St Martin, S.; Cao, L.; Falese, L.; Wechsler, T. Liver-targeted AAV gene therapy vectors produced by a clinical scale manu-facturing process result in high, continuous therapeutic levels of enzyme activity and effective sub-strate reduction in mouse model of Fabry disease. *Mol. Genet. Metab.* **2019**, *126*, S77. [CrossRef]
123. Kia, A.; McIntosh, J.; Rosales, C.; Hosseini, P.; Sheridan, R.; Spiewak, J.; Mills, K.; Corbau, R.; Nathwani, A.C. Efficacy Evaluation of Liver-Directed Gene Therapy in Fabry Mice. *Blood* **2018**, *132*, 2209. [CrossRef]
124. Zhu, X.; Yin, L.; Theisen, M.; Zhuo, J.; Siddiqui, S.; Levy, B.; Presnyak, V.; Frassetto, A.; Milton, J.; Salerno, T.; et al. Systemic mRNA Therapy for the Treatment of Fabry Disease: Preclinical Studies in Wild-Type Mice, Fabry Mouse Model, and Wild-Type Non-human Primates. *Am. J. Hum. Genet.* **2019**, *104*, 625–637. [CrossRef]
125. Sims, K.; Politei, J.; Banikazemi, M.; Lee, P. Stroke in Fabry disease frequently occurs before di-agnosis and in the absence of other clinical events: Natural history data from the Fabry Registry. *Stroke* **2009**, *40*, 788–794. [CrossRef]
126. Lairson, L.L.; Chiu, C.P.; Ly, H.D.; He, S.; Wakarchuk, W.W.; Strynadka, N.C.; Withers, S.G. Intermediate Trapping on a Mutant Retaining α-Galactosyltransferase Identifies an Unexpected Aspartate Residue. *J. Biol. Chem.* **2004**, *279*, 28339–28344. [CrossRef]
127. Persson, K. Crystal structure of the retaining galactosyltransferase LgtC from Neisseria men-ingitidis in complex with donor and acceptor sugar analogs. *Nat. Struct. Biol.* **2001**, *8*, 166–175. [CrossRef] [PubMed]
128. Ardèvol, A.; Rovira, C. Reaction Mechanisms in Carbohydrate-Active Enzymes: Glycoside Hy-drolases and Glycosyltransferases. Insights from ab Initio Quantum Mechanics/Molecular Mechan-ics Dynamic Simulations. *J. Am. Chem. Soc.* **2015**, *137*, 7528–7547. [CrossRef] [PubMed]
129. Ardèvol, A.; Rovira, C. The Molecular Mechanism of Enzymatic Glycosyl Transfer with Retention of Configuration: Evidence for a Short-Lived Oxocarbenium-Like Species. *Angew. Chem. Int. Ed.* **2011**, *50*, 10897–10901. [CrossRef] [PubMed]
130. Hughes, D.A.; Pastores, G.M. Eliglustat for Gaucher's disease: Trippingly on the tongue. *Lancet* **2015**, *385*, 2328–2330. [CrossRef]
131. Lukas, J.; Giese, A.-K.; Markoff, A.; Grittner, U.; Kolodny, E.; Mascher, H.; Lackner, K.J.; Meyer, W.; Wree, P.; Saviouk, V.; et al. Functional Characterisation of Alpha-Galactosidase A Mutations as a Basis for a New Classification System in Fabry Disease. *PLoS Genet.* **2013**, *9*, e1003632. [CrossRef] [PubMed]
132. Wennekes, T.; Berg, R.J.B.H.N.V.D.; Boot, R.G.; van der Marel, G.A.; Overkleeft, H.S.; Aerts, J.M. Glycosphingolipids-Nature, Function, and Pharmacological Modulation. *Angew. Chem. Int. Ed.* **2009**, *48*, 8848–8869. [CrossRef]
133. Steffensen, R.; Carlier, K.; Wiels, J.; Levery, S.B.; Stroud, M.; Cedergren, B.; Clausen, H. Cloning and Expression of the Histo-blood Group Pk UDP-galactose:Galbeta 1-4Glcbeta 1-Cer alpha 1,4-Galactosyltransferase. *J. Biol. Chem.* **2000**, *275*, 16723–16729. [CrossRef] [PubMed]
134. Kojima, Y.; Fukumoto, S.; Furukawa, K.; Okajima, T.; Wiels, J.; Yokoyama, K.; Suzuki, Y.; Urano, T.; Ohta, M.; Furukawa, K. Molecular Cloning of Globotriaosylceramide/CD77 Synthase, a Glycosyltransferase That Initiates the Synthesis of Globo Series Glycosphingolipids. *J. Biol. Chem.* **2000**, *275*, 15152–15156. [CrossRef] [PubMed]

135. Kaczmarek, R.; Duk, M.; Szymczak, K.; Korchagina, E.; Tyborowska, J.; Mikolajczyk, K.; Bovin, N.; Szewczyk, B.; Jaskiewicz, E.; Czerwinski, M. Human Gb3/CD77 synthase reveals specificity toward two or four different acceptors depending on amino acid at position 211, creating Pk, P1 and NOR blood group antigens. *Biochem. Biophys. Res. Commun.* **2016**, *470*, 168–174. [CrossRef]
136. Kaczmarek, R.; Mikolajewicz, K.; Szymczak, K.; Duk, M.; Majorczyk, E.; Krop-Watorek, A.; Buczkowska, A.; Czerwinski, M. Evaluation of an amino acid residue critical for the specificity and activity of human Gb3/CD77 synthase. *Glycoconj. J.* **2016**, *33*, 963–973. [CrossRef] [PubMed]
137. Hellberg, Å.; Schmidt-Melbye, A.-C.; Reid, M.E.; Olsson, M.L. Expression of a novel missense mutation found in the A4GALT gene of Amish individuals with the p phenotype. *Transfusion* **2008**, *48*, 479–487. [CrossRef]
138. Wang, Y.-C.; Chang, C.-F.; Lin, H.-C.; Lin, K.-S.; Lin, K.-T.; Hung, C.-M.; Lin, T.-M. Functional characterisation of a complex mutation in the α(1,4)galactosyltransferase gene in Taiwanese individuals with p phenotype. *Transfus. Med.* **2010**, *21*, 84–89. [CrossRef]
139. Reymond, D.; Karmali, M.A.; Clarke, I.; Winkler, M.; Petric, M. Comparison of the Western blot assay with the neutralizing-antibody and enzyme-linked immunosorbent assays for measuring anti-body to Verocytotoxin 1. *J. Clin. Microbiol.* **1997**, *35*, 609–613. [CrossRef] [PubMed]
140. Proulx, F.; Seidman, E.G.; Karpman, D. Pathogenesis of Shiga Toxin-Associated Hemolytic Uremic Syndrome. *Pediatr. Res.* **2001**, *50*, 163–171. [CrossRef] [PubMed]
141. Sandvig, K.; van Deurs, B. Endocytosis, intracellular transport, and cytotoxic action of Shiga tox-in and ricin. *Physiol. Rev.* **1996**, *346*, 99–102.
142. Cilmi, S.A.; Karalius, B.J.; Choy, W.; Smith, R.N.; Butterton, J.R. Fabry Disease in Mice Protects against Lethal Disease Caused by Shiga Toxin–Expressing EnterohemorrhagicEscherichia coli. *J. Infect. Dis.* **2006**, *194*, 1135–1140. [CrossRef]
143. Tian, S.; Muneeruddin, K.; Choi, M.Y.; Tao, L.; Bhuiyan, R.H.; Ohmi, Y.; Furukawa, K.; Furukawa, K.; Boland, S.; Shaffer, S.A.; et al. Genome-wide CRISPR screens for Shiga toxins and ricin reveal Golgi proteins critical for glycosylation. *PLoS Biol.* **2018**, *16*, e2006951. [CrossRef]
144. Yamaji, T.; Sekizuka, T.; Tachida, Y.; Sakuma, C.; Morimoto, K.; Kuroda, M.; Hanada, K. A CRISPR Screen Identifies LAPTM4A and TM9SF Proteins as Glycolipid-Regulating Factors. *iScience* **2019**, *11*, 409–424. [CrossRef] [PubMed]
145. Gloster, T.M.; Vocadlo, D.J. Developing inhibitors of glycan processing enzymes as tools for enabling glycobiology. *Nat. Chem. Biol.* **2012**, *8*, 683–694. [CrossRef]
146. Kamani, M.; Mylvaganam, M.; Tian, R.; Rigat, B.; Binnington, B.; Lingwood, C. Adamantyl Glycosphingolipids Provide a New Approach to the Selective Regulation of Cellular Glycosphingolipid Metabolism. *J. Biol. Chem.* **2011**, *286*, 21413–21426. [CrossRef] [PubMed]
147. Frantom, P.A.; Coward, J.K.; Blanchard, J.S. UDP-(5F)-GlcNAc acts as a slow-binding inhibitor of MshA, a retaining glycosyltransferase. *J. Am. Chem. Soc.* **2010**, *132*, 6626–6627. [CrossRef]
148. Hartman, M.C.T.; Jiang, S.; Rush, J.S.; Waechter, A.C.J.; Coward, J.K. Glycosyltransferase Mechanisms: Impact of a 5-Fluoro Substituent in Acceptor and Donor Substrates on Catalysis. *Biochemistry* **2007**, *46*, 11630–11638. [CrossRef] [PubMed]
149. Jamaluddin, H.; Tumbale, P.; Withers, S.G.; Acharya, K.R.; Brew, K. Conformational Changes Induced by Binding UDP-2F-galactose to α-1,3 Galactosyltransferase- Implications for Catalysis. *J. Mol. Biol.* **2007**, *369*, 1270–1281. [CrossRef] [PubMed]
150. Seo, K.-C.; Kwon, Y.-G.; Kim, D.-H.; Jang, I.-S.; Cho, J.-W.; Chung, S.-K. Chemoenzymatic syntheses of carbasugar analogues of nucleoside diphosphate sugars: UDP-carba-Gal, UDP-carba-GlcNAc, UDP-carba-Glc, and GDP-carba-Man. *Chem. Commun.* **2009**, *1733–1735*, 1733–1735. [CrossRef]
151. Mitchell, M.L.; Tian, F.; Lee, L.V.; Wong, C.H. Synthesis and evaluation of transition-state ana-logue inhibitors of α-1,3-fucosyltransferase. *Angew. Chem. Int. Ed.* **2002**, *114*, 3167–3170. [CrossRef]
152. Descroix, K.; Pesnot, T.; Yoshimura, Y.; Gehrke, S.S.; Wakarchuk, W.W.; Palcic, M.M.; Wagner, G.K. Inhibition of Galactosyltransferases by a Novel Class of Donor Analogues. *J. Med. Chem.* **2012**, *55*, 2015–2024. [CrossRef]
153. Schmidt, R.R.; Frische, K. A new galactosyl transferase inhibitor. *Bioorganic Med. Chem. Lett.* **1993**, *3*, 1747–1750. [CrossRef]
154. Wagstaff, B.A.; Rejzek, M.; Pesnot, T.; Tedaldi, L.M.; Caputi, L.; O'Neill, E.C.; Field, R. A Enzymatic synthesis of nucleobase-modified UDP-sugars: Scope and limita-tions. *Carbohydr. Res.* **2015**, *404*, 17–25. [CrossRef] [PubMed]
155. Pesnot, T.; Jørgensen, R.; Palcic, M.M.; Wagner, G.K. Structural and mechanistic basis for a new mode of glycosyltransferase inhibition. *Nat. Chem. Biol.* **2010**, *6*, 321–323. [CrossRef] [PubMed]

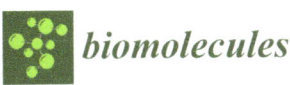

Article

Newborn Screening for Fabry Disease in Northeastern Italy: Results of Five Years of Experience

Vincenza Gragnaniello [1,†], Alessandro P Burlina [2,†], Giulia Polo [1], Antonella Giuliani [1], Leonardo Salviati [3], Giovanni Duro [4], Chiara Cazzorla [1], Laura Rubert [1], Evelina Maines [5], Dominique P Germain [6] and Alberto B Burlina [1,*]

[1] Division of Inherited Metabolic Diseases, Department of Diagnostic Services, University Hospital, 35129 Padua, Italy; vincenza.gragnaniello@aopd.veneto.it (V.G.); giulia.polo@aopd.veneto.it (G.P.); antonella.giuliani@aopd.veneto.it (A.G.); chiara.cazzorla@aopd.veneto.it (C.C.); laura.rubert@aopd.veneto.it (L.R.)
[2] Neurology Unit, St Bassiano Hospital, 36061 Bassano del Grappa, Italy; alessandro.burlina@aulss7.veneto.it
[3] Clinical Genetics Unit, Department of Diagnostic Services, University Hospital, 35128 Padua, Italy; leonardo.salviati@unipd.it
[4] Institute for Biomedical Research and Innovation, National Research Council of Italy (IRIB CNR), 90146 Palermo, Italy; giovanni.duro@ibim.cnr.it
[5] Division of Pediatrics, S. Chiara General Hospital, 38122 Trento, Italy; evelina.maines@apss.tn.it
[6] Division of Medical Genetics, University of Versailles and APHP Paris Saclay University, 92380 Garches, France; dominique.germain@uvsq.fr
* Correspondence: alberto.burlina@unipd.it; Tel.: +39-049-821-7462
† Both Vincenza Gragnaniello and Alessandro P Burlina contributed equally to the manuscript.

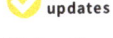

Abstract: Fabry disease (FD) is a progressive multisystemic lysosomal storage disease. Early diagnosis by newborn screening (NBS) may allow for timely treatment, thus preventing future irreversible organ damage. We present the results of 5.5 years of NBS for FD by α-galactosidase A activity and globotriaosylsphingosine (lyso-Gb$_3$) assays in dried blood spot through a multiplexed MS/MS assay. Furthermore, we report our experience with long-term follow-up of positive subjects. We screened more than 170,000 newborns and 22 males were confirmed to have a *GLA* gene variant, with an incidence of 1:7879 newborns. All patients were diagnosed with a variant previously associated with the later-onset phenotype of FD or carried an unclassified variant (four patients) or the likely benign p.Ala143Thr variant. All were asymptomatic at the last visit. Although lyso-Gb$_3$ is not considered a reliable second tier test for newborn screening, it can simplify the screening algorithm when its levels are elevated at birth. After birth, plasma lyso-Gb$_3$ is a useful marker for non-invasive monitoring of all positive patients. Our study is the largest reported to date in Europe, and presents data from long-term NBS for FD that reveals the current incidence of FD in northeastern Italy. Our follow-up data describe the early disease course and the trend of plasma lyso-Gb$_3$ during early childhood.

Keywords: Fabry disease; newborn screening; variant interpretation; second tier test; tandem mass spectrometry; lyso-Gb$_3$; dried blood spot; α-galactosidase A; *GLA* gene; globotriaosylsphingosine

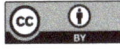

1. Introduction

Fabry disease (FD, OMIM 301500) is an X-linked lysosomal disorder (LSD) caused by a deficiency of α-galactosidase A (α-GAL A) activity that results in the progressive accumulation of globotriaosylceramide (Gb$_3$) and related glycosphingolipids, particularly in cellular lysosomes and body fluids [1,2]. The clinical phenotype includes a broad spectrum of clinical severity ranging from classic to later-onset FD. Male patients with the classic FD phenotype may present in childhood with acroparesthesias, angiokeratomas, corneal opacities, gastrointestinal symptoms, neuropathic pain, and hypohidrosis, followed in adulthood by renal failure, cardiac and cerebrovascular disease, and premature death [3,4]. Men with the later-onset phenotype of FD invariably present with cardiovascular involvement (hypertrophic cardiomyopathy with arrhythmias and conduction abnormalities), with very rare occurrences of renal (albuminuria, proteinuria) and cerebrovascular involvement [5]. In heterozygous females, clinical manifestations vary from asymptomatic to the classic severe phenotype, largely depending on X-chromosome inactivation [6]. Diagnosis in affected males can be achieved by the α-GAL A enzyme activity assay on several sample matrix types (dried blood spot DBS, peripheral white blood cells or plasma) and/or by molecular analysis [7,8]. α-GAL A enzyme activity levels may be normal in heterozygous females due to X-chromosome inactivation in blood cells, so that gene testing is necessary [1]. Analysis of biomarkers (e.g., Gb$_3$ and its deacylated form, lyso-Gb$_3$) in plasma, urine, and DBS are useful for both diagnosis and follow-up [9–11]. Enzyme replacement therapy (ERT) with agalsidase alfa or agalsidase beta [12,13] and chaperone therapy (for "amenable" *GLA* genetic variants) are available; expert panels have provided recommendations for clinical management [14,15]. Early intervention plays an important role in preventing irreversible damage due to disease progression [16].

Recently, pilot newborn screening (NBS) programs for FD, based on enzyme activity assay in DBS have been implemented worldwide using several analytical techniques. Initially, a fluorescent method with 4-methylumbelliferyl-D-galactopyranoside as a substrate was used [17]. Later, multiplexed techniques were developed using digital microfluidic fluorometric and MS/MS technology [18–21]. Several NBS programs in the USA (Washington State, Missouri, Illinois) [22–24], Europe (Hungary, Austria, Spain, Italy) [25–28], and East Asia (Taiwan, Japan) [29,30] showed that FD is surprisingly more prevalent than previously estimated (1:40,000) [31], especially the later-onset form, which may represent an important unrecognized genetic disease, although the caveats and difficulties of variant interpretation should be paid a lot of consideration [32]. A summary of available data on the known NBS programs for FD worldwide is presented in Table 1.

Table 1. Summary of the methods and results from pilot and regular screening programs for Fabry disease worldwide.

Publication Year	Study Period	Region	Method	Number of NBS Samples	Positive NBS/Patients Referred to Clinic	Confirmed Patients	Confirmed Male Patients	Reported Incidence *
2006	2003–2005	Italy [33]	Fluorometric enzyme assay	37,104 (only males)	12 (m)	12	12	1:3,100 (m)
2009	2006–2008	Taiwan [34]	Fluorometric enzyme assay	171,977 (m 90,288)	94 (m 91)	75	73	1:3821 (m 1:1237)
2017	2008	Spain [27]	Fluorometric enzyme assay	14,600 (m 7575)	106 (m 68)	37	20	1:394 (m 1:378) **
2009	2008–2009	Taiwan [35]	Fluorometric enzyme assay	110,027 (m 57,451)	67 (m 58)	45	42	1:2445 (m 1:1368)
2013	2007–2010	Japan [30]	Fluorometric enzyme assay	21,170 (m 10,827)	7 (m 5)	6	5	1:3,024 (m 1:2166)
2012	2010	Austria [26]	MS/MS	34,736 (deidentified)	28	9	6	1:3860
2012	2010–2011	Illinois [36]	Digital microfluidics	8012	11	7	6	1:1145
2012	2011	Hungary [25]	MS/MS	40,024	34	14	6	1:2858
2012	2010–2012	Italy [37]	Fluorometric enzyme assay	3403 (m 1702)	0	0	0	0
2014	2010–2013	Taiwan [38]	MS/MS	191,767	79	64	61	1:2996
2020	2011–2013	California [39]	MS/MS, immunocapture assay, digital microfluidics (comparative)	89,508 (deidentified) (m 44,664)	Variable based on method	50	46	1:1790 (m 1:970)

Table 1. Cont.

Publication Year	Study Period	Region	Method	Number of NBS Samples	Positive NBS/Patients Referred to Clinic	Confirmed Patients	Confirmed Male Patients	Reported Incidence *
2013	2013	Washington State [22]	MS/MS	108,905 (deidentified) (m 54,800)	16 (m 13)	7	7	1:15558 (m 1:7800)
2015	2013	Missouri [23]	Digital microfluidics	43,701	28	15	15	1:2913
2017	2007–2014	Japan [40]	Fluorometric enzyme assay	2443	2	2	2	1:1222
2018	2008–2014	Taiwan [41]	Fluorometric enzyme assay, then MS/MS	792,247 (m 412,299)	764 (m 425)	324	272	1:2445 (m 1:1515)
2016	2008–2015	Taiwan [42]	Fluorometric enzyme assay, then MS/MS	916,383 (m 476,909)	936 (m 505)	441	324	1:2078 (m 1:1472)
2017	2012–2016	Petroleos Mexicanos Health Services [43]	MS/MS	20,018 (m 10,241)	5	5	5	1:4003 (m 1:2048)
2017	2014–2016	Illinois [24]	MS/MS	219,793	107	32	32	1:6968
2016	2016	Washington [44]	MS/MS	43,000 (deidentified)	8	5	NA	1:8600
2018	2015–2017	Italy [28]	MS/MS	44,411	5	5	5	1:8882
2018	2017	Brazil [45]	Digital microfluidics	10,527	0	0	0	0
2020	2006–2018	Japan [46]	Fluorometric enzyme assay	599,711	138	108	64	1:5552
2019	2013–2019	New York [47]	MS/MS	65,605	31	7	7	1:9372
2020	2018–2019	Taiwan [48]	MS/MS	73,743	4	4	NA	1:18,436

m: males (if indicated); MS/MS: tandem mass spectrometry; NBS: newborn screening; * incidence as reported in the respective studies. It is difficult to make comparison among studies, especially because changes in the classification of variants over time, so that some previously pathogenic variants have been reclassified (e.g., p.Arg118Cys, p.Asp313Tyr and the debated variant p.Ala143Thr). Furthermore, regarding some unclassified variants, it is difficult to predict their pathogenicity (see text); ** only 1 known pathogenic variant, 11 variants of uncertain significance (VUS), 25 polymorphisms (see text).

2. Materials and Methods

2.1. Study Population

From September 2015 until March 2021, the DBS from 173,342 newborns were collected consecutively by the Regional North East Italy expanded neonatal screening program. The DBSs were assayed for the enzymes deficient in FD and three other lysosomal diseases (LSD-Pompe disease, Gaucher disease, mucopolysaccharidosis type I). Written informed consent was obtained from a parent. Proof of informed consent is available upon request. According to the NBS protocol, samples were collected between 36 and 48 h of life on the same card used for the other NBS tests; a second sample was required for premature newborns (<34 gestational weeks and/or weight <2000 g) and for sick newborns (those receiving transfusion or parenteral nutrition). DBS were analyzed on the day they were received, and the DBS cards were stored at −20 °C in plastic bags for at least five years after analysis. All analyses were performed in compliance with institutional review board guidelines.

2.2. Methods

α-GAL A enzyme activity was determined simultaneously with acid α-glucosidase (deficient in Pompe disease), β-glucosidase (deficient in Gaucher disease), and α-L-iduronidase (deficient in mucopolysaccharidosis type I) using a multiplex MS/MS assay (Perkin Elmer, Turku, Finland). Assay results were obtained after overnight incubation and enzyme activity was expressed as micromoles of substrate hydrolyzed per hour of incubation per liter of blood (μmol/L/h). Samples with low activities for several enzymes were repeated due to a suspected preanalytical error. For IDUA activity, an initial cut-off of 3.76 µmol/L/h was established using 0.2 multiples of the median (MOM); this was reset to 2.3 µmol/L/h after the first 9 months of screening [28]. Samples with α-GAL A activity below the cut-off were retested in duplicate. If the mean of the enzyme activity values was confirmed to be low, a second DBS was requested and assayed using the same cut-off. Newborns with abnormal enzyme results on the second round were referred to the Division of Inherited Metabolic Disease, Padua University Hospital, for confirmatory testing and clinical follow-up. DBS with low α-GAL A activity were also tested for lyso-Gb$_3$ using the LC-MS/MS method with a cut-off value of 1.3 nmol/L. This cut-off was established from the analysis of 253 anonymous healthy adult blood donors (n = 133) and pediatric patients (n = 120), and the 97.5 th percentile was considered [10].

Confirmatory testing included α-GAL A enzyme activity in peripheral lymphocytes, plasma lyso-Gb$_3$ measurement, and molecular analysis. Moreover, the mothers of confirmed newborns underwent *GLA* molecular testing. α-GAL A enzyme activity in lymphocytes was measured initially using a fluorometric method and more recently using a MS/MS assay. lyso-Gb$_3$ was measured in plasma samples using LC-MS/MS technology, as described in [10]. The *GLA* gene was sequenced using Next Generation Sequencing technology on genomic DNA isolated from peripheral leukocytes. Variants were classified according to published clinical reports and public databases including the International Fabry Disease Genotype-Phenotype Database and The Fabry Working Group Genotype Phenotype Database [49–51].

Patients were monitored every 12 months, with clinical evaluation: angiokeratomas, hypohidrosis, gastrointestinal symptoms, limb pain, kidney (eGFR according to Schwartz formula, microalbuminuria, proteinuria), and cardiac (electrocardiogram) assessments. Plasma lyso-Gb$_3$ was monitored as a specific marker of the disease.

3. Results

All results of the NBS program for FD are summarized in Table 2. Of the 173,342 newborns screened (89,485 males and 83,857 females) from September 2015 to March 2021, 53 (44 males and 9 females) had a low α-GAL A enzyme activity in the first DBS and were recalled for a second spot (recall rate 0.03%). Low α-GAL A activity was confirmed in 23 newborns (22 males and one female) at the second DBS and referred to our outpatient Clinical Unit for confirmatory testing. All 22 males from 20 families were confirmed to have a decreased α-GAL A enzyme activity in lymphocytes and a genetic variant in the *GLA* gene, with an incidence of one in 4068 males. The only female newborn with a measured low DBS α-GAL A activity was negative at molecular testing. Regarding the ethnicity of the 22 positive neonates, four were of African origin, two were of Asian origin, and the others were Caucasian. Patients #13 and #20 and patients #16 and #21 were brothers. None of the patients had a family history of a previous FD diagnosis or manifestations strongly suggestive of FD (e.g., angiokeratomas, cornea verticillata, end-stage renal failure). The clinical, biochemical, and molecular features of the patients are presented in Table 3.

Table 2. Results of the newborn screening program for Fabry disease in northeast Italy (September 2015 to March 2021).

	Males	Females	Total
Screened newborns	89,485	83,857	173,342
Newborns with decreased enzyme activity in the 1st DBS, after retesting in duplicate	44	9	53
Recall %	0.05%	0.01%	0.03%
Newborns with decreased enzyme activity in the 2nd DBS and referred to Clinic Unit for confirmatory testing	22	1	23
Newborns confirmed by low enzyme activity in lymphocytes and GLA gene mutation	22	0	22
Pathogenic classical variants	0	0	0
Pathogenic later-onset variants	13	0	13
Benign variants	1	0	1
False-positive results	0	1	1
Unclassified variants	4	0	4
p.Ala143Thr variant	4	0	4
Overall incidence	1:4068	0	1:7879
Pathogenic variants incidence	1:6883	0	1:13,334

Cut-off <0.2 MOM (multiple of median).

Table 3. Clinical, biochemical, and molecular results of the patients detected by newborn screening for Fabry disease: baseline and follow-up.

Case	Year of Birth	Gender	Ethnic Origin	DBS AGAL Activity *	DBS LysoGb$_3$ (nv < 1.13 nmol/L)	Lymphocytes AGAL Activity **	Plasma LysoGb$_3$ at First Visit (nv < 0.43 nmol/L)	cDNA Variation (Protein Variation)	Classification International Fabry Disease Genotype-Phenotype Database [49] ***	Age at Last Visit	Clinical Manifesta-tions	Plasma LysoGb$_3$ at the Last Visit (nv < 0.43 nmol/L)
1	2015	M	Europe	3.21	NA	100	0.53	c.427G>A (p.Ala143Thr)	Benign	5.5 years	No	0.54
2	2015	M	Europe	2.76	NA	9	0.12	c.427G>A (p.Ala143Thr)	Benign	4.5 years	No	0.48
3	2015	M	Europe	2.93	NA	354	0.31	c.427G>A (p.Ala143Thr)	Benign	4.5 years	No	0.35
4	2016	M	Europe	0.64	NA	0	1.07	c.644 A>G (p.Asn215Ser) + IVS2-77_81del5; IVS4-16A>G; IVS6-22C>T	Later-onset + NA ****	4.5 years	No	3.91
5	2016	M	Europe	2.25	1.02	355	0.19	-10C>T; IVS2-77_81del5; IVS4-16A>G; IVS6-22C>T	NA ****		Lost to follow-up	
6	2016	M	Europe	3.45	NA	346	0.27	c.737C>T (p.Thr246Ile)	NA	4.5 years	No	0.43
7	2016	M	East Asia	0.77	0.79	143	0.3	IVS4 + 919G>A	Later-onset	4 years	No	1.12
8	2016	M	North Africa	0.72	1.79	66	1.02	c.1088G>A (p.Arg363His)	Later-onset	4 years	No	1.91
9	2016	M	East Asia	1.16	0.62	222	0.54	IVS4 + 919G>A	Later-onset	4 years	No	1.7
10	2016	M	Europe	0.73	2.17	27	2.98	c.1066 C>G (p.Arg356Gly)	Likely later-onset	4 years	No	3.71
11	2017	M	Europe	2.05	0.54	316	0.36	c.427G>A (p.Ala143Thr) + IVS4-61_60delGT	Benign + NA	3.5 years	No	0.85
12	2017	M	Europe	1.37	1.25	NA	0.85	c.153G>A (p.Met51Ile)	Later-onset	3.5 years	No	0.82
13	2017	M	West Africa	1.51	0.96	0.73	0.26	c.1067G>A (p.Arg356Gln)	Later-onset	3 years	No	0.43

Table 3. Cont.

Case	Year of Birth	Gender	Ethnic Origin	DBS AGAL Activity *	DBS LysoGb3 (nv < 1.13 nmol/L)	Lymphocytes AGAL Activity **	Plasma LysoGb3 at First Visit (nv < 0.43 nmol/L)	cDNA Variation (Protein Variation)	Classification International Fabry Disease Genotype-Phenotype Database [49] ***	Age at Last Visit	Clinical Manifestations	Plasma LysoGb3 at the Last Visit (nv < 0.43 nmol/L)
14	2018	M	Europe	0.79	0.41	NA	0.2	c.868A>C (p.Met290Leu) + -10C>T; IVS2-77_81del5; IVS4-16A>G; IVS6-22C>T	Later-onset + NA ****		Lost to follow-up	
15	2018	M	Europe	0.87	0.73	0.82	0.35	c.347G>C (p.Gly116Ala) + c.376A>G (p.Ser126Gly) + -10C>T; IVS2-77_81del5; IVS4-16A>G; IVS6-22C>T	NA + likely benign + NA ****	2.5 years	No	0.92
16	2018	M	Europe	1.28	0.22	3.44	**0.49**	c.856C>G (p.Leu286Val)	NA	2 years	No	**0.43**
17	2019	M	Europe	0.63	0.5	1.84	**0.82**	c.644A>G (p.Asn215Ser)	Later-onset	1 year	No	**1.95**
18	2019	M	Europe	1.4	1.1	3.35	**1.32**	c.644A>G (p.Asn215Ser)	Later-onset	1.5 years	No	NA
19	2019	M	North Africa	0.77	**2.7**	2.41	**1**	c.1088G>A (p.Arg363His)	Later-onset	1.5 years	No	**1.49**
20	2019	M	West Africa	1.63	1.07	1.05	NA	c.1067G>A (p.Arg356Gln)	Later-onset	1 year	No	**0.56**
21	2020	M	Europe	1.12	1.07	2.18	0.41	c.856C>G (p.Leu286Val)	NA	10 d	No	0.41
22	2020	M	Europe	1.88	0.77	1.94	**0.44**	c.868A>C (p.Met290Leu)	Later-onset	6 m	No	**0.51**

AGAL: α-GAL A; DBS: dried blood spot; N/A: not available; nv: normal values; M: males; the pathological values are marked in bold. * First cut-off used until May 2016 (case number 6) 3.76 μmol/L/h, after 9 months of screening it was reset to 2.3 μmol/L/h; ** until June 2017 (case number 11) a fluorometric method was used (nv 360–1374 mU/L), then we used a MS/MS technology (in neonate nv < 4.38 nmol/h/mg protein); *** last accessed on 24 May 2021; **** IVS4-16A > G, IVS6-22C > T, -10C > T are classified as benign variants in other databases (e.g., Fabry-Gen-Phen [51]).

3.1. Enzyme Activity

The α-GAL A enzyme activities in DBS ranged from 0.63 to 3.45 µmol/L/h ($n = 22$, mean 1.54 µmol/L/h, SD 0.88). After confirmatory testing, we found that the α-GAL A enzyme activities of males with known pathogenic *GLA* variants ranged from 0.63 to 1.88 µmol/L/h ($n = 13$, mean 1.07 µmol/L/h, SD 0.43), whilst in males carrying unclassified *GLA* variants or the p.Ala143Thr variant, it ranged from 0.87 to 3.45 µmol/L/h ($n = 8$, mean 2.21 µmol/L/h, SD 1.02). This difference was statistically significant ($p = 0.003$, according to the Student's *t*-test).

3.2. Genetic Testing

Molecular analysis identified 13 newborns (including two brothers) carrying known pathogenic variants (11 had a missense variant, two had an intronic splicing variant) associated with the later-onset form of FD, four carrying previously unclassified GLA variants, four with the p.Ala143Thr variant, and one carrying a haplotype considered to be benign (patient #5). Among our patients, the most common variant was p.Ala143Thr (four patients), followed by p.Asn215Ser (three patients). This latter is a known pathogenic variant found in association with the later-onset cardiac form of FD [5,52], while the p.Ala143Thr, which had initially been classified as pathologic now has its pathogenicity of conflicting interpretation with a number of reports in favor of a likely benign variant [50,53]. Patients #7 and #9, unrelated newborns of Asiatic origin, carried the splicing variant IVS4 + 919G>A, which is common in the Taiwanese population and is associated with a later-onset cardiac phenotype [42]. Moreover, we found two unrelated patients from northern Africa carrying the p.Arg363His variant. Of note, we frequently found the benign complex allele −10 C > T + IVS2-77_81del5 + IVS4-16A > G + IVS6-22C > T polymorphism, in association with other variants. It was identified in the absence of other *GLA* variation in patient #5, who had near normal enzyme activity. All mothers carried the same *GLA* variant of their respective offspring.

3.3. DBS Lyso-Gb$_3$

We started DBS lyso-Gb$_3$ testing in 2016, and tested 17 out of the 22 positive newborns. The values ranged from 0.22 to 2.7 nmol/L (mean 1.04 nmol/L, SD 0.65). Levels were abnormal in five newborns (patients #8, #10, #12, #18, and #19), among the 12 tested patients carrying a known later-onset variant (mean 1.8 nmol/L, SD 0.70). No patient carrying unclassified or likely benign variants had abnormal levels of DBS lyso-Gb$_3$ at birth ($n = 5$, mean 0.72 nmol/L, SD 0.35). This difference was not statistically significant ($p = 0.188$, according to the Student's t-test), but this is likely due to the small number of samples. However, an inverse linear correlation was found between DBS α-GAL A activity and DBS lyso-Gb$_3$ at birth ($r = -0.28$).

3.4. Plasma Lyso-Gb$_3$

At the first visit, we evaluated plasma lyso-Gb$_3$ in all neonates (except in case #20 due to technical problems) and it ranged from 0.12 to 2.98 nmol/L (mean 0.66 nmol/L, SD 0.63). It was above the cut-off in 11/21 patients, nine of which had a known pathogenic variant. lyso-Gb$_3$ was only slightly increased in patient #1 (p.Ala143Thr variant) and in patient #16 (p.Leu286Val, unclassified variant), whilst the highest values were observed in patients with the known pathogenic variants p.Asn215Ser, p.Arg363His, and, interestingly, in patient #10 (p.Arg356Gly), which is listed as a likely later-onset form in the International Fabry Disease Genotype-Phenotype Database [49]. The mean of values for patients with known pathogenic variants was 0.90 ± 0.75 nmol/L, while for patients carrying unclassified variants or the likely benign p.Ala143Thr variant, it was 0.36 ± 0.13 nmol/L. This difference was not statistically significant ($p = 0.061$, according to Student's t-test). However, an inverse linear correlation, stronger than the one between DBS α-GAL A activity and DBS lyso-Gb$_3$, was found between DBS α-GAL A activity and plasma lyso-Gb$_3$ at first visit ($r = -0.41$).

3.5. Follow-Up

None of the patients showed clinical or biochemical abnormalities at the first visit. All patients participated in regular follow-up except patients #5 and #14, who were lost to follow-up because parents refused additional medical examinations. A summary of clinical and biochemical features at the first visit and during follow-up is reported in Table 3 and Table S1. All patients were asymptomatic at the latest follow-up visit at the age indicated in Table 3. None of the patients were receiving specific treatment for FD. The mean plasma lyso-Gb$_3$ level was 1.19 nmol/L SD 1.06 (range 0.35–3.91 nmol/L), with slightly elevated values in 17 patients at the latest visit (85%). Interestingly, plasma lyso-Gb$_3$ levels increased in most children (mean annual increase 0.21 ± 0.29 nmol/L; ranges between –0.024 nmol/L in case #16 and 1.13 nmol/L in case #17; Figure 1). Higher values were found in patients carrying a known pathogenic variant (n = 11, range 0.43–3.91 nmol/L, mean 1.65, SD 1.20, mean annually increase 0.32 ± 0.33 nmol/L) than in individuals carrying unclassified variants or the variant p.Ala143Thr (n = 7, range 0.4–0.92 nmol/L, mean 0.55, SD 0.21, mean annual increase 0.06 ± 0.09 nmol/L). This difference was statistically significant (p = 0.033, Student's t-test). The p.Asn215Ser variant appeared to be associated with greater increase. Of note, all three patients with this variant had a value of 1 nmol/L at birth, with values increasing with age. The older patient had a value of 3.91 nmol/L at the age of 4.5 years.

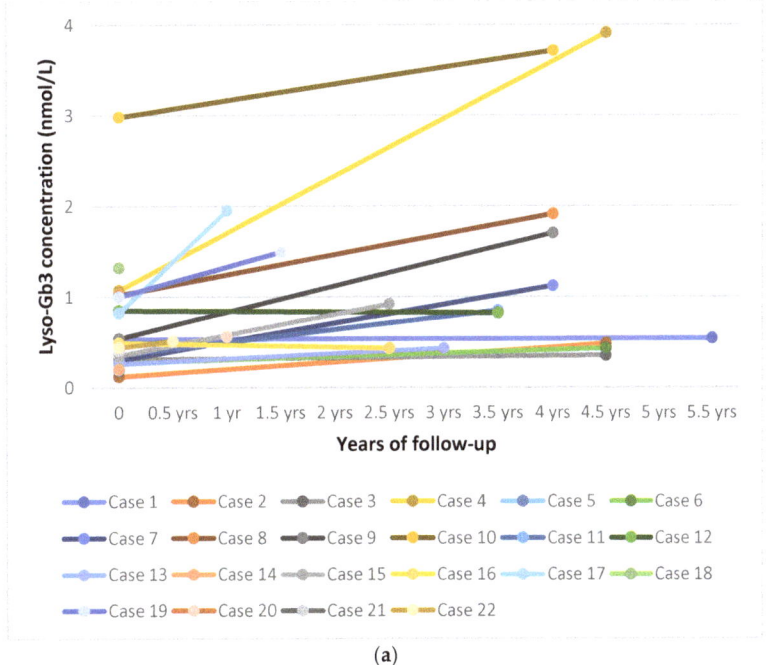

(a)

Figure 1. *Cont.*

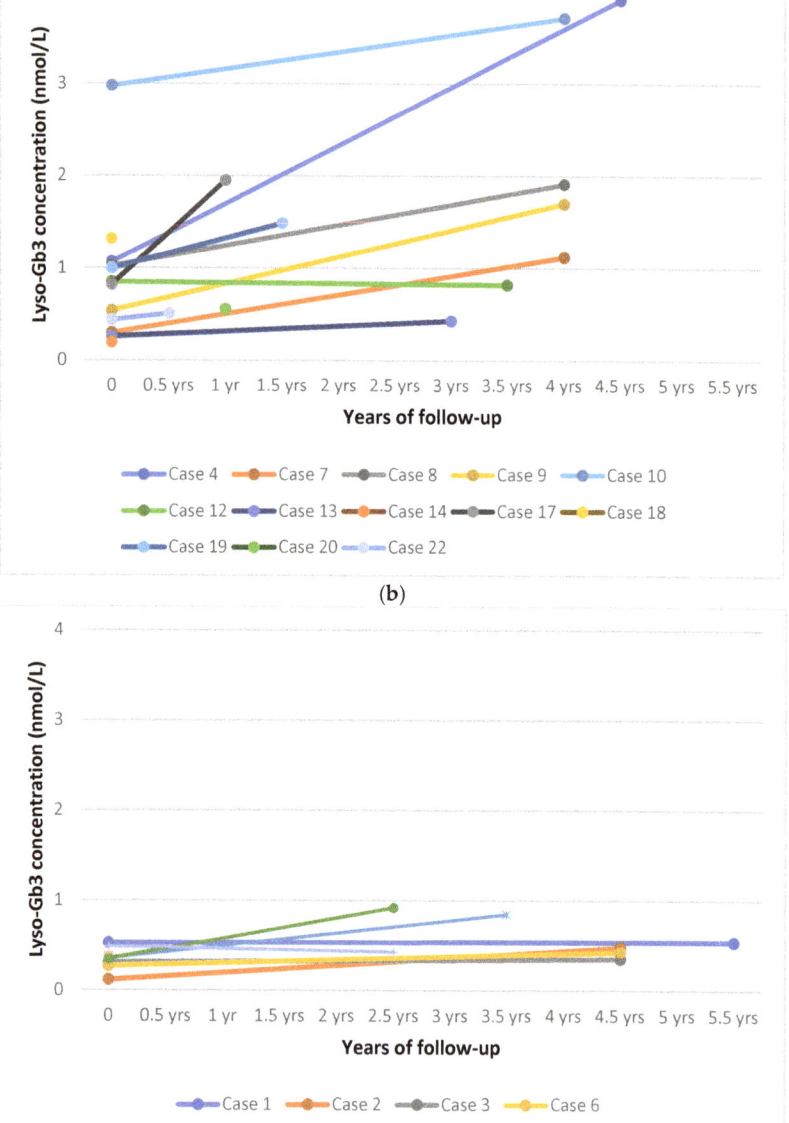

Figure 1. (a) Trend in plasma lyso-Gb$_3$ levels over time in all subjects positive for Fabry disease. (b) Plasma lyso-Gb$_3$ levels over time in patients carrying later-onset variants. (c) Plasma lyso-Gb$_3$ levels over time in subjects carrying benign and unclassified variants (including p.Ala143Thr). Abbreviation: yrs: years.

4. Discussion

Here, we report our results from more than five years of NBS for FD in northeast Italy, based on the determination of α-GAL A enzyme activity in DBS using a multiplex MS/MS assay.

4.1. Epidemiology

In the last 5.5 years, we screened 173,342 newborns (89,485 males and 83,857 females) for FD, which is the largest study reported to date in Europe. *GLA* variants were identified in 22 males, 13 of which were known pathogenic variants previously reported in association with a later-onset phenotype. One was a benign haplotype, four were unclassified variants, and four carried the p.Ala143Thr variant whose pathogenicity is debated. The four patients with the p.Ala143Thr variant did not appear to have classic FD, based on the clinical picture and biomarkers. Thus, the overall incidence of α-Gal A deficiency was of 1 in 7879 (1 in 4068 males), while the frequency of pathogenic variants was 1 in 6883 males. This incidence was similar to those detected in our previous pilot study, conducted from September 2015 to January 2017 on about 40,000 births (incidence 1:8,822 newborns) [28]. Moreover, this incidence was about six times higher than originally estimated from the clinical data (1:40,000) [31] but similar to previous reports from NBS programs. This is likely due to the recognition of previously undiagnosed later-onset forms of FD. Indeed, our incidence is comparable to those reported by a previous Italian study, conducted in north Italy from July 2003 to June 2005, using a fluorometric enzyme assay on 37,104 consecutive males. Twelve infants with *GLA* variants were found (incidence of 1:3100 males) and only one had a mutation known to cause the classic phenotype [33]. The incidence found in other studies is presented in Table 1. However, it is difficult to make comparisons among studies because there are differences in screening techniques, numbers of newborns, geographical/ethnical variation, and changes in the classification of variants over time as knowledge accumulates. This last point makes the comparison among studies particularly difficult, because some previously pathogenic variants have been reclassified over the years, based on associated clinical and biochemical features and their high incidence in the population (e.g., p.Arg118Cys, p.Asp313Tyr, and the debated variant p.Ala143Thr). Moreover, regarding some unclassified variants, it is difficult to predict their pathogenicity because FD may occur later in life. For example, a Spanish study reported a very high incidence of disease (1:394 births), but the number of screened newborns was low (*n* = 14,600). Moreover, only one patient had a known pathogenic variant, while 25/37 carried benign variants [27]. Conversely, a program conducted in Illinois on a newborn population similar in size to our study (nearly 220,000) and using similar methodology (MS/MS assay) reported an incidence of 1:6868 births [24], which is comparable to our result. However, different genetic backgrounds can also explain differences in incidence between countries. In Taiwan, screening of nearly one million newborns revealed an FD incidence of 1:2078, because of the high incidence and founder effect of the later-onset *GLA* splicing variant (IVS4 + 919G > A) (82% of patients) [35,42]. All studies including our NBS program show that even when non-pathogenic variants are discarded, FD is much more frequent than previously thought based on clinical estimates; it is the most frequent LSD screened. These findings, associated with available diagnostic methods and treatments, support the importance of NBS.

4.2. Interpretation of Genetic Variants

The lack of knowledge about the long-term course of the disease, especially for later-onset forms, complicates the establishment of clear correlations between genotype and phenotype in FD. Affected hemizygotes with the classic disease manifestations and no detectable α-GAL activity are associated with a variety of *GLA* variants including large and small gene rearrangements, splicing defects, and missense or nonsense variants. In contrast, most mildly affected atypical hemizygotes usually bears missense variants that express residual α-GAL A activity. However, most Fabry patients have private variants and attempts to predict the clinical phenotype based on the type or location of a variant may prove difficult. Moreover, the influence of modifier genes or other genetic factors on phenotype severity may be confounders since individuals with the same *GLA* variant may occasionally have variable phenotypes including within the same family. Thus, the clinical severity of private missense variants detected in Fabry families with few, or only young patients, is difficult to predict and requires more extensive clinical information from unrelated patients with the same FD genotype [50]. Furthermore, the burden of common risk factors (e.g., hypertension, high levels of cholesterol, diabetes) and the presence of concomitant diseases can be responsible for adjunctive signs and symptoms during aging [4,54].

Among the 12 different variants that we found (seven known pathogenic variants, four unclassified variants, and the debated p.Ala143Thr variant), there were 11 missense variants and one intronic splicing variant. The most frequent variant (p.Ala143Thr) was found in four patients (Pts. 1, 2, 3 and 11) and is more frequent in the Caucasian population. In a previous Italian study, three of six positive males carried this variant [33], and a similar frequency was found in Austria where it was found in three of six positive males [26]. Moreover, more recently, a California NBS study also reported a high frequency of the p.Ala143Thr variant among positive newborns (22/50) [39]. This variant, previously associated with both classic [55] and later-onset phenotype [56], was subsequently considered benign [53,57]. It is relatively frequent in the general population and a previous study in COS cells demonstrated a high residual enzyme activity of 36% [33]. Moreover, reported individuals with this variant showed unspecific symptoms, but no increase of plasma Gb$_3$ and lyso-Gb$_3$ [58] and no storage in tissue biopsies [53,57]. However, the significance of this variant is still controversial. A Fabry disease genotype-phenotype working group recently analyzed unclassified GLA variants in the Fabry registry through a five-stage iterative system based on expert clinical assessment, published literature, and clinical evidence of pathogenicity, but the expert panel did not reach a definitive conclusion, and classified it as a variant of uncertain significance [50]. Our patients carrying this variant had high residual enzyme activity (about 29% of mean normal activity). Of note, three of our patients (pts. 1, 2, and 3) were identified during the first phase of our screening program, before adjustment of the cut-off for the α-GAL A activity. The fourth patient (patient #11), who had lower α-GAL A activity (2.05 µmol/L/h), also carried an intronic unclassified variant (IVS4-61_60delGT). It is possible that the association of these two variants could produce a further reduction in enzyme activity. All our patients carrying the variant p.Ala143Thr maintained normal or very slightly increased levels of plasma lyso-Gb$_3$ during follow-up. Plasma lyso-Gb$_3$ was higher in the patient with p.Ala143Thr plus the intronic unclassified variant (pt. 11; mean lyso-Gb$_3$ 0.55 nmol/L, SD 0.21 at age 4.5 years); however, it was lower than the lyso-Gb$_3$ levels in patients carrying known pathogenic variants (mean 1.62 nmol/L, SD 1.20). In our opinion, the α-GAL A activity and the lyso-Gb$_3$ levels detected in the four babies with the genetic variant p.Ala143Thr are in favor of a likely benign classification of this variant. The high frequency of this variant in the gnomAD database (5.06×10^{-4}) is also in favor of a benign variant relatively frequent in the European population (found in 88 of 92,769 European alleles) [59].

Among the pathogenic variants, we found a high frequency of the mutation p.Asn215Ser (patients #4, #17, and #18), associated with very low enzyme activity in DBS (0.64, 0.63, and 1.4 µmol/L/h, respectively). This variant is reported in patients with predominant cardiac involvement [5,52]. Other variants seem to be correlated with ethnic origin. Two unrelated Eastern Asiatic infants (from South China) carried the IVS4 + 919G>A variant. Interestingly, the DBS α-GAL A activity values of patients carrying a known pathogenic variant were significantly lower than the values of the patients with an unclassified variant or the likely benign p.Ala143Thr variant ($p = 0.003$).

4.3. Clinical Follow-Up

All patients were monitored, except for two who did not want to come back to the hospital periodically. Because all our patients carried variants associated with the later-onset form or unclassified variants, we decided to follow them up every 12 months. The follow-up included clinical, instrumental, and biochemical assessments: the search for angiokeratomas, limb pain, hypohidrosis, gastrointestinal symptoms, renal, and cardiac evaluations (eGFR according to Schwartz formula, microalbuminuria, proteinuria, cardiologic visit with ECG) (Table S1). We detected four newborns with unclassified variants and followed their clinical outcomes. Patient #6, carrying the p.Thr246Ile variant, had a high DBS α-GAL A activity (3.45 µmol/L/h). Currently at age 4.5 years, he has no signs or symptoms of disease and plasma lyso-Gb$_3$ values correspond to the upper limit of the normal range (0.43 nmol/L), questioning pathogenicity of this variant. Patient #15 carried two variants (p.Gly116Ala) and the likely benign p.Ser126Gly and several benign intronic variants. He has no signs of disease at age 2.5 years, but plasma lyso-Gb3 level is slightly elevated (0.92 nmol/L), so that further follow-up visits are requested. Finally, two brothers (patients #16 and #21) carried the p.Leu286Val variant. The first brother is asymptomatic at two years of age, and has a plasma lyso-Gb$_3$ value that corresponds to the upper limit of normal range (0.43 nmol/L), while the second brother is a newborn. We will continue to monitor them. Because FD can undergo silent progression without evident clinical manifestations, especially with later-onset forms, we believe that long-term follow-up is important. Indeed, Hsu et al. demonstrated that cardiac damage could progress in silence, even when it becomes severe and irreversible (e.g., cardiac fibrosis) [42], whilst Öqvist et al. emphasized the importance of early diagnosis and NBS in FD-related nephropathy [60]. We also carefully assessed limb pain, which can manifest in boys at the age of three years [61,62].

Currently, after five years of NBS and follow-up, none of our patients with predicted later-onset forms (mean age at last visit: 3 years) have symptoms or signs of FD. However, further investigations are needed to find the best way for early detection of clinical manifestations in patients with unclassified and later-onset variants. This would allow us to establish an appropriate timing for specific treatments and avoid potential organ damage due to Gb$_3$ and lyso-Gb$_3$ accumulation. We have provided constant psychological support to the parents from diagnosis and during follow-up, especially to the mothers because this X-linked disease could be a major psychological burden on them [30]. The parents of newborns with later-onset forms were reassured that the newborn would have a normal childhood and that periodic evaluations would help us to determine when therapy is needed in the future.

4.4. Biomarkers and Biochemical

Biomarkers and biochemical follow-up show Lyso-Gb$_3$ (also known as globotriaosylsphingosine) is the N-deacylated form of Gb$_3$ that has been proposed as a specific biomarker for FD [63]. Lyso-Gb$_3$ can be measured in plasma or DBS by LC-MS/MS technology, as we have demonstrated [10]. Recently, we studied lyso-Gb$_3$ in a large cohort of Fabry patients ($n = 71$) where we observed high levels in males with the classic phenotype and mild-to-moderately elevated levels both in males with the later-onset phenotype and in heterozygous females with the classic phenotype [10]. Storage of Gb$_3$ begins in utero [64,65];

therefore, we evaluated the use of this biomarker as a second-tier test by measuring lyso-Gb$_3$ in DBS from neonates identified by NBS for FD. We found that only five patients, all with a later-onset pathogenic variant, had abnormal DBS lyso-Gb$_3$ at birth, among the 17 tested newborns (of which 12 carrying a pathogenic variant), indicating that a normal result cannot exclude FD and, therefore, cannot be used as a second tier test. At the first visit, plasma lyso-Gb$_3$ was abnormal in 11/21 patients, nine of them with a later-onset variant, one carried the p.Ala143Thr variant, and one had the unclassified p.Leu286Val variant. Interestingly, patient #10 had a very low α-GAL A activity (0.73 µmol/L/h) accompanied by the highest level of plasma lyso-Gb$_3$ that we found in our neonates (2.98 nmol/L). He carries the p.Arg356Gly variant, considered likely associated with a later-onset phenotype. Moreover, we found an inverse linear correlation between DBS lyso-Gb$_3$ /plasma lyso-Gb$_3$ and DBS α-GAL A activity at birth/first visit (r: −0.28 and −0.41, respectively). This finding suggests that lower enzyme activity corresponds to a higher storage from birth. Although a normal DBS lyso-Gb$_3$ value cannot rule out FD, its use as a specific marker in the diagnostic process is still valid. However, we believe that the use of lyso-Gb$_3$ as a second-tier test in newborn screening programs needs further evaluation.

In light of our five-year-experience with NBS for FD, we propose a new screening algorithm (Figure 2) that is simplified with respect to our previous protocol [28]. In the new algorithm, if the first DBS had a reduced α-GAL A activity and lyso-Gb$_3$ levels were above the cut-off, the newborn must be referred directly to a Pediatric Unit without requiring a second DBS. Moreover, biomarkers play an important role during follow-up. A recent case report showed that lyso-Gb$_3$ may be elevated in the first days of life and that it increases significantly during infancy in patients affected by a classic (severe) form of FD [66]. In our patients affected by later-onset FD, we found that the levels of plasma lyso-Gb$_3$ gradually increased with age, suggesting that there may be a progressive and insidious storage, even in milder forms (Figure 1a). At the last visit (between 0.5 months and 5.5 years of age), plasma lyso-Gb$_3$ was above the reference value in 17/19 patients, of which 11 had a later-onset form (all tested), three carried the p.Ala143Thr variant (very mild increase, except in patient #11 who also carried an intronic variant, with a higher although still moderate value of 0.85 nmol/L), and three carried unclassified variants (very slight increase, values in two of these infants were near the upper value of the normal range) (Figure 1a,b). A statistically significant difference was found between plasma lyso-Gb$_3$ values of patients carrying a known pathogenic variant (later-onset variant) and patients with unclassified variants or the p.Ala143Thr variant at last visit, but this difference was not statistically significant in the neonatal period. Of note, we found that all patients carrying the p.Asn215Ser variant (patients #4, #17, and #18) had plasma lyso-Gb$_3$ levels above the cut-off at birth. These values progressively increased and, interestingly, the highest value was found in the oldest patient (3.91 nmol/L at 4.5 years), suggesting progressive and insidious storage, even in an asymptomatic child. However, all our patients carrying unclassified variants had normal lyso-Gb$_3$ at birth and it remained in the normal range in three of four patients at the last visit. Only in case #15, carrying one previously unreported variant in cis with the likely benign p.S126G variant, showed a mild increase in plasma lyso-Gb$_3$ (0.92 nmol/L). Nevertheless, we believe that further studies are needed to assess the exact value of lyso-Gb$_3$ in neonates carrying unclassified variants. Whether a slight increase in lyso-Gb$_3$ has any clinical significance has not been proven and also warrants further studies.

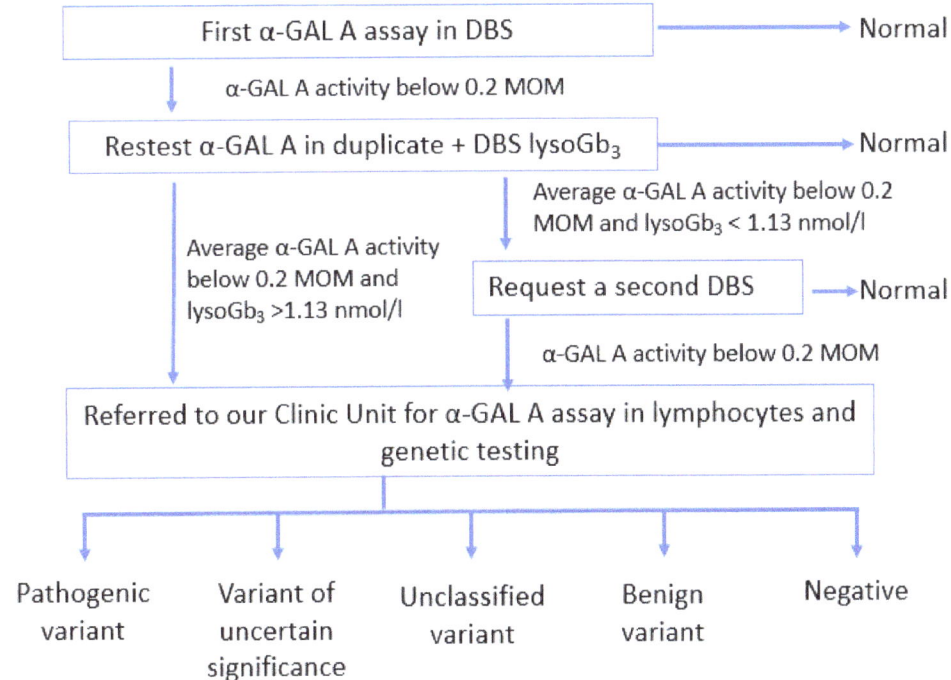

Figure 2. Proposal for a diagnostic algorithm of male newborn screening for Fabry disease. MOM: multiple of median; DBS: dried blood spot.

The high incidence of later-onset forms has raised ethical issues regarding the conduct of a NBS program. Detection in the newborn period may have a negative psychological impact on parents and carries the risk that these children, defined as "patient-in-waiting", are labelled and overmedicated. Moreover, it increases the costs for diagnostic laboratory testing and follow-up visits [67]. However, an early diagnosis of later-onset forms may also have several advantages. A significant number of patients with later-onset forms currently remain mis- or undiagnosed for many years. The implementation of NBS could avoid this "diagnostic odyssey", allowing timely treatment and subsequently better outcomes [24]. Interestingly, in a recent study, an interview among adult patients with lysosomal diseases was conducted on their opinion toward NBS. The majority of participants agreed with the implementation of NBS, in particular, all patients with FD were in favor of NBS because it may allow for the initiation of earlier treatment and prevent irreversible organ damage [68].

Moreover, their identification allows physicians to perform cascade genotyping in at risk family members and identify undiagnosed relatives [69]. Furthermore, NBS will help to better understand the natural course of the disease.

Our study on NBS for FD shows some limitations. Regarding the role of the biomarker lyso-Gb$_3$ as a second-tier test in NBS for FD, our experience confirms, as previously reported [70,71], that it is not reliable and cannot be used to reduce the recall rate. However, lyso-Gb$_3$, when elevated in DBS, makes the application of the diagnostic algorithm easier (Figure 2). During follow-up, plasma lyso-Gb$_3$ is very useful for the biochemical monitoring of patients.

We did not detect any heterozygotes among the 83,857 newborn females screened, which confirms that the current enzyme-based NBS approach misses most female carriers due to X-chromosome inactivation [72]. This is the major limitation of any enzymatic screening for FD [73]. These findings indicate that NBS for FD is more effective and cost beneficial when it is limited to male newborns. Some authors suggest first-tier screening with *GLA* gene sequencing in female newborns. This method was applied in Taiwan [29,74–76] where 21 variants account for approximately 98% of variants [76]. In Italy, mutational heterogeneity hampers the use of molecular analysis for high-throughput screening, which could also increase the number of variants of uncertain significance (VUS) [37]. Moreover, even when a GLA variant is known to be pathogenic, due to the X-chromosome inactivation, females might occasionally remain asymptomatic throughout life [6,77]. However, panels of genes may also be considered in the future, specifically due to improved technologies since they allow for the newborn screening of multiple diseases with the caveats of the difficulties in the interpretation of variants of unknown significance.

5. Conclusions

Our study confirms that NBS for Fabry disease is feasible through the measurement of α-GAL A enzyme activity in DBS and should be evaluated for inclusion in the national NBS program. Biomarkers like lyso-Gb$_3$ are useful in the NBS protocol for diagnosis and follow-up. In accordance with other NBS studies, FD appears to be more frequent than previously estimated clinically, therefore NBS may help to improve the diagnosis of many unrecognized patients. However, several issues still need further study: (1) the significance of mildly elevated plasma lyso-Gb$_3$; (2) the absence of a reliable second-tier test to reduce the recall rate; (3) poor detection of heterozygous females; (4) the clinical interpretation of unclassified and uncertain genetic variants; and (5) the impact of early diagnosis on patients with later-onset forms. Our overall experience in NBS for FD is positive, and the project is moving forward with the aim of gaining a better understanding of the disease and better care for the patients.

Supplementary Materials: The following are available online at https://www.mdpi.com/article/10.3390/biom11070951/s1, Table S1: Follow up of patients detected by newborn screening for Fabry disease.

Author Contributions: Conceptualization, A.B.B.; Methodology, G.P., A.G., L.S. and G.D.; Software, G.P.; Validation, G.P. and A.G.; Formal Analysis, A.P.B., D.P.G., A.B.B. and V.G.; Investigation, A.B.B., V.G., L.R., E.M. and C.C.; Resources, A.B.B.; Data Curation, A.B.B., A.P.B. and V.G.; Writing–Original Draft Preparation, A.B.B., A.P.B. and V.G.; Writing–Review & Editing, A.B.B., A.P.B., D.P.G. and V.G.; Supervision, A.B.B. and A.P.B.; Project Administration, A.B.B.; Funding Acquisition, A.B.B. All authors have read and agreed to the published version of the manuscript.

Funding: This work was supported by the Cometa A.S.M.M.E.—Associazione Studio Malattie Metaboliche Ereditarie—ONLUS.

Institutional Review Board Statement: Not applicable. The newborn screening program for lysosomal diseases has been approved by a Regional Law.

Informed Consent Statement: Informed consent was signed from parents of all subjects involved in the study.

Acknowledgments: We thank Richard Vernell, an independent medical writer, who provided medical writing support funded by Cometa A.S.M.M.E.—Associazione Studio Malattie Metaboliche Ereditarie—ONLUS.

Conflicts of Interest: The authors declare no conflict of interest.

References

1. Germain, D.P. Fabry disease. *Orphan J. Rare Dis.* **2010**, *5*, 30. [CrossRef]
2. Kok, K.; Zwiers, K.C.; Boot, R.G.; Overkleeft, H.S. Fabry Disease: Molecular Basis, Pathophysiology, Diagnostics and Potential Therapeutic Directions. *Biomolecules* **2021**, *11*, 271. [CrossRef] [PubMed]
3. Burlina, A.P.; Politei, J. Fabry disease. In *Neurometabolic Hereditary Diseases of Adults*; Burlina, A.P., Ed.; Springer: Berlin/Heidelberg, Germany, 2018; pp. 67–98.
4. Desnick, R.J.; Ioannou, Y.A.; Eng, C.M. *A-Galactosidase A Deficiency: Fabry Disease*; McGraw Hill: New York, NY, USA, 2021.
5. Germain, D.P.; Brand, E.; Burlina, A.; Cecchi, F.; Garman, S.C.; Kempf, J.; Laney, D.A.; Linhart, A.; Maródi, L.; Nicholls, K.; et al. Phenotypic Characteristics of the p.Asn215Ser (p.N215S) *GAL* Mutation in Male and Female Patients with Fabry Disease: A Multicenter Fabry Registry Study. *Mol. Genet. Genom. Med.* **2018**, *6*, 492–503. [CrossRef] [PubMed]

6. Echevarria, L.; Benistan, K.; Toussaint, A.; Dubourg, O.; Hagege, A.A.; Eladari, D.; Jabbour, F.; Beldjord, C.; De Mazancourt, P.; Germain, D.P. X-chromosome inactivation in female patients with Fabry disease. *Clin. Genet.* **2016**, *89*, 44–54. [CrossRef] [PubMed]
7. Massaccesi, L.; Burlina, A.; Baquero, C.J.; Goi, G.; Burlina, A.P.; Tettamanti, G. Whole-Blood Alpha-D-Galactosidase A Activity for the Identification of Fabry's Patients. *Clin. Biochem.* **2011**, *44*, 916–921. [CrossRef]
8. Gal, A.; Beck, M.; Höppner, W.; Germain, D.P. Clinical utility gene card for Fabry disease—Update 2016. *Eur. J. Hum. Genet.* **2017**, *25*, e1–e3. [CrossRef]
9. Rombach, S.M.; Dekker, N.; Bouwman, M.G.; Linthorst, G.E.; Zwinderman, A.H.; Wijburg, F.A.; Kuiper, S.; vd Bergh Weerman, M.A.; Groener, J.E.M.; Poorthuis, B.J.; et al. Plasma Globotriaosylsphingosine: Diagnostic Value and Relation to Clinical Manifestations of Fabry Disease. *Biochim. Biophys. Acta (BBA) Mol. Basis Dis.* **2010**, *1802*, 741–748. [CrossRef]
10. Polo, G.; Burlina, A.P.; Ranieri, E.; Colucci, F.; Rubert, L.; Pascarella, A.; Duro, G.; Tummolo, A.; Padoan, A.; Plebani, M.; et al. Plasma and Dried Blood Spot Lysosphingolipids for the Diagnosis of Different Sphingolipidoses: A Comparative Study. *Clin. Chem. Lab. Med.* **2019**, *57*, 1863–1874. [CrossRef]
11. Effraimidis, G.; Feldt-Rasmussen, U.; Rasmussen, Å.K.; Lavoie, P.; Abaoui, M.; Boutin, M.; Auray-Blais, C. Globotriaosylsphingosine (Lyso-Gb$_3$) and Analogues in Plasma and Urine of Patients with Fabry Disease and Correlations with Long-Term Treatment and Genotypes in a Nationwide Female Danish Cohort. *J. Med. Genet.* **2020**. [CrossRef]
12. Schiffmann, R.; Murray, G.J.; Treco, D.; Daniel, P.; Sellos-Moura, M.; Myers, M.; Quirk, J.M.; Zirzow, G.C.; Borowski, M.; Loveday, K.; et al. Infusion of alpha-Galactosidase A Reduces Tissue Globotriaosylceramide Storage in Patients with Fabry Disease. *Proc. Natl. Acad. Sci. USA* **2000**, *97*, 365–370. [CrossRef]
13. Eng, C.M.; Guffon, N.; Wilcox, W.R.; Germain, D.P.; Lee, P.; Waldek, S.; Caplan, L.; Linthorst, G.E.; Desnick, R.J. For The International Collaborative Fabry Disease Study Group: Safety and efficacy of recombinant human alphagalactosidase A—replacement therapy in Fabry's disease. *N. Engl. J. Med.* **2001**, *345*, 9–16. [CrossRef]
14. Germain, D.P.; Arad, M.; Burlina, A.; Elliott, P.M.; Falissard, B.; Feldt-Rasmussen, U.; Hilz, M.J.; Hughes, D.A.; Ortiz, A.; Wanner, C.; et al. The effect of enzyme replacement therapy on clinical outcomes in female patients with Fabry disease—A systematic literature review by a European panel of experts. *Mol. Genet. Metab.* **2018**, *126*, 224–235. [CrossRef] [PubMed]
15. Ortiz, A.; Germain, D.P.; Desnick, R.J.; Politei, J.; Mauer, M.; Burlina, A.; Eng, C.; Hopkin, R.J.; Laney, D.; Linhart, A.; et al. Fabry Disease Revisited: Management and Treatment Recommendations for Adult Patients. *Mol. Genet. Metab.* **2018**, *123*, 416–427. [CrossRef] [PubMed]
16. Germain, D.P.; Charrow, J.; Desnick, R.J.; Guffon, N.; Kempf, J.; Lachmann, R.H.; Lemay, R.; Linthorst, G.E.; Packman, S.; Scott, C.R.; et al. Ten-Year Outcome of Enzyme Replacement Therapy with Agalsidase Beta in Patients with Fabry Disease. *J. Med. Genet.* **2015**, *52*, 353–358. [CrossRef] [PubMed]
17. Chamoles, N.A.; Blanco, M.; Gaggioli, D. Fabry disease enzymatic diagnosis in dried blood spot on filter paper. *Clinica Chimica Acta* **2001**, *308*, 195–196. [CrossRef]
18. Gelb, M.H.; Turecek, F.; Scott, C.R.; Chamoles, N.A. Direct Multiplex Assay of Enzymes in Dried Blood Spots by Tandem Mass Spectrometry for the Newborn Screening of Lysosomal Storage Disorders. *J. Inherit. Metab Dis.* **2006**, *29*, 397–404. [CrossRef]
19. Zhang, X.K.; Elbin, C.S.; Chuang, W.-L.; Cooper, S.K.; Marashio, C.A.; Beauregard, C.; Keutzer, J.M. Multiplex Enzyme Assay Screening of Dried Blood Spots for Lysosomal Storage Disorders by Using Tandem Mass Spectrometry. *Clin. Chem.* **2008**, *54*, 1725–1728. [CrossRef]
20. Sista, R.S.; Eckhardt, A.E.; Wang, T.; Graham, C.; Rouse, J.L.; Norton, S.M.; Srinivasan, V.; Pollack, M.G.; Tolun, A.A.; Bali, D.; et al. Digital Microfluidic Platform for Multiplexing Enzyme Assays: Implications for Lysosomal Storage Disease Screening in Newborns. *Clin. Chem.* **2011**, *57*, 1444–1451. [CrossRef]
21. Mechtler, T.P.; Metz, T.F.; Müller, H.G.; Ostermann, K.; Ratschmann, R.; De Jesus, V.R.; Shushan, B.; Di Bussolo, J.M.; Herman, J.L.; Herkner, K.R.; et al. Short-Incubation Mass Spectrometry Assay for Lysosomal Storage Disorders in Newborn and High-Risk Population Screening. *J. Chromatogr. B* **2012**, *908*, 9–17. [CrossRef]
22. Scott, C.R.; Elliott, S.; Buroker, N.; Thomas, L.I.; Keutzer, J.; Glass, M.; Gelb, M.H.; Turecek, F. Identification of Infants at Risk for Developing Fabry, Pompe or Mucopolysaccharidosis-I from Newborn Blood Spots by Tandem Mass Spectrometry. *J. Pediatr.* **2013**, *163*, 498–503. [CrossRef]
23. Hopkins, P.V.; Campbell, C.; Klug, T.; Rogers, S.; Raburn-Miller, J.; Kiesling, J. Lysosomal Storage Disorder Screening Implementation: Findings from the First Six Months of Full Population Pilot Testing in Missouri. *J. Pediatr.* **2015**, *166*, 172–177. [CrossRef] [PubMed]
24. Burton, B.K. Newborn Screening for Lysosomal Storage Disorders in Illinois: The Initial 15-Month Experience. *J. Pediatr.* **2017**, *190*, 130–135. [CrossRef]
25. Wittmann, J.; Karg, E.; Turi, S.; Legnini, E.; Wittmann, G.; Giese, A.-K.; Lukas, J.; Gölnitz, U.; Klingenhäger, M.; Bodamer, O.; et al. Newborn Screening for Lysosomal Storage Disorders in Hungary. In *JIMD Reports—Case and Research Reports, 2012/3*; SSIEM, Ed.; JIMD Reports; Springer: Berlin/Heidelberg, Germany, 2012; Volume 6, pp. 117–125. [CrossRef]
26. Mechtler, T.P. Neonatal Screening for Lysosomal Storage Disorders: Feasibility and Incidence from a Nationwide Study in Austria. *Lancet* **2012**, *379*, 335–341. [CrossRef]
27. Colon, C.; Ortolano, S.; Melcon-Crespo, C.; Alvarez, J.V.; Lopez-Suarez, O.E.; Couce, M.L.; Fernández-Lorenzo, J.R. Newborn Screening for Fabry Disease in the North-West of Spain. *Eur. J. Pediatr.* **2017**, *176*, 1075–1081. [CrossRef]

28. Burlina, A.B.; Polo, G.; Salviati, L.; Duro, G.; Zizzo, C.; Dardis, A.; Bembi, B.; Cazzorla, C.; Rubert, L.; Zordan, R.; et al. Newborn Screening for Lysosomal Storage Disorders by Tandem Mass Spectrometry in North East Italy. *J. Inherit. Metab Dis.* **2018**, *41*, 209–219. [CrossRef]
29. Chien, Y.-H.; Lee, N.-C.; Chiang, S.-C.; Desnick, R.J.; Hwu, W.-L. Fabry Disease: Incidence of the Common Later-Onset α-Galactosidase A IVS4+919G→A Mutation in Taiwanese Newborns—Superiority of DNA-Based to Enzyme-Based Newborn Screening for Common Mutations. *Mol. Med.* **2012**, *18*, 780–784. [CrossRef]
30. Inoue, T.; Hattori, K.; Ihara, K.; Ishii, A.; Nakamura, K.; Hirose, S. Newborn Screening for Fabry Disease in Japan: Prevalence and Genotypes of Fabry Disease in a Pilot Study. *J. Hum. Genet.* **2013**, *58*, 548–552. [CrossRef]
31. Meikle, P.J. Prevalence of Lysosomal Storage Disorders. *JAMA* **1999**, *281*, 249. [CrossRef]
32. Richards, S.; Aziz, N.; Bale, S.; Bick, D.; Das, S.; Gastier-Foster, J.; Grody, W.W.; Hedge, M.; Lyon, E.; Spector, E.; et al. Standards and guidelines for the interpretation of sequence variants: A joint consensus recommendation of the American College of Medical Genetics and Genomics and the Association for Molecular Pathology. *Genet. Med.* **2015**, *17*, 405–424. [CrossRef] [PubMed]
33. Spada, M.; Pagliardini, S.; Yasuda, M.; Tukel, T.; Thiagarajan, G.; Sakuraba, H.; Ponzone, A.; Desnick, R.J. High Incidence of Later-Onset Fabry Disease Revealed by Newborn Screening. *Am. J. Hum. Genet.* **2006**, *79*, 31–40. [CrossRef] [PubMed]
34. Hwu, W.-L.; Chien, Y.-H.; Lee, N.-C.; Chiang, S.-C.; Dobrovolny, R.; Huang, A.-C.; Yeh, H.-Y.; Chao, M.-C.; Lin, S.-J.; Kitagawa, T.; et al. Newborn Screening for Fabry Disease in Taiwan Reveals a High Incidence of the Later-Onset *GLA* Mutation c.936+919G>A (IVS4+919G>A). *Hum. Mutat.* **2009**, *30*, 1397–1405. [CrossRef]
35. Lin, H.-Y.; Chong, K.-W.; Hsu, J.-H.; Yu, H.-C.; Shih, C.-C.; Huang, C.-H.; Lin, S.-J.; Chen, C.-H.; Chiang, C.-C.; Ho, H.-J.; et al. High Incidence of the Cardiac Variant of Fabry Disease Revealed by Newborn Screening in the Taiwan Chinese Population. *Circ. Cardiovasc. Genet.* **2009**, *2*, 450–456. [CrossRef]
36. Burton, B.; Charrow, J.; Angle, B.; Widera, S.; Waggoner, D. A pilot newborn screening program for lysosomal storage disease in Illinois. *Mol. Genet. Metab.* **2012**, *105*, S23–S24. [CrossRef]
37. Paciotti, S.; Persichetti, E.; Pagliardini, S.; Deganuto, M.; Rosano, C.; Balducci, C.; Codini, M.; Filocamo, M.; Menghini, A.R.; Pagliardini, V.; et al. First Pilot Newborn Screening for Four Lysosomal Storage Diseases in an Italian Region: Identification and Analysis of a Putative Causative Mutation in the GBA Gene. *Clin. Chim. Acta* **2012**, *5*, 1827–1831. [CrossRef] [PubMed]
38. Liao, H.-C.; Chiang, C.-C.; Niu, D.-M.; Wang, C.-H.; Kao, S.-M.; Tsai, F.-J.; Huang, Y.-H.; Liu, H.-C.; Huang, C.-K.; Gao, H.-J.; et al. Detecting Multiple Lysosomal Storage Diseases by Tandem Mass Spectrometry—A National Newborn Screening Program in Taiwan. *Clin. Chim. Acta* **2014**, *431*, 80–86. [CrossRef] [PubMed]
39. Sanders, K.A.; Gavrilov, D.K.; Oglesbee, D.; Raymond, K.M.; Tortorelli, S.; Hopwood, J.J.; Lorey, F.; Majumdar, R.; Kroll, C.A.; McDonald, A.M.; et al. A Comparative Effectiveness Study of Newborn Screening Methods for Four Lysosomal Storage Disorders. *IJNS* **2020**, *6*, 44. [CrossRef] [PubMed]
40. Chinen, Y.; Nakamura, S.; Yoshida, T.; Maruyama, H.; Nakamura, K. A New Mutation Found in Newborn Screening for Fabry Disease Evaluated by Plasma Globotriaosylsphingosine Levels. *Hum. Genome Var.* **2017**, *4*, 17002. [CrossRef]
41. Liao, H.-C.; Hsu, T.-R.; Young, L.; Chiang, C.-C.; Huang, C.-K.; Liu, H.-C.; Niu, D.-M.; Chen, Y.-J. Functional and Biological Studies of α-Galactosidase A Variants with Uncertain Significance from Newborn Screening in Taiwan. *Mol. Genet Metab.* **2018**, *123*, 140–147. [CrossRef] [PubMed]
42. Hsu, T.-R. Later Onset Fabry Disease, Cardiac Damage Progress in Silence. *J. Am. Coll. Cardiol.* **2016**, *68*, 2554–2563. [CrossRef]
43. Navarrete-Martínez, J.I.; Limón-Rojas, A.E.; Gaytán-García, M.d.J.; Reyna-Figueroa, J.; Wakida-Kusunoki, G.; Delgado-Calvillo, M.d.R.; Cantú-Reyna, C.; Cruz-Camino, H.; Cervantes-Barragán, D.E. Newborn Screening for Six Lysosomal Storage Disorders in a Cohort of Mexican Patients: Three-Year Findings from a Screening Program in a Closed Mexican Health System. *Mol. Genet. Metab.* **2017**, *121*, 16–21. [CrossRef] [PubMed]
44. Elliott, S.; Buroker, N.; Cournoyer, J.J.; Potier, A.M.; Trometer, J.D.; Elbin, C.; Schermer, M.J.; Kantola, J.; Boyce, A.; Turecek, F.; et al. Pilot Study of Newborn Screening for Six Lysosomal Storage Diseases Using Tandem Mass Spectrometry. *Mol. Genet. Metab.* **2016**, *118*, 304–309. [CrossRef]
45. Camargo Neto, E.; Schulte, J.; Pereira, J.; Bravo, H.; Sampaio-Filho, C.; Giugliani, R. Neonatal Screening for Four Lysosomal Storage Diseases with a Digital Microfluidics Platform: Initial Results in Brazil. *Genet. Mol. Biol.* **2018**, *41*, 414–416. [CrossRef]
46. Sawada, T.; Kido, J.; Yoshida, S.; Sugawara, K.; Momosaki, K.; Inoue, T.; Tajima, G.; Sawada, H.; Mastumoto, S.; Endo, F.; et al. Newborn Screening for Fabry Disease in the Western Region of Japan. *Mol. Genet. Metab. Rep.* **2020**, *22*, 100562. [CrossRef] [PubMed]
47. Wasserstein, M.P.; Caggana, M.; Bailey, S.M.; Desnick, R.J.; Edelmann, L.; Estrella, L.; Holzman, I.; Kelly, N.R.; Kornreich, R.; Kupchik, S.G.; et al. The New York Pilot Newborn Screening Program for Lysosomal Storage Diseases: Report of the First 65,000 Infants. *Genet. Med.* **2019**, *21*, 631–640. [CrossRef]
48. Chien, Y.-H. Newborn Screening for Morquio Disease and Other Lysosomal Storage Diseases: Results from the 8-Plex Assay for 70,000 Newborns. *Orphanet J. Rare Dis.* **2020**, *15*, 38. [CrossRef] [PubMed]
49. International Fabry Disease Genotype-Phenotype Database. Available online: www.dbfgp.org (accessed on 24 May 2021).
50. Germain, D.P.; Oliveira, J.P.; Bichet, D.G.; Yoo, H.-W.; Hopkin, R.J.; Lemay, R.; Politei, J.; Wanner, C.; Wilcox, W.R.; Warnock, D.G. Use of a Rare Disease Registry for Establishing Phenotypic Classification of Previously Unassigned *GLA* Variants: A Consensus Classification System by a Multispecialty Fabry Disease Genotype–Phenotype Workgroup. *J. Med. Genet.* **2020**, *57*, 542–551. [CrossRef]

51. Fabry-Gen-Phen: The Fabry Working Group Genotype Phenotype Database. Available online: http://fabrygenphen.com/ (accessed on 24 May 2021).
52. Lavalle, L.; Thomas, A.S.; Beaton, B.; Ebrahim, H.; Reed, M.; Ramaswami, U.; Elliott, P.; Mehta, A.B.; Hughes, D.A. Phenotype and Biochemical Heterogeneity in Late Onset Fabry Disease Defined by N215S Mutation. *PLoS ONE* **2018**, *13*, e0193550. [CrossRef] [PubMed]
53. Lenders, M.; Weidemann, F.; Kurschat, C.; Canaan-Kühl, S.; Duning, T.; Stypmann, J.; Schmitz, B.; Reiermann, S.; Krämer, J.; Blaschke, D.; et al. Alpha-Galactosidase A p.A143T, a Non-Fabry Disease-Causing Variant. *Orphanet J. Rare Dis.* **2016**, *11*, 54. [CrossRef] [PubMed]
54. Koca, S.; Tümer, L.; Okur, İ.; Erten, Y.; Bakkaloğlu, S.; Biberoğlu, G.; Kasapkara, Ç.; Küçükçongar, A.; Dalgıç, B.; Oktar, S.Ö.; et al. High Incidence of Co-Existing Factors Significantly Modifying the Phenotype in Patients with Fabry Disease. *Gene* **2019**, *687*, 280–288. [CrossRef]
55. Elliott, P.; Baker, R.; Pasquale, F.; Quarta, G.; Ebrahim, H.; Mehta, A.B.; Hughes, D.A.; On Behalf of the ACES Study Group. Prevalence of Anderson-Fabry Disease in Patients with Hypertrophic Cardiomyopathy: The European Anderson-Fabry Disease Survey. *Heart* **2011**, *97*, 1957–1960. [CrossRef] [PubMed]
56. Brabander, I.D. Phenotypical Characterization of α-Galactosidase A Gene Mutations Identified in a Large Fabry Disease Screening Program in Stroke in the Young. *Clin. Neurol. Neurosurg.* **2013**, *115*, 1088–1093. [CrossRef]
57. Terryn, W.; Vanholder, R.; Hemelsoet, D.; Leroy, B.P.; Van Biesen, W.; De Schoenmakere, G.; Wuyts, B.; Claes, K.; De Backer, J.; De Paepe, G.; et al. Questioning the Pathogenic Role of the GLA p.Ala143Thr "Mutation" in Fabry Disease: Implications for Screening Studies and ERT. In *JIMD Reports—Case and Research Reports, 2012/5*; Zschocke, J., Gibson, K.M., Brown, G., Morava, E., Peters, V., Eds.; JIMD Reports; Springer: Berlin/Heidelberg, Germany, 2012; Volume 8, pp. 101–108. [CrossRef]
58. Krüger, R.; Tholey, A.; Jakoby, T.; Vogelsberger, R.; Mönnikes, R.; Rossmann, H.; Beck, M.; Lackner, K.J. Quantification of the Fabry Marker LysoGb3 in Human Plasma by Tandem Mass Spectrometry. *J. Chromatogr. B* **2012**, *883–884*, 128–135. [CrossRef]
59. The Genome Aggregation Database. Available online: https://gnomad.broadinstitute.org (accessed on 24 May 2021).
60. Oqvist, B.; Brenner, B.M.; Oliveira, J.P.; Ortiz, A.; Schaefer, R.; Svarstad, E.; Wanner, C.; Zhang, K.; Warnock, D.G. Nephropathy in Fabry Disease: The Importance of Early Diagnosis and Testing in High-Risk Populations. *Nephrol. Dial. Transplant.* **2009**, *24*, 1736–1743. [CrossRef]
61. Ries, M.; Ramaswami, U.; Parini, R.; Lindblad, B.; Whybra, C.; Willers, I.; Gal, A.; Beck, M. The Early Clinical Phenotype of Fabry Disease: A Study on 35 European Children and Adolescents. *Eur. J. Pediatr.* **2003**, *162*, 767–772. [CrossRef]
62. Germain, D.P.; Fouilhoux, A.; Decramer, S.; Tardieu, M.; Pillet, P.; Fila, M.; Rivera, S.; Deschênes, G.; Lacombe, D. Consensus recommendations for diagnosis, management and treatment of Fabry disease in paediatric patients. *Clin. Genet.* **2019**, *96*, 107–117. [CrossRef] [PubMed]
63. Aerts, J.M.; Groener, J.E.; Kuiper, S.; Donker-Koopman, W.E.; Strijland, A.; Ottenhoff, R.; van Roomen, C.; Mirzaian, M.; Wijburg, F.A.; Linthorst, G.E.; et al. Elevated Globotriaosylsphingosine Is a Hallmark of Fabry Disease. *Proc. Natl. Acad. Sci. USA* **2008**, *105*, 2812–2817. [CrossRef]
64. Vedder, A.C.; Strijland, A.; Weerman, M.A.v.B.; Florquin, S.; Aerts, J.M.F.G.; Hollak, C.E.M. Manifestations of Fabry Disease in Placental Tissue. *J. Inherit. Metab. Dis.* **2006**, *29*, 106–111. [CrossRef] [PubMed]
65. Desnick, R.J. Prenatal Diagnosis of Fabry Disease. *Prenat. Diagn.* **2007**, *27*, 693–694. [CrossRef] [PubMed]
66. Spada, M.; Kasper, D.; Pagliardini, V.; Biamino, E.; Giachero, S.; Porta, F. Metabolic Progression to Clinical Phenotype in Classic Fabry Disease. *Ital. J. Pediatr.* **2017**, *43*, 1. [CrossRef] [PubMed]
67. Timmermans, S.; Buchbinder, M. Patients-in-waiting: Living between sickness and health in the genomics era. *J. Health Soc. Behav.* **2010**, *51*, 408–423. [CrossRef]
68. Lisi, E.; Ali, N. Opinions of adults affected with later-onset lysosomal storage diseases regarding newborn screening: A qualitative study. *J. Genet. Couns.* **2021**. [CrossRef] [PubMed]
69. Germain, D.P.; Moiseev, S.; Suárez-Obando, F.; Al Ismaili, F.; Al Khawaja, H.; Altarescu, G.; Barreto, F.C.; Haddoum, F.; Hadipour, F.; Maksimova, I.; et al. The benefits and challenges of family genetic testing in rare genetic diseases-lessons from Fabry disease. *Mol. Genet. Genomic Med.* **2021**, e1666. [CrossRef]
70. Burlina, A.B.; Polo, G.; Rubert, L.; Gueraldi, D.; Cazzorla, C.; Duro, G.; Salviati, L.; Burlina, A.P. Implementation of Second-Tier Tests in Newborn Screening for Lysosomal Disorders in North Eastern Italy. *IJNS* **2019**, *5*, 24. [CrossRef]
71. Johnson, B.; Mascher, H.; Mascher, D.; Legnini, E.; Hung, C.Y.; Dajnoki, A.; Chien, Y.-H.; Maródi, L.; Hwu, W.-L.; Bodamer, O.A. Analysis of Lyso-Globotriaosylsphingosine in Dried Blood Spots. *Ann. Lab. Med.* **2013**, *33*, 274–278. [CrossRef] [PubMed]
72. Hsu, T.-R.; Niu, D.-M. Fabry Disease: Review and Experience during Newborn Screening. *Trends Cardiovasc. Med.* **2018**, *28*, 274–281. [CrossRef]
73. Caudron, E.; Prognon, P.; Germain, D.P. Enzymatic diagnosis of Fabry disease using a fluorometric assay on dried blood spots: An alternative methodology. *Eur. J. Med. Genet.* **2015**, *58*, 681–684. [CrossRef]
74. Tai, C.-L.; Liu, M.-Y.; Yu, H.-C.; Chiang, C.-C.; Chiang, H.; Suen, J.-H.; Kao, S.-M.; Huang, Y.-H.; Wu, T.J.-T.; Yang, C.-F.; et al. The Use of High Resolution Melting Analysis to Detect Fabry Mutations in Heterozygous Females via Dry Bloodspots. *Clin. Chim. Acta* **2012**, *413*, 422–427. [CrossRef]
75. Lee, S.-H.; Li, C.-F.; Lin, H.-Y.; Lin, C.-H.; Liu, H.-C.; Tsai, S.-F.; Niu, D.-M. High-Throughput Detection of Common Sequence Variations of Fabry Disease in Taiwan Using DNA Mass Spectrometry. *Mol. Genet. Metab.* **2014**, *111*, 507–512. [CrossRef]

76. Lu, Y.-H.; Huang, P.-H.; Wang, L.-Y.; Hsu, T.-R.; Li, H.-Y.; Lee, P.-C.; Hsieh, Y.-P.; Hung, S.-C.; Wang, Y.-C.; Chang, S.-K.; et al. Improvement in the Sensitivity of Newborn Screening for Fabry Disease among Females through the Use of a High-Throughput and Cost-Effective Method, DNA Mass Spectrometry. *J. Hum. Genet.* **2018**, *63*, 1–8. [CrossRef] [PubMed]
77. MacDermot, K.D. Anderson-Fabry Disease: Clinical Manifestations and Impact of Disease in a Cohort of 60 Obligate Carrier Females. *J. Med. Genet.* **2001**, *38*, 769–775. [CrossRef]

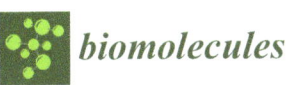

Review

Lysosomal Function and Axon Guidance: Is There a Meaningful Liaison?

Rosa Manzoli [1,2,†], Lorenzo Badenetti [1,3,4,†], Michela Rubin [1] and Enrico Moro [1,*]

1. Department of Molecular Medicine, University of Padova, 35121 Padova, Italy; rosa.manzoli@phd.unipd.it (R.M.); lorenzo.badenetti@phd.unipd.it (L.B.); michela.rubin@studenti.unipd.it (M.R.)
2. Department of Biology, University of Padova, 35121 Padova, Italy
3. Department of Women's and Children's Health, University of Padova, 35121 Padova, Italy
4. Pediatric Research Institute "Città della Speranza", 35127 Padova, Italy
* Correspondence: enrico.moro.1@unipd.it; Tel.: +39-04-98276341
† These authors contributed equally to this paper.

Abstract: Axonal trajectories and neural circuit activities strongly rely on a complex system of molecular cues that finely orchestrate the patterning of neural commissures. Several of these axon guidance molecules undergo continuous recycling during brain development, according to incompletely understood intracellular mechanisms, that in part rely on endocytic and autophagic cascades. Based on their pivotal role in both pathways, lysosomes are emerging as a key hub in the sophisticated regulation of axonal guidance cue delivery, localization, and function. In this review, we will attempt to collect some of the most relevant research on the tight connection between lysosomal function and axon guidance regulation, providing some proof of concepts that may be helpful to understanding the relation between lysosomal storage disorders and neurodegenerative diseases.

Keywords: axon guidance; lysosomal storage disorders; neuronal circuit

1. Introduction

The development of the central nervous system (CNS) occurs during embryonic stages in a strictly temporally and spatially regulated manner, to allow for the organization of a network of nervous fibers that progressively increase the range of functional neuronal interactions. The high degree of complexity is achieved through a balanced and controlled process of axonal remodeling, followed by the formation of specific synapses that cross-connect target neuronal populations in order to establish a dynamic system of integrated communication [1,2]. Axonal remodeling involves the elimination of "useless" connections and the formation and growth of new dendritic spines and axonal trajectories that enable brain plasticity and correct sensory responses to external stimuli. Impaired axonal remodeling and pathfinding lead to defective synaptic connectivity and aberrant neuronal circuit function, which characterize both congenital disorders and neurodegenerative conditions. While we know which extrinsic factors (that is, environmental stimuli, injury, and neuronal activity) may govern the ability to increase the axonal branching and pruning [3], we do not have a clear picture of which intrinsic factors (genetically encoded proteins, type of cell population) finely modulate the overall setting of the neuronal network during early embryogenesis. In addition, we still lack extensive knowledge of whether and how in certain cases (for instance, brain injuries and traumatic insults) axonal regeneration takes place and which molecules control this process. Understanding the cascade of molecular events occurring during both embryonic brain development and after brain injury could allow for the identification of druggable targets that may hamper neurodegenerative conditions and prevent the onset of irreversible cognitive decline in certain inherited disorders. In the past few years, lysosomes have attracted a remarkable interest for their key role in the autophagic process during axonal remodeling [4]. Besides, many lysosomal enzyme defects have been detected in neurodegenerative conditions [5]. A few years ago, a pioneering study revealed a tight association between lysosomal activity and axonal pruning [6]. More recently, Farfel-Becker and colleagues demonstrated that lysosomes are actively delivered to the distal termini, suggesting their pivotal function in axonal dynamics [7]. Therefore, an emerging role of lysosomal activity in axon growth and guidance is gaining attention, positing lysosomes as one of the top interests of neurobiologists. In this review, we will try to briefly summarize the current knowledge of up-to-date discovered axonal guidance cues, providing an inferential nexus between their impaired activity and the brain pathogenesis of lysosomal storage disorders (LSDs).

2. Axonal Guidance Cues

The term "axon guidance" refers to all mechanisms that allow a developing axon to elongate from the neuronal soma and reach its target tissues. A nascent axonal growth cone can indeed integrate and transduce a multitude of different stimuli it receives from the surrounding extracellular environment. This results in precise and predictable shaping of axonal routes in the developing nervous system. The striking concept of axonal pathfinding has traveled along centuries, from Ramón y Cajal and his studies of the embryonic chick spinal cord (1890), to the identification and characterization of axon guidance cues' major families (i.e., netrins, slits, semaphorins, and ephrins), together with morphogens, growth factors, glycoproteins, and cell adhesion molecules (CAMs) [8]. Axon guidance molecules can be divided into attractive and repulsive cues that act either diffusively over long distances or locally, in a contact-dependent manner. Cooperation between long-range and short-range guidance cues is required for the navigation of growing axons to their target cells (Figure 1).

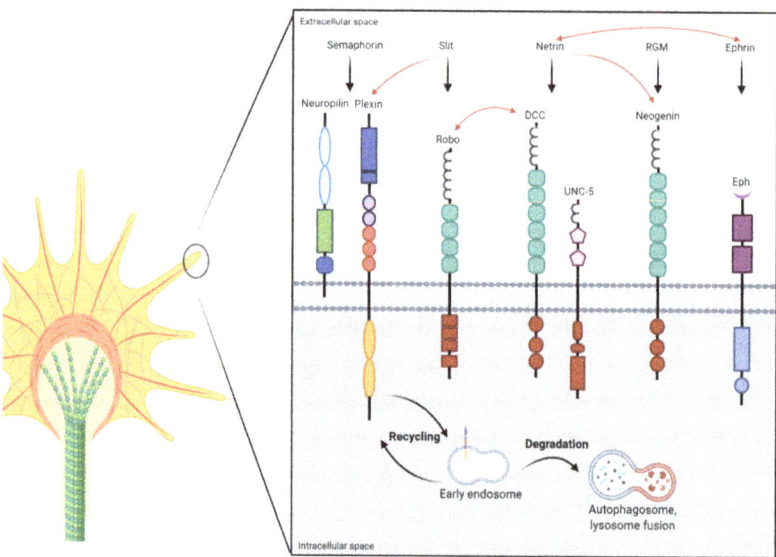

Figure 1. Axon guidance cues and endo-lysosomal pathway in the axonal growth cone. A schematic picture depicts the modular structure of major axonal guidance cue-related receptors and their respective ligands. Classical interactions are represented by black arrows, while red arrows indicate crosstalk between different axon guidance families. In the bottom part of the figure, the endosomal–lysosomal compartment is shown to mediate both receptor recycling and degradation. (created with BioRender.com).

2.1. Semaphorins

Semaphorins (SEMAs), first described in 1992 as "Fasciclin IV" by Kolodkin and colleagues, are a large family of proteins that can be either secreted, cell surface-attached, or membrane-bound [9]. Initially classified as repellents during axonal wiring, now it is known that some of them can also behave as attractants [10]. The growth-cone receptor PLEXIN is the most important protein involved in semaphorin signaling [11]. The interaction between semaphorin and PLEXIN can be direct or mediated by other membrane-associated proteins; for example, the SEMA3 class of semaphorin (except SEMA3E) interaction with PLEXIN is facilitated by neuropilins, type I transmembrane proteins located on the growth cone [12]. Cell adhesion molecules, such as Neuronal Cell Adhesion Molecule (Nr-CAM) and L1 cell adhesion molecule (L1-CAM) that associate with neuropilin receptors can be also required to mediate semaphorins' effects and transduce SEMA3-dependent signaling [13]. Additional receptors that directly bind semaphorins include, for example, integrins [14] and proteoglycans [15]. Besides their role in axon guidance modulation, the SEMA3 family of proteins has been demonstrated to play an important function in vascular homeostasis also. In particular, SEMA3F seems to be involved in endothelial barrier homeostasis and monocyte migration [16]. Finally, semaphorins are known modulators of cancer cell behavior, such as glioblastoma cell growth, survival, invasiveness, and angiogenesis [17].

2.2. Ephrins

Ephrins were first discovered and described in the context of retinotopic mapping [18]. They are membrane-related guidance cues categorized into two classes: Ephrin-As (Ephrin-A1–Ephrin-A5), which are glycophosphatidylinositol (GPI)-anchored to the membrane, and Ephrin-Bs (Ephrin-B1–Ephrin-B3), which have a transmembrane domain followed by a short cytoplasmic domain [19]. Ephrin ligands bind to erythropoietin-producing hepatoma (Eph) receptors that represent the largest subfamily among receptor tyrosine kinases (RTK). Although ephrin-dependent signaling was initially thought to mediate chemorepulsive interactions, later evidence showed that both attractive and repulsive responses can occur [20]. Since ephrins are anchored ligands, their interaction with Eph receptors is allowed only at sites of cell–cell contact, so that ephrin signaling becomes fundamental in axon choice points, where axons select between two alternative routes [21]. Here, the recognition between ligand and receptor triggers a peculiar cascade known as "bidirectional signaling"; unlike the classical unidirectional model characterized by ligand-mediated receptor activation and a downstream signaling cascade inside the receptor-expressing cell, the Eph–ephrin interaction induces a response both in ligand and receptor-harboring cells. Thus, traditionally what happens inside the Eph-expressing cell is called the "forward signal" and depends on Eph kinase activity, while the term "reverse signal" refers to the events inside the ligand-bearing cell mediated by Src family kinases [22]. Due to the fact that ephrins are extracellular GPI-anchored proteins, they require a transmembrane protein to mediate reverse signaling. Indeed, it has been shown that Ephrin-A interacts with different co-receptors, such as the p75 neurotrophin receptor (NTR) [23], TrkB [24], and Ret [25].

2.3. Repulsive Guidance Molecule (RGM)

The Repulsive Guidance Molecule (RGM) was identified by Monnier and colleagues in 2002 while studying chick growth cones of retinal axons [26]. RGM is a GPI-anchored glycoprotein that has been proven to interact with neogenin (NEO) and acts as a repulsive guidance molecule [27]. Indeed, the NEO–RGM interaction is also pivotal for embryonic neurodevelopment, as it is required for neural tube closure and neuroepithelial polarization [28,29]. Interestingly, RGM has been shown to be involved in the invasion by inflammatory cells of the CNS during autoimmune encephalomyelitis, thus establishing a link between axonal guidance and neuroinflammation [30]. Another key aspect is that RGMs have been shown to inhibit Bone Morphogenetic Protein (BMP) signaling through the interaction with Growth Differentiation Factor 5 (GDF5), providing direct proof of the close connection between axonal pathfinding and morphogens activity [31].

2.4. Netrins

Netrins are a family of laminin-related proteins that act in the extracellular compartment as chemotropic guidance cues during neuronal development. In mammals, both secreted Netrin-1, 3, and 4) and membrane-tethered GPI-linked Netrins (Netrin-G1 and G2) have been discovered [32]. Unlike classical netrins, Netrin-G1 does not bind to known netrin receptors, but instead interacts specifically with the Netrin-G ligand (NGL1, also known as LRRC4c) to modulate neurite elongation and the laminar organization of dendrites and induce the accumulation of microglial cells around axons [33–35]. The history of netrins began in the early 1990s, starting with the description of *Caenorhabditis elegans* (*C. elegans*) genes unc-5 (UNC5 in mammals), unc-6 (NTN1 in mammals), and unc-40 (DCC and NEO in mammals, frazzled in *Drosophila melanogaster*) [36]. The UNC5 protein is implicated in the repulsive netrin-mediated axon guidance through heterodimerization with Deleted in Colorectal Cancer (DCC) for long-range repulsion, and with Down syndrome cell adhesion molecule (DSCAM) for short-range repulsion [37]. Given the homology with the UNC family, mammalian DCC, originally identified as a tumor suppressor, was first proposed as a mediator of netrin pathways in 1996 [38]. DCC is a transmembrane receptor of the immunoglobulin superfamily highly expressed in spinal commissural neurons [38], retina [39], and many projection neurons of the forebrain and midbrain during embryonic development [40]. The netrin–DCC interaction can mediate both growth cone attraction and repulsion [37,38,41–44]. Moreover, Keino-Masu and colleagues discovered that NEO, a transmembrane protein strictly related to DCC, acts as a passive netrin receptor, serving as a stabilizer of the ligand gradient [38].

2.5. Slits

Slit is a secreted protein containing leucine-rich and Epidermal Growth Factor (EGF)-like repeats. First discovered in *Drosophila melanogaster* (*D. melanogaster*) by the end of the 1980s, slit is expressed in midline cells and required for normal development of midline structures [45]. Slit proteins are a class of single peptides of approximately 1500 amino acids. Invertebrates have only one slit, while vertebrates harbor three different variants, specifically SLIT1, SLIT2, and SLIT3 [46]. Slit proteins are cleaved by proteolytic enzymes between the fifth and sixth EGF-like domains to generate the long N-terminal Slit segment (SlitN) and the short C-terminal Slit segment (SlitC). These two domains have very different mediators; while SlitN can combine with the main slit interactors, Roundabout (ROBO) and DSCAM, to mediate axon guidance and branching extension, SlitC cannot bind ROBOs [47], but instead regulates axon guidance through its binding to PLEXIN, the main semaphorin receptor [48]. The first ROBO gene, ROBO1, was identified in *D. melanogaster* during an extensive screening focused on genes controlling the CNS midline crossing. [49]. The mammalian ROBO family is composed of four major components (ROBO1–4). While ROBO1 and ROBO2 mediate canonical slit signaling, ROBO3 and ROBO4 exhibit divergent features. ROBO3 cannot bind slits, but instead interacts with the Netrin-1–DCC complex [50]. Moreover, it antagonizes the SLIT2–ROBO1/2-induced repulsion by binding the diffusible factor NELL2. Recently, Pak and colleagues demonstrated the structural interplay between ROBO3 and NELL2, testing in vitro NELL preference towards ROBO3.1 binding [51]. On the other hand, ROBO4 cannot bind to slits directly, but interacts with the complex of SLIT2 and ROBO1 [52]. In addition, it can bind UNC5B, acting as a ligand to inhibit vascular endothelial growth factor (VEGF)-induced angiogenesis and vascular permeability [53]. It has been also proposed that ROBO4 transduces the downstream signaling through the interaction of a co-receptor and other molecules, such as ROBO1, with heparan sulfate proteoglycans (HSPGs) [54].

3. Axonal Guidance Cue Integration and Crosstalk

The high degree of complexity in studying axonal wiring is not due to the number of guidance cues, which are rather limited, but is likely derived from the combinatorial effect these cues induce at the growth cone. In fact, the axon guidance cue crosstalk, both in time and space, is fundamental for the proper shaping of axon-related molecular pathways. There are multiple mechanisms implicated in the mediation and regulation of axon guidance-induced responses, from alternative splicing, protein synthesis, and degradation to receptor trafficking and receptor–receptor interactions [55]. Moreover, during their "journey", axons are often guided by the epistatic influence of intermediate targets, which can switch from a repulsive to an attractive activity. This occurs, for instance, during the triggering of the SLIT/ROBO pathway, which inactivates the netrin-dependent attraction and drives the differential axonal preference in embryonic *Xenopus laevis* commissural spinal neurons [56]. Alternatively, another recent clear-cut example is the extracellular environment-mediated tuning of PLEXIN1a and ROBO1 receptors trafficking on the cell surface during the midline crossing of spinal cord commissural axons in chick embryos [57]. Synergistic crosstalk has also been reported for ephrin and netrin pathways in in vitro explants of chick spinal lateral motor column (LMC) neurons. It has been shown that Ephrin-A5, acting through its receptor EPHA4, induces sensitization to the Netrin-1 signal by increasing NEO abundance in motor neurons, probably acting on the receptor trafficking [58]. Therefore, through a selective combinatorial integration between different classes of axonal cues, a deep fine-tuning of neuronal modular patterning is achieved, allowing for the formation of the complex dynamic network of responses to environmental stimuli that shape the early brain embryonic development. The modular structure of major axonal guidance cue-related receptors and their respective ligands is depicted in Figure 1.

4. Lysosomal Function in Axonal Development

To correctly integrate signals coming from extracellular guidance cues, growing axons need to dynamically regulate the presence of receptor proteins available on the growth cone surface. Without considering the transcriptional aspect of this regulation, receptor presence and availability on the cell surface can be post-transcriptionally regulated by the endosomal–lysosomal pathway [59]. Endosomes participate in the dynamics of axonal growth, regulating the trafficking of endocytosed receptors [60]. Once inside the endosomes, receptors can be directed back to the cell membrane if they enter the recycling pathway, or they can be destined to degradation following the late endosomal–lysosomal pathway [61]. Indeed, endosomes can take part in the axonal guidance-related signaling cascades, being the host compartment for sorting signals [59]. For instance, the endolysosomal compartment is involved in guidance cue regulation of the EphA2 signaling cascade. In fact, it has been reported that an activated EphA2 receptor can be internalized by trans-endocytosis into endosomes and be recycled back to the plasma membrane or degraded into lysosomes. Moreover, in early endosomes, EphA2 can retain its active state and signal by recruiting and activating the Rac1-specific guanine nucleotide exchange factor (GEF) Tiam1, which seems to be implicated in neurite outgrowth [62,63]. Additionally, in commissural axons, ROBO levels are regulated by lysosomal degradation, thanks to the action of Commissureless (Comm), a late endosomal protein that targets ROBO to late endosomes/lysosomes, allowing the growing axon to cross the midline and reduce its sensibility towards slit-mediated repulsion [64]. The paramount importance of lysosomal function in axonal growth is also highlighted by the fact that inhibiting lysosome transport to the distal axon causes severe changes in size and dynamics of the growth cone [65]. As previously suggested, the impairment of lysosomal trafficking along the axon can affect growth cone homeostasis due to the lack of lysosomal degradative activity or a missing lysosomal-mediated delivery of signaling and adhesion molecules [65]. Moreover, it has been recently shown that RNA granules can also hitchhike on lysosomes to travel long distances in neurons, suggesting that the impairment of lysosomal movement could also imbalance local protein synthesis at the distal axon tip [66]. As a matter of fact, Corradi and colleagues reported that pre-miRNA can travel to the axon terminal, tagging late endosomes/lysosomes, and that SEMA3A signaling induces their maturation with consequent impact on growth cone dynamics [67]. Continuous anterograde transport of degradative active lysosomes and disrupted axon homeostasis due to lysosomal stalling have also been recently described by Farfel-Becker and colleagues, demonstrating that interference with lysosomal transport induces autophagic stress and accumulation of autophagosomes in the axons [7]. Local mitophagy has also been reported to occur in axons after induction of mitochondrial damage [68], further pointing out the relevance of lysosomal regulation and function in axons.

However, local degradation of cargos in axons is not the only mechanism by which lysosomes regulate waste removal and maintain homeostasis. As a matter of fact, retrograde transport of autophagosomes, together with their maturation and fusion with lysosomes, may suggest that the contribution of both local degradation and retrograde transport are mechanisms necessary to obtain efficient axonal clearance [69].

5. Brain Disorders with Axonal Guidance Defects

The correct assembly of neural circuits is crucial for cognitive development and interference of axonal growth, and pathfinding has been associated with the onset of neurodevelopmental disorders, such as autism, schizophrenia, and other, more rare conditions. Nonetheless, it has been progressively recognized that also in neurodegenerative disorders (for example, Parkinson's, Alzheimer's, and Huntington's disease), neural circuit impairments precede and carry over the progressive cognitive decline in affected patients [70–75]. In some inherited conditions (Table 1), a common pathological feature related to axon trajectories defects is the partial or complete agenesis of the corpus callosum (ACC), a peculiar placental mammalian-specific structure consisting of a large fiber tract that connects the two brain hemispheres [76]. Defects in corpus callosum formation and interhemispheric communication have been demonstrated in autism, schizophrenia, attention deficit hyperactivity disorders, and developmental language disorders [76]. In most cases, failure of contralateral callosal targeting, that is, the impairment of midline crossing and the contralateral positioning of the cortical callosal neurons projections, predispose subtle to gross behavioral abnormalities that severely affect diseased conditions, such as psychiatric disorders. Among identified molecular causes leading to aberrant axonal misrouting and corpus callosum agenesis or dysgenesis, mutations in the chemoattractant ligand netrin have been demonstrated to be detrimental and the leading cause of the congenital mirror movement (CMM) syndrome [77,78]. In these patients, the characteristic feature is synkinesis, that is, an involuntary movement occurring in one side of the body that mirrors intentional movements on the opposite side. This defect can also be diagnosed in patients harboring mutations in the DCC coding gene; in this latter case, partial or total ACC has been described [79,80]. While CMM abnormalities are not generally characterized by intellectual disabilities, the partial or complete ACC may be associated with mild to severe forms of developmental disabilities and cognitive impairment. Perturbed Netrin-1 signaling due to loss-of-function DCC mutations has been also described in the so-called "developmental split-brain syndrome" (DSBS), a severe neurological disease characterized by horizontal gaze palsy, scoliosis, ACC, and midline brain stem cleft [81]. In affected patients, biallelic homozygous mutations have been detected and associated with a complete absence of anterior and hippocampal commissures. Severe neurological abnormalities and intellectual disability have been also ascribed to mutations of the ROBO3 gene in the horizontal gaze palsy and progressive scoliosis (HGPPS) syndrome. In these patients, the cognitive impairment is associated with congenital absence of conjugate horizontal eye movements, preservation of vertical gaze and convergence, and progressive scoliosis developing in childhood and adolescence [82–85]. X-linked neurodevelopmental forms of intellectual disability have been also described in association with mutations of the L1CAM gene, coding for a neuronal cell adhesion molecule L1, which is involved in axon outgrowth and pathfinding, through interactions with various extracellular ligands and intracellular second messengers [86,87]. Although initially recognized as distinct clinical entities, several congenital forms characterized by L1CAM mutations are now classified as CRASH syndrome (Corpus callosum agenesis, Retardation, Adducted thumbs, Shuffling gait, and Hydrocephalus), a quite heterogeneous group of diseased conditions [88,89]. Aberrant corticospinal tract (CST) development, associated with mirror movement and hypogonadism, is due to defects in the ANOS1 gene in Kallmann syndrome. ANOS1 encodes anosmin, an extracellular glycoprotein important for the axonal guidance and migration of olfactory and Gonadotropin-Releasing Hormone (GnRH) neurons during brain development [90]. The activity of this protein has been largely investigated and has been recently shown to rely on the activation of the fibroblast growth factor (FGF) signaling pathway through a heparan sulfate-dependent mechanism [91]. A characteristic phenotypic feature related to impaired axonal guidance is also the aberrant decussation of nerve fibers. In Joubert syndrome and related disorders (JSRD), a reduced decussation of the superior cerebellar peduncles has been tied to the onset of social disabilities and synkinetic mirror movements [92,93]. The syndrome is associated with defects in several genes (at least 30), most of which play a role in the function of the primary cilium [93]. Among them, the gene ADP-ribosylation factor-like protein 13B (ARL13B) codes a small GTPase, which regulates Sonic Hedgehog (Shh) signaling, and its inactivation results in defective commissural axon guidance in vivo [94]. Another featured example of disorders of misguided axonal branching is the Duane retraction syndrome (DRS), a congenital form of strabismus caused by mutations of the α2-Chimerin [95]. This gene codes for a Rac1 GTPase-activating protein, a cytoskeletal-related protein involved in Ephrin-A-mediated spine morphogenesis [96] and required for oculomotor axon guidance targeting [97,98]. Dysgenesis of the corpus callosum and anterior commissure have been identified in patients harboring mutations in the TUBB3 gene, which cause two distinct clinical entities, named Cortical Dysplasia, Complex, with other Brain Malformations 1 (CDCBM1) and Congenital Fibrosis of the Extraocular Muscles 3 (CFEOM3) [98,99]. In both cases, the loss of function occurring in the third (III) member of the beta-tubulin protein family (TUBB3) leads to microtubule instability and axonal guidance defects in commissural axons and cranial nerves that result in intellectual and behavioral impairments and aberrant eye movement [100]. Additional *corpus callosum* defects, although with minimal or undetectable intellectual disability, have been described in the Craniofrontonasal syndrome (CFNS), in which loss-of-function Ephrin-B mutations primarily affect the boundaries of the coronal cranial suture, leading to pathological craniosinostosis [101]. While no direct evidence of abnormal decussation or impaired commissures formation has been detected in patients affected by lysosomal storage disorders, recent investigations have suggested the potential implication of axonal guidance defects in the onset of neurological abnormalities in Mucopolysaccharidosis (MPS) type II (Hunter syndrome), type IIIb (Sanfilippo syndrome), and type VII (Sly syndrome) [102–104]. In MPSII and MPSIIIb, the aberrant heparan sulfate catabolism associated with the onset of progressive severe neurological abnormalities have been tied to neuronal dysfunction and misexpression of axonal guidance cues [102,103]. Future studies will enable us to verify whether the cognitive decline observed in these and other LSD diseases is tightly related to axonal guidance-related abnormalities.

Table 1. Brain disorders in which axon guidance alterations have been described or inferred.

Disorder	Human Gene	Axon Guidance-Related Defect	Symptoms	Reference
Congenital mirror movements (CMM) and partial or complete agenesis of the *corpus callosum*	NETRIN1 (NTN1)	Corticospinal tract (CST) abnormality	Involuntary movements of one hand that mirror intentional movements of the opposite hand	[77,78]
Congenital mirror movements (CMM) and/or isolated agenesis of the *corpus callosum*	Deleted in colorectal cancer (DCC)	Decreased crossing of descending corticospinal tract projections	Variable range of intellectual disabilities, cognitive impairment, language delay, and visual and spatial deficits	[79,80]
Developmental split-brain syndrome (gaze palsy, familial horizontal, with progressive scoliosis 2, with impaired intellectual development)	Deleted in colorectal cancer (DCC)	Agenesis of the *corpus callosum* and absence of the anterior and hippocampal commissures	Neurological abnormalities, horizontal gaze palsy, intellectual disability, and progressive scoliosis	[81]
Horizontal gaze palsy with progressive scoliosis (HGPPS)	Roundabout guidance receptor 3 (ROBO3)	Abnormal flattening of the basis pontis and hypoplasia in the pontine tegmentum; anomalous innervations of the lateral rectus muscle of the eye by the abducens supranuclear nerve	Horizontal gaze palsy, intellectual disability and progressive scoliosis	[82–85]
CRASH syndrome (*Corpus callosum* agenesis, Retardation, Adducted thumbs, Shuffling gait, and Hydrocephalus)	L1CAM	Agenesis of the *corpus callosum* and corticospinal tract	Microcephaly, mental retardation, spastic paraparesis	[86,87]
Kallman syndrome (X-linked)	ANOS1 (KAL1)	Defective olfactory axon guidance and migration	Congenital anosmia, hypogonadotropic hypogonadism, mirror movements, and aberrant corticospinal tract	[89,90]
Joubert syndrome and related disorders (JSRD)	Multiple genes (AHI1, NPHP1, CEP290, TMEM67, RPGRIP1, ARL13B, CC2D2A)	Hypotonia, ataxia, mental retardation, altered respiratory patterns, social disabilities, and synkinetic mirror movements	Cerebellar vermian hypoplasia, reduction in pontine neurons, and reduced decussation of the superior cerebellar peduncles.	[92,93]
Duane retraction syndrome (DRS)	α2-CHIMERIN	Absence of *abducens* motor neurons and nerves; aberrant innervation of the lateral rectus muscle by the oculomotor nerve	Restricted horizontal gaze and ocular synkinesis	[95,96]
Cortical dysplasia, complex, with other brain malformations 1 (CDCBM1)	Beta tubulin protein family member TUBB3	Thin *corpus callosum*, hypoplastic brainstem, and dysplastic cerebellar vermis	Severe mental retardation, strabismus, axial hypotonia, and spasticity	[99]
Congenital fibrosis of the extraocular muscles 3 (CFEOM3)	Beta tubulin protein family member TUBB3	Dysgenesis of the *corpus callosum* and anterior commissure (AC), and internal capsule; generalized loss of white matter; basal ganglia dysmorphisms	Aberrant eye movements, facial weakness, axonal peripheral neuropathy, contractures of the wrist and fingers, delayed development, and learning disabilities	[100]
Craniofrontonasal syndrome (CFNS)	Ephrin B1(EFNB1)	Dysgenesis or agenesis of the *corpus callosum*	Variable difficulties in speech and language, limited or no intellectual disabilities, facial asymmetry, skeletal and dermatological abnormalities	[101]
Mucopolysaccharidosis type II (Hunter syndrome)	Iduronate sulfatase (IDS)	Indirect experimental observation	Mental retardation, language delay, cognitive impairment	[103]
Mucopolysaccharidosis type IIIb (Sanfilippo Syndrome)	α-N-acetylglucosaminidase (NAGLU)	Indirect experimental observation	Mental retardation, cognitive decline, dysphagia, sleep problems, seizures	[102]
Mucopolysaccharidosis type VII (Sly syndrome)	β-glucuronidase (GUSB)	Indirect experimental observation	developmental Delay, speech delay, intellectual disability of variable degree	[104]

6. Concluding Remarks

In light of the recent discoveries, the contribution of lysosomes to the process of axonal guidance and remodeling has gained substantial interest. The utmost importance of correct lysosomal hydrolases activity and, more in general, of lysosomal trafficking and function, pinpoints and justifies increasing research efforts towards the study of these organelles in the context of neurological disorders. Bearing in mind that lysosomal storage disorders often exhibit severe neurological abnormalities, starting from early childhood, it appears to be groundbreaking in the investigation of the functional relationship between axonal guidance and lysosomal protein activity. A more detailed understanding of this hypothetical epistatic interaction would encourage the development of more targeted therapies against neurological defects in both lysosomal disorders and neurodegenerative conditions.

Author Contributions: Conceptualization, E.M., R.M. and L.B.; writing—original draft preparation, E.M., R.M. and L.B.; writing—review and editing, E.M., R.M., L.B. and M.R.; visualization, E.M.; supervision, E.M.; project administration, E.M.; funding acquisition, E.M. All authors were involved in the reviewing and editing of the manuscript. All authors approved the final version. All authors have read and agreed to the published version of the manuscript.

Funding: This work was supported by the contribution of the National MPS Society 2019 to E.M.

Acknowledgments: We apologize for the papers that were not mentioned in the text or included in the References of the present manuscript.

Conflicts of Interest: The authors declare no conflict of interest.

References

1. Purves, D.; Lichtman, J.W. Elimination of synapses in the developing nervous system. *Science* **1980**, *210*, 153–157. [CrossRef] [PubMed]
2. Yaron, A.; Schuldiner, O. Common and Divergent Mechanisms in Developmental Neuronal Remodeling and Dying Back Neurodegeneration. *Curr. Biol.* **2016**, *26*, R628–R639. [CrossRef] [PubMed]
3. Gibson, D.A.; Ma, L. Developmental regulation of axon branching in the vertebrate nervous system. *Development* **2011**, *138*, 183–195. [CrossRef] [PubMed]
4. Yue, Z.; Friedman, L.; Komatsu, M.; Tanaka, K. The cellular pathways of neuronal autophagy and their implication in neurodegenerative diseases. *Biochim. Biophys. Acta* **2009**, *1793*, 1496–1507. [CrossRef] [PubMed]
5. Hou, X.; Watzlawik, J.O.; Fiesel, F.C.; Springer, W. Autophagy in Parkinson's Disease. *J. Mol. Biol.* **2020**, *432*, 2651–2672. [CrossRef] [PubMed]
6. Song, J.W.; Misgeld, T.; Kang, H.; Knecht, S.; Lu, J.; Cao, Y.; Cotman, S.L.; Bishop, D.L.; Lichtman, J.W. Lysosomal activity associated with developmental axon pruning. *J. Neurosci.* **2008**, *28*, 8993–9001. [CrossRef]
7. Farfel-Becker, T.; Roney, J.C.; Cheng, X.T.; Li, S.; Cuddy, S.R.; Sheng, Z.H. Neuronal Soma-Derived Degradative Lysosomes Are Continuously Delivered to Distal Axons to Maintain Local Degradation Capacity. *Cell Rep.* **2019**, *28*, 51–64.e54. [CrossRef]
8. O'Donnell, M.; Chance, R.K.; Bashaw, G.J. Axon growth and guidance: Receptor regulation and signal transduction. *Annu. Rev. Neurosci.* **2009**, *32*, 383–412. [CrossRef]
9. Kolodkin, A.L.; Matthes, D.J.; O'Connor, T.P.; Patel, N.H.; Admon, A.; Bentley, D.; Goodman, C.S. Fasciclin IV: Sequence, expression, and function during growth cone guidance in the grasshopper embryo. *Neuron* **1992**, *9*, 831–845. [CrossRef]
10. Polleux, F.; Morrow, T.; Ghosh, A. Semaphorin 3A is a chemoattractant for cortical apical dendrites. *Nature* **2000**, *404*, 567–573. [CrossRef]
11. Tamagnone, L.; Artigiani, S.; Chen, H.; He, Z.; Ming, G.I.; Song, H.; Chedotal, A.; Winberg, M.L.; Goodman, C.S.; Poo, M.; et al. Plexins are a large family of receptors for transmembrane, secreted, and GPI-anchored semaphorins in vertebrates. *Cell* **1999**, *99*, 71–80. [CrossRef]
12. Fujisawa, H. Discovery of semaphorin receptors, neuropilin and plexin, and their functions in neural development. *J. Neurobiol.* **2004**, *59*, 24–33. [CrossRef] [PubMed]
13. Sharma, A.; Verhaagen, J.; Harvey, A.R. Receptor complexes for each of the Class 3 Semaphorins. *Front. Cell Neurosci.* **2012**, *6*, 28. [CrossRef] [PubMed]
14. Pasterkamp, R.J.; Peschon, J.J.; Spriggs, M.K.; Kolodkin, A.L. Semaphorin 7A promotes axon outgrowth through integrins and MAPKs. *Nature* **2003**, *424*, 398–405. [CrossRef] [PubMed]
15. Cho, J.Y.; Chak, K.; Andreone, B.J.; Wooley, J.R.; Kolodkin, A.L. The extracellular matrix proteoglycan perlecan facilitates transmembrane semaphorin-mediated repulsive guidance. *Genes Dev.* **2012**, *26*, 2222–2235. [CrossRef]
16. Zhang, H.; Vreeken, D.; Junaid, A.; Wang, G.; Sol, W.; de Bruin, R.G.; van Zonneveld, A.J.; van Gils, J.M. Endothelial Semaphorin 3F Maintains Endothelial Barrier Function and Inhibits Monocyte Migration. *Int. J. Mol. Sci.* **2020**, *21*, 1471. [CrossRef] [PubMed]
17. Angelucci, C.; Lama, G.; Sica, G. Multifaceted Functional Role of Semaphorins in Glioblastoma. *Int. J. Mol. Sci.* **2019**, *20*, 2144. [CrossRef]
18. Cheng, H.J.; Nakamoto, M.; Bergemann, A.D.; Flanagan, J.G. Complementary gradients in expression and binding of ELF-1 and Mek4 in development of the topographic retinotectal projection map. *Cell* **1995**, *82*, 371–381. [CrossRef]
19. Egea, J.; Klein, R. Bidirectional Eph-ephrin signaling during axon guidance. *Trends Cell Biol.* **2007**, *17*, 230–238. [CrossRef]
20. Klein, R. Eph/ephrin signalling during development. *Development* **2012**, *139*, 4105–4109. [CrossRef]

21. Chenaux, G.; Henkemeyer, M. Forward signaling by EphB1/EphB2 interacting with ephrin-B ligands at the optic chiasm is required to form the ipsilateral projection. *Eur. J. Neurosci.* **2011**, *34*, 1620–1633. [CrossRef] [PubMed]
22. Pasquale, E.B. Eph receptors and ephrins in cancer: Bidirectional signalling and beyond. *Nat. Rev. Cancer.* **2010**, *10*, 165–180. [CrossRef] [PubMed]
23. Lim, Y.S.; McLaughlin, T.; Sung, T.C.; Santiago, A.; Lee, K.F.; O'Leary, D.D. p75(NTR) mediates ephrin-A reverse signaling required for axon repulsion and mapping. *Neuron* **2008**, *59*, 746–758. [CrossRef]
24. Marler, K.J.; Becker-Barroso, E.; Martínez, A.; Llovera, M.; Wentzel, C.; Poopalasundaram, S.; Hindges, R.; Soriano, E.; Comella, J.; Drescher, U. A TrkB/EphrinA interaction controls retinal axon branching and synaptogenesis. *J. Neurosci.* **2008**, *28*, 12700–12712. [CrossRef]
25. Bonanomi, D.; Chivatakarn, O.; Bai, G.; Abdesselem, H.; Lettieri, K.; Marquardt, T.; Pierchala, B.A.; Pfaff, S.L. Ret is a multifunctional coreceptor that integrates diffusible- and contact-axon guidance signals. *Cell* **2012**, *148*, 568–582. [CrossRef]
26. Monnier, P.P.; Sierra, A.; Macchi, P.; Deitinghoff, L.; Andersen, J.S.; Mann, M.; Flad, M.; Hornberger, M.R.; Stahl, B.; Bonhoeffer, F.; et al. RGM is a repulsive guidance molecule for retinal axons. *Nature* **2002**, *419*, 392–395. [CrossRef]
27. Rajagopalan, S.; Deitinghoff, L.; Davis, D.; Conrad, S.; Skutella, T.; Chedotal, A.; Mueller, B.K.; Strittmatter, S.M. Neogenin mediates the action of repulsive guidance molecule. *Nat. Cell Biol.* **2004**, *6*, 756–762. [CrossRef] [PubMed]
28. Kee, N.; Wilson, N.; De Vries, M.; Bradford, D.; Key, B.; Cooper, H.M. Neogenin and RGMa control neural tube closure and neuroepithelial morphology by regulating cell polarity. *J. Neurosci.* **2008**, *28*, 12643–12653. [CrossRef]
29. Lah, G.J.; Key, B. Novel roles of the chemorepellent axon guidance molecule RGMa in cell migration and adhesion. *Mol. Cell Biol.* **2012**, *32*, 968–980. [CrossRef]
30. Muramatsu, R.; Kubo, T.; Mori, M.; Nakamura, Y.; Fujita, Y.; Akutsu, T.; Okuno, T.; Taniguchi, J.; Kumanogoh, A.; Yoshida, M.; et al. RGMa modulates T cell responses and is involved in autoimmune encephalomyelitis. *Nat. Med.* **2011**, *17*, 488–494. [CrossRef] [PubMed]
31. Malinauskas, T.; Peer, T.V.; Bishop, B.; Mueller, T.D.; Siebold, C. Repulsive guidance molecules lock growth differentiation factor 5 in an inhibitory complex. *Proc. Natl. Acad. Sci. USA* **2020**, *117*, 15620–15631. [CrossRef]
32. Lai Wing Sun, K.; Correia, J.P.; Kennedy, T.E. Netrins: Versatile extracellular cues with diverse functions. *Development* **2011**, *138*, 2153–2169. [CrossRef] [PubMed]
33. Lin, J.C.; Ho, W.H.; Gurney, A.; Rosenthal, A. The netrin-G1 ligand NGL-1 promotes the outgrowth of thalamocortical axons. *Nat. Neurosci.* **2003**, *6*, 1270–1276. [CrossRef] [PubMed]
34. Nishimura-Akiyoshi, S.; Niimi, K.; Nakashiba, T.; Itohara, S. Axonal netrin-Gs transneuronally determine lamina-specific subdendritic segments. *Proc. Natl. Acad. Sci. USA* **2007**, *104*, 14801–14806. [CrossRef] [PubMed]
35. Fujita, Y.; Nakanishi, T.; Ueno, M.; Itohara, S.; Yamashita, T. Netrin-G1 Regulates Microglial Accumulation along Axons and Supports the Survival of Layer V Neurons in the Postnatal Mouse Brain. *Cell Rep.* **2020**, *31*, 107580. [CrossRef] [PubMed]
36. Hedgecock, E.M.; Culotti, J.G.; Hall, D.H. The unc-5, unc-6, and unc-40 genes guide circumferential migrations of pioneer axons and mesodermal cells on the epidermis in C. elegans. *Neuron* **1990**, *4*, 61–85. [CrossRef]
37. Finci, L.I.; Kruger, N.; Sun, X.; Zhang, J.; Chegkazi, M.; Wu, Y.; Schenk, G.; Mertens, H.D.T.; Svergun, D.I.; Zhang, Y.; et al. The crystal structure of netrin-1 in complex with DCC reveals the bifunctionality of netrin-1 as a guidance cue. *Neuron* **2014**, *83*, 839–849. [CrossRef]
38. Keino-Masu, K.; Masu, M.; Hinck, L.; Leonardo, E.D.; Chan, S.S.; Culotti, J.G.; Tessier-Lavigne, M. Deleted in Colorectal Cancer (DCC) encodes a netrin receptor. *Cell* **1996**, *87*, 175–185. [CrossRef]
39. Gad, J.M.; Keeling, S.L.; Shu, T.; Richards, L.J.; Cooper, H.M. The spatial and temporal expression patterns of netrin receptors, DCC and neogenin, in the developing mouse retina. *Exp. Eye Res.* **2000**, *70*, 711–722. [CrossRef]
40. Shu, T.; Valentino, K.M.; Seaman, C.; Cooper, H.M.; Richards, L.J. Expression of the netrin-1 receptor, deleted in colorectal cancer (DCC), is largely confined to projecting neurons in the developing forebrain. *J. Comp. Neurol.* **2000**, *416*, 201–212. [CrossRef]
41. Hamelin, M.; Zhou, Y.; Su, M.W.; Scott, I.M.; Culotti, J.G. Expression of the UNC-5 guidance receptor in the touch neurons of C. elegans steers their axons dorsally. *Nature* **1993**, *364*, 327–330. [CrossRef] [PubMed]
42. Kolodziej, P.A.; Timpe, L.C.; Mitchell, K.J.; Fried, S.R.; Goodman, C.S.; Jan, L.Y.; Jan, Y.N. frazzled encodes a Drosophila member of the DCC immunoglobulin subfamily and is required for CNS and motor axon guidance. *Cell* **1996**, *87*, 197–204. [CrossRef]
43. Fazeli, A.; Dickinson, S.L.; Hermiston, M.L.; Tighe, R.V.; Steen, R.G.; Small, C.G.; Stoeckli, E.T.; Keino-Masu, K.; Masu, M.; Rayburn, H.; et al. Phenotype of mice lacking functional Deleted in colorectal cancer (Dcc) gene. *Nature* **1997**, *386*, 796–804. [CrossRef] [PubMed]
44. Colavita, A.; Krishna, S.; Zheng, H.; Padgett, R.W.; Culotti, J.G. Pioneer axon guidance by UNC-129, a C. elegans TGF-beta. *Science* **1998**, *281*, 706–709. [CrossRef] [PubMed]
45. Rothberg, J.M.; Hartley, D.A.; Walther, Z.; Artavanis-Tsakonas, S. Slit: An EGF-homologous locus of D. melanogaster involved in the development of the embryonic central nervous system. *Cell* **1988**, *55*, 1047–1059. [CrossRef]
46. Dickson, B.J.; Gilestro, G.F. Regulation of commissural axon pathfinding by slit and its Robo receptors. *Annu. Rev. Cell Dev. Biol.* **2006**, *22*, 651–675. [CrossRef]
47. Nguyen Ba-Charvet, K.T.; Brose, K.; Ma, L.; Wang, K.H.; Marillat, V.; Sotelo, C.; Tessier-Lavigne, M.; Chedotal, A. Diversity and specificity of actions of Slit2 proteolytic fragments in axon guidance. *J. Neurosci.* **2001**, *21*, 4281–4289. [CrossRef]

48. Delloye-Bourgeois, C.; Jacquier, A.; Charoy, C.; Reynaud, F.; Nawabi, H.; Thoinet, K.; Kindbeiter, K.; Yoshida, Y.; Zagar, Y.; Kong, Y.; et al. PlexinA1 is a new Slit receptor and mediates axon guidance function of Slit C-terminal fragments. *Nat. Neurosci.* **2015**, *18*, 36–45. [CrossRef]
49. Kidd, T.; Brose, K.; Mitchell, K.J.; Fetter, R.D.; Tessier-Lavigne, M.; Goodman, C.S.; Tear, G. Roundabout controls axon crossing of the CNS midline and defines a novel subfamily of evolutionarily conserved guidance receptors. *Cell* **1998**, *92*, 205–215. [CrossRef]
50. Zelina, P.; Blockus, H.; Zagar, Y.; Peres, A.; Friocourt, F.; Wu, Z.; Rama, N.; Fouquet, C.; Hohenester, E.; Tessier-Lavigne, M.; et al. Signaling switch of the axon guidance receptor Robo3 during vertebrate evolution. *Neuron* **2014**, *84*, 1258–1272. [CrossRef]
51. Pak, J.S.; DeLoughery, Z.J.; Wang, J.; Acharya, N.; Park, Y.; Jaworski, A.; Ozkan, E. NELL2-Robo3 complex structure reveals mechanisms of receptor activation for axon guidance. *Nat. Commun.* **2020**, *11*, 1489. [CrossRef] [PubMed]
52. Morlot, C.; Thielens, N.M.; Ravelli, R.B.; Hemrika, W.; Romijn, R.A.; Gros, P.; Cusack, S.; McCarthy, A.A. Structural insights into the Slit-Robo complex. *Proc. Natl. Acad. Sci. USA* **2007**, *104*, 14923–14928. [CrossRef] [PubMed]
53. Koch, A.W.; Mathivet, T.; Larrivee, B.; Tong, R.K.; Kowalski, J.; Pibouin-Fragner, L.; Bouvree, K.; Stawicki, S.; Nicholes, K.; Rathore, N.; et al. Robo4 maintains vessel integrity and inhibits angiogenesis by interacting with UNC5B. *Dev. Cell* **2011**, *20*, 33–46. [CrossRef] [PubMed]
54. Fukuhara, N.; Howitt, J.A.; Hussain, S.A.; Hohenester, E. Structural and functional analysis of slit and heparin binding to immunoglobulin-like domains 1 and 2 of Drosophila Robo. *J. Biol. Chem.* **2008**, *283*, 16226–16234. [CrossRef] [PubMed]
55. Gorla, M.; Bashaw, G.J. Molecular mechanisms regulating axon responsiveness at the midline. *Dev. Biol.* **2020**, *466*, 12–21. [CrossRef] [PubMed]
56. Stein, E.; Tessier-Lavigne, M. Hierarchical organization of guidance receptors: Silencing of netrin attraction by slit through a Robo/DCC receptor complex. *Science* **2001**, *291*, 1928–1938. [CrossRef] [PubMed]
57. Pignata, A.; Ducuing, H.; Boubakar, L.; Gardette, T.; Kindbeiter, K.; Bozon, M.; Tauszig-Delamasure, S.; Falk, J.; Thoumine, O.; Castellani, V. A Spatiotemporal Sequence of Sensitization to Slits and Semaphorins Orchestrates Commissural Axon Navigation. *Cell Rep.* **2019**, *29*, 347–362.e345. [CrossRef]
58. Croteau, L.P.; Kao, T.J.; Kania, A. Ephrin-A5 potentiates netrin-1 axon guidance by enhancing Neogenin availability. *Sci. Rep.* **2019**, *9*, 12009. [CrossRef]
59. Pasterkamp, R.J.; Burk, K. Axon guidance receptors: Endocytosis, trafficking and downstream signaling from endosomes. *Prog. Neurobiol.* **2020**, 101916. [CrossRef]
60. Winckler, B.; Yap, C.C. Endocytosis and endosomes at the crossroads of regulating trafficking of axon outgrowth-modifying receptors. *Traffic* **2011**, *12*, 1099–1108. [CrossRef]
61. Szymanska, E.; Budick-Harmelin, N.; Miaczynska, M. Endosomal "sort" of signaling control: The role of ESCRT machinery in regulation of receptor-mediated signaling pathways. *Semin. Cell Dev. Biol.* **2018**, *74*, 11–20. [CrossRef]
62. Boissier, P.; Chen, J.; Huynh-Do, U. EphA2 signaling following endocytosis: Role of Tiam1. *Traffic* **2013**, *14*, 1255–1271. [CrossRef] [PubMed]
63. Tanaka, M.; Ohashi, R.; Nakamura, R.; Shinmura, K.; Kamo, T.; Sakai, R.; Sugimura, H. Tiam1 mediates neurite outgrowth induced by ephrin-B1 and EphA2. *EMBO J.* **2004**, *23*, 1075–1088. [CrossRef] [PubMed]
64. Keleman, K.; Rajagopalan, S.; Cleppien, D.; Teis, D.; Paiha, K.; Huber, L.A.; Technau, G.M.; Dickson, B.J. Comm sorts robo to control axon guidance at the Drosophila midline. *Cell* **2002**, *110*, 415–427. [CrossRef]
65. Farias, G.G.; Guardia, C.M.; De Pace, R.; Britt, D.J.; Bonifacino, J.S. BORC/kinesin-1 ensemble drives polarized transport of lysosomes into the axon. *Proc. Natl. Acad. Sci. USA* **2017**, *114*, E2955–E2964. [CrossRef] [PubMed]
66. Liao, Y.C.; Fernandopulle, M.S.; Wang, G.; Choi, H.; Hao, L.; Drerup, C.M.; Patel, R.; Qamar, S.; Nixon-Abell, J.; Shen, Y.; et al. RNA Granules Hitchhike on Lysosomes for Long-Distance Transport, Using Annexin A11 as a Molecular Tether. *Cell* **2019**, *179*, 147–164.e120. [CrossRef]
67. Corradi, E.; Dalla Costa, I.; Gavoci, A.; Iyer, A.; Roccuzzo, M.; Otto, T.A.; Oliani, E.; Bridi, S.; Strohbuecker, S.; Santos-Rodriguez, G.; et al. Axonal precursor miRNAs hitchhike on endosomes and locally regulate the development of neural circuits. *EMBO J.* **2020**, *39*, e102513. [CrossRef] [PubMed]
68. Ashrafi, G.; Schlehe, J.S.; LaVoie, M.J.; Schwarz, T.L. Mitophagy of damaged mitochondria occurs locally in distal neuronal axons and requires PINK1 and Parkin. *J. Cell Biol.* **2014**, *206*, 655–670. [CrossRef]
69. Maday, S.; Wallace, K.E.; Holzbaur, E.L. Autophagosomes initiate distally and mature during transport toward the cell soma in primary neurons. *J. Cell Biol.* **2012**, *196*, 407–417. [CrossRef]
70. Canter, R.G.; Penney, J.; Tsai, L.H. The road to restoring neural circuits for the treatment of Alzheimer's disease. *Nature* **2016**, *539*, 187–196. [CrossRef]
71. Caligiore, D.; Helmich, R.C.; Hallett, M.; Moustafa, A.A.; Timmermann, L.; Toni, I.; Baldassarre, G. Parkinson's disease as a system-level disorder. *NPJ Parkinsons Dis.* **2016**, *2*, 16025. [CrossRef] [PubMed]
72. Busche, M.A.; Konnerth, A. Impairments of neural circuit function in Alzheimer's disease. *Philos. Trans. R. Soc. Lond. B Biol. Sci.* **2016**, *371*. [CrossRef] [PubMed]
73. McGregor, M.M.; Nelson, A.B. Circuit Mechanisms of Parkinson's Disease. *Neuron* **2019**, *101*, 1042–1056. [CrossRef] [PubMed]
74. Blumenstock, S.; Dudanova, I. Cortical and Striatal Circuits in Huntington's Disease. *Front. Neurosci.* **2020**, *14*, 82. [CrossRef]
75. Harris, S.S.; Wolf, F.; De Strooper, B.; Busche, M.A. Tipping the Scales: Peptide-Dependent Dysregulation of Neural Circuit Dynamics in Alzheimer's Disease. *Neuron* **2020**, *107*, 417–435. [CrossRef]

76. Fenlon, L.R.; Richards, L.J. Contralateral targeting of the *crpus callosum* in normal and pathological brain function. *Trends Neurosci.* 2015, *38*, 264–272. [CrossRef]
77. Meneret, A.; Franz, E.A.; Trouillard, O.; Oliver, T.C.; Zagar, Y.; Robertson, S.P.; Welniarz, Q.; Gardner, R.J.M.; Gallea, C.; Srour, M.; et al. Mutations in the netrin-1 gene cause congenital mirror movements. *J. Clin. Investig.* 2017, *127*, 3923–3936. [CrossRef]
78. Srour, M.; Riviere, J.B.; Pham, J.M.; Dube, M.P.; Girard, S.; Morin, S.; Dion, P.A.; Asselin, G.; Rochefort, D.; Hince, P.; et al. Mutations in DCC cause congenital mirror movements. *Science* 2010, *328*, 592. [CrossRef]
79. Marsh, A.P.; Heron, D.; Edwards, T.J.; Quartier, A.; Galea, C.; Nava, C.; Rastetter, A.; Moutard, M.L.; Anderson, V.; Bitoun, P.; et al. Mutations in DCC cause isolated agenesis of the *Corpus callosum* with incomplete penetrance. *Nat. Genet.* 2017, *49*, 511–514. [CrossRef]
80. Marsh, A.P.L.; Edwards, T.J.; Galea, C.; Cooper, H.M.; Engle, E.C.; Jamuar, S.S.; Meneret, A.; Moutard, M.L.; Nava, C.; Rastetter, A.; et al. DCC mutation update: Congenital mirror movements, isolated agenesis of the *Corpus callosum*, and developmental split brain syndrome. *Hum. Mutat.* 2018, *39*, 23–39. [CrossRef]
81. Jamuar, S.S.; Schmitz-Abe, K.; D'Gama, A.M.; Drottar, M.; Chan, W.M.; Peeva, M.; Servattalab, S.; Lam, A.N.; Delgado, M.R.; Clegg, N.J.; et al. Biallelic mutations in human DCC cause developmental split-brain syndrome. *Nat. Genet.* 2017, *49*, 606–612. [CrossRef] [PubMed]
82. Jen, J.C.; Chan, W.M.; Bosley, T.M.; Wan, J.; Carr, J.R.; Rub, U.; Shattuck, D.; Salamon, G.; Kudo, L.C.; Ou, J.; et al. Mutations in a human ROBO gene disrupt hindbrain axon pathway crossing and morphogenesis. *Science* 2004, *304*, 1509–1513. [CrossRef] [PubMed]
83. Chan, W.M.; Traboulsi, E.I.; Arthur, B.; Friedman, N.; Andrews, C.; Engle, E.C. Horizontal gaze palsy with progressive scoliosis can result from compound heterozygous mutations in ROBO3. *J. Med. Genet.* 2006, *43*, e11. [CrossRef] [PubMed]
84. Volk, A.E.; Carter, O.; Fricke, J.; Herkenrath, P.; Poggenborg, J.; Borck, G.; Demant, A.W.; Ivo, R.; Eysel, P.; Kubisch, C.; et al. Horizontal gaze palsy with progressive scoliosis: Three novel ROBO3 mutations and descriptions of the phenotypes of four patients. *Mol. Vis.* 2011, *17*, 1978–1986. [PubMed]
85. Xiu, Y.; Lv, Z.; Wang, D.; Chen, X.; Huang, S.; Pan, M. Introducing and Reviewing a Novel Mutation of ROBO3 in Horizontal Gaze Palsy with Progressive Scoliosis from a Chinese Family. *J. Mol. Neurosci.* 2020. [CrossRef] [PubMed]
86. Wong, E.V.; Kenwrick, S.; Willems, P.; Lemmon, V. Mutations in the cell adhesion molecule L1 cause mental retardation. *Trends Neurosci.* 1995, *18*, 168–172. [CrossRef]
87. Fransen, E.; Van Camp, G.; Vits, L.; Willems, P.J. L1-associated diseases: Clinical geneticists divide, molecular geneticists unite. *Hum. Mol. Genet.* 1997, *6*, 1625–1632. [CrossRef]
88. Engle, E.C. Human genetic disorders of axon guidance. *Cold Spring Harb. Perspect. Biol.* 2010, *2*, a001784. [CrossRef]
89. Dode, C.; Hardelin, J.P. Clinical genetics of Kallmann syndrome. *Ann. Endocrinol. (Paris)* 2010, *71*, 149–157. [CrossRef]
90. Soussi-Yanicostas, N.; de Castro, F.; Julliard, A.K.; Perfettini, I.; Chedotal, A.; Petit, C. Anosmin-1, defective in the X-linked form of Kallmann syndrome, promotes axonal branch formation from olfactory bulb output neurons. *Cell* 2002, *109*, 217–228. [CrossRef]
91. Gonzalez-Martinez, D.; Kim, S.H.; Hu, Y.; Guimond, S.; Schofield, J.; Winyard, P.; Vannelli, G.B.; Turnbull, J.; Bouloux, P.M. Anosmin-1 modulates fibroblast growth factor receptor 1 signaling in human gonadotropin-releasing hormone olfactory neuroblasts through a heparan sulfate-dependent mechanism. *J. Neurosci.* 2004, *24*, 10384–10392. [CrossRef] [PubMed]
92. Guo, J.; Otis, J.M.; Suciu, S.K.; Catalano, C.; Xing, L.; Constable, S.; Wachten, D.; Gupton, S.; Lee, J.; Lee, A.; et al. Primary Cilia Signaling Promotes Axonal Tract Development and Is Disrupted in Joubert Syndrome-Related Disorders Models. *Dev. Cell.* 2019, *51*, 759–774.e755. [CrossRef] [PubMed]
93. Parisi, M.A. The molecular genetics of Joubert syndrome and related ciliopathies: The challenges of genetic and phenotypic heterogeneity. *Transl. Sci. Rare Dis.* 2019, *4*, 25–49. [CrossRef] [PubMed]
94. Ferent, J.; Constable, S.; Gigante, E.D.; Yam, P.T.; Mariani, L.E.; Legue, E.; Liem, K.F., Jr.; Caspary, T.; Charron, F. The Ciliary Protein Arl13b Functions Outside of the Primary Cilium in Shh-Mediated Axon Guidance. *Cell Rep.* 2019, *29*, 3356–3366.e3353. [CrossRef] [PubMed]
95. Miyake, N.; Chilton, J.; Psatha, M.; Cheng, L.; Andrews, C.; Chan, W.M.; Law, K.; Crosier, M.; Lindsay, S.; Cheung, M.; et al. Human CHN1 mutations hyperactivate alpha2-chimaerin and cause Duane's retraction syndrome. *Science* 2008, *321*, 839–843. [CrossRef] [PubMed]
96. Nugent, A.A.; Park, J.G.; Wei, Y.; Tenney, A.P.; Gilette, N.M.; DeLisle, M.M.; Chan, W.M.; Cheng, L.; Engle, E.C. Mutant alpha2-chimaerin signals via bidirectional ephrin pathways in Duane retraction syndrome. *J. Clin. Investig.* 2017, *127*, 1664–1682. [CrossRef]
97. Ferrario, J.E.; Baskaran, P.; Clark, C.; Hendry, A.; Lerner, O.; Hintze, M.; Allen, J.; Chilton, J.K.; Guthrie, S. Axon guidance in the developing ocular motor system and Duane retraction syndrome depends on Semaphorin signaling via alpha2-chimaerin. *Proc. Natl. Acad. Sci. USA* 2012, *109*, 14669–14674. [CrossRef]
98. Clark, C.; Austen, O.; Poparic, I.; Guthrie, S. Alpha2-Chimaerin regulates a key axon guidance transition during development of the oculomotor projection. *J. Neurosci.* 2013, *33*, 16540–16551. [CrossRef]
99. Poirier, K.; Saillour, Y.; Bahi-Buisson, N.; Jaglin, X.H.; Fallet-Bianco, C.; Nabbout, R.; Castelnau-Ptakhine, L.; Roubertie, A.; Attie-Bitach, T.; Desguerre, I.; et al. Mutations in the neuronal ss-tubulin subunit TUBB3 result in malformation of cortical development and neuronal migration defects. *Hum. Mol. Genet.* 2010, *19*, 4462–4473. [CrossRef]

100. Tischfield, M.A.; Baris, H.N.; Wu, C.; Rudolph, G.; Van Maldergem, L.; He, W.; Chan, W.M.; Andrews, C.; Demer, J.L.; Robertson, R.L.; et al. Human TUBB3 mutations perturb microtubule dynamics, kinesin interactions, and axon guidance. *Cell* **2010**, *140*, 74–87. [CrossRef]
101. Twigg, S.R.F.; Kan, R.; Babbs, C.; Bochukova, E.G.; Robertson, S.P.; Wall, S.A.; Morriss-Kay, G.M.; Wilkie, A.O.M. Mutations of ephrin-B1 (EFNB1), a marker of tissue boundary formation, cause craniofrontonasal syndrome. *Proc. Natl. Acad. Sci. USA* **2004**, *101*, 8652–8657. [CrossRef] [PubMed]
102. Lemonnier, T.; Blanchard, S.; Toli, D.; Roy, E.; Bigou, S.; Froissart, R.; Rouvet, I.; Vitry, S.; Heard, J.M.; Bohl, D. Modeling neuronal defects associated with a lysosomal disorder using patient-derived induced pluripotent stem cells. *Hum. Mol. Genet.* **2011**, *20*, 3653–3666. [CrossRef] [PubMed]
103. Salvalaio, M.; D'Avanzo, F.; Rigon, L.; Zanetti, A.; D'Angelo, M.; Valle, G.; Scarpa, M.; Tomanin, R. Brain RNA-Seq Profiling of the Mucopolysaccharidosis Type II Mouse Model. *Int. J. Mol. Sci.* **2017**, *18*, 1072. [CrossRef] [PubMed]
104. Parente, M.K.; Rozen, R.; Cearley, C.N.; Wolfe, J.H. Dysregulation of gene expression in a lysosomal storage disease varies between brain regions implicating unexpected mechanisms of neuropathology. *PLoS ONE* **2012**, *7*, e32419. [CrossRef] [PubMed]

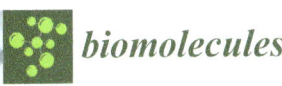

Article

Visual System Impairment in a Mouse Model of Krabbe Disease: The Twitcher Mouse

Ilaria Tonazzini [1,†], Chiara Cerri [2,3,†], Ambra Del Grosso [1], Sara Antonini [1], Manuela Allegra [2,4], Matteo Caleo [2,5] and Marco Cecchini [1,*]

1 NEST, Istituto Nanoscienze-CNR and Scuola Normale Superiore, Piazza San Silvestro 12, 56127 Pisa, Italy; ilaria.tonazzini@sns.it (I.T.); ambra.delgrosso@sns.it (A.D.G.); sara.antonini@gmail.com (S.A.)
2 Istituto Neuroscienze-CNR, Via G. Moruzzi 1, 56124 Pisa, Italy; chiara.cerri@unipi.it (C.C.); manuela.allegra84@gmail.com (M.A.); matteo.caleo@unipd.it (M.C.)
3 Department of Pharmacy, University of Pisa, Via Bonanno Pisano 6, 56126 Pisa, Italy
4 Department of Neuroscience, Institut Pasteur, 25 Rue du Dr Roux, 75015 Paris, France
5 Department of Biomedical Sciences, University of Padua, Viale G. Colombo 3, 35131 Padua, Italy
* Correspondence: marco.cecchini@nano.cnr.it
† These authors equally contributed to the work.

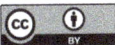

Citation: Tonazzini, I.; Cerri, C.; Del Grosso, A.; Antonini, S.; Allegra, M.; Caleo, M.; Cecchini, M. Visual System Impairment in a Mouse Model of Krabbe Disease: The Twitcher Mouse. *Biomolecules* **2021**, *11*, 7. https://dx.doi.org/10.3390/biom11010007

Received: 11 November 2020
Accepted: 19 December 2020
Published: 23 December 2020

Publisher's Note: MDPI stays neutral with regard to jurisdictional claims in published maps and institutional affiliations.

Copyright: © 2020 by the authors. Licensee MDPI, Basel, Switzerland. This article is an open access article distributed under the terms and conditions of the Creative Commons Attribution (CC BY) license (https://creativecommons.org/licenses/by/4.0/).

Abstract: Krabbe disease (KD, or globoid cell leukodystrophy; OMIM #245200) is an inherited neurodegenerative condition belonging to the class of the lysosomal storage disorders. It is caused by genetic alterations in the gene encoding for the enzyme galactosylceramidase, which is responsible for cleaving the glycosydic linkage of galatosylsphingosine (psychosine or PSY), a highly cytotoxic molecule. Here, we describe morphological and functional alterations in the visual system of the Twitcher (TWI) mouse, the most used animal model of Krabbe disease. We report in vivo electrophysiological recordings showing defective basic functional properties of the TWI primary visual cortex. In particular, we demonstrate a reduced visual acuity and contrast sensitivity, and a delayed visual response. Specific neuropathological alterations are present in the TWI visual cortex, with reduced myelination, increased astrogliosis and microglia activation, and around the whole brain. Finally, we quantify PSY content in the brain and optic nerves by high-pressure liquid chromatography-mass spectrometry methods. An increasing PSY accumulation with time, the characteristic hallmark of KD, is found in both districts. These results represent the first complete characterization of the TWI visual system. Our data set a baseline for an easy testing of potential therapies for this district, which is also dramatically affected in KD patients.

Keywords: Krabbe disease; Twitcher mouse; psychosine; visual system; visual cortex; astrogliosis

1. Introduction

Krabbe disease (KD, or globoid cell leukodystrophy; OMIM #245200) is an inherited neurodegenerative condition belonging to the class of the lysosomal storage disorders (LSDs). It is caused by multiple genetic alterations in the gene encoding for the enzyme galactosylceramidase (GALC; EC 3.2.1.46) or, in some rare cases, for the Sphingolipid activator protein saposin A (SapA) [1]. The deficiency of GALC or SapA does not allow the proper functioning of the complex sphingolipid cell pathway, which is especially crucial for myelinating cells [2]. More specifically, the GALC-SapA complex is also responsible for cleaving the glycosydic linkage of galatosylsphingosine (psychosine or PSY), a highly cytotoxic molecule which is able to insert into the cell membrane, disrupt raft architecture, and presumably deregulate multiple cell signaling cascades [3,4]. Still, the exact mechanism through which this deadly molecule exerts its cytotoxicity has not been completely elucidated yet [5], even if the PSY hypothesis has been recently confirmed [6]. The most proved explanations about KD molecular pathogenesis sustain that PSY primarily causes a massive death of oligodendrocytes and Schwann cells with consequent demyelination of central and peripheral nervous system (CNS and PNS), which is followed by neurodegeneration owing to the disruption of the neuronal-glial homeostasis [7]. Widespread cell death also leads to activation of the inflammatory cascade, which recruits macrophages and activates microglia, amplifying the production of cytotoxic molecules [8]. The inflammatory response to demyelination is then followed by astrocytic gliosis [9]. In the areas of active demyelination, furthermore, multinucleated macrophages, called globoid cells, are often clustered around blood vessels [10,11]. The only available treatment for presymptomatic human patients is hematopoietic stem cell transplantation (HSCT) [10], which in a few cases could delay the symptoms onset and progression. However, at the moment no effective cure exists for KD. Available options are symptomatic and supportive only [12]. The first hallmarks of the disease are generally alteration of neuronal conduction and neurological dysfunctions. Four different clinical forms of KD are usually described according to symptom onset: infantile, late infantile, juvenile, and adult. The infantile phenotype (95% of the known cases) has usually onset within first 6 months of life and leads to death by age of 2–4 years [13–15]. Hyperirritability, hypersensitivity to the external environment, stiffness of the limbs, and episodic fever of unknown origin are firstly reported. The psychomotor functions deteriorate quickly with marked hypertonicity, and the backward bent head. At the latest stage of the disease, the infants are in a decerebrate posture and become blind and unresponsive of their surroundings. The late infantile form, instead, has onset between 6 months to 3 years. Irritability, psychomotor regression, stiffness, ataxia, and loss of vision are frequent initial symptoms. The course is progressive and results in death approximately 2 or 3 years after the onset. The juvenile form presents onset between 3 and 8 years. Patients commonly develop loss of vision, hemiparesis, ataxia, and psychomotor regression [16,17]. Adult form, whose onset is after 20 years, has a milder phenotype and a slower rate of progression, allowing sometimes a normal life span to patients. Some individuals remain stable for long periods of time, while others show a steady decline in a vegetative state and death [18]. Patients usually experience a progressive decline of their visual skills culminating with blindness.

An anatomical characteristic of KD patients visual system is an extensive demyelination of the optic nerve [19] that coexists with an early stage optic nerve enlargement due to the presence of numerous globoid cells [20,21]. Demyelination was also found in the white matter of postmortem KD brain that additionally displayed a massive gliosis [19]. Beside the general white matter volume loss in the brain of children with KD disease, alterations of visual system in KD patients have been reported in the clinic also in terms of functionality. Indeed, electroencephalographic recordings upon visual stimulation showed abnormal visual evoked potential (VEP) response in KD patients [15,22].

As evident, common features of all clinical KD forms are defects of the visual system. However, although visual system impairment is a significant hallmark of KD, it has not yet received much attention from the scientific community, and has not yet been sufficiently characterized. For example, a detailed analysis of which visual response parameters are compromised in KD is still lacking and almost nothing has been investigated about the visual system in the most used mouse model, the Twitcher mouse (TWI). The TWI mouse presents an autosomal recessive mutation in the GALC gene with no counterpart in humans [23], and pathological phenotype closely recapitulates human pathology [24,25]. TWI mice are the most used animal model for the testing of experimental therapies for KD, such as enzyme replacement therapies or gene therapy [26,27]. With the disease progression animals experience severe tremors, paralysis of hind legs and neck muscles, important weight loss, and demyelization, and lifespan rarely extends beyond PND40 [9,23]. Rather than for KD, visual defects have been broadly studied and found in animal models of other LSDs, such as the Cystinosis (CTSN) [28,29], Sandhoff and GM1 gangliosidosis [30], and Mucopolysaccharidosis type IIIA [31].

In the present study, for the first time, we investigate the visual system of the TWI mouse. We report in vivo electrophysiological recordings of the basic functional properties (acuity, contrast sensitivity, and visual evoked potentials latency) of the primary visual cortex of TWI mice (PND 30-36). In parallel, we investigate the presence of neuropathological alterations in TWI CNS tissues, as possible biomarkers of TWI condition, and quantify the PSY content in brain and optic nerves.

2. Materials and Methods

2.1. Animals

Twitcher heterozygous mice (TWI$^{+/-}$ C57BL6 mice; Jackson Labs), kindly donated by Dr. A. Biffi (San Raffaele Telethon Institute for Gene Therapy, Milan, Italy), were used as breeder pairs to generate homozygous TWI$^{-/-}$ mice (TWI). Animals were maintained under standard housing conditions and used according to the protocols and ethical guidelines approved by the Ministry of Health (Permit Numbers: CBS-not. 0517, approved the 04/01/2018; 535/2018-PR, approved 09/07/2018). For genotyping purpose, mice genomic DNA was extracted from clipped tails by Proteinase K digestion and subsequent genomic DNA extraction (EUROGOLD Tissue-DNA Mini Kit, EuroClone), as previously reported. The genetic status of each mouse was later determined from the genome analysis of the TWI mutation, as reported from [9,32]. TWI and WT (TWI$^{+/+}$) littermate animals at postnatal day (PND) between PND20 and PND43 were used for experiments, while the heterozygous (TWI$^{+/-}$) littermates were retained for the colony maintenance.

2.2. Visual Cortex Recording

Electrophysiological recordings were performed as described previously [33,34]. Mice were anesthetized with Hypnorm/Hypnovel (in water; 0.3 mL/20 g; VetaPharma, Leeds, UK) and placed in a stereotaxic apparatus. A portion of the skull overlying the binocular visual cortex was drilled on one side. A tungsten electrode (1 MΩ; FHC, Bowdoin, ME, USA) was mounted on a three-axis motorized micromanipulator (Scientifica, Uckfield East Sussex, UK) and inserted into the binocular portion of the visual cortex (approximately 2.9 mm lateral from midline and in correspondence with lambda in PND30-36 mice). VEPs were recorded from 3 to 4 penetrations/animal and the electrode was positioned at 100 and 400 µm depth within the cortex. Electrical signals were amplified (10,000-fold), band-pass filtered (0.3–100 Hz), digitized, and averaged in synchrony with the stimulus contrast reversal (temporal frequency, 1 Hz). Analysis of the amplitude of VEP responses was performed blind to animal genotype. Visual stimuli were gratings of various spatial frequencies and contrast generated by a VSG2/5 card (Cambridge Research Systems, Rochester, UK) on a display (Sony Multiscan G500; Sony Europe B.V., Milano, Italy; mean luminance, 15 cd/m^2) that was positioned 20–30 cm in front of the mouse eyes to include the central visual field (110 × 85° of visual angle).

The visual response was measured as the peak to through amplitude (µV). We also collected the responses to 0% contrast (blank stimuli) to measure noise level. Visual acuity (c/deg) was assessed after presentation of gratings of variable spatial frequencies (90% contrast). Contrast threshold was determined via the presentation of gratings of different contrasts and fixed spatial frequency (0.06 c/deg). Visual acuity and contrast threshold were determined as the highest spatial frequency and lowest contrast that evoked a VEP response greater than the mean value of the noise. We used $n = 7$ TWI and $n = 6$ WT mice, age range PND30-36.

2.3. Immunohistochemistry and Confocal Imaging

TWI and WT mice ($n = 4$ for each genotype, PND21-36) were deeply anesthetized and perfused transcardially with phosphate buffer saline (PBS) and subsequently with 4% paraformaldehyde (PFA). After perfusion, the brains were stored at 4 °C in a 4% PFA solution for minimum 2 days. Consecutive coronal sections of the visual cortex, 50 µm thick, were cut with a microtome (VT 1000 S, Leica BIOSYSTEM, Buccinasco (MI), Italy) Sections were maintained at 4 °C in PBS until use. For the immunohistochemistry staining [35], sections were transferred in a 24 well cell culture plate (maximum of 3 sections per well) and incubated with blocking solution (3% bovine serum albumin, 0.3% Triton X-100 in

PBS; 1 mL per well) for 1 h at room temperature (RT). Then, the blocking solution was removed and the primary antibody mix (1% BSA, 0.3% Triton X-100, antibody at the optimal dilution and PBS to reach 1 mL) was added to the well and left overnight at 4° under gentle shaking. We used the following antibodies: anti-GFAP (ab7260 Abcam, 1:1000), anti-MBP (ab980 Merck Millipore, 1:500), and anti-Iba-1 (Wako 019/1974, 1:500). The next morning, primary antibody solution was removed and 3 washes with 1 mL of PBS were made (10 min each). Then, secondary antibody solution was added (BSA 1%, Triton X-100 0.3%, antimouse, or antirabbit Alexa 647 1:1000, antimouse or anti-rabbit Alexa 488 1:000 and PBS to reach 1 mL total volume). After 2 h of incubation at RT, other 3 washes with PBS were made. Sections were then stained with a Hoechst solution for 1 min and then mounted on SUPERFROST Microscope Slides (Thermo Scientific Waltham, MA, USA) with Vectashield Antifade Mounting Medium (VECTOR LABORATORIES), also with DAPI. Finally, slides were sealed and stored at 4 °C until confocal imaging.

Cortical sections were examined with a Leica Confocal microscope, Buccinasco (MI), Italy using a 10× air objective. For each section, confocal series of a step size of 2 µm were obtained throughout the whole section thickness (50 µm) and collapsed as an average. Acquisition parameters of each labeling (width along the z-axes, laser intensity, photomultiplier gain, and pinhole size) were kept constant for both experimental groups (TWI and WT mice).

2.4. Western Blot

Western blot analysis on brain lysates was performed to assess the levels of MBP, GFAP, and Iba-1 proteins, such as biomarkers of demyelination, astrogliosis, and microglia-macrophages activation, respectively. For mouse tissues, the extracted brains (without olfactory bulbs and cerebellum) were lysed on ice in RIPA buffer (Merck KGaA, Darmstadt, Germany R0278) containing protease and phosphatase inhibitors cocktail (cOmplete and PhosSTOP, Roche Diagnostics, Basel, Switzerland). Brain lysates were centrifuged (15,000× g for 25 min, 4 °C), and then, the supernatants were tested for protein concentration by a protein assay kit (Micro BCA™, Thermo Scientific Pierce). The samples were mixed with Laemmli buffer containing β-mercapto-ethanol (5% final concentration), boiled for 5 min, and used for gel electrophoresis (or kept at −80 °C). Brain lysates (60 µg/lane) were processed by immunoblot, as in [26,36]. Briefly, samples were resolved by gel electrophoresis (SDS-PAGE) using Gel Criterion XT-Precast polyacrylamide gel 4–12% Bis-Tris (Bio-Rad, Hercules, CA, USA), transferred to nitrocellulose membranes, and probed overnight at 4 °C with primary antibodies. We used the following antibodies against: GFAP (1:1000; Synaptic Systems #173211), MBP (1:1000; Abcam, ab62631), Iba-1 (1:1000; Sigma, MABN92), Tubulin (1:2000; Merck, T6074), and GAPDH (1:3000; Merck, G8795). Membranes, after incubation with the appropriate peroxidase-linked secondary antibodies (goat anti-Rabbit/Mouse IgG-HRP Conjugate, Bio-Rad; 1:2500), were developed by the ClarityTM (Bio-Rad, 170-5060) enhanced chemiluminescent (ECL) substrates. The chemiluminescent signal was acquired by ImageQuant LAS400 scanner (GE Healthcare Life Sciences, Uppsala, Sweden). The density of immunoreactive bands was quantified by ImageJ; the results were normalized to the relative total GAPDH or Tubulin protein levels (according to the more appropriate molecular weight) and reported in percentage with respect to WT levels. At least 18 mice were analyzed for each genotype; age range was PND29-43 for WT mice, and PND30-40 for TWI mice.

2.5. Psychosine and GALC Activity Quantification in TWI Tissues

Brain and optic nerve lysates, prepared as above, were used to measure the content of psychosine (PSY) in TWI mice, as in [5].

For lipid extraction, a mixture was prepared combining each lysate, N,N-dimethylsphingosine 1.250 µM (N,N-DMS, the selected internal standard for LC/MS-MS; SML0311-5MG; Merck KGaA, Darmstadt, Germany and Milli-Q water. Then, a chloroform/methanol solution (2:1) was added. Samples were vortexed, left at RT for 10 min, and supplemented with NaCl 0.9% w/v in Milli-Q water. The biphasic mixture was centrifuged at 800 g for 30 min, and the lower layer was collected and evaporated to dryness under vacuum at 30 °C. The residue was dissolved in 50 µL of methanol/formic acid 100/0.1 and processed for HPLC/MS.

HPLC/MS quantitation was performed on a Shimadzu Nexera UHPLC chromatograph (Shimadzu Europa GmbH, Duisburg, Germany) interfaced with an AB Sciex 3200 mass spectrometer (AB SCIEX). HPLC analyses were performed on a Vydac C4 1 × 250 mm column (particle size 4 µm), using water/methanol/isopropanol/formic acid 40/55/5/0.1 (A) and methanol/isopropanol/formic acid 95/5/0.1 (B) as mobile phases at 0.1 mL/min flow. Runs were performed under a 45 min linear gradient from 0% to 100% of solvent B, followed by a 5 min purge step at 100% of B and by a 10-min re-equilibration step to the starting conditions. MRM analyses were performed under the following conditions: ion spray voltage: 5000 V, source temperature 350 °C, declustering potential 50 V, collision energy variable (see value in parentheses), ion source gas 20 L/min, curtain gas: 25 L/min. The following transitions were monitored (acquisition time 150 msec/transition): (i) N,N-dimethylsphingosine (Q1/Q3, m/z, CE in parenthesis): 328.2/310.2 (26 V), 328.2/280.2 (32 V), and 328.2/110.2 (42 V) and (ii) PSY (Q1/Q3, m/z, CE in parenthesis): 462.5/444 (25 V), 462.5/282 (30 V);462.5/264 (27 V), and 462.5/252 (39 V). Transitions 328.2/310.2 (N,N-dimethylsphingosine) and 462.5/282 (PSY) were used for quantitation purposes.

We considered mice within PND= 28 such as "early stage" (PND20-28) and mice after PND = 30 such as "late stage" (PND30-38). We used $n = 7$ mice at early stage and $n = 12$ at late stage for brain analysis, while $n = 7$ mice at early stage and $n = 8$ at late stage for optic nerves.

Brain and optic nerve lysates were used also to measure GALC activity in WT and TWI mice, as reported in [26]. Results were expressed in unit per microgram ((U/ug) = unit of enzyme per microgram of cell lysate; unit (U) = amount of enzyme that catalyzes 1 nmol of substrate per hour) and reported in percentage of the activity of the WT-early. Here, we considered mice at PND = 18–21 such as "early stage" and mice after PND = 30 such as "late stage" (PND30-34).

2.6. Statistical Analysis

Data are reported as average value ± the standard error of the mean (mean ± SEM), if not differently stated. All the experiments were repeated at least three times independently for each reported dataset ($n \geq 3$ independent samples for each condition), if not differently stated. Data were statistically analyzed by GraphPad PRISM 5.00 (GraphPad Software, San Diego, CA, USA). For parametric data (the mean values obtained in each repeated experiment were assumed to be normally distributed about the true mean), Student's t-test (unpaired, two-tailed) analyses were used, if not differently stated. Statistical significance refers to the results where $p < 0.05$.

3. Results
3.1. Functional Alterations in the Visual System of the Twitcher Mouse

In order to assess the functional impairments of the TWI mouse visual system, we performed visual evoked potential (VEP) recordings and measured the basic physiological parameters of the primary visual cortex. VEPs from the binocular visual cortex were recorded in vivo in PND30-P36 mice, blind to genotype at a depth of 100 or 400 µm into the cortex in response to patterned stimuli. Cortical spatial resolution (visual acuity) and contrast sensitivity, well-established measures of overall rodent as well as human visual function [37–39], were both impaired in the primary visual cortex of TWI mice (Figure 1). Indeed, we found a lower visual acuity (Figure 1A) and an increased contrast threshold (Figure 1B) in TWI mice in comparison to age-matched WT animals. As demyelination is expected to result in slower conduction of visual afferent input to the cortex, the VEP latency was also measured. As expected, we found that visual responses were significantly delayed in TWI mice compared to those measured in control mice (Figure 1C). VEP amplitudes were not significantly different between the two groups (data not shown). Thus, the GALC deficiency induced an immature functional visual system in TWI mice.

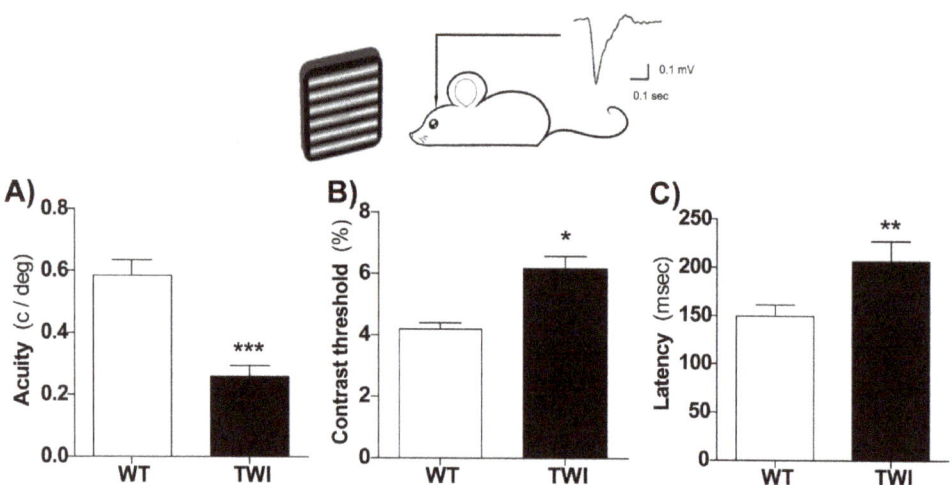

Figure 1. Altered functional properties of the visual cortex in Twitcher (TWI) mice. In vivo electrophysiological visual evoked potential (VEP) recordings from the primary visual cortex at postnatal day (PND)30-36 revealed reduced visual acuity ((**A**) Student' t-test, *** $p < 0.001$), higher contrast threshold ((**B**) t-test, ** $p < 0.01$), and latency of visual responses ((**C**) t-test, * $p < 0.05$) in TWI mice ($n = 7$, black) compared to wild type (WT, white) control littermates ($n = 6$). Bars represent mean ± SEM.

3.2. Demyelination and Gliosis in Twitcher Mice

In order to investigate the relationship between visual functional dysfunction and structural alterations, we analyzed the anatomical features of the mouse visual cortex. We qualitatively assessed the levels of myelination (myelin basic protein, MBP), astrogliosis (glial-fibrillary acidic protein, GFAP), and microglia/macrophages activation (Iba-1), which are commonly associated to neuroinflammation. At the neuroanatomical level, in the primary visual cortex of the TWI mouse (PND34), we found a very clear reduction in the myelin specific marker MBP labelling (Figure 2A, left panel) and a corresponding robust increase in the density of astrocytes and microglial cells, immunostained for GFAP and Iba-1, respectively (Figure 2A middle and right panels).

In parallel, we found an overall reduction in MBP labelling and an increase in GFAP-positive astrocytosis in the whole TWI brain (Figure 2B), suggesting that the degeneration of the visual cortex is comparable with the degeneration present in other brain areas (e.g., motor cortex and corpus callosum). We also quantified the amount of these protein markers in total brain lysates from TWI brains by Western blot (Figure 2C). The protein markers of demyelination, astrogliosis, and microglia activation showed the same trend visualized in the TWI visual cortex. We found a significant increase in GFAP ($p < 0.001$ WT vs. TWI, Student's t-test) and a reduced MBP level ($p < 0.05$ WT vs. TWI, Student's t-test) in the TWI samples compared to WT littermates (Figure 2C).

Overall, demyelination and gliosis are particularly evident in the TWI visual cortex. These data demonstrate and confirm specific neuropathological alterations in the visual system of TWI mice.

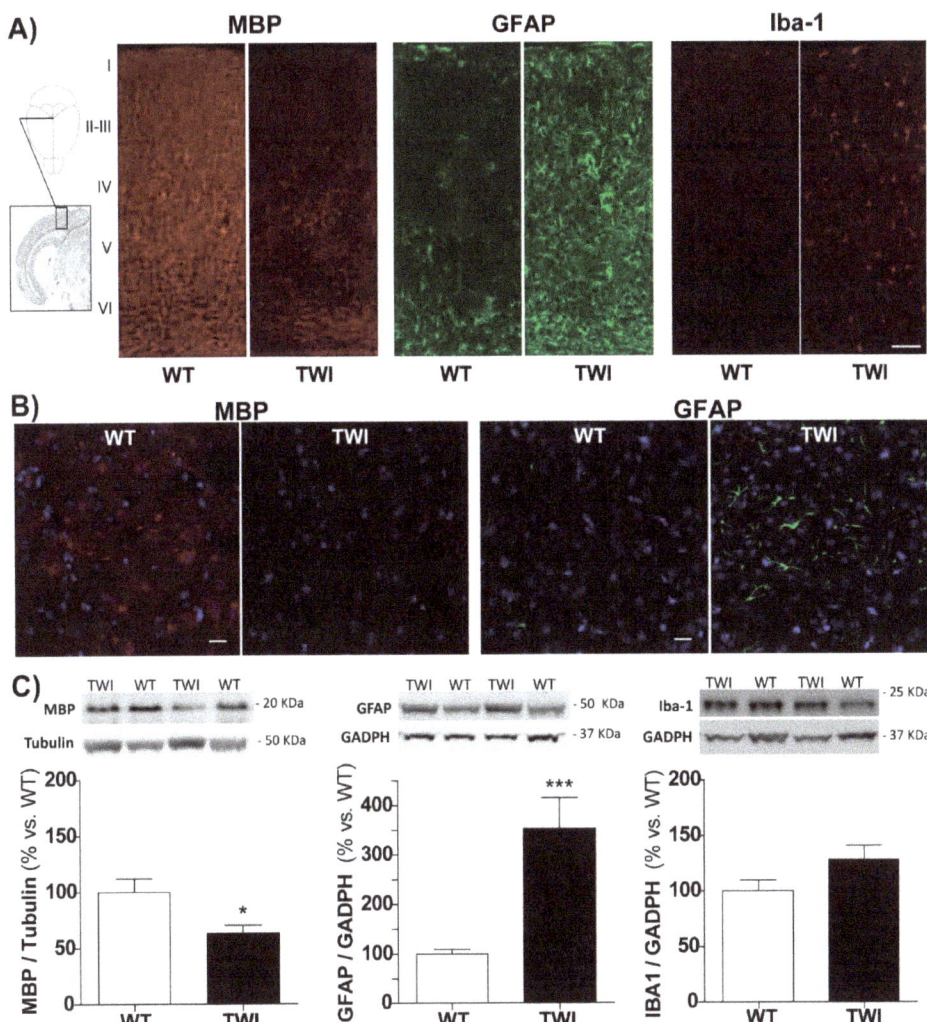

Figure 2. (**A**) Coronal sections through the visual cortex (inset) of representative WT (left) and TWI (right) mice (PND34) immunostained with antibodies against myelin basic protein (MBP) (marker of myelination), glial-fibrillary acidic protein (GFAP) (marker of astrogliosis), and Iba-1 (Ionized calcium-binding adaptor molecule 1, marker of microglia/macrophages). Cortical layers are indicated by Roman numbers on the left. Notice reduced myelin staining and robust gliosis in the visual cortex of TWI mice. Scale bars = 100 µm. (**B**) Representative confocal images of WT (left) and TWI (right) mouse brain (i.e., motor cortex) immunostained for MBP (marker of myelination, in red) and GFAP (marker of astrogliosis, in green), together with nuclei (DAPI, in blue): the overall degeneration status is comparable with the one of visual cortex. Scale bars = 20 µm. (**C**) Representative Western blot panels and blot analysis of MBP, GFAP, and Iba-1 levels in brain tissue lysates from WT (white) and TWI (black columns) mice. Results (normalized to Tubulin or GAPDH, Glyceraldehyde-3-phosphate Dehydrogenase, levels) were reported in % with respect to WT levels. */*** $p < 0.05/0.001$ WT vs. TWI; Student's t-test. Data= mean ± SEM, $n \geq 18$; WT mice: age range PND29-43; TWI mice: age range PND30-40.

3.3. Psychosine Accumulation in Twitcher Tissues

We successfully setup an analytical method for the quantitation of PSY in mouse tissue extracts [5,26]. We used a LC-ESI-tandem-MS method showing excellent sensitivity and specificity. Detection and quantitation limits were 5.2 and 8.3 ng PSY/mg protein (11.3 and 18.0 pmol/mg protein), respectively. These values allowed us to quantify PSY levels in the brain and optic nerve of TWI mice at different disease-time progression (Figure 3A).

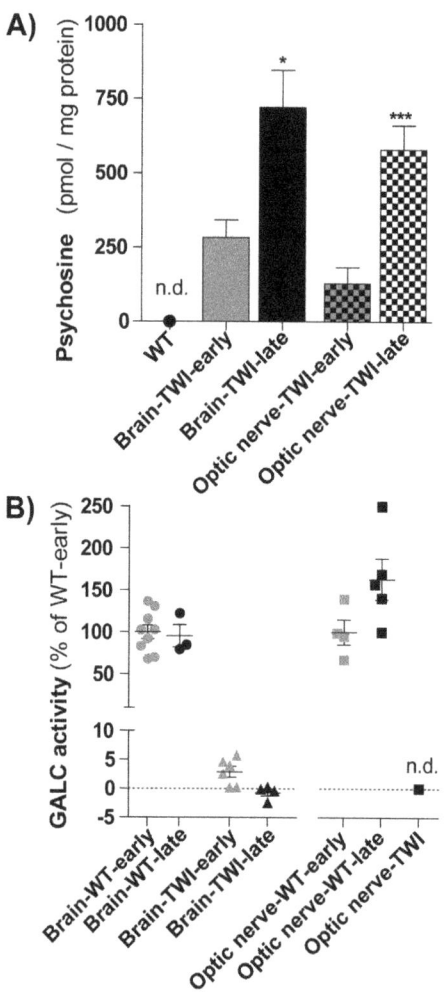

Figure 3. (**A**) Psychosine (PSY) quantification. PSY content was measured in brains (full-filled color columns) and optic nerves (squared columns) of TWI mice in the early stage of disease (early: PND20-28, $n = 7$) and in the late stage of the disease (late: PND30-38, $n = 12$ for brain and $n = 8$ for optic nerve). */*** $p < 0.05/0.001$ early vs. late, Student's t-test. PSY was not detectable (n.d.) in WT mice, in both districts. Data = mean ± SEM. (**B**) Galactosylceramidase (GALC) quantification. GALC activity (reported in percentage in respect to the respective WT-early) was measured in brains (left; circles and triangles) and optic nerves (right; squares) of WT and TWI mice in the early stage of disease (early, in grey: PND20-21 for brains, PDN18 for optic nerves) and in the late stage of the disease (late, in black: PND30-38). GALC was not detectable (n.d.) in the optic nerves of TWI mice. Each point represents a mouse; data= mean ± SEM.

We found that PSY accumulated with age progression in both the brain and optic nerve of TWI mice. In details, in the brain tissue, PSY levels increased from 284 ± 60 pmol/mg protein in TWI mice at early stage of the disease (within PND28) to 720 ± 130 pmol/mg protein at late stage (from PND30) ($p < 0.05$, Student' t-test). Similarly, in optic nerves, PSY levels increased from 130 ± 50 pmol/mg protein in TWI at early stage to 580 ± 80 pmol/mg protein at late stage of disease ($p < 0.001$, Student' t-test). As comparison, the PSY level in the correspondent WT tissues was not detectable in the same analysis conditions. In parallel, we quantified also GALC activity (Figure 3B). In both the brain and the optic nerve, GALC activity did not changed with age progression in WT mice, while it was, as expected, negligible in TWI mice (Figure 3B).

These data show that PSY accumulated in the brain and optic nerves of TWI mice already at early stages of the disease and further increased with time progression. PSY is a characteristic hallmark of KD, also at the level of visual system.

4. Discussion

In the present work, we analyzed the visual system functionality and the myelination status of visual cortical neurons in the Twitcher mouse, as a model of Krabbe disease. The in vivo electrophysiological recordings showed defective basic functional properties of the TWI primary visual cortex. In particular, we found a reduced visual acuity as well as contrast sensitivity and a delayed visual response. Specific neuropathological alterations were present in the visual cortex of the TWI mouse. We found reduced myelination, astrogliosis, and microglia activation, as showed by the biomarkers for myelin (MBP), astrocytes (GFAP), and microglia/macrophages (Iba-1), respectively, by both immunostaining and Western blot. Moreover, we quantified the evolution of the PSY accumulation in brain and optic nerves by high-pressure liquid chromatography-mass spectrometry methods. PSY, the characteristic hallmark of KD, started accumulating already at the early stage of the disease, both at brain and optic nerve level, and increased with time in both districts.

To the best of our knowledge, this study provides the first report about functional and structural defects of the visual system in the TWI mouse. Only recently, VEPs have been investigated in KD patients, with the first evidence in literature in 2000. It has been found that VEPs are abnormal in KD children and VEPS have been suggested as helpful early sentinel signs and tests for the objective evaluation of KD patients [22,40]. Here, for the first time, we found VEPs abnormalities also in TWI mice: the increased latency registered in TWI mice is in line with the neuronal demyelination that we observed histologically in the visual cortex and that leads to a slower signal conductance.

We here further suggest that visual acuity and contrast sensitivity might also be impaired in KD. In fact, we found that these features are deteriorated in TWI mouse primary visual cortex, likely because the visual cortex has not developed properly. For a complete evaluation of KD patients and as a diagnostic marker, the acuity and contrast sensitivity measurements could also be exploited in the clinic. In support of this, the usefulness of visual response analysis for the monitoring of functional alterations in children with severe disabilities was recently described in a study where abnormal VEPs and visual acuity deterioration were identified as biomarkers for another pediatric disease, the Rett Syndrome [41]. Noteworthy visual acuity as well contrast sensitivity can be easily assessed in children with various methods [37], including behavioral ones (electrophysiological that are technically more difficult to implement in a child).

At structural level, we confirmed demyelination as a typical neuroanatomical hallmark of the KD CNS. In addition, we found astrogliosis and microglia activation in the TWI visual cortex and whole brain, in agreement with the literature and the inflammatory profile of KD [8].

Little is known regarding the molecular progression of KD. The most obvious candidate as a molecular catalyst for KD is psychosine, even if its mechanism of action remains elusive. Here, PSY levels are increased in both the brain and the optic nerve of TWI mice. We found that PSY accumulation correlates with the reduced myelination in TWI mouse CNS and this is in line with the causative effect of PSY on oligodendrocytes death that it has been suggested in literature [7]. Thus, the visual functional defects we observed in

TWI mice visual cortex might be due to the increased levels of PSY, at least concerning the visual response latency. At the best of our knowledge, we did not find any measurements about the PSY levels in TWI optic nerves, although its accumulation was already proposed as possible cause of the optic nerve structural anomaly in a human KD patient in 1978 [42]. It has been recently reported that neuronal GALC is required for proper brainstem development and that the deficiency of GALC is critical for KD pathogenesis [43]. In parallel to psychosine analysis, we quantified also GALC activity in the brain and optic nerves, GALC activity did not changed with age progression in WT mice, while it was, as expected, negligible or not detectable in TWI mice.

Overall, our results suggest that the visual system is an optimal and accessible model for studying KD. Moreover, our results may have important implications for KD research since we identified visual system parameters useful for the preclinical evaluations of new therapeutic strategies in the TWI mouse.

For example, recent studies suggest that gene therapy might be a valid option for KD treatment and gene technology constantly develops [13]. The visual system might be exploited as the preferential field of investigation to examine the impact of gene therapy even that of last generation, on brain defects due to KD. In particular, it might be useful to establish the adequate dose of gene therapy, able to completely correct KD impairments. In support of this, a recent study showed that low but not high-dose gene therapy-treated dogs had visual system deficits [44].

Importantly, visual defects have been similarly reported also in animal models of other LSDs. In a mouse model of Cystinosis (CTSN), for example, an LSD characterized by abnormal accumulation of cystine, the eye is one of the first organs affected, with visual impairment in the second decade of life. The tempo spatial pattern of cystine accumulation in CTSN mice parallels that of patients, validating CTSN mice as a model for the visual anomalies of CTSN and for the testing of novel ocular cystine-depleting therapies [28,29]. Visual abnormality has also been well characterized in model of Sandhoff (SD) and GM1 gangliosidosis mice. Although electroretinograms appeared normal in the SD and the GM1 mice, VEP were subnormal in both these mutants, indicating clear visual impairments [30]. Additionally, visual system degeneration and impairment have been demonstrated also in a mouse model for Mucopolysaccharidosis type IIIA (MPS-IIIA, Sanfilippo A), a severe LSD caused by the inherited deficiency of sulfamidase, and in parallel in MPS-IIIA patients [31].

The importance to acquire a deep knowledge about the visual system of LSD mouse models with visual impairment is further supported by the fact that the acquired knowledge can be further exploited for monitoring human patients. In this regard, the visual system might represent a new target for monitoring the effect of the currently standard of care for presymptomatic patients, the HSCT, that has been shown to effectively treat the CNS but not the PNS [13]. In addition, the importance of visual system studies in KD disease is highlighted by the fact that the eye can be also used as an administration route for testing experimental therapies [45].

Overall, these results constitute the first complete characterization of the TWI visual systems. Our data set a baseline for an easy testing of potential therapies for this district, which is also dramatically affected in KD patients. The new knowledge might also be further translated in human patients to shorten the KD diagnosis process.

Author Contributions: I.T. and C.C. performed experiments and analyzed data; I.T. wrote the manuscript; A.D.G. and S.A. performed PSY and GALC experiments; M.A. performed in vivo recordings; M.C. (Matteo Caleo) planned experiments, analyzed data and critically read the manuscript; M.C. (Marco Cecchini) planned experiments, analyzed data and wrote the manuscript; all authors critically read the manuscript. All authors have read and agreed to the published version of the manuscript.

Funding: This research was supported by European Leukodystrophy Association (ELA) International, under the framework of the following projects: 1. "nanoERT–Nanoparticle based Enzyme Replacement Therapy for the treatment of Krabbe disease: a pre-clinical study in the Twitcher Mouse", Grant no. ELA 2019-008I2; 2. "Pre-clinical testing of single and combined autophagy modulation by Lithium and Rapamycin in Globoid Cell Leukodystrophy", Grant no. ELA 2018-008F2.

Institutional Review Board Statement: The study was approved by the Ministry of Health (Permit Numbers: CBS-not. 0517, approved the 04/01/2018; 535/2018-PR, approved 09/07/2018).

Data Availability Statement: Data is contained within the article.

Conflicts of Interest: The authors declare no conflict of interest

References

1. Calderwood, L.; Wenger, D.A.; Matern, D.; Dahmoush, H.; Watiker, V.; Lee, C. Rare Saposin A deficiency: Novel variant and psychosine analysis. *Mol. Genet. Metab.* **2020**, *129*, 161–164. [CrossRef]
2. Giussani, P.; Prinetti, A.; Tringali, C. The role of Sphingolipids in myelination and myelin stability and their involvement in childhood and adult demyelinating disorders. *J. Neurochem.* **2020**, 1–12. [CrossRef]
3. White, A.B.; Givogri, M.I.; Lopez-Rosas, A.; Cao, H.; Van Breemen, R.; Thinakaran, G. Psychosine accumulates in membrane microdomains in the brain of Krabbe patients, disrupting the raft architecture. *J. Neurosci.* **2009**, *29*, 6068–6077. [CrossRef] [PubMed]
4. White, A.B.; Givogri, M.I.; Lopez-Rosas, A.; Cao, H.; van Breemen, R.; Thinakaran, G.; Bongarzone, E.R. Persistence of psychosine in brain lipid rafts is a limiting factor in the therapeutic recovery of a mouse model for Krabbe disease. *J. Neurosci. Res.* **2011**, *89*, 6068–6077. [CrossRef] [PubMed]
5. Del Grosso, A.; Antonini, S.; Angella, L.; Tonazzini, I.; Signore, G.; Cecchini, M. Lithium improves cell viability in psychosine-treated MO3.13 human oligodendrocyte cell line via autophagy activation. *J. Neurosci. Res.* **2016**, *94*, 1246–1260. [CrossRef] [PubMed]
6. Li, Y.; Xu, Y.; Benitez, B.A.; Nagree, M.S.; Dearborn, J.T.; Jiang, X.; Guzman, M.A.; Woloszynek, J.C.; Giaramita, A.; Yip, B.K.; et al. Genetic ablation of acid ceramidase in Krabbe disease confirms the psychosine hypothesis and identifies a new therapeutic target. *Proc. Natl. Acad. Sci. USA* **2019**, *116*, 20097–20103. [CrossRef]
7. Cantuti-Castelvetri, L.; Bongarzone, E.R. Synaptic failure: The achilles tendon of sphingolipidoses. *J. Neurosci. Res.* **2016**, *94*, 1031–1036. [CrossRef]
8. Voccoli, V.; Tonazzini, I.; Signore, G.; Caleo, M.; Cecchini, M. Role of extracellular calcium and mitochondrial oxygen species in psychosine-induced oligodendrocyte cell death. *Cell. Death Dis.* **2014**, *5*, e1529. [CrossRef]
9. de Vito, G.; Cappello, V.; Tonazzini, I.; Cecchini, M.; Piazza, V. RP-CARS reveals molecular spatial order anomalies in myelin of an animal model of Krabbe disease. *J. Biophotonics* **2017**, *10*, 385–389. [CrossRef]
10. Graziano, A.C.E.; Cardile, V. History, genetic, and recent advances on Krabbe disease. *Gene* **2015**, *555*, 2–13. [CrossRef]
11. Parlanti, P.; Cappello, V.; Brun, F.; Tromba, G.; Rigolio, R.; Tonazzini, I.; Cecchini, M.; Piazza, V.; Gemmi, M. Size and specimen-dependent strategy for x-ray micro-ct and tem correlative analysis of nervous system samples. *Sci. Rep.* **2017**, *7*, 1–12. [CrossRef] [PubMed]
12. Megha, J.; De Jesus, O. "Krabbe Disease." StatPearls. 2020. Available online: https://pubmed.ncbi.nlm.nih.gov/32965986 (accessed on 23 December 2020).
13. Wenger, D.A.; Rafi, M.A.; Luzi, P. Krabbe disease: One Hundred years from the bedside to the bench to the bedside. *J. Neurosci. Res.* **2016**, *94*, 982–989. [CrossRef] [PubMed]
14. Hagberg, B.; Sourander, P.; Svennerholm, L. Diagnosis of Krabbe's infantile leucodystrophy. *J. Neurol. Neurosurg Psychiatry* **1963**, *26*, 195–198. [CrossRef] [PubMed]
15. Beltran-Quintero, M.L.; Bascou, N.A.; Poe, M.D.; Wenger, D.A.; Saavedra-Matiz, C.A.; Nichols, M.J.; Escolar, M.L. Early progression of Krabbe disease in patients with symptom onset between 0 and 5 months. *Orphanet J. Rare Dis.* **2019**, *14*, 1–13. [CrossRef]
16. Lyon, G.; Hagberg, B.; Evrard, P.; Allaire, C.; Pavone, L.; Vanier, M. Symptomatology of late onset krabbe's leukodystrophy: The european experience. *Dev Neurosci.* **1991**, *13*, 240–244. [CrossRef]
17. Bascou, N.; Derenzo, A.; Poe, M.D.; Escolar, M.L. A prospective natural history study of Krabbe disease in a patient cohort with onset between 6 months and 3 years of life. *Orphanet J. Rare Dis.* **2018**, *13*, 1–17. [CrossRef]
18. Debs, R.; Froissart, R.; Aubourg, P.; Papeix, C.; Douillard, C.; Degos, B.; Fontaine, B.; Audoin, B.; Lacour, A.; Said, G.; et al. Krabbe disease in adults: Phenotypic and genotypic update from a series of 11 cases and a review. *J. Inherit. Metab. Dis.* **2013**, *36*, 859–868. [CrossRef]
19. Emery, J.M.; Green, W.R.; Huff, D.S. Krabbe's disease. Histopathology and ultrastructure of the eye. *Am. J. Ophthalmol.* **1972**, *74*, 400–406. [CrossRef]
20. Milton Lima Garcia, A.; Martins Menezes Morais, N.; Ohlweiler, L.; Isabel Bragatti Winckler, M.; Ranzan, J.; Alfonso Pinto Artigalás, O.; Pinto, P.L.; Netto, C.B.; Ashton-Prolla, P.; Vedolin, L.; et al. Optic nerve enlargement and leukodystrophy An unusual finding of the infantile form of Krabbe disease EspEssamEnto dE vias ópticAs E LEuCodistrofia: Um aChado pouCo frEqüEntE da forma infantiL. *Arq. Neuropsiquiatr.* **2010**, *68*, 816–818. [CrossRef]
21. Brodsky, M.C.; Hunter, J.S. Positional ocular flutter and thickened optic nerves as sentinel signs of Krabbe disease. *J. AAPOS* **2011**, *15*, 595–597. [CrossRef]
22. Aldosari, M.; Altuwaijri, M.; Husain, A.M. Brain-stem auditory and visual evoked potentials in children with Krabbe disease. *Clin. Neurophysiol.* **2004**, *115*, 1653–1656. [CrossRef] [PubMed]

23. Suzuki, K.; Suzuki, K. The Twitcher Mouse: A Model for Krabbe Disease and for Experimental Therapies. *Brain Pathol.* **1995**, *5*, 249–258. [CrossRef] [PubMed]
24. Olmstead, C.E. Neurological and neurobehavioral development of the mutant "twitcher" mouse. *Behav. Brain Res.* **1987**, *25*, 143–153. [CrossRef]
25. Suzuki, K.; Suzuki, K. Myelin Pathology in the Twitcher Mouse. *Ann. N. Y. Acad. Sci.* **1990**, *605*, 313–324. [CrossRef]
26. Grosso, A.; Galliani, M.; Angella, L.; Santi, M.; Tonazzini, I.; Parlanti, G.; Signore, G.; Cecchini, M. Brain-targeted enzyme-loaded nanoparticles: A breach through the blood-brain barrier for enzyme replacement therapy in Krabbe disease. *Sci. Adv.* **2019**, *5*, eaax7462. [CrossRef] [PubMed]
27. Marshall, M.S.; Issa, Y.; Jakubauskas, B.; Stoskute, M.; Elackattu, V.; Marshall, J.N.; Bogue, W.; Nguyen, D.; Hauck, Z.; Rue, E.; et al. Long-Term Improvement of Neurological Signs and Metabolic Dysfunction in a Mouse Model of Krabbe's Disease after Global Gene Therapy. *Mol. Ther.* **2018**, *26*, 874–889. [CrossRef]
28. Kalatzis, V. The ocular anomalies in a cystinosis animal model mimic disease pathogenesis (Pediatric Research 62, (156–162)). *Pediatr. Res.* **2007**, *62*, 558. [CrossRef]
29. Simpson, J.; Nien, C.J.; Flynn, K.; Jester, B.; Cherqui, S.; Jester, J. Quantitative in vivo and ex vivo confocal microscopy analysis of corneal cystine crystals in the Ctns -/- knockout mouse. *Mol. Vis.* **2011**, *17*, 2212–2220.
30. Denny, C.A.; Alroy, J.; Pawlyk, B.S.; Sandberg, M.A.; D'Azzo, A.; Seyfried, T.N. Neurochemical, morphological, and neurophysiological abnormalities in retinas of Sandhoff and GM1 gangliosidosis mice. *J. Neurochem.* **2007**, *101*, 1294–1302. [CrossRef]
31. Intartaglia, D.; Giamundo, G.; Marrocco, E.; Maffia, V.; Salierno, F.G.; Nusco, E. Retinal Degeneration in MPS-IIIA Mouse Model. *Front. Cell Dev. Biol.* **2020**, *8*, 1–12. [CrossRef]
32. Sakai, N.; Inui, K.; Tatsumi, N.; Fukushima, H.; Nishigaki, T.; Taniike, M.; Nishimoto, J.; Tsukamoto, H.; Yanagihara, I.; Ozono, K.; et al. Molecular cloning and expression of cDNA for murine galactocerebrosidase and mutation analysis of the twitcher mouse, a model of Krabbe's disease. *J. Neurochem.* **1996**, *66*, 1118–1124. [CrossRef] [PubMed]
33. Pinto, L.; Drechsel, D.; Schmid, M.T.; Ninkovic, J.; Irmler, M.; Brill, M.S.; Restani, L.; Gianfranceschi, L.; Cerri, C.; Weber, S.N.; et al. AP2γ regulates basal progenitor fate in a region- and layer-specific manner in the developing cortex. *Nat. Neurosci.* **2009**, *12*, 1229–1237. [CrossRef] [PubMed]
34. Allegra, M.; Genovesi, S.; Maggia, M.; Cenni, M.C.; Zunino, G.; Sgadò, P.; Caleo, M.; Bozzi, Y. Altered GABAergic markers, increased binocularity and reduced plasticity in the visual cortex of engrailed-2 knockout mice. *Front. Cell Neurosci.* **2014**, *8*, 1–15. [CrossRef] [PubMed]
35. Del Grosso, A.; Angella, L.; Tonazzini, I.; Moscardini, A.; Giordano, N.; Caleo, M.; Rocchiccioli, S.; Cecchini, M. Dysregulated autophagy as a new aspect of the molecular pathogenesis of Krabbe disease. *Neurobiol. Dis.* **2019**, *129*, 195–207. [CrossRef]
36. Tonazzini, I.; Van Woerden, G.M.; Masciullo, C.; Mientjes, E.J.; Elgersma, Y.; Cecchini, M. The role of ubiquitin ligase E3A in polarized contact guidance and rescue strategies in UBE3A-deficient hippocampal neurons. *Mol. Autism.* **2019**, *10*, 1–18. [CrossRef]
37. Leat, S.J.; Yadav, N.K.; Irving, E.L. Development of visual acuity and contrast sensitivity in children. *J. Optom.* **2009**, *2*, 19–26. [CrossRef]
38. Gianfranceschi, L.; Fiorentini, A.; Maffei, L. Behavioural visual acuity of wild type and bcl2 transgenic mouse. *Vis. Res.* **2000**, *39*, 569–574. [CrossRef]
39. Porciatti, V.; Pizzorusso, T.; Maffei, L. The visual physiology of the wild type mouse determined with pattern VEPs. *Vis. Res.* **1999**, *39*, 3071–3081. [CrossRef]
40. Al-Essa, M.A.; Bakheet, S.M.; Patay, Z.J.; Powe, J.E.; Ozand, P.T. Clinical and cerebral FDG PET scan in a patient with Krabbe's disease. *Pediatr. Neurol.* **2000**, *22*, 44–47. [CrossRef]
41. LeBlanc, J.J.; DeGregorio, G.; Centofante, E.; Vogel-Farley, V.K.; Barnes, K.; Kaufmann, W.E.; Fagiolini, M.; Nelson, C.A. Visual evoked potentials detect cortical processing deficits in Rett syndrome. *Ann. Neurol.* **2015**, *78*, 775–786. [CrossRef]
42. Brownstein, S. Optic Nerve in Globoid Leukodystrophy (Krabbe's Disease). *Arch. Ophthalmol.* **1978**, *96*, 864. [CrossRef] [PubMed]
43. Weinstock, N.I.; Kreher, C.; Favret, J.; Nguyen, D.; Bongarzone, E.R.; Wrabetz, L.; Feltri, M.L.; Shin, D. Brainstem development requires galactosylceramidase and is critical for pathogenesis in a model of Krabbe disease. *Nat. Commun.* **2020**, *11*, 1–16. [CrossRef] [PubMed]
44. Bradbury, A.M.; Bagel, J.H.; Nguyen, D.; Lykken, E.A.; Salvador, J.P.; Jiang, X.; Swain, G.P.; Assenmacher, C.A.; Hendricks, I.J.; Miyadera, K.; et al. Krabbe disease successfully treated via monotherapy of intrathecal gene therapy. *J. Clin. Investig.* **2020**, *130*, 4906–4920. [CrossRef] [PubMed]
45. Hennig, A.K.; Levy, B.; Ogilvie, J.M.; Vogler, C.A.; Galvin, N.; Bassnett, S.; Sands, M.S. Intravitreal gene therapy reduces lysosomal storage in specific areas of the CNS in mucopolysaccharidosis VII mice. *J. Neurosci.* **2003**, *23*, 3302–3307. [CrossRef]

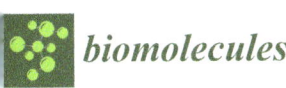

Review

Mucopolysaccharidosis Type I: Current Treatments, Limitations, and Prospects for Improvement

Christiane S. Hampe [1,*], Jacob Wesley [1], Troy C. Lund [2], Paul J. Orchard [2], Lynda E. Polgreen [3], Julie B. Eisengart [2], Linda K. McLoon [4], Sebahattin Cureoglu [5], Patricia Schachern [5] and R. Scott McIvor [6,7]

1. Immusoft Corp., Seattle, WA 98103, USA; jake.wesley@immusoft.com
2. Department of Pediatrics, University of Minnesota, Minneapolis, MN 55455, USA; lundx072@umn.edu (T.C.L.); orcha001@umn.edu (P.J.O.); eisen139@umn.edu (J.B.E.)
3. The Lundquist Institute at Harbor, UCLA Medical Center, Torrance, CA 90502, USA; lpolgreen@lundquist.org
4. Department of Ophthalmology and Visual Neurosciences, University of Minnesota, Minneapolis, MN 55455, USA; mcloo001@umn.edu
5. Department of Otolaryngology, Head and Neck Surgery, University of Minnesota, Minneapolis, MN 55455, USA; cureo003@umn.edu (S.C.); schac002@umn.edu (P.S.)
6. Immusoft Corp, Minneapolis, MN 55413, USA; mcivo001@umn.edu
7. Department of Genetics, Cell Biology and Development and Center for Genome Engineering, University of Minnesota, Minneapolis, MN 55455, USA
* Correspondence: chris.hampe@immusoft.com; Tel.: +1-206-5549181

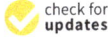

Abstract: Mucopolysaccharidosis type I (MPS I) is a lysosomal disease, caused by a deficiency of the enzyme alpha-L-iduronidase (IDUA). IDUA catalyzes the degradation of the glycosaminoglycans dermatan and heparan sulfate (DS and HS, respectively). Lack of the enzyme leads to pathologic accumulation of undegraded HS and DS with subsequent disease manifestations in multiple organs. The disease can be divided into severe (Hurler syndrome) and attenuated (Hurler-Scheie, Scheie) forms. Currently approved treatments consist of enzyme replacement therapy (ERT) and/or hematopoietic stem cell transplantation (HSCT). Patients with attenuated disease are often treated with ERT alone, while the recommended therapy for patients with Hurler syndrome consists of HSCT. While these treatments significantly improve disease manifestations and prolong life, a considerable burden of disease remains. Notably, treatment can partially prevent, but not significantly improve, clinical manifestations, necessitating early diagnosis of disease and commencement of treatment. This review discusses these standard therapies and their impact on common disease manifestations in patients with MPS I. Where relevant, results of animal models of MPS I will be included. Finally, we highlight alternative and emerging treatments for the most common disease manifestations.

Keywords: mucopolysaccharidosis type I; Hurler syndrome; enzyme replacement therapy; hematopoietic stem cell transplantations; animal models; experimental therapies

1. Introduction

Mucopolysaccharidosis type I (MPS I) is a lysosomal disease, caused by a deficiency of the enzyme alpha-L-iduronidase (IDUA). Currently approved treatments consist of enzyme replacement therapy (ERT) and/or hematopoietic stem cell transplantation (HSCT). While these treatments significantly improve disease manifestations and prolong life, a considerable burden of disease remains. Both treatments may at best prevent the development or worsening of abnormal function and somatic complications but cannot revert already existing symptoms. Therefore, treatment must commence as early as possible for maximum effect and diagnostic delay-due to the nonspecific nature of early symptoms-limits treatment success [1]. To overcome this limitation, implementation of MPS I in newborn screening programs is strongly recommended [2,3].

Moreover, the therapeutic effect in some systems appears to wear off after several years. Bones, eyes, and heart valves prove to be especially resistant to treatment. A number of experimental strategies are currently under development to reduce the remaining burden of disease.

2. Standard Therapies for MPS I

2.1. Allogeneic HSCT

Allogeneic HSCT is considered the gold standard for treatment of Hurler syndrome and can alleviate a number of disease symptoms and increase the patient's life span, especially when performed before the age of 2 years and prior to cognitive impairment [4–8]. Clinical effect is evident in reduced facial coarseness, joint mobility, and reduction in sleep apnea, cardiac disease, and hearing loss [9–11]. Overall, survival is significantly prolonged [4,12,13], and when initiated early, decline of neurocognition can be stabilized [8]. However, clinical benefit varies, both between patients and between different organs in the same patient. Interpatient variation is mainly due to differential effectiveness of engraftment and is governed by such variables as genotype, age at transplantation, and donor specifications [14]. Tissue specific improvement is caused by different accessibility of tissues, such as heart, eyes, and bones, to circulating enzyme. Notably, HSCT can prevent, but not significantly improve, clinical manifestations in bone, cornea, cardiac valves, and CNS [15,16], resulting in residual disease burden in the majority of patients.

2.1.1. Mortality Rates and Conditioning Regimens

Improved myeloablative conditioning regimens, donor matching availability, and improved supportive care have greatly reduced mortality rates associated with HSCT for MPS I during the last decades at experienced centers [5]. Viral infections, graft rejection, pulmonary hemorrhage, and graft-versus-host disease (GvHD) remain the most common causes of death and are most commonly seen in the first several months after transplant, but can occur within the first year post-transplantation [13,17]. These complications may be related to the immunologic responses of the recipient to the donor cells or vice versa, or may be due to the conditioning chemotherapy regimen, with use of agents such as busulfan and cyclophosphamide [5,18]. Conditioning is necessary for successful engraftment, allowing complete donor chimerism and creation of niches for the incoming donor stem cells. Myeloablative conditioning and reduced-intensity conditioning regimens are available. In the early era of HSCT, patients were subjected to total body irradiation (TBI) with severe side-effects, including neurocognitive impairment, stunted growth, and a higher risk of hypothyroidism and cataracts, especially in very young children [19,20]. Long-term effects of myeloablative conditioning regimens are infertility in both females and males [21,22]. Comparing infertility risks associated with treatment in pre-puberty (1–12 years) with treatment after the age of 13 revealed opposite trends in males and females. While pre-pubertal treatment in males was associated with increased risk for infertility, females treated at a younger age had a lower risk for infertility [23]. Busulfan-based treatment was associated with higher infertility in females but not in males, and TBI increased risk of infertility in males, but not in females [23]. Fertility preservation needs to be addressed in patients prior to HSCT [24].

Recent transplant regimens utilize non-TBI based preparative conditioning regimens. Current regimens are generally based on a combination of busulfan and fludarabine or cyclophosphamide [5,25,26]. While the use of busulfan is an important agent to achieve successful transplants with high chimerism, the myeloablative drug is associated with significant toxicity [20,27]. Reduced intensity conditioning regimens may decrease toxicity, but are associated with an increased risk for graft failure [17]. Antibody based therapy, such as anti-thymocyte globulin (ATG) or anti-CD52 antibody therapy are being utilized as a means of decreasing toxicity in combination with reduced intensity regimens [28], and continuing research is ongoing to optimize an approach that achieves full donor chimerism while minimizing side-effects.

2.1.2. Effectiveness of HSCT

Achieving the best outcomes in patients treated by HSCT depends on a variety of factors, including the age of the recipient, existing disease manifestations, the availability of a well matched donor, donor status (carrier or non-affected), and tissue source of HSCT [29]. Different biochemical parameters can be used to evaluate success of HSCT, such as glycosaminoglycan (GAG) levels in blood, spinal fluid, and urine, IDUA activity levels in blood [30,31], and leukocyte lysates [32]. Umbilical cord blood has largely replaced BM as donor cell sources in young patients with MPS I. Umbilical cord blood presents an attractive alternative because of the less stringent requirements for donor HLA-matching and ease of availability [7,33].

The level of enzyme activity directly correlates with donor chimerism and the use of a non-carrier donor [5,31,33]. In patients with full donor chimerism normal IDUA activity can be measured in blood cell lysates, but delivery of enzyme to the tissues is more difficult to ascertain [34]. Rapid reduction of heparan sulfate and dermatan sulfate in blood and urine is observed in the majority of patients [1,11,31,35–37]. This reduction is long-lived and continues for years after transplantation. However, GAG levels typically remain above reference levels [36], although normal leukocyte lysate enzyme levels are observed for the majority of patients [1,36,37]. The lack of normalization of blood and urine levels may be a consequence of partial GAG degradation in difficult-to-reach organs. Remaining GAGs will diffuse from these organs into the circulation and will eventually be excreted in the urine [36]. In support of this, dermatan sulfate stems predominantly from hard-to-reach organs and tissues, such as bone, cartilage, and heart valves [38,39] and dermatan sulfate levels tend to remain relatively elevated compared to heparan sulfate [36].

Animal studies further confirmed that IDUA expression and GAG level reduction differ between tissues. HSCT performed in young MPS I cats resulted in significant increases in IDUA activity in liver, spleen, lung, and thyroid, but not in kidney, brain, or heart. GAG levels were reduced in liver, lung, thyroid, kidney, and heart. The reduction of GAG levels in the absence of detectable IDUA activity in kidney and heart may indicate that IDUA levels below the sensitivity of the activity assay were sufficient to reduce GAG levels [40]. In neonatal MPS I mice HSCT resulted in significant increases of IDUA activity, most prominently in the spleen, followed by liver and kidneys, heart, and lungs. While IDUA activity also varies between tissues in wild-type animals, IDUA levels after HSCT reached up to 70% of normal in the spleen but only 10% of normal in the lungs and heart. Consequently, reduction in GAG levels were also found to be tissue dependent. While GAG levels in spleen and liver were normalized overall, they were only partially reduced in kidneys, heart, and lungs [41,42].

This tissue specificity is probably a consequence of differential donor cell engraftment and differentiation to resident cells, and diffusion or lack thereof of circulating enzyme. Donor monocytes can leave the blood stream and infiltrate into peripheral organs, where they differentiate into tissue-specific macrophages [29]. Enzyme produced by engrafted donor cells can be transferred to the recipient's cells via cross-correction. Enzyme is released by donor macrophages and leukocytes and is taken up by the recipient's cells, where GAGs are metabolized [43,44].

Thus, organs with higher vascularization, such as liver, and spleen, show higher numbers of engrafted donor cells, while tissues with less vascularization, including cartilage and corneas, will benefit less from the transplanted cells. The brain poses a unique situation, where donor monocytes differentiate into microglia or brain macrophages after crossing the blood brain barrier (BBB) [45]. Replacement of the recipients' microglia by donor-derived cells takes up to one year [46,47]. During the first posttransplant year, deterioration in intellect and development may continue, emphasizing the importance of early treatment to prevent cognitive impairment [11,48–50].

2.2. Enzyme Replacement Therapy (ERT)

ALDURAZYME (laronidase) is a recombinant variant of the human IDUA produced in a Chinese hamster ovary cell line. The ~82 kD glycoprotein contains mannose-6-phosphate (M6P) residues that enable the binding of the enzyme by cell surface M6P receptors. Subsequent uptake directs the enzyme to the lysosomes. Intravenous infusions with laronidase are administered weekly. Complications are rare, and ERT is considered safe overall [51]. Weekly intravenous infusions of 0.58 mg/kg of laronidase led to a significant drop in urinary GAG levels [51–54] accompanied by a reduction in hepatosplenomegaly [51,52,54,55]. ERT also improved upper airway restrictions, physical performance, and resulted in some improvement in left ventricular hypertrophy [56–58].

While ERT for patients with MPS I is well tolerated with no serious adverse events, the infusions require several hours every week, adding to the disease burden of patients and families. Another major drawback lays in the enzyme's low level of BBB penetration and inefficient delivery to avascular tissues [59,60]. Consequently, cognitive function, skeletal deformities, and visual acuity do not improve when it is the sole therapy [61–66]. Moreover, the majority of patients (up to 90%) produce IgG antibodies to laronidase in response to ERT [65], which can interfere with enzyme activity and uptake [65,67]. Studies investigating the effect of ERT-induced IDUA antibodies on biochemical markers and clinical parameters gave conflicting results [56]. While all studies concluded that ERT led to the development of IDUA antibodies and poorer urinary GAG reduction [30,51,65,67], one study found no effect on clinical outcome in patients receiving only ERT [65]. Another study found a higher incidence of sleep disordered breathing in ERT-treated patients with or without HSCT, probably caused by IDUA antibody development [32]. Interestingly, these antibodies diminish over time despite continuous ERT [51,65,68].

Contradictory results were reported when development of antibodies to IDUA were examined. In some cases post-transplant ERT was associated with the development of IDUA antibodies, which were inhibitory and were accompanied with an increase in heparan sulfate excretion [67,69] and poorer endurance as established by the 6-min-walk-test [67]. However, in the absence of inhibitory antibodies, ERT post-HSCT had a beneficial effect on the 6-min walk test [67]. Therefore, efforts are currently focused on the induction of tolerance to exogenous IDUA [70–72].

While ERT is not recommended as the sole treatment for Hurler syndrome, a combination of ERT with HSCT may have benefits over each treatment alone [73–75]. Peri-transplant ERT appears to have beneficial effects on the clinical condition of the patient [7,31,48,50,58,67,73,74,76]. ERT can bridge the time until a suitable donor for HSCT has been identified, and therefore ERT is often initiated at time of diagnosis [31]. Importantly, ERT was not associated with a reduced engraftment rate [48,73,76,77], and subsequent HSCT attenuated the formation of neutralizing IDUA antibodies [78]. Moreover, GAG-reduction due to peri-transplant ERT appeared to improve HSCT engraftment [73,75,79]. Continuous ERT post-transplant has been reported to improve residual disease burden [48,56,65,72,74]. Recent studies in neonatal MPS I mice allowed an in-depth analysis of the combined treatment [80]. Animals receiving both HSCT and ERT showed higher IDUA levels in the spleen, lower plasma GAG levels, and improved bone architecture compared to animals receiving either treatment alone [80]. Beneficial effects of combined HSCT/ERT treatment pertaining to specific manifestations are discussed in the appropriate sections below.

3. Impact of HSCT and ERT on Tissue-Specific Disease Manifestations

The effect of HSCT, ERT, and the combination of both treatments on different disease manifestations is summarized in Table 1.

Table 1. Effect of HSCT and ERT on clinical manifestations in MPS I.

Clinical Manifestation	HSCT	ERT	HSCT + ERT
Partial improvement with added benefit of combination therapy			
Cognitive function	Stabilization	No effect	Improvement
Pulmonary function	Limited improvement	Improvement	Improvement
Skeletal manifestations	• Minimal effect of linear growth • Improved facial features and odontoid hypoplasia	No effect	Improved growth rate
Partial improvement			
Upper respiratory	Improvement	Improvement	Improvement
Joint mobility	Improved range of motion	Improved range of motion (shoulder)	NA
Cardiac function	• Improved cardiac hypertrophy and coronary artery narrowing • No effect on valve insufficiencies	• Improved cardiac hypertrophy and ventricular function • No significant effect on cardiac valve thickening	Improvement
Limited effect			
Hearing loss	Improvement/stabilization	No effect	NA
Corneal clouding	Limited stabilization	No effect	NA
Retinal dysfunction	No effect	No effect	NA
Hearing loss	Improvement/stabilization	No effect	NA

3.1. Ocular Manifestations

Ocular manifestations of MPS I include corneal clouding, retinal degeneration, optic nerve damage, and glaucoma. The effects of HSCT on ocular manifestations are complex. The cornea is an avascular structure, and in general not protected by HSCT. A multinational study of over 200 patients with MPS I, with a follow-up period of over 9 years, showed stabilization or improvement of corneal clouding for the majority of patients [5]. While several earlier studies supported this finding [81–83], others showed onset of corneal clouding despite HSCT [64,84,85]. A recent longitudinal analysis of 24 patients with MPS I indicated stabilization of corneal clouding during the first years post HSCT, after which corneal clouding reappeared [86]. The differences in outcomes may be due to sample size, length of follow-up, success of engraftment, and post-transplant enzyme levels. Both Aldenhoven et al. [5] and Javed et al. [84] noticed a strong correlation between outcome, age at transplant, level of engraftment, and post-transplant IDUA levels. Recent studies detected large numbers of myofibroblasts in the cornea of a MPS I patient after HSCT, indicating that continuous or reappearing of corneal clouding may be caused by the transformation of keratocytes into myofibroblasts, which would not be affected by HSCT [87].

While initial analyses of ocular symptoms other than corneal clouding showed promising effects [82], the majority of later studies reported continued loss of visual acuity and increased retinal dysfunction despite HSCT [11,35,81,85,86,88,89]. As the retina is part of the central nervous system, it is protected from blood cell entry by the blood-retinal barrier. Thus, over time after HSCT treatment, visual acuity declined and retinal pathology visible on OCT examination developed [64].

Animal studies revealed species-specific responses in the eye to both HSCT and ERT. In dogs, HSCT resulted in greatly reduced development of ocular manifestations, including corneal clouding [90,91]. Dogs also demonstrated a beneficial effect of ERT on GAG accumulation in the cornea [92], while no significant effect on ocular manifestations in patients with MPS I or mice was noted in response to ERT [93,94]. Results from ERT in MPS I cats were largely inconclusive, as corneal clouding was reduced in only one of two cats treated with high-dose ERT [54].

One possible reason for the lack of ocular responsiveness to ERT may be due to insufficient delivery of enzyme to the eye. Low levels of IDUA in tear film indicate poor enzyme transport from the circulation to multiple tissues within the orbit [95].

It is important to note that there is a great deal of variability in the ocular pathology in individuals with MPS I [96]. Due to the inability of HSCT and ERT to prevent retinal and corneal pathology, it is critical to detect and treat patients with MPS as early as possible in order to improve their eyesight long-term [97].

3.2. Respiratory System

Upper airway obstructions often result in sleep disordered breathing (SDB), including obstructive sleep apnea syndrome (OSAS). HSCT appeared to improve SDB, including OSAS, through reduction in adenoid hyperplasia, tongue, and maxillary constrictions [32,98–101]. However, a long-term follow-up study of 10 years indicated that the beneficial effect of HSCT may be only temporary [102]. Similar to other disease manifestations, effectiveness of HSCT on respiratory function depended on non-carrier donor and enzyme levels one year post HSCT [32]. Improvement of respiratory symptoms, even if only temporary, benefited airway management during anesthesia [98,103,104], although some studies report ongoing difficulties with intubation despite ERT and HSCT [105] especially in older patients [106]. These difficulties may be due to continued musculoskeletal issues and MPS-related pathology. Beneficial effects of HSCT exceed those of ERT, postulated to be the result of developing inhibitory IDUA antibodies, as patients without high levels of such antibodies showed significant clinical improvement [98]. However, ERT reduced the frequency of upper airway infections and improved sleep apnea [51,52,107–109]. Results from a case study demonstrated that relapse in respiratory function could be treated by weekly ERT with good clinical outcome [110].

Few studies address the effect of treatment on pulmonary function. A large retrospective study of patients treated with ERT and/or HSCT showed improvement or stabilization of pulmonary function in the majority of patients for the duration of over 12 years. However, residual restrictive lung disease remained in all patients and 1/3 of the patients experienced progressive loss of pulmonary function despite treatment [111]. Other studies reported ongoing overnight hypoxia, suggesting incomplete resolution of pulmonary insufficiency [29]. Patients with MPS I are at an increased risk of developing pulmonary complications following HSCT. ERT alone resulted in improved lung function [51,107,112]; however, this appeared to be only a temporary effect [51]. Part of the improved pulmonary function was thought to result from reduction in liver and/or spleen size after HSCT and ERT, as this would reduce pressure on the diaphragm. It remains to be seen whether the variety of responses were caused by donor/recipient specific factors or by the persistent disease-associated skeletal deformities of the thoracic cage, which are not affected by either treatment. Combined HSCT and ERT therapy had beneficial outcomes on pulmonary manifestations [76].

To date few studies have evaluated the effect of treatment on respiratory issues in animal models of MPS I [113], possibly due to the often challenging assays involved.

3.3. Hearing Loss

Hearing loss is one of the most common manifestations in patients with MPS I. Hearing loss can be neurosensorial, conductive, or present as a mixture of both. Some improvement or stabilization of hearing loss was observed for the majority of children treated by

HSCT, especially in children receiving the transplant at an early age [11,85,114–116]. This improvement was attributed predominantly to improved sensorineural hearing [85,115]. A longitudinal follow-up study of 28 patients with MPS I post-HSCT investigated hearing loss using auditory brainstem response and pure tone audiometry [117]. While some improvement was noted, none of the patients recovered normal hearing. Importantly, the authors discovered that initially improved hearing was due to improved air conduction thresholds, possibly by a reduction in GAG deposits in the middle ear, and reduced frequency of chronic otitis. However, bone conduction worsened over time and resulted in an overall loss of hearing, which became apparent 10 years after transplantation. These results confirmed the finding of Aldenhoven reporting overall hearing loss in a large MPS I cohort 10 years post HSCT [29].

The effect of ERT on hearing loss is unclear. Case studies reported stabilized sensorineural hearing loss in one patient and improved conductive hearing loss in the other [118], or progressive sensorineural hearing loss [119]. A larger longitudinal study of 15 patients with MPS I treated with ERT reported continuous hearing loss over 2.5 years [120].

3.4. Skeletal Manifestations

Skeletal manifestations in MPS I are notoriously resistant to treatment, necessitating patients with MPS I to undergo surgeries including correction of genua valga, odontoid hypoplasia, hip dysplasia, and thoracolumbar kyphosis. As discussed in other parts of this review, remaining bone deformities may cause other complications such as limiting pulmonary function due to severe kyphosis and/or scoliosis.

The first report investigating musculoskeletal manifestations after HSCT showed promising results [35] and following studies indicated normalized longitudinal growth for the first year after HSCT [121]. Eventually, however, long-term follow-up studies revealed that the initial normalization of the growth rate was followed by a subsequent growth failure [11,29,34,85,122–124]. For example, while the longitudinal growth in children with MPS I receiving HSCT was better as compared to non-treated historic controls, it remained significantly lower when compared to CDC growth charts [125]. The reason for eventual decline in growth rate is unknown. It has been posited to be due to a reduced ability of enzyme to penetrate the epiphyseal growth plate as chondrocytes differentiate and become ossified [122]. Reduced trunk growth with continuous kyphosis can contribute to short stature [85,122,123,126], although poor growth was described irrespective of kyphosis [11].

Aside from impaired longitudinal growth, hip dysplasia [61,63,127,128], genu valgum [63,129], thoracolumbar kyphosis, and scoliosis [61,63,129–131] progress despite HSCT. Human ex vivo data is limited to a single publication [132] where two patients were briefly described, and histologic evidence was provided for correction of chondrocytes from the lumbar spine in a patient with MPS I treated with HSCT. The lack of effectiveness on skeletal manifestations through ERT and HSCT has been attributed to several factors. It is possible that the amount of enzyme that reaches ossification centers may simply be too low to overcome the accumulation of GAG and associated defects [86,122]. Moreover, cultured mouse osteoblasts, derived from a mouse calvaria immortalized precursor cell line, have decreased uptake of exogenous IDUA compared to mouse fibroblasts [133].

Remarkably, disease manifestations in facial bones [85,122] and the odontoid process showed improvement following HSCT. The typical coarse facial features were alleviated, the head circumference normalized [11,29], and prevalence of odontoid hypoplasia was reduced [63,126,129,134–136], with much desired relief of spinal cord compression. It is unclear why these bones responded to HSCT treatment compared to the bony skeleton. However, the distinct difference between facial and cranial bones versus long bones and vertebrae is that they form through intramembranous ossification versus endochondral ossification.

ERT alone has minimal effects on skeletal manifestations, especially in patients with Hurler syndrome [112,137]. Better outcomes were reported in patients with attenuated MPS I, where early initiation of ERT treatment prevented or delayed development of skeletal manifestations [138,139].

Combination of HSCT and ERT may provide the best outcome. In a recent clinical trial the effect of ERT post-HSCT was evaluated and resulted in improved growth rate, particularly in young patients [67]. Peri-HSCT ERT resulted in improved odontoid process morphology and reduced spinal cord compression in a 10-year old girl treated with HSCT and ERT at age 18 months [74].

In animal models of MPS I, treatment with HSCT showed overall more promising outcomes, especially when performed in neonatal animals. Less severe skeletal manifestations were observed in MPS I cats and dogs post-HSCT [40,90]. Transplantation of neonatal MPS I mice with umbilical cord blood or BM prevented the development of dysostosis multiplex altogether [41,42]. Notably, these studies corrected for busulfan-associated effects by including busulfan-treated wildtype mice that received wildtype HSCT. Dimensions of skull and leg bones, and cortical and trabecular bone architecture of treated animals were similar to that of wild-type control mice. On the cellular level, osteocytes showed fewer and smaller GAG deposits, and the growth plates appeared more organized as compared to untreated animals [41]. Transplantation at a later age (8 weeks) resulted in overcorrection of the reduced osteoclastogenesis described in untreated IDUA-deficient mice, which was corrected with combined HSCT and ERT [140]. ERT in neonatal MPS I mice was not accompanied by any improved bone manifestations compared to non-treated animals [141], while in MPS I dogs ERT attenuated skeletal manifestations, especially when administered to neonatal animals [136]. Particular benefit was reported regarding cervical spine disease.

3.5. Joint Mobility

Restriction of joint range of motion (JROM) of upper and lower limbs is present in many patients with MPS I and restricts their mobility [142–144]. Some studies reported that HSCT had a beneficial effect on JROM. It remains to be determined whether all joints benefit from HSCT [11,29,63,122,145]. Specifically, the effect on shoulder mobility varied between different studies. Notably, range of motion of the shoulder joint responded positively to ERT, while other joints showed little effect [51,54,57,146]. The effect of HSCT on development of carpal tunnel syndrome remains unclear, with some studies indicating partial improvement after HSCT, especially if performed at a young age [147], while others found no effect of HSCT with or without ERT on the development of carpal tunnel syndrome [148]. Studies in mice found no benefit of ERT on joint disease [141].

3.6. Cardiac Function

Cardiac manifestations in patients with MPS I involve mainly valvular heart disease and coronary artery narrowing. However, occlusion of the abdominal aorta and renal arteries and associated systemic hypertension have also been described. Animal models showed aortic dilation as well.

HSCT improved some of the underlying cardiac manifestations, including cardiac hypertrophy [15,149–151] and coronary artery narrowing [10,152]. However, mitral and aortic valve insufficiencies persisted [7,15,153], causing progressive valvular dysfunction, including stenosis and regurgitation [7,15]. Similar to changes in skeletal manifestations and corneal clouding, insufficient correction of valvular disease was likely due to inadequate supply of the heart with enzyme in patients. In contrast to these findings in patients, BMT in MPS I dogs resulted in partial correction of mitral and aortic valve abnormalities and correction of aortic root dilation [90,154]. The differences in response are not understood.

ERT had a positive effect on cardiac hypertrophy and stabilized or even improved systolic ventricular function [53,155–157]. However, ERT did not prevent progression of cardiac valve thickening [51,155,156,158–160], although some studies reported stabilization or improvement of cardiac valve function [51,107,141,161]. Similar results were reported in MPS I dogs receiving ERT after a tolerization regimen comprising cyclosporine A with azathioprine and low-dose IDUA [162].

3.7. Cognitive Function

HSCT remains the standard treatment for severe MPS I because it can stabilize cognitive function and prevent progressive developmental decline [16,83,163–165]. However, HSCT cannot restore cognitive function. Consequently, neurodevelopmental outcome is predicted by baseline function and age at HSCT. Typically, cognitive function declines in the first year post-HSCT, after which it stabilizes [8,50,153], possibly due to a delay in infiltration and engraftment of donor cells in the CNS. The relative long lag-time between treatment and possible effect on cognitive function poses a challenge for clinical trials, which is also augmented by the interpatient variability of cognitive manifestations.

ERT on its own is not expected to provide neurocognitive benefit due to the inability of the enzyme to cross the BBB. However, there is a single case report of a girl with Hurler syndrome who was treated with only ERT starting before age 2, showing a significantly extended course of normal neurocognitive function, unpredicted by the natural history of the disease; the authors speculated that ERT was a critical factor in this finding [50,66]. Further, in MPS I mice, treatment with doses of ERT at levels higher than the clinical standard dose was accompanied by an increase of IDUA activity and reduction in GAG accumulation in the brain [141,166,167]. It is interesting that the treatment not only prevented the development of cognitive impairment in neonatal animals, but also resulted in a significant improvement when administered up to 10 weeks of age. However, older animals with established cognitive impairment, at 6 months or older, did not show improved neurobehavior [161].

The observation that high-dose ERT resulted in an increase of IDUA activity in the brain may indicate that the BBB is not impermeable to enzyme, but that the amount of enzyme delivered under clinical dosages is insufficient to yield detectable changes. Combined HSCT and ERT was associated with better short-term cognitive function in patients with MPS I [50]. The mechanism remains unclear; however, it has been posed that conditioning may increase BBB permeability [168], thereby allowing entry of IDUA into the CNS.

4. Experimental Therapies

The residual disease burden in patients with MPS I is caused mainly by insufficient enzyme levels in the CNS, the eyes, heart, and bones. Different experimental therapies have been developed to address this shortcoming, and some preclinical treatments have been translated into clinical trials (Table 2).

Table 2. Clinical Trials for MPS I.

Drug	Clinical Trials
Anti-inflammatory therapy	
Adalimumab	Phase I/II: NCT02437253: completed NCT03153319: recruiting
In utero ERT	
laronidase	Phase I: NCT04532047: not yet recruiting
Intrathecal delivery	
laronidase	Phase I: NCT00215527, NCT00786968: terminated due to slow enrolment) Phase not applicable: NCT00852358: completed NCT02232477: terminated due to COVID-19
laronidase with HSCT	Phase I: NCT00638547: completed

Table 2. Cont.

Drug	Clinical Trials
BBB-crossing IDUA-fusion proteins	
AGT-181 (fusion to Insulin receptor monoclonal antibody)	Phase I/II: NCT03071341, NCT03053089, NCT02597114: completed
JR-171 (Undisclosed fusion partner)	Phase I/II: NCT04227600, NCT04453085: not yet recruiting
Ex vivo gene transfer	
Autologous HSPC transduced with IDUA	Phase I/II: NCT03488394: recruiting
ISP-001 (B cells transposed with IDUA)	Phase I/II: NCT04284254: not yet recruiting
In vivo gene transfer	
RGX-111 (AAV9-mediated)	Phase I/II: NCT03580083: recruiting
SB-318 (Genome editing ZFN)	Phase I/II: NCT02702115: active, not recruiting

4.1. Substrate Reduction

While the majority of current therapies focus on the delivery of IDUA, a different approach is taken in substrate deprivation therapy. Treatment of 4 week old MPS I mice with weekly IV injections of the GAG synthesis inhibitor Rhodamine B resulted in prevention of some skeletal manifestations and better cognitive function as evaluated by a water cross maze [169].

4.2. Accelerated GAG Degradation

A different approach was taken by stimulating autophagy in order to accelerate GAG degradation [170]. Resveratrol is a stilbenoid polyphenol with many biological properties, including acceleration of autophagy, which may reduce GAG accumulation in patients with MPS I. Importantly, Resveratrol crosses the blood brain barrier. However, the short half-life of the drug and its rapid degradation in the liver limits its applicability as a long-term treatment. Jupiter Orphan Therapeutics reported that administration of their formulation of Resveratrol (JOTROL™) to rats led to an increase of IDUA levels in plasma and brain [171].

4.3. Anti-Inflammatory Therapy

Subcutaneous injections of the anti-inflammatory drug pentosan polysulfate (PPS) in MPS I dogs not only reduced inflammatory markers, but resulted in reduced GAG concentrations, increased luminal openings, and reduced intimal media thickening in the carotid arteries and aortas of MPS I dogs [172]. In a subsequent study of patients with attenuated MPS I, this treatment resulted in reduced urinary GAG excretion, improved joint mobility, and reduced pain [173]. Treatment of one patient with MPS I with the anti-inflammatory adalimumab resulted in improved range-of-motion and reduced bodily pain (NCT02437253) [174]. A phase 1/2 trial (NCT03153319) is currently recruiting patients with MPS I to evaluate safety and efficacy of adalimumab.

4.4. Intracerebroventricular and Intrathecal Delivery ERT

Direct delivery of enzyme by intrathecal (IT) ERT in dogs was associated with partial correction of pathological manifestations as assessed by neuroimaging [175]. Similar to direct enzyme delivery, transplantation of HSCT into the cerebral ventricle of neonatal immunodeficient MPS I mice resulted in improved motor function as assessed by rotarod test [176].

A number of small clinical trials are currently underway to test IT ERT on cognitive function in patients with MPS I. The first intrathecal ERT in patients with MPS I resulted in some improvement in endurance and pulmonary function [177]. IT ERT in one patient with attenuated MPS I resulted in significantly improved memory and adaptive functioning and mildly improved attention and IQ [66]. IT IDUA administration in five patients with MPS I (NCT00215527, NCT00786968) resulted in subjective improvement reported in the three subjects that completed the study. However, objective outcome measures including the 6 min-walk-test did not support this finding [178]. Similar findings were seen in a follow-up study of 16 patients with MPS I (NCT00852358) [179]; however, the authors argued that the lack of effect may have been due to the relatively older age, normal cognitive function of the participants, and the short study period of 2 years. More promising results were reported when children with MPS I were infused intrathecally with Laronidase prior to and following HSCT (NCT00638547). Here, improvement was also reflected in decreased CSF opening pressure and levels of biomarkers of disease activity and inflammation. Notably, some of these changes occurred after ERT-IT, but prior to HSCT. Further, this study reported a significant relationship between biomarker change and neurocognitive outcome, in that a reduction in a heparan sulfate-derived part of the GAG was associated with a more favorable IQ trajectory [180].

4.5. In Utero ERT Treatment

Treatment in utero was attempted in the canine MPS I disease model, where fetal pups were injected either with retroviral vector containing the IDUA encoding sequence, or with HSC retrovirally transduced with IDUA. While transduction and cell engraftment were observed, no IDUA activity or IDUA transcripts were detected; consequently there was no evidence of disease amelioration [181,182]. A clinical phase I study is planned to establish safety and feasibility of in utero ERT to induce tolerance and improved neurodevelopmental outcomes (NCT04532047).

4.6. Shuttling of Enzyme Across the BBB

Tissue-specific delivery of IDUA to the brain was attempted by targeting receptors present on the luminal side of the BBB. Fusion of the IDUA molecule to ApoE-derived receptor-binding peptides enabled the enzyme to cross the BBB of MPS I mice resulting in increased brain IDUA activity and normalized brain GAG levels [183]. The treatment correlated with normalization of behavioral performance as assessed by repeated open-field tests [167]. The same receptor pathway was targeted by an Angiopep-2-IDUA fusion protein, developed by Angiochem Inc. An unusual delivery pathway was selected by fusing IDUA to the plant lectin ricin B chain (RTB). Peripheral delivery of RBT-IDUA led to a significant increase in enzyme activity and normalization of GAG levels in the brain and improved cognitive function in MPS I mice [184]. BioStrategies LC is developing the RTB-IDUA drug as a delivery option to treat bone and connective tissue in MPS I. Finally, fusion of IDUA to a monoclonal antibody targeting the human insulin receptor [185] allowed transport of IDUA across the BBB in animal models [186,187]. The effect of this approach on cognitive function was investigated in a 52-week clinical trial enrolling children with MPS I with severe neurocognitive impairment (NCT03071341). An additional trial (NCT03053089) enrolled patients with attenuated MPS I. Treatment stabilized CNS function as assessed by cognitive testing and total grey matter volume [188].

Another IDUA fusion protein targeted to cross the BBB was developed by JCR Pharmaceuticals Co Ltd. (JR 171). A phase 1/2 clinical trial (NCT04227600) was concluded in July 2020; however, results are unpublished. An additional phase 1/2 trial NCT04453085 is planned, but not yet recruiting. While the exact nature of the modification is proprietary, it is likely that the fusion protein consists of IDUA fused to anti-human transferrin receptor analogous to the company's drug JR-141, a fusion protein of anti-human transferrin receptor and iduronate-2-sulfate [189]. The human transferrin receptor was also targeted by the transferrin-IDUA fusion protein [190], developed as Txb4-Ls1 by Ossianix.

4.7. Molecular Therapies

4.7.1. Nonsense Suppression and mRNA Engineering

The most common mutation in MPS I is the W402X nonsense mutation, which introduces a premature stop codon. Nonsense suppression therapy aims at the suppression of the nonsense mutation, thereby enabling continuous translation into a full-length protein. Suppression can be achieved using specific drugs [191]. The aminoglycoside derivative NB84 partially restored IDUA activity in MPS I mice carrying the murine nonsense mutation (W392X mice) and resulted in partial prevention of cardiac, skeletal, and behavioral abnormalities [192]. The effect on behavioral manifestations was likely due to aminoglycosides entering the CNS at ~10–20% of their serum concentration.

Therapeutic RNA editing aims to correct a mutation within the mRNA. In one approach, a synthetic antisense RNA complementary to the mutated sequence forms a double-stranded RNA, which activates the deamination of adenosine-to-inosine (A-to-I), resulting in a read-through of the stop-codon. The deamination is carried out by endogenous adenosine deaminase acting on RNA (ADAR) enzymes, which act on double stranded RNAs.

To date, results for therapeutic RNA editing to correct the TGG>TAG nonsense mutation within the IDUA gene have been published only in abstract format and will be discussed briefly here. The Leveraging Endogenous ADAR for Programmable Editing of RNA (LEAPER) program uses ADAR recruiting (ar) RNA, which targets the enzyme to the TGG>TAG nonsense mutation. Administration of arRNA packaged into AAV vectors in MPS I mice carrying the W392X mutation resulted in higher IDUA enzymatic activity [193]. This approach is currently under investigation for its applicability as an MPS I therapeutic by EdiGene Inc. A similar approach is used by RNA Editing for Specific C-to-U Exchange (RESCUE), which fuses the inactive Cas13 (dCas13) protein to the ADAR deaminase domain (ADARdd). Delivery of this fusion protein and guide RNA via AAV into W392X mice resulted in correction of 15% of total IDUA mRNA and a significant increase of IDUA activity in the liver [194]. In a slightly different strategy, exogenous adenosine deaminases were introduced into the host. Fusion of two monomers of E.coli tRNA-specific adenosine deaminase with inactive Cas9 protein gives rise to the Adenine Base Editor (ABEmax). AAV9 mediated co-delivery of guide RNA and ABEmax into neonatal W392X mice resulted in durable enzyme expression alongside reduction of accumulation of GAGs in tissues [195].

Systemic delivery of suppressor tRNA therapy by AAV vectors into W392X mice resulted in prolonged restoration of low serum and liver IDUA activity (1–3% of the normal level) [196].

4.7.2. Ex Vivo Gene Transfer

Stable genetic complementation of IDUA deficiency in autologous HSC has the potential to address some of the complications of allotransplant, such as graft-vs-host disease, while at the same time engineering a much higher level of enzyme expression and delivery and maintaining access to the CNS [197,198]. Transplantation of HSPCs transduced ex vivo with IDUA-lentivirus vector into 8 week old MPS I mice resulted in the correction of disease manifestations, including cognitive impairment, hearing deficits, skeletal deformities, and retinopathy [197]. Results from studies investigating this approach in MPS I dogs using murine gamma-retroviral vector were less compelling [199,200]. While the engineered cells showed high IDUA expression and transplanted cells engrafted successfully in the animals, enzyme expression in vivo was undetectable. This gene deactivation was caused by cellular and humoral immune responses against the transduced cells and the resultant protein.

The ex vivo gene therapy approach is currently being tested in a small clinical trial, where patients with severe MPS I received HSPCs transduced with lentiviral vector encoding IDUA (NCT03488394). Preliminary data after 1 year suggested stabilization of cognitive function and improvement of skeletal deficits [201].

Transplantation of 6–8 week old immune-deficient MPS I mice with HSCPs edited via the CRISPR-Cas9 approach for insertion of the IDUA coding sequence into the CCR5 locus resulted in IDUA activity in serum, liver, spleen, and brain together with normalization of skeletal parameters and improved cognitive function [202].

The Sleeping beauty (SB) transposon system presents another alternative to viral genetic therapy for stable gene transfer and expression. The SB system uses the SB transposase to integrate gene sequences in co-delivered transposons into host chromosomal DNA. Hydrodynamic co-delivery of SB transposase and the SB transposon encoding IDUA into MPS I mice or MPS I dogs resulted in successful expression of the enzyme in the liver. However, the animals' immune response resulted in the subsequent decline of IDUA levels [203,204]. Immunosuppression or the use of immunodeficient NOD/SCID-MPS I mice allowed prolonged expression of IDUA in the liver, reduction of GAG accumulation, and correction of some skeletal manifestations [205]. Immusoft Corp is currently developing the SB approach as a cell-based therapy for IDUA deficiency using autologous human B cells. Infusions of immunodeficient NSG-MPS I mice with IDUA-transposed B cells resulted in substantial plasma IDUA activity and reduction of tissue GAG storage [206]. A similar approach was taken using a combination of CRISPR/Cas9 and rAAV vector to integrate the IDUA gene into B cells. Transplantation of these IDUA-positive B cells into NSG-MPS I mice resulted in a significant increase in IDUA enzyme activity [207].

Sigilon Therapeutics Inc is currently developing their Shielded Living Therapeutics approach as a strategy to protect therapeutic human cells that have been engineered to express high levels of IDUA from the host's immune response. Administration of this shielded IDUA-secreting human cell line (SIG-005) into MPS I mice resulted in GAG reduction in plasma and tissues [208].

4.7.3. In Vivo Gene Transfer

In vivo gene therapy using AAV vector can take advantage of varying tropisms conferred by different AAV serotypes to direct transduction to a desired tissue. However, AAV rarely integrates into the host genome, so these vectors are most applicable to target tissues where there is limited cell division, such as the CNS. Intrastromal delivery of AAV8G9-vector encoding IDUA resulted in lasting reversal of corneal clouding in MPS I dogs [209]. Administration of AAV2 vector encoding IDUA in neonatal mice partially ameliorated bone defects and behavioral abnormalities as assessed in an open field test [210]. There was only a moderate level of IDUA detected in brain tissues, so these findings suggest that even small amounts of enzyme in the CNS can have a significant impact on cognitive function. Much higher levels of enzyme were expressed in the brain after ICV infusion of neonatal MPS I mice with AA8 vector encoding human IDUA, preventing emergence of neurocognitive deficits as determined in the Morris water maze [211]. Intranasal administration of IDUA-encoding AAV9 vector to adult MPS I mice resulted in normalized IDUA enzyme activity and reduction of GAG accumulation in the brain. Moreover, neurocognitive function was corrected as assessed in the Barnes maze [212]. AAV9 vector encoding IDUA corrected CNS pathology after intrathecal delivery in MPS I cats [213]. IDUA transduction using AAV9 vector was tested for safety and expression in non-human primates after intrathecal suboccipital delivery to the CSV [214]. REGENXBIO is currently testing intracisternally administered rAAV9 vector encoding IDUA in a clinical trial for MPS I (NCT03580083).

Administration of gamma-retroviral vector encoding IDUA into neonatal MPS I mice prevented development of ocular and hearing impairments, aortic insufficiencies, and skeletal defects [215] and resulted in improved outcomes in adult mice as well [216].

In vivo gene therapy using the CRISPR-Cas9 strategy was first tested in neonatal MPS I mice, where the ubiquitously expressed ROSA26 locus was targeted as the transgene insertion site. A long-term, modest increase in IDUA activity in serum and all organs (except for brain) was observed using this approach [113]. Pulmonary function was normalized, bone defects were prevented, and elastin breaks in the aorta were partially reduced. However, heart valves and brain showed no functional improvement [113]. A

Zinc Finger Nuclease (ZFN) mediated gene editing approach was used to insert the IDUA coding sequence into the albumin locus for high-level protein expression [217]. Delivery of the construct by AAV8 vector to hepatocytes in 4–10 week old MPS I mice resulted in significant increases in IDUA activity and GAG reduction in blood and peripheral tissues and in the brain. Development of neurobehavioral deficits was prevented as assessed by Barnes maze. An ongoing phase 1/2 clinical trial involving patients with mild forms of MPS I with no CNS involvement is being sponsored by Sangamo Therapeutics (NCT02702115).

5. Conclusions

The current approved treatment options for MPS I consist of HSCT, ERT, or combinations of both therapies. While these treatments significantly improve disease manifestations and prolong life, a considerable burden of disease remains in the treated children and adults. Both treatments may at best prevent the development or worsening of abnormal function and somatic complications but cannot revert already existing symptoms. Therefore, treatment must commence as early as possible for maximum effect. Even when conducted under optimal conditions, such as early age and matching non-carrier donor for the HSCT, the therapeutic effect in some systems appears to wear off after several years. Some organs are altogether resistant to treatment. The most resistant organs/tissues are the bones, eyes, and heart valves.

A number of experimental strategies are currently under development to reduce the burden of disease further. Some molecular therapies target nonsense mutations at the mRNA level through nonsense suppression, mRNA editing, and suppressor tRNAs. Gene transfer is being tested both ex vivo by engineering HSCPs and human B cells prior to transplantation and in vivo using both viral and non-viral approaches. Other therapies address GAG accumulation by enhancing autophagy or inhibiting GAG synthesis. The effect of delivering IDUA to the CNS via direct infusion, shuttling pathways, or targeted viral delivery is currently under investigation in small clinical trials. With concentrated efforts, the prospect for significantly improving the long-term outcome for these children is within our grasp.

Author Contributions: C.S.H.; writing-review and editing, C.S.H., J.W., T.C.L., P.J.O., L.E.P., J.B.E., L.K.M., S.C., P.S., R.S.M. All authors have read and agreed to the published version of the manuscript.

Funding: This research received no external funding.

Conflicts of Interest: C.S.H., J.W. and R.S.M. are employees of Immusoft Corporation. T.C.L. is a paid consultant of Immusoft Corporation.

References

1. Kuiper, G.A.; Meijer, O.L.M.; Langereis, E.J.; Wijburg, F.A. Failure to shorten the diagnostic delay in two ultra-orphan diseases (mucopolysaccharidosis types I and III): Potential causes and implications. *Orphanet J. Rare Dis.* **2018**, *13*, 1–13. [CrossRef] [PubMed]
2. Clarke, L.A.; Dickson, P.; Ellinwood, N.M.; Klein, T.L. Newborn screening for mucopolysaccharidosis I: Moving forward learning from experience. *Int. J. Neonatal Screen.* **2020**, *6*, 91. [CrossRef] [PubMed]
3. Donati, M.A.; Pasquini, E.; Spada, M.; Polo, G.; Burlina, A. Newborn screening in mucopolysaccharidoses. *Ital. J. Pediatr.* **2018**, *44*. [CrossRef] [PubMed]
4. Eisengart, J.B.; Rudser, K.D.; Xue, Y.; Orchard, P.; Miller, W.; Lund, T.; Van der Ploeg, A.; Mercer, J.; Jones, S.; Mengel, K.E.; et al. Long-term outcomes of systemic therapies for Hurler syndrome: An international multicenter comparison. *Genet. Med.* **2018**, *20*, 1423–1429. [CrossRef]
5. Aldenhoven, M.; Jones, S.A.; Bonney, D.; Borrill, R.E.; Coussons, M.; Mercer, J.; Bierings, M.B.; Versluys, B.; van Hasselt, P.M.; Wijburg, F.A.; et al. Hematopoietic Cell Transplantation for Mucopolysaccharidosis Patients Is Safe and Effective: Results after Implementation of International Guidelines. *Biol. Blood Marrow Transplant.* **2015**, *21*, 1106–1109. [CrossRef]
6. Boelens, J.J.; Van Hasselt, P.M. Neurodevelopmental outcome after hematopoietic cell transplantation in inborn errors of metabolism: Current considerations and future perspectives. *Neuropediatrics* **2016**, *47*, 285–292. [CrossRef]

7. Lum, S.H.; Stepien, K.M.; Ghosh, A.; Broomfield, A.; Church, H.; Mercer, J.; Jones, S.; Wynn, R. Long term survival and cardiopulmonary outcome in children with Hurler syndrome after haematopoietic stem cell transplantation. *J. Inherit. Metab. Dis.* **2017**, *40*, 455–460. [CrossRef]
8. Shapiro, E.G.; Nestrasil, I.; Rudser, K.; Delaney, K.; Kovac, V.; Ahmed, A.; Yund, B.; Orchard, P.J.; Eisengart, J.; Niklason, G.R.; et al. Neurocognition across the spectrum of mucopolysaccharidosis type I: Age, severity, and treatment. *Mol. Genet. Metab.* **2015**, *116*, 61–68. [CrossRef]
9. Peters, C.; Steward, C.G. Hematopoietic cell transplantation for inherited metabolic diseases: An overview of outcomes and practice guidelines. *Bone Marrow Transplant.* **2003**, *31*, 229–239. [CrossRef]
10. Braunlin, E.A.; Rose, A.G.; Hopwood, J.J.; Candel, R.D.; Krivit, W. Coronary artery patency following long-term successful engraftment 14 years after bone marrow transplantation in the Hurler syndrome. *Am. J. Cardiol.* **2001**, *88*, 1075–1077. [CrossRef]
11. Souillet, G.; Guffon, N.; Maire, I.; Pujol, M.; Taylor, P.; Sevin, F.; Bleyzac, N.; Mulier, C.; Durin, A.; Kebaili, K.; et al. Outcome of 27 patients with Hurler's syndrome transplanted from either related or unrelated haematopoietic stem cell sources. *Bone Marrow Transplant.* **2003**, *31*, 1105–1117. [CrossRef] [PubMed]
12. Moore, D.; Connock, M.J.; Wraith, E.; Lavery, C. The prevalence of and survival in Mucopolysaccharidosis I: Hurler, Hurler-Scheie and Scheie syndromes in the UK. *Orphanet J. Rare Dis.* **2008**, *3*, 24. [CrossRef] [PubMed]
13. Rodgers, N.J.; Kaizer, A.M.; Miller, W.P.; Rudser, K.D.; Orchard, P.J.; Braunlin, E.A. Mortality after hematopoietic stem cell transplantation for severe mucopolysaccharidosis type I: The 30-year University of Minnesota experience. *J. Inherit. Metab. Dis.* **2017**, *40*, 271–280. [CrossRef] [PubMed]
14. Peters, B.C.; Shapiro, E.G.; Anderson, J.; Henslee-downey, P.J.; Klemperer, M.R.; Cowan, M.J.; Saunders, E.F.; Pedro, A.; Twist, C.; Nachman, J.B.; et al. Hurler syndrome: II. Outcome of HLA-genotypically identical sibling and HLA-haploidentical related donor bone marrow transplantation in fifty-four children. *Blood* **1998**, *91*, 2601–2608. [CrossRef]
15. Braunlin, E.A.; Stauffer, N.R.; Peters, C.H.; Bass, J.L.; Berry, J.M.; Hopwood, J.J.; Krivit, W. Usefulness of bone marrow transplantation in the Hurler syndrome. *Am. J. Cardiol.* **2003**, *92*, 882–886. [CrossRef]
16. Kunin-Batson, A.S.; Shapiro, E.G.; Rudser, K.D.; Lavery, C.A.; Bjoraker, K.J.; Jones, S.A.; Wynn, R.F.; Vellodi, A.; Tolar, J.; Orchard, P.J. Long-term cognitive and functional outcomes in children with mucopolysaccharidosis (MPS)-IH (Hurler syndrome) treated with hematopoietic cell transplantation. *JIMD Rep.* **2016**, *29*, 95–102.
17. Boelens, J.J.; Wynn, R.F.; O'Meara, A.; Veys, P.; Bertrand, Y.; Souillet, G.; Wraith, J.E.; Fischer, A.; Cavazzana-Calvo, M.; Sykora, K.W.; et al. Outcomes of hematopoietic stem cell transplantation for Hurler's syndrome in Europe: A risk factor analysis for graft failure. *Bone Marrow Transplant.* **2007**, *40*, 225–233. [CrossRef]
18. Ansari, M.; Théoret, Y.; Rezgui, M.A.; Peters, C.; Mezziani, S.; Desjean, C.; Vachon, M.F.; Champagne, M.A.; Duval, M.; Krajinovic, M.; et al. Association between busulfan exposure and outcome in children receiving intravenous busulfan before hematopoietic stem cell transplantation. *Ther. Drug Monit.* **2014**, *36*, 93–99. [CrossRef]
19. Giorgiani, G.; Bozzola, M.; Locatelli, F.; Picco, P.; Zecca, M.; Cisternino, M.; Dallorso, S.; Bonetti, F.; Dini, G.; Borrone, C. Role of busulfan and total body irradiation on growth of prepubertal children receiving bone marrow transplantation and results of treatment with recombinant human growth hormone. *Blood* **1995**, *86*, 825–831. [CrossRef]
20. Allewelt, H.; El-Khorazaty, J.; Mendizabal, A.; Taskindoust, M.; Martin, P.L.; Prasad, V.; Page, K.; Sanders, J.; Kurtzberg, J. Late effects after umbilical cord blood transplantation in very young children after busulfan-based, myeloablative conditioning. *Biol. Blood Marrow Transpl.* **2016**, *22*, 1627–1635. [CrossRef]
21. Vatanen, A.; Wilhelmsson, M.; Borgström, B.; Gustafsson, B.; Taskinen, M.; Saarinen-Pihkala, U.M.; Winiarski, J.; Jahnukainen, K. Ovarian function after allogeneic hematopoietic stem cell transplantation in childhood and adolescence. *Eur. J. Endocrinol.* **2014**, *170*, 211–218. [CrossRef] [PubMed]
22. Tichelli, A.; Rovó, A. Fertility issues following hematopoietic stem cell transplantation. *Expert Rev. Hematol.* **2013**, *6*, 375–388. [CrossRef] [PubMed]
23. Borgmann-Staudt, A.; Rendtorff, R.; Reinmuth, S.; Hohmann, C.; Keil, T.; Schuster, F.R.; Holter, W.; Ehlert, K.; Keslova, P.; Lawitschka, A.; et al. Fertility after allogeneic haematopoietic stem cell transplantation in childhood and adolescence. *Bone Marrow Transplant.* **2012**, *47*, 271–276. [CrossRef] [PubMed]
24. Dalle, J.H.; Lucchini, G.; Balduzzi, A.; Ifversen, M.; Jahnukainen, K.; MacKlon, K.T.; Ahler, A.; Jarisch, A.; Ansari, M.; Beohou, E.; et al. State-of-the-art fertility preservation in children and adolescents undergoing haematopoietic stem cell transplantation: A report on the expert meeting of the Paediatric Diseases Working Party (PDWP) of the European Society for Blood and Marrow Transplantation (EBMT) in Baden, Austria, 29–30 September 2015. *Bone Marrow Transplant.* **2017**, *52*, 1029–1035. [CrossRef]
25. Bartelink, I.H.; van Reij, E.M.L.; Gerhardt, C.E.; van Maarseveen, E.M.; de Wildt, A.; Versluys, B.; Lindemans, C.A.; Bierings, M.B.; Boelens, J.J. Fludarabine and exposure-targeted busulfan compares favorably with busulfan/cyclophosphamide-based regimens in pediatric hematopoietic cell transplantation: Maintaining efficacy with less toxicity. *Biol. Blood Marrow Transpl.* **2014**, *20*, 345–353. [CrossRef]
26. Ben-Barouch, S.; Cohen, O.; Vidal, L.; Avivi, I.; Ram, R. Busulfan fludarabine vs busulfan cyclophosphamide as a preparative regimen before allogeneic hematopoietic cell transplantation: Systematic review and meta-analysis. *Bone Marrow Transplant.* **2016**, *51*, 232–240. [CrossRef]
27. Gyurkocza, B.; Sandmaier, B.M. Conditioning regimens for hematopoietic cell transplantation: One size does not fit all. *Blood* **2014**, *124*, 344–353. [CrossRef]

28. Hansen, M.D.; Filipovich, A.H.; Davies, S.M.; Mehta, P.; Bleesing, J.; Jodele, S.; Hayashi, R.; Barnes, Y.; Shenoy, S. Allogeneic hematopoietic cell transplantation (HCT) in Hurler's syndrome using a reduced intensity preparative regimen. *Bone Marrow Transplant.* **2008**, *41*, 349–353. [CrossRef]
29. Aldenhoven, M.; Wynn, R.F.; Orchard, P.J.; O'Meara, A.; Veys, P.; Fischer, A.; Valayannopoulos, V.; Neven, B.; Rovelli, A.; Prasad, V.K.; et al. Long-term outcome of Hurler syndrome patients after hematopoietic cell transplantation: An international multicenter study. *Blood* **2015**, *125*, 2164–2172. [CrossRef]
30. Langereis, E.J.; van Vlies, N.; Church, H.J.; Geskus, R.B.; Hollak, C.E.M.; Jones, S.A.; Kulik, W.; van Lenthe, H.; Mercer, J.; Schreider, L.; et al. Biomarker responses correlate with antibody status in mucopolysaccharidosis type I patients on long-term enzyme replacement therapy. *Mol. Genet. Metab.* **2015**, *114*, 129–137. [CrossRef]
31. Wynn, R.; Wraith, E.; Mercer, J.; O'Meara, A.; Tylee, K.; Thornley, M.; Church, H.; Bigger, B. Improved metabolic correction in patients with lysosomal storage disease treated with hematopoietic stem cell transplant compared with enzyme replacement therapy. *J. Pediatr.* **2009**, *154*, 609–611. [CrossRef] [PubMed]
32. Pal, A.R.; Langereis, E.J.; Saif, M.A.; Mercer, J.; Church, H.J.; Tylee, K.L.; Wynn, R.F.; Wijburg, F.A.; Jones, S.A.; Bruce, I.A.; et al. Sleep disordered breathing in mucopolysaccharidosis I: A multivariate analysis of patient, therapeutic and metabolic correlators modifying long term clinical outcome. *Orphanet J. Rare Dis.* **2015**, *10*, 1–13. [CrossRef]
33. Boelens, J.J.; Aldenhoven, M.; Purtill, D.; Ruggeri, A.; Defor, T.; Wynn, R.; Wraith, E.; Cavazzana-Calvo, M.; Rovelli, A.; Fischer, A.; et al. Outcomes of transplantation using various hematopoietic stem cell sources in children with Hurler syndrome after myeloablative conditioning. *Blood* **2013**, *121*, 3981–3987. [CrossRef] [PubMed]
34. Staba, S.L.; Escolar, M.L.; Poe, M.; Kim, Y.; Martin, P.L.; Szabolcs, P.; Allison-Thacker, J.; Wood, S.; Wenger, D.A.; Rubinstein, P.; et al. Cord-blood transplants from unrelated donors in patients with Hurler's syndrome. *N. Engl. J. Med.* **2004**, *350*, 1960–1969. [CrossRef]
35. Hobbs, J.; Hugh-Jones, K.; Barrett, A.; Byrom, N.; James, D.C.O.; Lucas, C.F. Reversal of clinical features of Hurler's disease and biochemical improvement after treatment by bone-marrow transplantation. *Lancet* **1981**, *2*, 709–712. [CrossRef]
36. Kuiper, G.A.; van Hasselt, P.M.; Boelens, J.J.; Wijburg, F.A.; Langereis, E.J. Incomplete biomarker response in mucopolysaccharidosis type I after successful hematopoietic cell transplantation. *Mol. Genet. Metab.* **2017**, *122*, 86–91. [CrossRef] [PubMed]
37. Church, H.; Tylee, K.; Cooper, A.; Thornley, M.; Mercer, J.; Wraith, E.; Carr, T.; O'Meara, A.; Wynn, R.F. Biochemical monitoring after haemopoietic stem cell transplant for Hurler syndrome (MPSIH): Implications for functional outcome after transplant in metabolic disease. *Bone Marrow Transplant.* **2007**, *39*, 207–210. [CrossRef] [PubMed]
38. Poole, A.; Webber, C.; Pidoux, I.; Choi, H.; Rosenberg, L. Localization of a Dermatan Sulfate Proteoglycan (DS-PGII) in Cartilage and the Presence of an Immunologically Related Species in Other Tissues. *J. Histochem. Cytochem.* **1986**, *34*, 619–625. [CrossRef] [PubMed]
39. Grande-Allen, K.J.; Clabro, A.; Gupta, V.; Wight, T.N.; Hascall, V.C.; Vesely, I. Glycosaminoglycans and proteoglycans in normal mitral valve leaflets and chordae: Association with regions of tensile and compressive loading. *Glycobiology* **2004**, *14*, 621–633. [CrossRef]
40. Ellinwood, N.M.; Colle, M.A.; Weil, M.A.; Casal, M.L.; Vite, C.H.; Wiemelt, S.; Hasson, C.W.; O'Malley, T.M.; He, X.; Prociuk, U.; et al. Bone marrow transplantation for feline mucopolysaccharidosis I. *Mol. Genet. Metab.* **2007**, *91*, 239–250. [CrossRef]
41. Pievani, A.; Azario, I.; Antolini, L.; Shimada, T.; Patel, P.; Remoli, C.; Rambaldi, B.; Valsecchi, M.; Riminucci, M.; Biondi, A.; et al. Neonatal bone marrow transplantation prevents bone pathology in a mouse model of mucopolysaccharidosis type I. *Blood* **2014**, *124*. [CrossRef]
42. Azario, I.; Pievani, A.; Del Priore, F.; Antolini, L.; Santi, L.; Corsi, A.; Cardinale, L.; Sawamoto, K.; Kubaski, F.; Gentner, B.; et al. Neonatal umbilical cord blood transplantation halts skeletal disease progression in the murine model of MPS-I. *Sci. Rep.* **2017**, *7*, 1–13. [CrossRef] [PubMed]
43. Hoogerbrugge, P.M.; Brouwer, O.F.; Bordigoni, P.; Cornu, G.; Kapaun, P.; Ortega, J.J.; O'Meara, A.; Souillet, G.; Frappaz, D.; Blanche, S.; et al. Allogeneic bone marrow transplantation for lysosomal storage diseases. *Lancet* **1995**, *345*, 1398–1402. [CrossRef]
44. Prasad, V.K.; Kurtzberg, J. Emerging trends in transplantation of inherited metabolic diseases. *Bone Marrow Transplant.* **2008**, *41*, 99–108. [CrossRef] [PubMed]
45. Cronk, J.C.; Filiano, A.J.; Louveau, A.; Marin, I.; Marsh, R.; Ji, E.; Goldman, D.H.; Smirnov, I.; Geraci, N.; Acton, S.; et al. Peripherally derived macrophages can engraft the brain independent of irradiation and maintain an identity distinct from microglia. *J. Exp. Med.* **2018**, *215*, 1627–1647. [CrossRef] [PubMed]
46. Unger, E.; Sung, J.; Manivel, J.C.; Chenggis, M.; Blazar, B.; Krivit, W. Male donor-derived cells in the brain of female sex-mismatched bone marrow transplant recipients: A y-chromosome specific in situ hybridization study. *J. Neuropathol. Exp. Neurol.* **1993**, *52*, 460–470. [CrossRef]
47. Araya, K.; Sakai, N.; Mohri, I.; Kagitani-Shimono, K.; Okinaga, T.; Hashii, Y.; Ohta, H.; Nakamichi, I.; Aozasa, K.; Taniike, M.; et al. Localized donor cells in brain of a Hunter disease patient after cord blood stem cell transplantation. *Mol. Genet. Metab.* **2009**, *98*, 255–263. [CrossRef]
48. de Ru, M.H.; Boelens, J.J.; Das, A.M.; Jones, S.A.; van der Lee, J.H.; Mahlaoui, N.; Mengel, E.; Offringa, M.; O'Meara, A.; Parini, R.; et al. Enzyme Replacement Therapy and/or Hematopoietic Stem Cell Transplantation at diagnosis in patients with Mucopolysaccharidosis type I: Results of a European consensus procedure. *Orphanet J. Rare Dis.* **2011**, *6*, 55. [CrossRef]

49. Krivit, W.; Sung, J.; Shapiro, E.G.; Lockman, L.A. Microglia: The effector cell for reconstitution of the central nervous system following bone marrow transplantation for lysosomal and peroxisomal storage diseases. *Cell Transpl.* **1995**, *4*, 385–392. [CrossRef]
50. Eisengart, J.; Rudser, K.; Tolar, J.; Orchared, P.; Kivisto, T.; Ziegler, R.S.; Whitley, C.; Shapiro, E. Enzyme replacement is associated with better cognitive outcomes after transplant in Hurler syndrome. *J. Pediatrics* **2013**, *162*, 375–380. [CrossRef]
51. Clarke, L.A.; Wraith, J.E.; Beck, M.; Kolodny, E.H.; Pastores, G.M.; Muenzer, J.; Rapoport, D.M.; Berger, K.I.; Sidman, M.; Kakkis, E.D.; et al. Long-term efficacy and safety of laronidase in the treatment of mucopolysaccharidosis I. *Pediatrics* **2009**, *123*, 229–240. [CrossRef] [PubMed]
52. Sifuentes, M.; Doroshow, R.; Hoft, R.; Mason, G.; Walot, I.; Diament, M.; Okazaki, S.; Huff, K.; Cox, G.F.; Swiedler, S.J.; et al. A follow-up study of MPS I patients treated with laronidase enzyme replacement therapy for 6 years. *Mol. Genet. Metab.* **2007**, *90*, 171–180. [CrossRef] [PubMed]
53. Wraith, J.E.; Beck, M.; Lane, R.; van der Ploeg, A.; Shapiro, E.; Xue, Y.; Kakkis, E.D.; Guffon, N. Enzyme replacement therapy in patients who have mucopolysaccharidosis I and are younger than 5 years: Results of a multinational study of recombinant human alpha-L-iduronidase (laronidase). *Pediatrics* **2007**, *120*, e37–e46. [CrossRef]
54. Kakkis, E.; Muenzer, J.; Tiller, G.E.; Waber, L.; Belmont, J.; Passage, M.; Izykowski, B.; Phillips, J.; Doroshow, R.; Walot, I.; et al. Enzyme-replacement therapy in mucopolysaccharidosis I. *N. Engl. J. Med.* **2001**, *344*, 182–188. [CrossRef] [PubMed]
55. Giugliani, R.; Rojas, V.M.; Martins, A.M.; Valadares, E.R.; Clarke, J.T.; Goes, J.E.; Kakkis, E.D.; Worden, M.A.; Sidman, M.; Cox, G.F. A dose-optimization trial of laronidase (Aldurazyme) in patients with mucopolysaccharidosis I. *Mol. Genet. Metab.* **2009**, *96*, 13–19. [CrossRef]
56. Parini, R.; Deodato, F. Intravenous enzyme replacement therapy in mucopolysaccharidoses: Clinical effectiveness and limitations. *Int. J. Mol. Sci.* **2020**, *21*, 2975. [CrossRef]
57. Tylki-Szymanska, A.; Marucha, J.; Jurecka, A.; Syczewska, M.; Czartoryska, B. Efficacy of recombinant human α-L-iduronidase (laronidase) on restricted range of motion of upper extremities in mucopolysaccharidosis type I patients. *J. Inherit. Metab. Dis.* **2010**, *33*, 151–157. [CrossRef]
58. Wiseman, D.H.; Mercer, J.; Tylee, K.; Malaiya, N.; Bonney, D.K.; Jones, S.A.; Wraith, J.E.; Wynn, R.F. Management of mucopolysaccharidosis type IH (Hurler's syndrome) presenting in infancy with severe dilated cardiomyopathy: A single institution's experience. *J. Inherit. Metab. Dis.* **2013**, *36*, 263–270. [CrossRef]
59. Muenzer, J. Early initiation of enzyme replacement therapy for the mucopolysaccharidoses. *Mol. Genet. Metab.* **2014**, *111*, 63–72. [CrossRef]
60. Sawamoto, K.; Stapleton, M.; Alméciga-Díaz, C.J.; Espejo-Mojica, A.J.; Losada, J.C.; Suarez, D.A.; Tomatsu, S. *Therapeutic Options for Mucopolysaccharidoses: Current and Emerging Treatments*; Springer International Publishing: Berlin/Heidelberg, Germany, 2019; Volume 79, ISBN 4026501901147.
61. White, K.K. Orthopaedic aspects of mucopolysaccharidoses. *Rheumatology* **2011**, *50*, 26–33. [CrossRef]
62. Spina, V.; Barbuti, D.; Gaeta, A.; Palmucci, S.; Soscia, E.; Grimaldi, M.; Leone, A.; Manara, R.; Polonara, G. The role of imaging in the skeletal involvement of mucopolysaccharidoses. *Ital. J. Pediatr.* **2018**, *44*, 1–6. [CrossRef] [PubMed]
63. Schmidt, M.; Breyer, S.; Löbel, U.; Yarar, S.; Stücker, R.; Ullrich, K.; Müller, I.; Muschol, N. Musculoskeletal manifestations in mucopolysaccharidosis type I (Hurler syndrome) following hematopoietic stem cell transplantation. *Orphanet J. Rare Dis.* **2016**, *11*, 1–13. [CrossRef] [PubMed]
64. Teär Fahnehjelm, K.; Olsson, M.; Chen, E.; Hengstler, J.; Naess, K.; Winiarski, J. Children with mucopolysaccharidosis risk progressive visual dysfunction despite haematopoietic stem cell transplants. *Acta Paediatr. Int. J. Paediatr.* **2018**, *107*, 1995–2003. [CrossRef] [PubMed]
65. Xue, Y.; Richards, S.M.; Mahmood, A.; Cox, G.F. Effect of anti-laronidase antibodies on efficacy and safety of laronidase enzyme replacement therapy for MPS I: A comprehensive meta-analysis of pooled data from multiple studies. *Mol. Genet. Metab.* **2016**, *117*, 419–426. [CrossRef] [PubMed]
66. Eisengart, J.B.; Jarnes, J.; Ahmed, A.; Nestrasil, I.; Ziegler, R.; Delaney, K.; Shapiro, E.; Whitley, C. Long-term cognitive and somatic outcomes of enzyme replacement therapy in untransplanted Hurler syndrome. *Mol. Genet. Metab. Rep.* **2017**, *13*, 64–68. [CrossRef] [PubMed]
67. Polgreen, L.E.; Lund, T.C.; Braunlin, E.; Tolar, J.; Miller, B.S.; Fung, E.; Whitley, C.B.; Eisengart, J.B.; Northrop, E.; Rudser, K.; et al. Clinical trial of laronidase in Hurler syndrome after hematopoietic cell transplantation. *Pediatr. Res.* **2019**. [CrossRef]
68. Kakavanos, R.; Turner, C.T.; Hopwood, J.J.; Kakkis, E.D.; Brooks, D.A. Immune tolerance after long-term enzyme-replacement therapy among patients who have mucopolysaccharidosis I. *Lancet* **2003**, *361*, 1608–1613. [CrossRef]
69. Lund, T.C.; Miller, W.P.; Liao, A.Y.; Tolar, J.; Shanley, R.; Pasquali, M.; Sando, N.; Bigger, B.W.; Polgreen, L.E.; Orchard, P.J. Post-transplant laronidase augmentation for children with Hurler syndrome: Biochemical outcomes. *Sci. Rep.* **2019**, *9*, 5–10. [CrossRef]
70. Giugliani, R.; Vieira, T.A.; Carvalho, C.G.; Munoz-Rojas, M.V.; Semyachkina, A.N.; Voinova, V.Y.; Richards, S.; Cox, G.F.; Xue, Y. Immune tolerance induction for laronidase treatment in mucopolysaccharidosis I. *Mol. Genet. Metab. Rep.* **2017**, *10*, 61–66. [CrossRef]
71. Ghosh, A.; Liao, A.; O'Leary, C.; Mercer, J.; Tylee, K.; Goenka, A.; Holley, R.; Jones, S.A.; Bigger, B.W. Strategies for the Induction of Immune Tolerance to Enzyme Replacement Therapy in Mucopolysaccharidosis Type I. *Mol. Ther. Methods Clin. Dev.* **2019**, *13*, 321–333. [CrossRef]

72. Kakkis, E.; Lester, T.; Yang, R.; Tanaka, C.; Anand, V.; Lemontt, J.; Peinovich, M.; Passage, M. Successful induction of immune tolerance to enzyme replacement therapy in canine mucopolysaccharidosis I. *Proc. Natl. Acad. Sci. USA* **2004**, *101*, 829–834. [CrossRef] [PubMed]
73. Cox-Brinkman, J.; Boelens, J.J.; Wraith, J.E.; O'Meara, A.; Veys, P.; Wijburg, F.A.; Wulffraat, N.; Wynn, R.F. Haematopoietic cell transplantation (HCT) in combination with enzyme replacement therapy (ERT) in patients with Hurler syndrome. *Bone Marrow Transplant.* **2006**, *38*, 17–21. [CrossRef] [PubMed]
74. Ferrara, G.; Maximova, N.; Zennaro, F.; Gregori, M.; Tamaro, P. Hematopoietic stem cell transplantation effects on spinal cord compression in Hurler. *Pediatr. Transplant.* **2014**, *18*, 2–5. [CrossRef] [PubMed]
75. Ghosh, A.; Miller, W.; Orchard, P.J.; Jones, S.A.; Mercer, J.; Church, H.J.; Tylee, K.; Lund, T.; Bigger, B.W.; Tolar, J.; et al. Enzyme replacement therapy prior to haematopoietic stem cell transplantation in Mucopolysaccharidosis Type I: 10 year combined experience of 2 centres. *Mol. Genet. Metab.* **2016**, *117*, 373–377. [CrossRef] [PubMed]
76. Tolar, J.; Grewal, S.S.; Bjoraker, K.J.; Whitley, C.B.; Shapiro, E.G.; Charnas, L.; Orchard, P.J. Combination of enzyme replacement and hematopoietic stem cell transplantation as therapy for Hurler syndrome. *Bone Marrow Transplant.* **2008**, *41*, 531–535. [CrossRef]
77. Grewal, S.S.; Wynn, R.; Abdenur, J.E.; Burton, B.K.; Gharib, M.; Haase, C.; Hayashi, R.J.; Shenoy, S.; Sillence, D.; Tiller, G.E.; et al. Safety and efficacy of enzyme replacement therapy in combination with hematopoietic stem cell transplantation in Hurler syndrome. *Genet. Med.* **2005**, *7*, 143–146. [CrossRef]
78. Saif, M.A.; Bigger, B.W.; Brookes, K.E.; Mercer, J.; Tylee, K.L.; Church, H.J.; Bonney, D.K.; Jones, S.; Wraith, J.E.; Wynn, R.F. Hematopoietic stem cell transplantation improves the high incidence of neutralizing allo-antibodies observed in Hurler's syndrome after pharmacological enzyme replacement therapy. *Haematologica* **2012**, *97*, 1320–1328. [CrossRef]
79. Watson, H.A.; Holley, R.J.; Langford-Smith, K.J.; Wilkinson, F.L.; Van Kuppevelt, T.H.; Wynn, R.F.; Wraith, J.E.; Merry, C.L.R.; Bigger, B.W. Heparan sulfate inhibits hematopoietic stem and progenitor cell migration and engraftment in mucopolysaccharidosis I. *J. Biol. Chem.* **2014**, *289*, 36194–36203. [CrossRef]
80. Santi, L.; De Ponti, G.; Dina, G.; Pievani, A.; Corsi, A.; Riminucci, M.; Khan, S.; Sawamoto, K.; Antolini, L.; Gregori, S.; et al. Neonatal combination therapy improves some of the clinical manifestations in the Mucopolysaccharidosis type I murine model. *Mol. Genet. Metab.* **2020**, *130*, 197–208. [CrossRef]
81. Fahnehjelm, K.T.; Törnquist, A.L.; Malm, G.; Winiarski, J. Ocular findings in four children with mucopolysaccharidosis I-Hurler (MPS I-H) treated early with haematopoietic stem cell transplantation. *Acta Ophthalmol. Scand.* **2006**, *84*, 781–785. [CrossRef]
82. Summers, C.G.; Purple, R.L.; Krivit, W.; Pineda, R.; Copland, G.T.; Ramsay, N.K.C.; Kersey, J.H.; Whitley, C.B. Ocular changes in the mucopolysaccharidoses after bone marrow transplantation: A preliminary report. *Ophthalmology* **1989**, *96*, 977–985. [CrossRef]
83. Coletti, H.Y.; Aldenhoven, M.; Yelin, K.; Poe, M.D.; Kurtzberg, J.; Escolar, M.L. Long-term functional outcomes of children with hurler syndrome treated with unrelated umbilical cord blood transplantation. *JIMD Rep.* **2015**, *20*, 77–86. [CrossRef] [PubMed]
84. Javed, A.; Aslam, T.; Jones, S.A.; Ashworth, J. Objective quantification of changes in corneal clouding over time in patients with mucopolysaccharidosis. *Investig. Ophthalmol. Vis. Sci.* **2017**, *58*, 954–958. [CrossRef] [PubMed]
85. Guffon, N.; Souillet, G.; Maire, I.; Straczek, J.; Guibaud, P. Follow-up of nine patients with Hurler syndrome after bone marrow transplantation. *J. Pediatr.* **1998**, *133*, 119–125. [CrossRef]
86. Van Den Broek, B.T.A.; Van Doorn, J.; Hegeman, C.V.; Nierkens, S.; Lindemans, C.A.; Verhoeven-Duif, N.; Boelens, J.J.; Van Hasselt, P.M. Hurdles in treating Hurler disease: Potential routes to achieve a "real" cure. *Blood Adv.* **2020**, *4*, 2837–2849. [CrossRef]
87. Yuan, C.; Bothun, E.; Hardten, D.; Tolar, J.; McLoon, L. A novel explanation of corneal clouding in a bone marrow transplant-treated patient with Hurler syndrome. *Exp. Eye Res.* **2016**, *148*, 83–89. [CrossRef]
88. Gullingsrud, E.O.; Krivit, W.; Summers, C.G. Ocular abnormalities in the mucopolysaccharidoses after bone marrow transplantation. Longer follow-up. *Ophthalmology* **1998**, *105*, 1099–1105. [CrossRef]
89. Tomatsu, S.; Pitz, S.; Hampel, U. Ophthalmological Findings in Mucopolysaccharidoses. *J. Clin. Med.* **2019**, *8*, 1467. [CrossRef]
90. Breider, M.A.; Shull, R.M.; Constantopoulos, G. Long-term effects of bone marrow transplantation in dogs with mucopolysaccharidosis I. *Am. J. Pathol.* **1989**, *134*, 677–692.
91. Constantopoulos, G.; Scott, J.A.; Shull, R.M. Corneal opacity in canine MPS I. Changes after bone marrow transplantation. *Investig. Ophthalmol. Vis. Sci.* **1989**, *30*, 1802–1807.
92. Newkirk, K.M.; Atkins, R.M.; Dickson, P.I.; Rohrbach, B.W.; McEntee, M.F. Ocular lesions in canine mucopolysaccharidosis I and response to enzyme replacement therapy. *Investig. Ophthalmol. Vis. Sci.* **2011**, *52*, 5130–5135. [CrossRef]
93. Pitz, S.; Ogun, O.; Bajbouj, M.; Arash, L.; Schulze-Frenking, G.; Beck, M. Ocular changes in patients with mucopolysaccharidosis I receiving enzyme replacement therapy: A 4-year experience. *Arch. Ophthalmol.* **2007**, *125*, 1353–1356. [CrossRef] [PubMed]
94. Gonzalez, E.A.; Visioli, F.; Pasqualim, G.; de Souza, C.F.M.; Marinho, D.R.; Giugliani, R.; Matte, U.; Baldo, G. Progressive eye pathology in mucopolysaccharidosis type I mice and effects of enzyme replacement therapy. *Clin. Exp. Ophthalmol.* **2020**, *48*, 334–342. [CrossRef] [PubMed]
95. van Doorn, J.; van den Broek, B.T.A.; Geboers, A.J.; Kuiper, G.A.; Boelens, J.J.; van Hasselt, P.M. Salivary α-Iduronidase activity as a potential new biomarker for the diagnosis and monitoring the effect of therapy in mucopolysaccharidosis type I. *Biol. Blood Marrow Transplant.* **2018**, *24*, 1808–1813. [CrossRef] [PubMed]
96. Sornalingam, K.; Javed, A.; Aslam, T.; Sergouniotis, P.; Jones, S.; Ghosh, A.; Ashworth, J. Variability in the ocular phenotype in mucopolysaccharidosis. *Br. J. Ophthalmol.* **2019**, *103*, 504–510. [CrossRef]

97. Ferrari, S.; Ponzin, D.; Ashworth, J.L.; Fahnehjelm, K.T.; Summers, C.G.; Harmatz, P.R.; Scarpa, M. Diagnosis and management of ophthalmological features in patients with mucopolysaccharidosis. *Br. J. Ophthalmol.* **2011**, *95*, 613–619. [CrossRef]
98. Belani, K.G.; Krivit, W.; Carpenter, B.L.; Braunlin, E.; Buckley, J.J.; Liao, J.C.; Floyd, T.; Leonard, A.S.; Summers, C.G.; Levine, S.; et al. Children with mucopolysaccharidosis: Perioperative care, morbidity, mortality, and new findings. *J. Pediatr. Surg.* **1993**, *28*, 403–410. [CrossRef]
99. Yeung, A.H.; Cowan, M.J.; Horn, B.; Rosbe, K.W. Airway management in children with mucopolysaccharidoses. *Arch. Otolaryngol. Head Neck Surg.* **2009**, *135*, 73–79. [CrossRef]
100. Koehne, T.; Müller-Stöver, S.; Köhn, A.; Stumpfe, K.; Lezius, S.; Schmid, C.; Lukacs, Z.; Kahl-Nieke, B.; Muschol, N. Obstructive sleep apnea and craniofacial appearance in MPS type I-Hurler children after hematopoietic stem cell transplantation. *Sleep Breath.* **2019**, *23*, 1315–1321. [CrossRef]
101. Malone, B.N.; Whitley, C.B.; Duvall, A.J.; Belani, K.; Sibley, R.K.; Ramsay, N.K.; Kersey, J.H.; Krivit, W.; Berlinger, N.T. Resolution of obstructive sleep apnea in Hurler syndrome after bone marrow transplantation.; *Int. J. Pediatr. Otorhinolaryngol.* **1988**, *15*, 23–31. [CrossRef]
102. Moreau, J.; Brassier, A.; Amaddeo, A.; Neven, B.; Caillaud, C.; Chabli, A.; Fernandez-Bolanos, M.; Olmo, J.; Valayannopoulos, V.; Fauroux, B. Obstructive sleep apnea syndrome after hematopoietic stem cell transplantation in children with mucopolysaccharidosis type I. *Mol. Genet. Metab.* **2015**, *116*, 275–280. [CrossRef] [PubMed]
103. Kirkpatrick, K.; Ellwood, J.; Walker, R.W. Mucopolysaccharidosis type I (Hurler syndrome) and anesthesia: The impact of bone marrow transplantation, enzyme replacement therapy, and fiberoptic intubation on airway management. *Paediatr. Anaesth.* **2012**, *22*, 745–751. [CrossRef] [PubMed]
104. Frawley, G.; Fuenzalida, D.; Donath, S.; Yaplito-Lee, J.; Peters, H. A retrospective audit of anesthetic techniques and complications in children with mucopolysaccharidoses. *Paediatr. Anaesth.* **2012**, *22*, 737–744. [CrossRef] [PubMed]
105. Megens, J.H.; de Wit, M.; van Hasselt, P.M.; Boelens, J.J.; van der Werff, D.B.; de Graaff, J.C. Perioperative complications in patients diagnosed with mucopolysaccharidosis and the impact of enzyme replacement therapy followed by hematopoietic stem cell transplantation at early age. *Paediatr. Anaesth.* **2014**, *24*, 521–527. [CrossRef]
106. Madoff, L.U.; Kordun, A.; Cravero, J.P. Airway management in patients with mucopolysaccharidoses: The progression toward difficult intubation. *Paediatr. Anaesth.* **2019**, *29*, 620–627. [CrossRef]
107. Laraway, S.; Mercer, J.; Jameson, E.; Ashworth, J.; Hensman, P.; Jones, S.A. Outcomes of long-term treatment with laronidase in patients with mucopolysaccharidosis type I. *J. Pediatr.* **2016**, *178*, 219–226. [CrossRef]
108. Jezela-Stanek, A.; Chorostowska-Wynimko, J.; Tylki-Szymańska, A. Pulmonary involvement in selected lysosomal storage diseases and the impact of enzyme replacement therapy: A state-of-the art review. *Clin. Respir. J.* **2020**, *14*, 422–429. [CrossRef]
109. Dualibi, A.P.; Martins, A.M.; Moreira, G.A.; de Azevedo, M.F.; Fujita, R.R.; Pignatari, S.S. The impact of laronidase treatment in otolaryngological manifestations of patients with mucopolysaccharidosis. *Braz. J. Otorhinolaryngol.* **2016**, *82*, 522–528. [CrossRef]
110. Valayannopoulos, V.; Wijburg, F.A. Therapy for the mucopolysaccharidoses. *Rheumatology* **2011**, *50*, 49–59. [CrossRef]
111. Broomfield, A.; Sims, J.; Mercer, J.; Hensman, P.; Ghosh, A.; Tylee, K.; Stepien, K.M.; Oldham, A.; Prathivadi Bhayankaram, N.; Wynn, R.; et al. The evolution of pulmonary function in childhood onset Mucopolysaccharidosis type I. *Mol. Genet. Metab.* **2020**, 1. [CrossRef]
112. Wraith, J.E.; Clarke, L.A.; Beck, M.; Kolodny, E.H.; Pastores, G.M.; Muenzer, J.; Rapoport, D.M.; Berger, K.I.; Swiedler, S.J.; Kakkis, E.D.; et al. Enzyme replacement therapy for mucopolysaccharidosis I: A randomized, double-blinded, placebo-controlled, multinational study of recombinant human alpha-L-iduronidase (laronidase). *J. Pediatr.* **2004**, *144*, 581–588. [CrossRef] [PubMed]
113. Schuh, R.S.; Gonzalez, E.A.; Tavares, A.M.V.; Seolin, B.G.; Elias, L.; de Sr. Vera, L.N.P.; Kubaski, F.; Poletto, E.; Giugliani, R.; Teixeira, H.F.; et al. Neonatal nonviral gene editing with the CRISPR/Cas9 system improves some cardiovascular, respiratory, and bone disease features of the mucopolysaccharidosis I phenotype in mice. *Gene Ther.* **2019**. [CrossRef] [PubMed]
114. Papsin, B.C.; Vellodi, A.; Bailey, C.M.; Ratcliffe, P.C.; Leighton, S.E.J. Otologic and laryngologic manifestations of mucopolysaccharidoses after bone marrow transplantation. *Otolaryngol. Head Neck Surg.* **1998**, *118*, 30–36. [CrossRef]
115. Da Costa, V.; O'Grady, G.; Jackson, L.; Kaylie, D.; Raynor, E. Improvements in sensorineural hearing loss after cord blood transplant in patients with mucopolysaccharidosis. *Arch. Otolaryngol. Head Neck Surg.* **2012**, *138*, 1071–1076. [CrossRef] [PubMed]
116. Wang, J.; Luan, Z.; Jiang, H.; Fang, J.; Qin, M.; Lee, V.; Chen, J. Allogeneic hematopoietic stem cell transplantation in thirty-four pediatric cases of mucopolysaccharidosis—a ten-year report from the China children transplant group. *Biol. Blood Marrow Transplant.* **2016**, *22*, 2104–2108. [CrossRef]
117. van den Broek, B.T.A.; Smit, A.L.; Boelens, J.J.; van Hasselt, P.M. Hearing loss in patients with mucopolysaccharidoses-1 and -6 after hematopoietic cell transplantation: A longitudinal analysis. *J. Inherit. Metab. Dis.* **2020**. [CrossRef]
118. Tokic, V.; Barisic, I.; Huzjak, N.; Petkovic, G.; Fumic, K.; Paschke, E. Enzyme replacement therapy in two patients with an advanced severe (Hurler) phenotype of mucopolysaccharidosis I. *Eur. J. Pediatr.* **2007**, *166*, 727–732. [CrossRef]
119. Mercimek-Mahmutoglu, S.; Reilly, C.; Human, D.; Waters, P.J.; Stoeckler-Ipsiroglu, S. Progression of organ manifestations upon enzyme replacement therapy in a patient with mucopolysaccharidosis type I/Hurler. *World J. Pediatr.* **2009**, *5*, 319–321. [CrossRef]
120. Dornelles, A.D.; Lapagesse, L.; Pinto, D.C.; Paula, A.C.; de Eduardo, C.; Lourenço, C.M.; Kim, C.A.; Dain, D.; Horovitz, G.; Marques, E.; et al. Enzyme replacement therapy for Mucopolysaccharidosis Type I among patients followed within the MPS Brazil Network. *Genet. Mol. Biol.* **2014**, *37*, 23–29. [CrossRef]

121. Hugh-Jones, K. Psychomotor development of children with mucopolysaccharidosis type 1-H following bone marrow transplantation. *Birth Defects Orig. Artic. Ser.* **1986**, *22*, 25–29.
122. Field, R.; Buchanan, J.; Copplemans, M.; Aichroth, P. Bone-marrow transplantation in Hurler's syndrome. Effect on skeletal development. *J. Bone Jt. Surg. Br.* **1994**, *76*, 975–981. [CrossRef]
123. Vellodi, A.; Young, E.P.; Cooper, A.; Wraith, J.E.; Winchester, B.; Meaney, C.; Ramaswami, U.; Will, A.; Marrow, B. Bone marrow transplantation for mucopolysaccharidosis type I: Experience of two British centres. *Arch. Dis. Child* **1997**, *76*, 92–99. [CrossRef] [PubMed]
124. Polgreen, L.; Plog, M.; Schwender, J.; Tolar, J.; Thomas, W.; Orchard, P.; Miller, B.; Petryk, A. Short-term growth hormone treatment in children with Hurler syndrome after hematopoietic cell transplantation. *Bone Marrow Transplant.* **2009**, *44*, 279–285. [CrossRef]
125. Polgreen, L.; Tolar, J.; Plog, M.; Himes, J.; Orchard, P.; Whitley, C.; Miller, B.; Petryk, A. Growth and endocrine function in patients with Hurler syndrome after hematopoietic stem cell transplantation. *Bone Marrow Transplant.* **2008**, *41*, 1005–1011. [CrossRef] [PubMed]
126. Tandon, V.; Williamson, J.B.; Cowie, R.A.; Wraith, J.E. Spinal problems in mucopolysaccharidosis I (Hurler syndrome). *J. Bone Jt. Surg. Br.* **1996**, *78*, 938–944. [CrossRef]
127. Langereis, E.J.; den Os, M.M.; Breen, C.; Jones, S.A.; Knaven, O.C.; Mercer, J.; Miller, W.P.; Kelly, P.M.; Kennedy, J.; Ketterl, T.G.; et al. Progression of hip dysplasia in mucopolysaccharidosis type I hurler after successful hematopoietic stem cell transplantation. *J. Bone Jt. Surg.* **2016**, *98*, 386–395. [CrossRef]
128. Thawrani, D.P.; Walker, K.; Polgreen, L.; Tolar, J.; Orchard, P.J. Hip dysplasia in patients with Hurler syndrome (mucopolysaccharidosis type 1H). *J. Pediatr. Orthop.* **2013**, *33*, 635–643. [CrossRef]
129. Stoop, F.; Kruyt, M.; van der Linden, M.; Sakkers, R.; van Hasselt, P.; Casterlein, R. Prevalence and development of orthopaedic symptoms in the Dutch hurler patient population after haematopoietic stem cell transplantation. *JIMD Rep.* **2012**, 17–29. [CrossRef]
130. Yasin, M.N.; Sacho, R.; Oxborrow, N.J.; Wraith, J.E.; Williamson, J.B.; Siddique, I. Thoracolumbar kyphosis in treated mucopolysaccharidosis 1 (hurler syndrome). *Spine* **2014**, *39*, 381–387. [CrossRef]
131. Abelin Genevois, K.; Garin, C.; Solla, F.; Guffon, N.; Kohler, R. Surgical management of thoracolumbar kyphosis in mucopolysaccharidosis type 1 in a reference center. *J. Inherit. Metab. Dis.* **2014**, *37*, 69–78. [CrossRef]
132. Tomatsu, S.; Alméciga-Díaz, C.J.; Montaño, A.; Yabe, H.; Tanaka, A.; Dung, V.; Giugliani, R.; Kubaski, F.; Mason, R.W.; Yasuda, E.; et al. Therapies for the bone in mucopolysaccharidoses. *Mol. Genet. Metab.* **2015**, *114*, 94–109. [CrossRef] [PubMed]
133. Tsukimura, T.; Tajima, Y.; Kawashima, I.; Fukushige, T.; Kanzaki, T.; Kanekura, T.; Ikekita, M.; Sugawara, K.; Suzuki, T.; Togawa, T.; et al. Uptake of a recombinant human α-L-iduronidase (laronidase) by cultured fibroblasts and osteoblasts. *Biol. Pharm. Bull.* **2008**, *31*, 1691–1695. [CrossRef] [PubMed]
134. Hite, S.; Peters, C.; Krivit, W. Correction of odontoid dysplasia following bone-marrow transplantation and engraftment (in Hurler syndrome MPS 1H). *Pediatr. Radiol.* **2000**, *30*, 464–470. [CrossRef] [PubMed]
135. Miebach, E. Management of infusion-related reactions to enzyme replacement therapy in a cohort of patients with mucopolysaccharidosis disorders. *Int. J. Clin. Pharmacol. Ther.* **2009**, *47* (Suppl. 1), S100–S106. [CrossRef] [PubMed]
136. Chiaro, J.A.; O'Donnell, P.; Shore, E.M.; Malhotra, N.R.; Ponder, K.P.; Haskins, M.E.; Smith, L.J. Effects of neonatal enzyme replacement therapy and simvastatin treatment on cervical spine disease in mucopolysaccharidosis I dogs. *J. Bone Min. Res.* **2014**, *29*, 2610–2617. [CrossRef]
137. Opoka-Winiarska, V.; Jurecka, A.; Emeryk, A.; Tylki-Szymanska, A. Osteoimmunology in mucopolysaccharidoses type I, II, VI and VII. Immunological regulation of the osteoarticular system in the course of metabolic inflammation. *Osteoarthritis Cartil.* **2013**, *21*, 1813–1823. [CrossRef]
138. Gabrielli, O.; Clarke, L.A.; Ficcadenti, A.; Santoro, L.; Zampini, L.; Volpi, N.; Coppa, G. V 12 year follow up of enzyme-replacement therapy in two siblings with attenuated mucopolysaccharidosis I: The important role of early treatment. *BMC Med. Genet.* **2016**, *17*, 19. [CrossRef]
139. Al-Sannaa, N.A.; Bay, L.; Barbouth, D.S.; Benhayoun, Y.; Goizet, C.; Guelbert, N.; Jones, S.A.; Kyosen, S.O.; Martins, A.M.; Phornphutkul, C.; et al. Early treatment with laronidase improves clinical outcomes in patients with attenuated MPS I: A retrospective case series analysis of nine sibships. *Orphanet J. Rare Dis.* **2015**, *10*, 1–9. [CrossRef]
140. Kuehn, S.C.; Koehne, T.; Cornils, K.; Markmann, S.; Riedel, C.; Pestka, J.M.; Schweizer, M.; Baldauf, C.; Yorgan, T.A.; Krause, M.; et al. Impaired bone remodeling and its correction by combination therapy in a mouse model of mucopolysaccharidosis-I. *Hum. Mol. Genet.* **2015**, *24*, 7075–7086. [CrossRef]
141. Baldo, G.; Mayer, F.Q.; Martinelli, B.Z.; de Carvalho, T.G.; Meyer, F.S.; de Oliveira, P.G.; Meurer, L.; Tavares, Â.; Matte, U.; Giugliani, R. Enzyme replacement therapy started at birth improves outcome in difficult-to-treat organs in mucopolysaccharidosis I mice. *Mol. Genet. Metab.* **2013**, *109*, 33–40. [CrossRef]
142. Clarke, L.A. Pathogenesis of skeletal and connective tissue involvement in the mucopolysaccharidoses: Glycosaminoglycan storage is merely the instigator. *Rheumatology* **2011**, *50*, 13–18. [CrossRef] [PubMed]
143. Simonaro, C.M.; D'Angelo, M.; He, X.; Eliyahu, E.; Shtraizent, N.; Haskins, M.E.; Schuchman, E.H. Mechanism of glycosaminoglycan-mediated bone and joint disease: Implications for the mucopolysaccharidoses and other connective tissue diseases. *Am. J. Pathol.* **2008**, *172*, 112–122. [CrossRef] [PubMed]

144. Neufeld, E.F.; Muenzer, I. *The Metabolic & Molecular Basis of Inherited Disease, 8th ed*; Scriver, C.R., Beudet, A.L., Sly, W.S., Valle, D., Eds.; McGraw-Hill: New York, NY, USA, 2001; Volume 3.
145. Weisstein, J.S.; Delgado, E.; Steinbach, L.S.; Hart, K.; Packman, S. Musculoskeletal manifestations of Hurler syndrome: Long-term follow-up after bone marrow transplantation. *J. Pediatr. Orthop.* **2004**, *24*, 97–101. [CrossRef] [PubMed]
146. Matos, M.A.; Barreto, R.; Acosta, A.X. Evaluation of motor response in mucopolysaccharidosis patients treated with enzyme replacement therapy. *Ortop. Traumatol. Rehabil.* **2013**, *15*, 389–393. [CrossRef] [PubMed]
147. Khanna, G.; Van Heest, A.E.; Agel, J.; Bjoraker, K.; Grewal, S.; Abel, S.; Krivit, W.; Peters, C.; Orchard, P.J. Analysis of factors affecting development of carpal tunnel syndrome in patients with Hurler syndrome after hematopoietic cell transplantation. *Bone Marrow Transplant.* **2007**, *39*, 331–334. [CrossRef]
148. Wyffels, M.L.; Orchard, P.J.; Shanley, R.M.; Miller, W.P.; Van Heest, A.E. The frequency of carpal tunnel syndrome in hurler syndrome after peritransplant enzyme replacement therapy: A retrospective comparison. *J. Hand Surg. Am.* **2017**. [CrossRef] [PubMed]
149. Guffon, N.; Bertrand, Y.; Forest, I.; Fouilhoux, A.; Froissart, R. Bone marrow transplantation in children with hunter syndrome: Outcome after 7 to 17 Years. *J. Pediatr.* **2009**, *154*, 733–737. [CrossRef]
150. Gatzoulis, M.A.; Vellodi, A.; Redington, A.N. Cardiac involvement in mucopolysaccharidoses: Effects of allogeneic bone marrow transplantation. *Arch. Dis. Child.* **1995**, *73*, 259–260. [CrossRef]
151. Viñallonga, X.; Sanz, N.; Balaguer, A.; Miro, L.; Ortega, J.J.; Casaldaliga, J. Hypertrophic cardiomyopathy in mucopolysaccharidoses: Regression after bone marrow transplantation. *Pediatr. Cardiol.* **1992**, *13*, 107–109. [CrossRef]
152. Orchard, P.J.; Blazar, B.R.; Wagner, J.; Charnas, L.; Krivit, W.; Tolar, J. Hematopoietic cell therapy for metabolic disease. *J. Pediatr.* **2007**, *151*, 340–346. [CrossRef]
153. Malm, G.; Gustafsson, B.; Berglund, G.; Lindström, M.; Naess, K.; Borgström, B.; Von Döbeln, U.; Ringdén, O. Outcome in six children with mucopolysaccharidosis type IH, hurler syndrome, after haematopoietic stem cell transplantation (HSCT). *Acta Paediatr. Int. J. Paediatr.* **2008**, *97*, 1108–1112. [CrossRef] [PubMed]
154. Gompf, R.E.; Shull, R.; Breider, M.A.; Scott, J.A.; Constantopoulos, G.C. Cardiovascular changes after bone marrow transplantation in dogs with mucopolysaccharidosis I. *Am. J. Vet. Res.* **1990**, *51*, 2054–2060. [PubMed]
155. Lin, H.Y.; Chan, W.C.; Chen, L.J.; Lee, Y.C.; Yeh, S.I.; Niu, D.M.; Chiu, P.C.; Tsai, W.H.; Hwu, W.L.; Chuang, C.K.; et al. Ophthalmologic manifestations in Taiwanese patients with mucopolysaccharidoses. *Mol. Genet. Genomic Med.* **2019**, *7*, 1–14. [CrossRef] [PubMed]
156. Braunlin, E.A.; Berry, J.M.; Whitley, C.B. Cardiac findings after enzyme replacement therapy for mucopolysaccharidosis type I. *Am. J. Cardiol.* **2006**, *98*, 416–418. [CrossRef]
157. Okuyama, T.; Tanaka, A.; Suzuki, Y.; Ida, H.; Tanaka, T.; Cox, G.F.; Eto, Y.; Orii, T. Japan Elaprase Treatment (JET) study: Idursulfase enzyme replacement therapy in adult patients with attenuated Hunter syndrome (Mucopolysaccharidosis II, MPS II). *Mol. Genet. Metab.* **2010**, *99*, 18–25. [CrossRef]
158. Brands, M.M.; Frohn-Mulder, I.M.; Hagemans, M.L.; Hop, W.C.; Oussoren, E.; Helbing, W.A.; van der Ploeg, A.T. Mucopolysaccharidosis: Cardiologic features and effects of enzyme-replacement therapy in 24 children with MPS I, II and VI. *J. Inherit. Metab. Dis.* **2013**, *36*, 227–234. [CrossRef]
159. Fesslová, V.; Corti, P.; Sersale, G.; Rovelli, A.; Russo, P.; Mannarino, S.; Butera, G.; Parini, R. The natural course and the impact of therapies of cardiac involvement in the mucopolysaccharidoses. *Cardiol. Young* **2009**, *19*, 170–178. [CrossRef]
160. Braunlin, E.; Miettunen, K.; Lund, T.; Luquette, M.; Orchard, P. Hematopoietic cell transplantation for severe MPS I in the first six months of life: The heart of the matter. *Mol. Genet. Metab.* **2019**, *126*, 117–120. [CrossRef]
161. Pasqualim, G.; Baldo, G.; de Carvalho, T.G.; Tavares, A.M.V.; Giugliani, R.; Matte, U. Effects of enzyme replacement therapy started late in a murine model of mucopolysaccharidosis type I. *PLoS ONE* **2015**, *10*, e0117271. [CrossRef]
162. Dickson, P.; Peinovich, M.; McEntee, M.; Lester, T.; Le, S.; Krieger, A.; Manuel, H.; Jabagat, C.; Passage, M.; Kakkis, E.D. Immune tolerance improves the efficacy of enzyme replacement therapy in canine mucopolysaccharidosis I. *J. Clin. Investig.* **2008**, *118*, 2868–2876. [CrossRef]
163. Bjoraker, K.J.; Delaney, K.; Peters, C.; Krivit, W.; Shapiro, E.G. Long-term outcomes of adaptive functions for children with mucopolysaccharidosis I (Hurler syndrome) treated with hematopoietic stem cell transplantation. *J. Dev. Behav. Pediatr.* **2006**, *27*, 290–296. [CrossRef] [PubMed]
164. Shapiro, E.; Guler, O.E.; Rudser, K.; Delaney, K.; Bjoraker, K.; Whitley, C.; Tolar, J.; Orchard, P.; Provenzale, J.; Thomas, K.M. An exploratory study of brain function and structure in mucopolysaccharidosis type I: Long term observations following hematopoietic cell transplantation (HCT). *Mol. Genet. Metab.* **2012**, *107*, 116–121. [CrossRef]
165. Poe, M.D.; Chagnon, S.L.; Escolar, M.L. Early treatment is associated with improved cognition in Hurler syndrome. *Ann. Neurol.* **2014**, *76*, 747–753. [CrossRef] [PubMed]
166. Ou, L.; Herzog, T.L.; Wilmot, C.M.; Whitley, C.B. Standardization of α-L-iduronidase enzyme assay with Michaelis-Menten kinetics. *Mol. Genet. Metab.* **2014**, *111*, 113–115. [CrossRef] [PubMed]
167. El-Amouri, S.S.; Dai, M.; Han, J.F.; Brady, R.O.; Pan, D. Normalization and improvement of CNS deficits in mice with hurler syndrome after long-term peripheral delivery of BBB-targeted iduronidase. *Mol. Ther.* **2014**, *22*, 2028–2037. [CrossRef] [PubMed]

168. Vogler, C.; Levy, B.; Grubb, J.H.; Galvin, N.; Tan, Y.; Kakkis, E.; Pavloff, N.; Sly, W.S. Overcoming the blood-brain barrier with high-dose enzyme replacement therapy in murine mucopolysaccharidosis VII. *Proc. Natl. Acad. Sci. USA* **2005**, *102*, 14777–14782. [CrossRef]
169. Derrick-Roberts, A.; Jackson, M.; Pyragius, C.; Byers, S. Substrate Deprivation Therapy to Reduce Glycosaminoglycan Synthesis Improves Aspects of Neurological and Skeletal Pathology in MPS I Mice. *Diseases* **2017**, *5*, 5. [CrossRef]
170. Rintz, E.; Pierzynowska, K.; Podlacha, M.; Węgrzyn, G. Has resveratrol a potential for mucopolysaccharidosis treatment? *Eur. J. Pharmacol.* **2020**, *888*. [CrossRef]
171. JOTROLTM Pre-Clinical Studies. Available online: http://www.jupiterorphan.com/jotroltrade8203-pre-clinical-studies.html (accessed on 15 December 2020).
172. Simonaro, C.M.; Tomatsu, S.; Sikora, T.; Kubaski, F.; Frohbergh, M.; Guevara, J.M.; Wang, R.Y.; Vera, M.; Kang, J.L.; Smith, L.J.; et al. Pentosan polysulfate: Oral versus subcutaneous injection in mucopolysaccharidosis type I dogs. *PLoS ONE* **2016**, *11*, 1–18. [CrossRef]
173. Hennermann, J.B.; Gökce, S.; Solyom, A.; Mengel, E.; Schuchman, E.H.; Simonaro, C.M. Treatment with pentosan polysulphate in patients with MPS I: Results from an open label, randomized, monocentric phase II study. *J. Inherit. Metab. Dis.* **2016**, *39*, 831–837. [CrossRef]
174. Polgreen, L.E.; Kunin-Batson, A.; Rudser, K.; Vehe, R.K.; Utz, J.J.; Whitley, C.B.; Dickson, P. Pilot study of the safety and effect of adalimumab on pain, physical function, and musculoskeletal disease in mucopolysaccharidosis types I and II. *Mol. Genet. Metab. Rep.* **2017**, *10*, 75–80. [CrossRef] [PubMed]
175. Vite, C.H.; Nestrasil, I.; Mlikotic, A.; Jens, J.K.; Snella, E.; Gross, W.; Shapiro, E.G.; Kovac, V.; Provenzale, J.M.; Chen, S.; et al. Features of brain MRI in dogs with treated and untreated mucopolysaccharidosis type I. *Comp. Med.* **2013**, *63*, 163–173. [PubMed]
176. Nan, Z.; Shekels, L.; Ryabinin, O.; Evavold, C.; Nelson, M.S.; Khan, S.A.; Deans, R.J.; Mays, R.W.; Low, W.C.; Gupta, P. Intracerebroventricular transplantation of human bone marrow-derived multipotent progenitor cells in an immunodeficient mouse model of mucopolysaccharidosis type I (MPS-I). *Cell Transplant.* **2012**, *21*, 1577–1593. [CrossRef]
177. Munoz-Rojas, M.V.; Vieira, T.; Costa, R.; Fagondes, S.; John, A.; Jardim, L.B.; Vedolin, L.M.; Raymundo, M.; Dickson, P.I.; Kakkis, E.; et al. Intrathecal enzyme replacement therapy in a patient with mucopolysaccharidosis type I and symptomatic spinal cord compression. *Am. J. Med. Genet. A* **2008**, *146A*, 2538–2544. [CrossRef] [PubMed]
178. Dickson, P.I.; Kaitila, I.; Harmatz, P.; Mlikotic, A.; Chen, A.H.; Victoroff, A.; Passage, M.B.; Madden, J.; Le, S.Q.; Naylor, D.E.; et al. Safety of laronidase delivered into the spinal canal for treatment of cervical stenosis in mucopolysaccharidosis I. *Mol. Genet. Metab.* **2015**, *116*, 69–74. [CrossRef]
179. Chen, A.H.; Harmatz, P.; Nestrasil, I.; Eisengart, J.B.; King, K.E.; Rudser, K.; Kaizer, A.M.; Svatkova, A.; Wakumoto, A.; Le, S.Q.; et al. Intrathecal enzyme replacement for cognitive decline in mucopolysaccharidosis type I, a randomized, open-label, controlled pilot study. *Mol. Genet. Metab.* **2020**, *129*, 80–90. [CrossRef]
180. Eisengart, J.B.; Pierpont, E.I.; Kaizer, A.M.; Rudser, K.D.; King, K.E.; Pasquali, M.; Polgreen, L.E.; Dickson, P.I.; Le, S.Q.; Miller, W.P.; et al. Intrathecal enzyme replacement for Hurler syndrome: Biomarker association with neurocognitive outcomes. *Genet. Med.* **2019**, *21*, 2552–2560. [CrossRef]
181. Lutzko, C.; Omori, F.; Abrams-Ogg, A.C.G.; Shull, R.; Li, L.; Lau, C.; Ruedy, C.; Nanji, S.; Gartley, C.; Dobson, H.; et al. Gene therapy for canine α-L-iduronidase deficiency: In utero adoptive transfer of genetically corrected hematopoietic progenitors results in engraftment but not amelioration of disease. *Hum. Gene Ther.* **1999**, *10*, 1521–1532. [CrossRef]
182. Meertens, L.; Kohn, D.; Kruth, S.; Hough, M.R.; Dubé, I.D.; Zhao, Y.; Rosic-Kablar, S.; Li, L.; Chan, K.; Dobson, H.; et al. In utero injection of α-L-iduronidase-carrying retrovirus in canine mucopolysaccharidosis type I: Infection of multiple tissues and neonatal gene expression. *Hum. Gene Ther.* **2002**, *13*, 1809–1820. [CrossRef]
183. Wang, D.; El-Amouri, S.S.; Dai, M.; Kuan, C.-Y.; Hui, D.; Brady, R.O.; Pan, D. Engineering a lysosomal enzyme with a derivative of receptor-binding domain of apoE enables delivery across the blood-brain barrier. *Proc. Natl. Acad. Sci. USA* **2013**, *110*, 2999–3004. [CrossRef]
184. Ou, L.; Przybilla, M.; Koniar, B.; Whitley, C.B. RTB lectin-mediated delivery of lysosomal α-L-iduronidase mitigates disease manifestations systemically including the central nervous system. *Mol. Genet. Metab.* **2018**, *123*, 105–111. [CrossRef] [PubMed]
185. Boado, R.J.; Zhang, Y.Y.; Xia, C.; Wang, Y.; Pardridge, W.M. Genetic engineering of a lysosomal enzyme fusion protein for targeted delivery across the human blood-brain barrier. *Biotechnol. Bioeng.* **2008**, *99*, 475–484. [CrossRef] [PubMed]
186. Boado, R.J.; Hui, E.K.-W.; Lu, J.Z.; Zhou, Q.-H.; Pardridge, W.M. Reversal of lysosomal storage in brain of adult MPS-I mice with intravenous Trojan horse-iduronidase fusion protein. *Mol. Pharm.* **2011**, *8*, 1342–1350. [CrossRef] [PubMed]
187. Boado, R.J.; Lu, J.Z.; Hui, E.K.-W.; Lin, H.; Pardridge, W.M. Insulin receptor antibody-alpha-N-acetylglucosaminidase fusion protein penetrates the primate blood-brain barrier and reduces glycosoaminoglycans in sanfilippo type B fibroblasts. *Mol. Pharm.* **2016**, *13*, 1385–1392. [CrossRef] [PubMed]
188. Giugliani, R.; Dalla Corte, A.; Poswar, F.; Vanzella, C.; Horovitz, D.; Riegel, M.; Baldo, G.; Vairo, F. Intrathecal/Intracerebroventricular enzyme replacement therapy for the mucopolysaccharidoses: Efficacy, safety, and prospects. *Expert Opin. Orphan Drugs* **2018**, *6*, 403–411. [CrossRef]
189. Okuyama, T.; Eto, Y.; Sakai, N.; Minami, K.; Yamamoto, T.; Sonoda, H.; Yamaoka, M.; Tachibana, K.; Hirato, T.; Sato, Y. Iduronate-2-sulfatase with anti-human transferrin receptor antibody for neuropathic mucopolysaccharidosis II: A phase 1/2 Trial. *Mol. Ther.* **2019**, *27*, 456–464. [CrossRef]

190. Osborn, M.J.; McElmurry, R.T.; Peacock, B.; Tolar, J.; Blazar, B.R. Targeting of the CNS in MPS-IH using a nonviral transferrin-α-L-iduronidase fusion gene product. *Mol. Ther.* **2008**, *16*, 1459–1466. [CrossRef]
191. Lee, H.L.R.; Dougherty, J.P. Pharmaceutical therapies to recode nonsense mutations in inherited diseases. *Pharmacol. Ther.* **2012**, *136*, 227–266. [CrossRef]
192. Gunn, G.; Dai, Y.; Du, M.; Belakhov, V.; Kandasamy, J.; Schoeb, T.R.; Baasov, T.; Bedwell, D.M.; Keeling, K.M. Long-term nonsense suppression therapy moderates MPS I-H disease progression. *Mol. Genet. Metab.* **2014**, *111*, 374–381. [CrossRef]
193. Liu, N. A novel oligonucleotide-based RNA base editing therapeutic approach for the treatment of Hurler syndrome. *Mol. Ther.* **2020**, *28*, 18.
194. Wang, J.; Ren, L.; Li, J.; Gao, G.; Wang, D. dCas13-Mediated Therapeutic RNA Base Editing for In Vivo Gene Therapy. *Mol. Ther.* **2020**, *28*, R3–R14.
195. Osborn, M.J.; Levy, J.M.; Newby, G.A.; McElroy, A.N.; Nielsen, S.A.; Liu, D.R.; Tolar, J. In vivo base editing to correct a murine model of mucopolysaccharidosis type IH. *Mol. Ther.* **2020**, *28*, 1177–1189.
196. Mendonca, C.; Ren, L.; Li, J.; Zhang, Y.; Min, J.; Wang, J.; Su, Q.; Gao, G.; Wang, D. In vivo suppressor tRNA mediated readthrough therapy for nonsense mutations. *Mol. Ther.* **2020**, *28*, 120.
197. Visigalli, I.; Delai, S.; Politi, L.S.; Di Domenico, C.; Cerri, F.; Mrak, E.; D'Isa, R.; Ungaro, D.; Stok, M.; Sanvito, F.; et al. Gene therapy augments the efficacy of hematopoietic cell transplantation and fully corrects mucopolysaccharidosis type I phenotype in the mouse model. *Blood* **2010**, *116*, 5130–5139. [CrossRef]
198. Wang, D.; Zhang, W.; Kalfa, T.; Grabowski, G.; Davies, S.; Malik, P.; Pan, D. Reprogramming erythroid cells for lysosomal enzyme production leads to visceral and CNS cross-correction. *Proc. Natl. Acad. Sci. USA* **2009**, *106*, 19958–19963. [CrossRef]
199. Shull, R.; Lu, X.; Dubé, I.; Lutzko, C.; Kruth, S.; Abrams-Ogg, A.; Kiem, H.P.; Goehle, S.; Schuening, F.; Millan, C.; et al. Humoral immune response limits gene therapy in canine MPS I. *Blood* **1996**, *88*, 377–379. [CrossRef]
200. Lutzko, C.; Kruth, S.; Abrams-Ogg, A.; Lau, K.; Clark, B.; Ruedy, C.; Nanji, S.; Foster, R.; Kohn, D.; Shull, R.; et al. Genetically corrected autologous stem cells engraft, but host immune responses limit their utility in canine alpha-L-iduronidase deficiency. *Blood* **1999**, *93*, 1895–1905.
201. Gentner, B.; Bernardo, M.E.; Tucci, F.; Zonari, E.; Fumagalli, F.; Pontesilli, S.; Acquati, S.; Silvani, P.; Ciceri, F.; Rovelli, A.; et al. Extensive metabolic correction of hurler disease by hematopoietic stem cell-based gene therapy: Preliminary results from a phase I/II trial. *Blood* **2019**, *134*, 607. [CrossRef]
202. Gomez-Ospina, N.; Scharenberg, S.G.; Mostrel, N.; Bak, R.O.; Mantri, S.; Quadros, R.M.; Gurumurthy, C.B.; Lee, C.; Bao, G.; Suarez, C.J.; et al. Human genome-edited hematopoietic stem cells phenotypically correct Mucopolysaccharidosis type I. *Nat. Commun.* **2019**, *10*, 1–14. [CrossRef]
203. Aronovich, E.L.; Bell, J.B.; Belur, L.R.; Gunther, R.; Erickson, D.C.C.; Schachern, P.A.; Matise, I.; McIvor, R.S.; Whitley, C.B.; Hackett, P.B.; et al. Prolonged expression of a lysosomal enzyme in mouse liver after Sleeping Beauty transposon-mediated gene delivery: Implications for non-viral gene therapy of mucopolysaccharidoses. *J. Gene Med.* **2007**, *9*, 403–415. [CrossRef]
204. Aronovich, E.L.; Hyland, K.A.; Hall, B.C.; Bell, J.B.; Olson, E.R.; Rusten, M.U.; Hunter, D.W.; Ellinwood, N.M.; McIvor, R.S.; Hackett, P.B. Prolonged expression of secreted enzymes in dogs after liver-directed delivery of sleeping beauty transposons: Implications for non-viral gene therapy of systemic disease. *Hum. Gene Ther.* **2017**, *28*, 551–564. [CrossRef] [PubMed]
205. Aronovich, E.L.; Bell, J.B.; Khan, S.A.; Belur, L.R.; Gunther, R.; Koniar, B.; Schachern, P.A.; Parker, J.B.; Carlson, C.S.; Whitley, C.B.; et al. Systemic correction of storage disease in MPS I NOD/SCID mice using the sleeping beauty transposon system. *Mol. Ther.* **2009**, *17*, 1136–1144. [CrossRef] [PubMed]
206. Hampe, C.S.; Olson, E.; de Laat, R.; Meeker, K.; Lund, T.C.; Swietlicka, M.; Wesley, J.; Xu, M.; Grandea, G.; Scholz, M.; et al. Sleeping beauty IDUA transposed human plasma cells for long-term treatment of an immunodeficient murine model of mucopolysaccharidosis Type I. *Mol. Ther.* **2020**, *28*, 580–589.
207. Laoharawee, K.; Johnson, M.; Peterson, J.; Yamamoto, K.; Lahr, W.; Webber, B.R.; Moriarity, B.S. Engineered B cells as a novel and sustainable cell-based enzyme replacement therapy for Hurler/Scheie syndrome. *Mol. Ther.* **2020**, *28*, 178–187.
208. Donovan, M.; Makino, E.; Fluharty, B.; Tietz, D.; Pearson, E.; Jansen, L.; Barney, L.; Sewel, J.; Huang, J.; Corzo, D.; et al. Preclinical development of SIG-005 for treatment of MPS I. *Mol. Genet. Metab.* **2019**, *129*, S50. [CrossRef]
209. Miyadera, K.; Conatser, L.; Llanga, T.A.; Carlin, K.; O'Donnell, P.; Bagel, J.; Song, L.; Kurtzberg, J.; Samulski, R.J.; Gilger, B.; et al. Intrastromal gene therapy prevents and reverses advanced corneal clouding in a canine model of mucopolysaccharidosis I. *Mol. Ther.* **2020**, *28*, 1455–1463. [CrossRef]
210. Hartung, S.D.; Frandsen, J.L.; Pan, D.; Koniar, B.L.; Graupman, P.; Gunther, R.; Low, W.C.; Whitley, C.B.; McIvor, R.S. Correction of metabolic, craniofacial, and neurologic abnormalities in MPS I mice treated at birth with adeno-associated virus vector transducing the human alpha-L-iduronidase gene. *Mol. Ther.* **2004**, *9*, 866–875. [CrossRef]
211. Wolf, D.A.; Lenander, A.W.; Nan, Z.; Belur, L.R.; Whitley, C.B.; Gupta, P.; Low, W.C.; McIvor, R.S. Direct gene transfer to the CNS prevents emergence of neurologic disease in a murine model of mucopolysaccharidosis type I. *Neurobiol. Dis.* **2011**, *43*, 123–133. [CrossRef]
212. Belur, L.R.; Temme, A.; Podetz-Pedersen, K.M.; Riedl, M.; Vulchanova, L.; Robinson, N.; Hanson, L.R.; Kozarsky, K.F.; Orchard, P.J.; Frey, W.H., 2nd; et al. Intranasal adeno-associated virus mediated gene delivery and expression of human iduronidase in the central nervous system: A noninvasive and effective approach for prevention of neurologic disease in mucopolysaccharidosis type I. *Hum. Gene Ther.* **2017**, *28*, 576–587. [CrossRef]

213. Hinderer, C.; Bell, P.; Gurda, B.L.; Wang, Q.; Louboutin, J.-P.; Zhu, Y.; Bagel, J.; O'Donnell, P.; Sikora, T.; Ruane, T.; et al. Liver-directed gene therapy corrects cardiovascular lesions in feline mucopolysaccharidosis type I. *Proc. Natl. Acad. Sci. USA* **2014**, *111*, 14894–14899. [CrossRef]
214. Hordeaux, J.; Hinderer, C.; Buza, E.L.; Louboutin, J.P.; Jahan, T.; Bell, P.; Chichester, J.A.; Tarantal, A.F.; Wilson, J.M. Safe and sustained expression of human iduronidase after intrathecal administration of adeno-associated virus serotype 9 in infant rhesus monkeys. *Hum. Gene Ther.* **2019**, *30*, 957–966. [CrossRef] [PubMed]
215. Liu, Y.; Xu, L.; Hennig, A.K.; Kovacs, A.; Fu, A.; Chung, S.; Lee, D.; Wang, B.; Herati, R.S.; Mosinger Ogilvie, J.; et al. Liver-directed neonatal gene therapy prevents cardiac, bone, ear, and eye disease in mucopolysaccharidosis I mice. *Mol. Ther.* **2005**, *11*, 35–47. [CrossRef] [PubMed]
216. Ma, X.; Liu, Y.; Tittiger, M.; Hennig, A.; Kovacs, A.; Popelka, S.; Wang, B.; Herati, R.; Bigg, M.; Ponder, K.P. Improvements in mucopolysaccharidosis I mice after adult retroviral Vector-mediated gene therapy with immunomodulation. *Mol. Ther.* **2007**, *15*, 889–902. [CrossRef] [PubMed]
217. Ou, L.; De Kelver, R.C.; Rohde, M.; Tom, S.; Radeke, R.; St. Martin, S.J.; Santiago, Y.; Sproul, S.; Przybilla, M.J.; Koniar, B.L.; et al. ZFN-mediated in vivo genome editing corrects murine hurler syndrome. *Mol. Ther.*. [CrossRef] [PubMed]

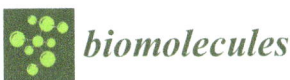

Article

Proteomic Analysis of Mucopolysaccharidosis IIIB Mouse Brain

Valeria De Pasquale [1,†], Michele Costanzo [1,2,†], Rosa Anna Siciliano [3], Maria Fiorella Mazzeo [3], Valeria Pistorio [1], Laura Bianchi [4], Emanuela Marchese [2,5], Margherita Ruoppolo [1,2], Luigi Michele Pavone [1,*] and Marianna Caterino [1,2]

1. Department of Molecular Medicine and Medical Biotechnology, School of Medicine, University of Naples Federico II, 80131 Naples, Italy; valeria.depasquale@unina.it (V.D.P.); michele.costanzo@unina.it (M.C.); valeria.pistorio@unina.it (V.P.); margherita.ruoppolo@unina.it (M.R.); marianna.caterino@unina.it (M.C.)
2. CEINGE-Biotecnologie Avanzate scarl, 80145 Naples, Italy; emanuela.marchese89@gmail.com
3. Institute of Food Sciences, CNR, 83100 Avellino, Italy; rosa.siciliano@isa.cnr.it (R.A.S.); fiorella.mazzeo@isa.cnr.it (M.F.M.)
4. Laboratory of Functional Proteomics, Department of Life Sciences, University of Siena, 53100 Siena, Italy; bianchi12@unisi.it
5. Department of Mental Health and Preventive Medicine, University of Campania Luigi Vanvitelli, 80138 Naples, Italy
* Correspondence: luigimichele.pavone@unina.it; Tel.: +39-081-7463043
† These authors equally contributed to this work.

Received: 24 November 2019; Accepted: 24 February 2020; Published: 26 February 2020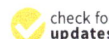

Abstract: Mucopolysaccharidosis IIIB (MPS IIIB) is an inherited metabolic disease due to deficiency of α-N-Acetylglucosaminidase (NAGLU) enzyme with subsequent storage of undegraded heparan sulfate (HS). The main clinical manifestations of the disease are profound intellectual disability and neurodegeneration. A label-free quantitative proteomic approach was applied to compare the proteome profile of brains from MPS IIIB and control mice to identify altered neuropathological pathways of MPS IIIB. Proteins were identified through a bottom up analysis and 130 were significantly under-represented and 74 over-represented in MPS IIIB mouse brains compared to wild type (WT). Multiple bioinformatic analyses allowed to identify three major clusters of the differentially abundant proteins: proteins involved in cytoskeletal regulation, synaptic vesicle trafficking, and energy metabolism. The proteome profile of NAGLU$^{-/-}$ mouse brain could pave the way for further studies aimed at identifying novel therapeutic targets for the MPS IIIB. Data are available via ProteomeXchange with the identifier PXD017363.

Keywords: mucopolysaccharidosis IIIB; quantitative proteomics; NAGLU; lysosomes

1. Introduction

Mucopolysaccharidosis type IIIB (MPS IIIB) is an inherited metabolic disease caused by the deficiency of the enzyme α-N-Acetylglucosaminidase (NAGLU, EC: 3.2.1.50) required for the degradation of the glycosaminoglycan (GAG) heparan sulfate (HS) [1,2]. The undigested HS accumulates in different tissues leading to progressive cellular damage and organ dysfunction, with the central nervous system (CNS) being the primary site of the pathology [3–7]. The CNS pathology in MPS IIIB patients comprises hydrocephalus, behavioral disorders, sleep disturbances, vision and progressive hearing loss, learning delay, and intellectual disability [8,9]. Although different pathophysiological mechanisms have been investigated both in the brain of MPS IIIB patients and in animal models of the disease [9], the etiology of the neurological dysfunction in MPS IIIB is still unclear. The characteristic pathological changes include white matter abnormalities, cortical and corpus callosum atrophy [10,11], cerebellar atrophy with loss of Purkinje cells [12,13], retinal epithelium pigmentation loss, and photoreceptor degeneration [14]. Accumulation of specific HS glycoforms in neurons and glial cells in the brain of MPS IIIB mouse model has been associated with increased expression of HS biosynthetic enzymes, may contributing to the neuropathology of MPS IIIB by exacerbating the lysosomal HS storage. [15,16]. Secondary accumulation of gangliosides in the brain of patients and MPS IIIB mice has also been documented [17,18]. The molecular mechanisms underlying the neuropathology in MPS IIIB appear to imply a complex interplay between the activation of glial cells, alterations of the oxidative status, as well as neuroinflammation [19–21]. However, there are still many issues to be elucidated.

In this study, a comparative analysis of the proteome profiles of MPS IIIB and wild type (WT) mouse brains was performed using a quantitative proteomic approach [22–25], which allowed us to identify 204 proteins that were significantly differentially expressed in the brain of MPS IIIB versus WT mice. Multiple bioinformatic analyses using PANTHER [26], REACTOME, [27] STRING [28] and MetaCore [29] databases allowed a functional classification of the detected proteins and highlighted the biological pathways perturbed in MPS IIIB brains. These results might provide useful tools for further studies aimed to identify molecular targets for therapies.

2. Material and Methods

2.1. Animal Description

MPS IIIB knockout mice (NAGLU$^{-/-}$) available to us were generated by Prof. Elizabeth Neufeld, University of California, Los Angeles (UCLA), by insertion of neomycin resistance gene into exon 6 of NALGU gene on the C57/BL6 background [30]. NAGLU$^{-/-}$ and WT mice were genotyped by PCR [31]. Mice were housed with no more than four per cage, maintained under identical conditions of temperature (21 ± 1 °C), humidity (60% ± 5%) and light/dark cycle, and had free access to normal mouse chow. All animal experiments were in compliance with the ARRIVE (Animal Research: Reporting of in vivo Experiments) guidelines and were carried out in accordance with the EU Directive 2010/63/EU for animal experiments. All mouse care and handling procedures were approved by the rules of the Institutional Animal Care and Use Committee (IACUC) of the Centre of Biotechnologies A.O.R.N. "Antonio Cardarelli" (Naples 80131, Italy).

2.2. Sample Collection and Preparation

Whole mouse brains were collected from five MPS IIIB and five WT male mice (8-month old) for further analysis [32,33]. Brain tissues were lysed in ice-cold lysis buffer containing 7 M urea, 2 M thiourea, 4% cholamidopropyl dimethylammonio 1 propanesulfonate (CHAPS), 30 mM Tris-HCl pH = 7.8 supplemented with protease inhibitor cocktail (Roche, Indianapolis, IN, USA) [34]. Mechanical disruption of tissues was performed on ice using 2 mL Dounce homogenizer applying ten strokes per brain sample [35]. Lysed tissues were centrifuged for 20 min at 13,000 rpm; supernatants were collected and protein concentration was quantified by Bradford assay using Bio-Rad Protein Assay Dye Reagent Concentrate (Hercules, CA, USA). Protein extract aliquots (50 µg) from the five biological replicates for each condition (NAGLU$^{-/-}$ and WT) were fractionated on 10% SDS–PAGE. The resolved proteins were stained using Gel Code Blue Stain Reagent (Thermo Fisher Scientific, Waltham, MA, USA) and each gel lane was divided into five pieces and hydrolyzed by in situ trypsin digestion as previously described [36–38].

2.3. LC–MS/MS Analysis

Peptide mixtures were dissolved in 0.2% HCOOH and analyzed by LC–MS/MS using a Q-Exactive^{TM} mass spectrometer (Thermo Scientific, Bremen, Germany) coupled with an UltiMate 3000 RSLC nanoLC system (Thermo Scientific). The peptide mixture was desalted by a precolumn (Acclaim PepMap C18, 300 µm × 5 mm nanoViper, 5 µm, 100 Å, Thermo Scientific), in 0.05% formic acid and 2% acetonitrile. Finally, the peptide mixture was fractionated on a reverse phase capillary column (Acclaim Easy Spray PepMap RSLC C18, 75 µm × 15cm nanoViper, 3µm, 100 Å, Thermo Scientific) and eluted by a nonlinear gradient: 4% B for 5 min, from 4% to 40% B in 45 min and from 40% to 90% B in 1 min at flow rate of 300 nL/min. (Eluent A, 0.1% formic acid; Eluent B, 80% acetonitrile, 0.08% formic acid). MS analysis was setup as follows: data dependent full MS/ddMS2; ten most intense precursor ions fragmentation; 30 sec dynamic exclusion; MS resolution 70,000; MS/MS resolution 17,500 [39,40].

2.4. Protein Identification and Data Processing

The identification of proteins in brain samples from WT and MPS IIIB mice was performed using the platform Thermo Proteome Discoverer™ (version 1.3.0.339, Thermo Scientific, Bremen, Germany), combined with the use of the SEQUEST HT Search Engine server (University of Washington, Seattle, WA, USA).

The peak lists were processed according to the follow parameters: (I) Spectrum Selector. Minimum Precursor Mass: 350 Da, Maximum Precursor Mass: 5000 Da, Minimum Peak Count: 1; (II) SEQUEST HT: 1. Input Data. Protein Database: Swiss-Prot, Enzyme: Trypsin, Maximum Missed Cleavage Sites: 2, Instrument: Electrospray Ionization Fourier Transform Ion Cyclotron Resonance Mass Spectrometer (ESI FT-ICR MS), Taxonomy: *Mus Musculus*. 2. Tolerances. Precursor Mass Tolerance: 5 ppm, Fragment Mass Tolerance: 0.8 Da. 3. Dynamic Modification. Methionine Oxidation, N-terminal Glutamine cyclization to Pyroglutamic Acid, N-terminal protein Acetylation. 4. Static modification: Cysteine Carboamidomethylation; (III) Target Decoy/PSM validator: 1. Maximum Delta Cn: 0.05; 2. Target false discovery rate (FDR) (strict): 0.01; 3. Target FDR (relaxed): 0.05. Proteins identified by a minimum of three peptides along the replicates were accepted. The dataset has been deposited to ProteomeXchange via the PRIDE database (PXD017363).

2.5. Quantitative Label-Free Proteomic Analysis

The relative abundances of proteins within the proteomic datasets were compared between the two groups, NAGLU$^{-/-}$ and WT murine brains, according to the spectral counting approach [34]. The quantitative analysis was performed by calculating the Normalized Spectral Abundance Factor (NSAF) as the number of spectral counts (SpCs) of each protein divided by protein length (SAF) and normalized for the sum of SAFs in a given lane. A Student's t test was used to select proteins showing significant changes between the analyzed datasets, resulting in two-tailed p values. The value of $p < 0.05$ was considered to be statistically significant. In order to measure the relative abundance for each identified protein and significantly represented into the two datasets, Fold$_{NSAF}$ was calculated as log2 (NSAF1/NSAF2), where NSAF1 was referred to the mean of NAGLU$^{-/-}$ samples NSAF, and NSAF2 to the mean of WT samples, respectively. Fold$_{NSAF}$ was reported as abundance index [38].

2.6. Western Blot Analysis

The total protein extract (50 µg) from NAGLU$^{-/-}$ and WT murine brains was analyzed by Western blotting with the rabbit monoclonal antibody anti-Gfap (ab-68428, Abcam). Mouse anti-β-actin monoclonal antibody (G043) from Abm was used to ensure equal loading of proteins in all lanes.

2.7. Bioinformatic Analysis

To investigate the molecular pathways influenced by NAGLU depletion in murine brain tissues, the identified proteomic dataset was analyzed by using the PANTHER (Protein ANalysis THrough Evolutionary Relationship) database available online at http://www.pantherdb.org [41–43] and the REACTOME database available online at https://www.reactome.org. Results of the PANTHER analyses for the biological process enrichment and pathway enrichment were expressed as percentage of protein listed in each category. The deregulated protein dataset was also processed using STRING (Search Tool for the Retrieval of Interacting Genes) functional protein association networks (http://string-db.org/) in order to identify protein networks linked to the differentially expressed proteins. The identified networks were evaluated by a significant score as negative logarithm of the p-value. The differentially expressed proteome dataset (n = 204 proteins) was further analyzed by the MetaCore™ resource (Clarivate Analytics, London, UK) in order to investigate protein functional interconnections. To facilitate the software processing, protein differences were processed using their corresponding EntrezGene IDs. The EntrezGene ID list was imported into MetaCore and processed for functional enrichment by "diseases by biomarkers" and "process networks" ontologies using the Functional Ontology Enrichment tool. While the "diseases by biomarkers" enrichment analysis allows for clustering proteins that were annotated as statistically significant biomarkers in characterized pathologies, the "process networks" analysis visualizes the involvement of experimental proteins in biochemical and molecular processes of biological systems. The differentially abundant proteins that characterize NAGLU$^{-/-}$ mouse brains were also investigated by using the MetaCore Network Building tool software that functionally crosslinks proteins under processing and builds protein networks. The Shortest Path algorithm was selected to highlight tight functional correlation existing among experimental proteins. It actually allows for inclusion in the same net only those proteins that directly interact or that are functionally correlated by a further factor not present in the processed protein list, but that is known to act as a molecular functional bridge between them. The relevant obtained pathway maps are indeed prioritized according to their statistical significance ($p \leq 0.001$) and graphically visualized as nodes (proteins) and edges (interconnections among proteins). All annotations used by the MetaCore tools are from an in-house database, periodically updated and built by extrapolating information from highly reliable scientific sources.

3. Results

3.1. SDS–PAGE and Protein Identification in Brain Samples from MPS IIIB and WT Mice

Brain samples from five MPS IIIB and five WT mice were collected in order to identify differentially expressed proteins through a label-free proteomic analysis and their protein extracts were independently fractionated by SDS–PAGE (Figure 1). Each gel lane was divided into five pieces and each piece was hydrolyzed by in situ trypsin digestion.

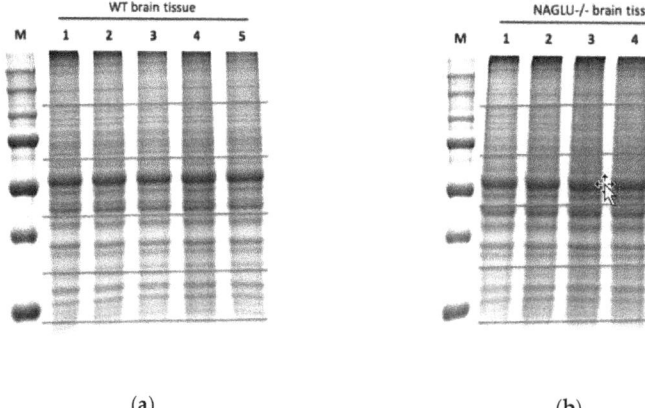

(a)   (b)

Figure 1. SDS–PAGE of proteins from murine WT (wild type) and NAGLU$^{-/-}$ (α-N-Acetylglucosaminidase) brain tissues. Proteins from five murine WT brains (**a**) and five murine NAGLU$^{-/-}$ brains (**b**) were resolved on a 10% SDS–polyacrylamide gel and stained by a gel code blue stain reagent. Each gel lane was fractionated at the level of the blue horizontal bars in order to obtain five gel bands per sample.

Peptide mixtures from each of the five biological replicates were analyzed two times by LC–MS/MS with a Q-Exactive mass spectrometer coupled with a nanoLC system. From the two MS analyses, we obtained ten protein datasets for NAGLU$^{-/-}$ and ten protein datasets for WT mice. The MS details of protein identifications are listed in Table S1.

Proteins identified by a minimum of two peptides in the 70% (7/10) of the analyzed replicates were included in the dataset that underwent further quantitative analysis.

3.2. Quantitative Analysis of Differentially Expressed Proteins in Brain Samples from MPS IIIB and WT Mice

The spectral count abundance parameter NSAF was calculated for each protein. Its variability was evaluated within the technical replicates into the same biological replicate by linear regression of the correlation (Supplemental Figure S1). The R-squared values for WT 1, WT 2, WT 3, WT 4, WT 5, and NAGLU$^{-/-}$ 1, NAGLU$^{-/-}$ 2, NAGLU$^{-/-}$ 3, NAGLU$^{-/-}$ 4, NAGLU$^{-/-}$ 5, were 0.983, 0.994, 0.993, 0.993, 0.995, and 0.989, 0.986, 0.983, 0.990, 0.991, respectively. These results show that the data have a high quantitative reproducibility. Normal distribution of the NSAF parameter both in WT and NAGLU$^{-/-}$ dataset was verified (Supplemental Figure S2A). Moreover, similarities in the WT and NAGLU$^{-/-}$ proteomes was evaluated by using multivariate analysis PCA (Supplemental Figure S2B). No outliers are found in plots of PCA scores. Finally, the overall sample correlation matrix is shown in Supplemental Figure S2C.

Protein relative abundance was then calculated by a spectral counting approach using the FoldNSAF, and Table 1 shows the list of these significant differentially abundant proteins. Table 1 includes the Swiss-Prot accession code, gene name, protein description, Fold$_{NSAF}$ value, p value, and subcellular localization (Uniport database) for each protein. The volcano plot analysis of the global proteome comparison between NAGLU$^{-/-}$ and WT is shown in Supplemental Figure S3.

Table 1. Dysregulated proteins in NAGLU$^{-/-}$ mouse brains compared to WT.

Swiss-Prot Code	Gene Name	Protein Description	Fold NSAF	p Value	Subcellular Localization
Q545B6	Stmn1	Stathmin	−12.6	0.00002	CK
Q9QYX7	Pclo	Protein piccolo	−8.4	0.00101	CK, GA
Q6P9K8	Caskin1	Caskin-1	−3.8	0.00262	CK
A8DUK2	Hbbt1	Beta-globin	−3.4	0.00008	C
Q4VAE3	Tmem65	Transmembrane protein 65	−3.3	0.00374	M, PM
Q8CHF1	mKIAA0531	Kinesin-like protein (Fragment)	−3.2	0.00232	CK
P17563	Selenbp1	Selenium-binding protein 1	−3.2	0.00046	CK, N
Q4KMM3	Oxr1	Oxidation resistance protein 1	−3	0.00036	M, N
A2AS98	Nckap1	Nck-associated protein 1	−2.9	0.00209	CK, PM
C7G3P1	Ppfia3	MKIAA0654 protein (Fragment)	−2.6	0.00328	CK
Q8BVQ5	Ppme1	Protein phosphatase methylesterase 1	−2.5	0.00345	N
Q3UVN5	Nsfl1c	Putative uncharacterized protein	−2.5	0.00002	CK, GA, N
Q9R0Q6	Arpc1a	Actin-related protein 2/3 complex subunit 1A	−2.4	0.00036	CK, N, PM
Q3TF14	Ahcy	Adenosylhomocysteinase	−2.4	0.00329	CK, N
Q9CX86	Hnrnpa0	Heterogeneous nuclear ribonucleoprotein A0	−2.4	0.00165	N
Q9Z1B3	Plcb1	1-phosphatidylinositol 4,5-bisphosphate phosphodiesterase beta-1	−2.4	0.00671	CK, N, PM
O54991	Cntnap1	Contactin-associated protein 1	−2.3	0.00626	PM
B0V2P5	Dmxl2	DmX-like protein 2	−2.3	0.01109	PM
E9Q8N8	Slc4a4	Anion exchange protein	−2.3	0.0011	PM
B1AQX9	Srcin1	SRC kinase-signaling inhibitor 1	−2.3	0.0004	CK
P24472	Gsta4	Glutathione S-transferase A4	−2.3	0.00125	M
Q3UK83	Hnrnpa1	Putative uncharacterized protein	−2.2	0.00047	ERS, N
D3Z4J3	Myo5a	Unconventional myosin-Va	−2.2	0.00636	CK, C, ER, En, GA, Ly, Pe
Q61411	Hras	GTPase HRas	−2.2	0.00583	C, GA, N, PM
Q9Z0X1	Aifm1	Apoptosis-inducing factor 1, mitochondrial	−2.1	0.00398	CK, M, N
B2L107	Vsnl1	Visinin-like protein 1	−2.1	0.00018	C
Q9DBF1	Aldh7a	Alpha-aminoadipic semialdehyde dehydrogenase	−2.1	0.02264	C, M, N
Q3TJF2	Ola1	Obg-like ATPase 1	−2.1	0.00001	CK, C, N
Q8VDD5	Myh9	Myosin-9	−2	0.01358	C, CK, N, PM
Q9JJK2	Lancl2	LanC-like protein 2	−2	0.00232	C, CK, N, PM
E9Q2L2	Dlg2	Disks large homolog 2	−2	0.00218	PM
Q91VR5	Ddx1	ATP-dependent RNA helicase DDX1	−2	0.00216	C, M, N
Q9JHU4	Dync1h1	Cytoplasmic dynein 1 heavy chain 1	−2	0.00407	CK, N

Table 1. Cont.

Swiss-Prot Code	Gene Name	Protein Description	Fold NSAF	p Value	Subcellular Localization
Q99PU5	Acsbg1	Long-chain-fatty-acid–CoA ligase ACSBG1	−1.9	0.01942	ER, PM
Q64010	Crk	Adapter molecule crk	−1.9	0.0031	CK, PM
P14733	Lmnb1	Lamin-B1	−1.9	0.02293	CK, N
P54775	Psmc4	26S protease regulatory subunit 6B	−1.9	0.03099	CK, N
A0A1S6GWI0	Ndufa8	NADH dehydrogenase (Ubiquinone) 1 alpha subcomplex, 8	−1.8	0.00156	M
Q3U741	Ddx17	DEAD (Asp-Glu-Ala-Asp) box polypeptide 17, isoform CRA_a	−1.8	0.00085	C, N
Q3TIQ2	Rpl12	Putative uncharacterized protein	−1.8	0.01139	C, N
P70168	Kpnb1	Importin subunit beta-1	−1.7	0.00011	C, M, N
Q80TZ3	Dnajc6	Putative tyrosine-protein phosphatase auxilin	−1.7	0.00164	C
Q5DTG0	Atp8a1	Phospholipid-transporting ATPase (Fragment)	−1.7	0.00428	ER, GA, PM
Q9QXS1	Plec	Plectin	−1.7	0.00377	C, CK, PM
Q921F2	Tardbp	TAR DNA-binding protein 43	−1.7	0.00786	N
B2RX08	Sptb	Spectrin beta chain	−1.7	0.00319	C, CK, PM
Q3TKG4	Psmc3	Putative uncharacterized protein (Fragment)	−1.6	0.00396	N
Q3UH59	Myh10	Myosin-10	−1.6	0.02527	C, CK, PM
Q9JM76	Arpc3	Actin-related protein 2/3 complex subunit 3	−1.6	0.01437	C, N
A0A1S6GWJ8		Uncharacterized protein	−1,5	0.02713	
Q3UN60	Mpp6	Membrane protein, palmitoylated 6 (MAGUK p55 subfamily member 6), isoform CRA_b	−1.5	0.00085	PM
Q91XV3	Basp1	Brain acid soluble protein 1	−1.5	0.00001	N, PM
Q07076	Anxa7	Annexin A7	−1.5	0.01183	C, ER, ERS, N, PM
Q3UY05	Ndufs8	Putative uncharacterized protein	−1.4	0.00008	M
A0A0R4J0Q5	Lmnb2	Lamin-B2	−1.4	0.03275	CK, N
Q4FJX9	Sod2	Superoxide dismutase	−1.4	0.01379	M
Q91VN4	Chchd6	MICOS complex subunit Mic25	−1.4	0.01573	C, M
O88737	Bsn	Protein bassoon	−1.3	0.00915	C, GA
Q3UWW9	Psmd11	Putative uncharacterized protein	−1.3	0.01386	C, N
O08788	Dctn1	Dynactin subunit 1	−1.3	0.01243	CK, C, ERS, N
A0A0R4J275	Ndufa12	NADH dehydrogenase [ubiquinone] 1 alpha subcomplex subunit 12	−1.3	0.0197	C, M
Q63932	Map2k2	Dual specificity mitogen-activated protein kinase kinase 2	−1.3	0.01951	CK, C, ER, En, GA, M, N, PM
Q61361	Bcan	Brevican core protein	−1.3	0.01264	ERS
Q3V117	Acly	ATP-citrate synthase	−1.3	0.0078	C, M, N, PM
Q8R570	Snap47	Synaptosomal-associated protein 47	−1.3	0.00248	C, PM
Q9DCS9	Ndufb10	NADH dehydrogenase [ubiquinone] 1 beta subcomplex subunit 10	−1.2	0.01688	M
P14824	Anxa6	Annexin A6	−1.2	0.01378	C, En, ERS, Ly, M, N, PM
P54071	Idh2	Isocitrate dehydrogenase [NADP], mitochondrial	−1.2	0.00039	C, M, Pe
Q7TSJ2	Map6	Microtubule-associated protein 6	−1.2	0.00159	CK, GA
Q8BGN3	Enpp6	Ectonucleotide pyrophosphatase/phosphodiesterase family member 6	−1.2	0.03099	ERS, PM
Q9CZD3	Gars	Glycine–tRNA ligase	−1.2	0.01474	C, ERS, M
A0A0R4J083	Acadl	Long-chain-specific acyl-CoA dehydrogenase, mitochondrial	−1.2	0.03611	M
Q8CGK3	Lonp1	Lon protease homolog, mitochondrial	−1.1	0.01936	C, M, N
E9Q7Q3	Tpm3	Tropomyosin alpha-3 chain	−1.1	0.00355	CK, C
Q8BWT1	Acaa2	3-ketoacyl-CoA thiolase, mitochondrial	−1.1	0.04478	M
P61226	Rap2b	Ras-related protein Rap-2b	−1.1	0.03025	C, En, ERS, PM
Q8R5C5	Actr1b	Beta-centractin	−1.1	0.00172	CK
E9Q0J5	Kif21a	Kinesin-like protein KIF21A	−1.1	0.04345	CK, C, PM
B9EKR1	Ptprz1	Receptor-type tyrosine-protein phosphatase zeta	−1.1	0.01214	ERS, PM
Q6ZQ38	Cand1	Cullin-associated NEDD8-dissociated protein 1	−1	0.00177	C, GA, N
Q9JI91	Actn2	Alpha-actinin-2	−1	0.00286	CK, PM
P68040	Rack1	Receptor of activated protein C kinase 1	−1	0.03823	CK, M, N, PM
E9PUL5	Prrt2	Proline-rich transmembrane protein 2	−1	0.0411	PM
F6SEU4	Syngap1	Ras/Rap GTPase-activating protein SynGAP	−1	0.03268	PM
Q8CHG1	Dclk1	MKIAA0369 protein (Fragment)	−1	0.02306	PM
Q61490	Alcam	CD166 antigen	−1	0.03414	PM
D3Z656	Synj1	Synaptojanin-1	−1	0.02126	PM
H3BIV5	Akap5	A-kinase anchor protein 5	−1	0.01709	CK, PM

Table 1. Cont.

Swiss-Prot Code	Gene Name	Protein Description	Fold NSAF	p Value	Subcellular Localization
Q8VD37	Sgip1	SH3-containing GRB2-like protein 3-interacting protein 1	−1	0.04017	CK, PM
W6PPR4	Ank3	480-kDa ankyrinG	−1	0.00579	CK, C, PM
Q9CWS0	Ddah1	N(G),N(G)-dimethylarginine dimethylaminohydrolase 1	−0.9	0.04649	M
Q11011	Npepps	Puromycin-sensitive aminopeptidase	−0.9	0.00505	C, N
Q3TXE5	Canx	Putative uncharacterized protein	−0.9	0.00488	ER, PM
Q3UAG2	Pgd	6-phosphogluconate dehydrogenase, decarboxylating	−0.9	0.02403	C
Q99JX6	Anxa6	Annexin	−0.9	0.04313	C, En, ERS, Ly, M, N, PM
A0A0G2JEG8	Amph	Amphiphysin	−0.9	0.00912	CK, PM
Q99P72	Rtn4	Reticulon-4	−0.9	0.01061	ER, N, PM
Q49S98	Slc32a1	Putative uncharacterized protein	−0.9	0.04098	PM
B2RQQ5	Map1b	Microtubule-associated protein 1B	−0.9	0.03443	CK, C, PM
D3Z2H9	Tpm3	Uncharacterized protein	−0.9	0.02982	CK, C
Q6ZQ61	Matr3	MCG121979, isoform CRA_c (Fragment)	−0.8	0.01811	N
Q3TE45	Sdhb	Succinate dehydrogenase [ubiquinone] iron-sulfur subunit, mitochondrial	−0.8	0.01667	M, N, PM
Q0VF55	Atp2b3	Calcium-transporting ATPase	−0.8	0.03416	PM
Q3UEG9	Flot2	Putative uncharacterized protein	−0.8	0.02632	CK, En, PM
Q91V61	Sfxn3	Sideroflexin-3	−0.8	0.00937	M
P61164	Actr1a	Alpha-centractin	−0.8	0.03531	CK
Q571M2	Hspa4	MKIAA4025 protein (Fragment)	−0.7	0.00487	C, ERS, N
Q9Z2Y3	Homer1	Homer protein homolog 1	−0.7	0.01584	C, PM
E9Q455	Tpm1	Tropomyosin alpha-1 chain	−0.7	0.04225	C
A2A5Y6	Mapt	Microtubule-associated protein	−0.7	0.04838	CK, C, N, PM
A0A1S6GWH1		Uncharacterized protein	−0,7	0.02404	
P35486	Pdha1	Pyruvate dehydrogenase E1 component subunit alpha, somatic form, mitochondrial	−0.6	0.00552	M, N
Q8CC13	Ap1b1	AP complex subunit beta	−0.6	0.03216	C, GA
E9Q2W9	Actn4	Alpha-actinin-4 (Fragment)	−0.6	0.00847	CK, C, N
Q8BVE3	Atp6v1h	V-type proton ATPase subunit H	−0.6	0.02175	C, Ly
A0A0A6YY91	Ncam1	Neural cell adhesion molecule 1 (Fragment)	−0.6	0.0182	CK, PM
Q3TYK4	Prkar1a	Putative uncharacterized protein	−0.6	0.01177	CK, C, PM
P12960	Cntn1	Contactin-1	−0.6	0.02931	PM
Q3TPZ5	Dctn2	Dynactin 2	−0.6	0.00054	CK, C
A0A1L1SV25	Actn4	Alpha-actinin-4	−0.6	0.0286	CK, C, N
P19246	Nefh	Neurofilament heavy polypeptide	−0.5	0.04106	CK, M, N, PM
A0A0R4J117	Igsf8	Immunoglobulin superfamily member 8	−0.5	0.04908	PM
Q68FG2	Sptbn2	Spectrin beta chain	−0.5	0.04372	CK, C, ER, En, GA
Q80YU5	Mog	Myelin oligodendrocyte glycoprotein (Fragment)	−0.5	0.02477	C, ER, M, PM
E9QB01	Ncam1	Neural cell adhesion molecule 1	−0.5	0.03648	C, PM
Q01853	Vcp	Transitional endoplasmic reticulum ATPase	−0.5	0.03249	C, ER, N
P09041	Pgk2	Phosphoglycerate kinase 2	−0.4	0.03696	C
Q7TPR4	Actn1	Alpha-actinin-1	−0.4	0.01557	CK, N, PM
P63011	Rab3a	Ras-related protein Rab-3A	−0.4	0.0162	C, En, Ly, PM
P09411	Pgk1	Phosphoglycerate kinase 1	−0.3	0.01617	C, ERS, PM
O08599	Stxbp1	Syntaxin-binding protein 1	0.1	0.03134	CK, C, M, PM
A0A0A0MQA5	Tuba4a	Tubulin alpha chain (Fragment)	0.2	0.01472	CK
P68369	Tuba1a	Tubulin alpha-1A chain	0.2	0.02299	CK, En
Q52L87	Tuba1c	Tubulin alpha chain	0.3	0.0146	CK, N
P50396	Gdi1	Rab GDP dissociation inhibitor alpha	0.3	0.03464	GA
P60710	Actb	Actin, cytoplasmic 1	0.3	0.02793	CK, C, N, PM
Q9CZU6	Cs	Citrate synthase, mitochondrial	0.3	0.00075	M
P05202	Got2	Aspartate aminotransferase, mitochondrial	0.3	0.03387	M, PM
P63038	Hspd1	60 kDa heat shock protein, mitochondrial	0.3	0.02215	CK, ER, En, ERS, GA, M, PM
E9Q912	Rap1gds1	RAP1, GTP-GDP dissociation stimulator 1	0.3	0.00467	CK, ER, M
B2CSK2		Heat shock protein 1-like protein	0.3	0.00172	
O88935	Syn1	Synapsin-1	0.3	0.03624	CK, C, GA, N
P68033	Actc1	Actin, alpha cardiac muscle 1	0.3	0.00986	CK
P08249	Mdh2	Malate dehydrogenase, mitochondrial	0.3	0.00731	M
Q03265	Atp5a1	ATP synthase subunit alpha, mitochondrial	0.3	0.00169	M, N, PM
Q99KI0	Aco2	Aconitate hydratase, mitochondrial	0.3	0.00087	C, M
P17879	Hspa1b	Heat shock 70 kDa protein 1B	0.4	0.00362	CK, C, M, N, PM
O08553	Dpysl2	Dihydropyrimidinase-related protein 2	0.4	0.00004	CK, C, M, PM
Q5FW97	EG433182	Enolase 1, alpha non-neuron	0.4	0.00346	C
Q64332	Syn2	Synapsin-2	0.4	0.01708	PM
Q3TQ70	Gnb1	Beta1 subunit of GTP-binding protein	0.4	0.01897	PM

Table 1. Cont.

Swiss-Prot Code	Gene Name	Protein Description	Fold NSAF	p Value	Subcellular Localization
P62631	Eef1a2	Elongation factor 1-alpha 2	0.4	0.00011	N
P80316	Cct5	T-complex protein 1 subunit epsilon	0.4	0.04942	CK, C
Q8CE19	Syn2	Putative uncharacterized protein	0.4	0.02198	PM
Q3UA81	Eef1a1	Elongation factor 1-alpha	0.4	0.00003	CK, C, M, PM
Q8C2Q7	Hnrnph1	Heterogeneous nuclear ribonucleoprotein H	0.4	0.01261	C, N
Q9D6F9	Tubb4a	Tubulin beta-4A chain	0.4	0.00031	CK
P17751	Tpi1	Triosephosphate isomerase	0.4	0.00008	C
P48774	Gstm5	Glutathione S-transferase Mu 5	0.4	0.01045	C, ERS
P18872	Gnao1	Guanine nucleotide-binding protein G(o) subunit alpha	0.4	0.00334	PM
Q3UYK6	Slc1a2	Amino acid transporter	0.4	0.03711	PM
Q8BVI4	Qdpr	Dihydropteridine reductase	0.4	0.02048	C, M
Q9D2G2	Dlst	Dihydrolipoyllysine-residue succinyltransferase component of 2-oxoglutarate dehydrogenase complex, mitochondrial	0.4	0.00639	M, N, PM
Q3UD06	Atp5c1	ATP synthase subunit gamma	0.4	0.00728	M
P68372	Tubb4b	Tubulin beta-4B chain	0.4	0.00008	CK
P99024	Tubb5	Tubulin beta-5 chain	0.4	0.00005	CK, C, M
P56480	Atp5b	ATP synthase subunit beta, mitochondrial	0.4	0.00166	M, PM
E9QKR0	Gnb2	Guanine nucleotide-binding protein G(I)/G(S)/G(T) subunit beta-2	0.4	0.0162	PM
B2RSN3	Tubb2b	Tubulin beta chain	0.4	0.00013	CK
Q7TMM9	Tubb2a	Tubulin beta-2A chain	0.4	0.0001	CK
P63017	Hspa8	Heat shock cognate 71 kDa protein	0.4	0.0001	CK, C, En, ERS, Ly, N, PM
Q3TIC8	Uqcrc1	Putative uncharacterized protein	0.4	0.00014	C, M
P26443	Glud1	Glutamate dehydrogenase 1, mitochondrial	0.4	0.00008	M
Q3TYV5	Cnp	2′,3′-cyclic-nucleotide 3′-phosphodiesterase	0.5	0.00001	ERS
B7U582		Heat shock protein 70-2	0.5	0.00001	
Q8BH95	Echs1	Enoyl-CoA hydratase, mitochondrial	0.5	0.03689	M
Q6P1J1	Crmp1	Crmp1 protein	0.5	0.00045	CK, C, N
B2CY77	Rpsa	Laminin receptor (Fragment)	0.5	0.01872	C, ERS, N, PM
Q922F4	Tubb6	Tubulin beta-6 chain	0.5	0.00002	CK
Q9ERD7	Tubb3	Tubulin beta-3 chain	0.5	0.00003	CK
Q60930	Vdac2	Voltage-dependent anion-selective channel protein 2	0.5	0.00247	M
P14152	Mdh1	Malate dehydrogenase, cytoplasmic	0.5	0.00092	C, M
A6ZI44	Aldoa	Fructose-bisphosphate aldolase	0.5	0.00156	CK, C, ERS, M, N, PM
Q80X68	Csl	Citrate synthase	0.5	0.00001	N
A2AQ07	Tubb1	Tubulin beta-1 chain	0.5	0.00009	CK
P01831	Thy1	Thy-1 membrane glycoprotein	0.6	0.00272	C, ER, PM
A0A1S6GWG6		Uncharacterized protein	0,6	0.00144	
Q3UBZ3	Capza2	Putative uncharacterized protein	0.6	0.03767	CK
Q9D6M3	Slc25a22	Mitochondrial glutamate carrier 1	0.6	0.02851	M
O08749	Dld	Dihydrolipoyl dehydrogenase, mitochondrial	0.6	0.00293	M, N
Q91VA7	Idh3b	Isocitrate dehydrogenase [NAD] subunit, mitochondrial	0.6	0.0105	M
O88712	Ctbp1	C-terminal-binding protein 1	0.6	0.00177	N
Q8C3L6	Atp6v1b1	Putative uncharacterized protein	0.6	0.04137	PM
P70333	Hnrnph2	Heterogeneous nuclear ribonucleoprotein H2	0.6	0.00158	N
P14094	Atp1b1	Sodium/potassium-transporting ATPase subunit beta-1	0.7	0.00001	PM
O55100	Syngr1	Synaptogyrin-1	0.7	0.03643	PM
Q9R0P9	Uchl1	Ubiquitin carboxyl-terminal hydrolase isozyme L1	0.7	0.00142	C, ER, PM
P05063	Aldoc	Fructose-bisphosphate aldolase C	0.7	0.00002	C, M
Q61990	Pcbp2	Poly(rC)-binding protein 2	0.8	0.03331	C, N
Q8R464	Cadm4	Cell adhesion molecule 4	0.8	0.01837	PM
P21279	Gnaq	Guanine nucleotide-binding protein G(q) subunit alpha	0.9	0.04159	C, N, PM
Q00898	Serpina1	Alpha-1-antitrypsin 1-5	1.2	0.04259	ER, ERS, GA
P63330	Ppp2ca	Serine/threonine-protein phosphatase 2A catalytic subunit alpha isoform	1.4	0.00163	CK, C, N, PM
P03995	Gfap	Glial fibrillary acidic protein	1.4	0.00001	CK, Ly

CK, Cytoskeleton; C, Cytosol; ER, Endoplasmic reticulum; En, Endosome; ERS, Extracellular region or secreted; GA, Golgi apparatus; Ly, Lysosome; M, Mitochondrion; N, Nucleus; Pe, Peroxisome PM, Plasma Membrane.

Overall, the NAGLU$^{-/-}$ brain proteome dataset showed 130 under-represented and 74 over-represented proteins compared to WT mice. For technical validation of the label-free quantitative proteomic analysis, Gfap (P03995) differential abundance was proved by Western blotting analysis using an independent set of brain sample from NAGLU$^{-/-}$ and WT mice (Figure S4).

3.3. Bioinformatic Analysis of Differentially Abundant Proteins

In order to elucidate the biological implications of the differentially abundant proteins in NAGLU$^{-/-}$ brain tissue, the whole proteome profile containing the upregulated and downregulated proteins were analyzed by the PANTHER database, which allows classification and identification of protein functions. The PANTHER enrichment analysis allowed for clustering differentially abundant proteins with respect to cellular pathways (Figure 2 and Table S2) and biological processes (Figure 3 and Table S3).

Figure 2 shows the graphical enrichment of cellular pathways in the deregulated dataset, expressed as the log of fractional difference (observed vs. expected): (number of genes for the category − number of genes expected) / (number of genes expected). The most significant and enriched processes (enrichment threshold > 20) are shown in Figure 2 as "TCA cycle" (81.7, p 1.99 × 10^{-8}), "Pyruvate metabolism" (59.9, p 1.54 × 10^{-6}), "ATP Synthesis" (44.9, p 1.33 × 10^{-3}), "Cytoskeletal regulation by Rho GTPase" (27.0, p 1.19 × 10^{-13}), "Synaptic vesicle trafficking" (25.7, p 2.84 × 10^{-5}), and "Glycolysis" (23.4, p 3.91 × 10^{-4}) (Table S2).

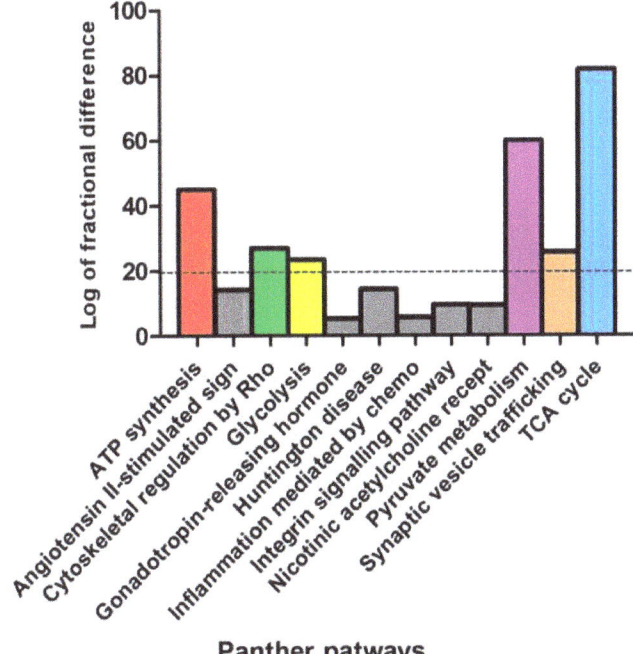

Figure 2. PANTHER pathways classification of murine NAGLU$^{-/-}$ brain tissue proteome. The dysregulated proteins in NAGLU$^{-/-}$ brain versus murine WT brain proteomes were clustered according to their cellular pathways using the Protein Analysis Through Evolutionary Relationship (PANTHER) software. The PANTHER pathways graphical enrichment (y-axis) was associated to each cellular pathway (x axis). The PANTHER cellular pathways were listed according to enriched values, expressed as the log of fractional difference (observed vs expected): (number of genes for the category − number of genes expected) / (number of genes expected).

Figure 3 and Table S3 show the most significant biological processes in our dataset. Among the significant categories the most interesting processes are the "tricarboxylic acid cycle" (53.9% enriched value) and "gluconeogenesis" (33.7% enriched value). Interestingly, a variety of pathways resulted deregulated in the MPS IIIB mouse brains, indicating the complexity of the pathogenesis for the disease.

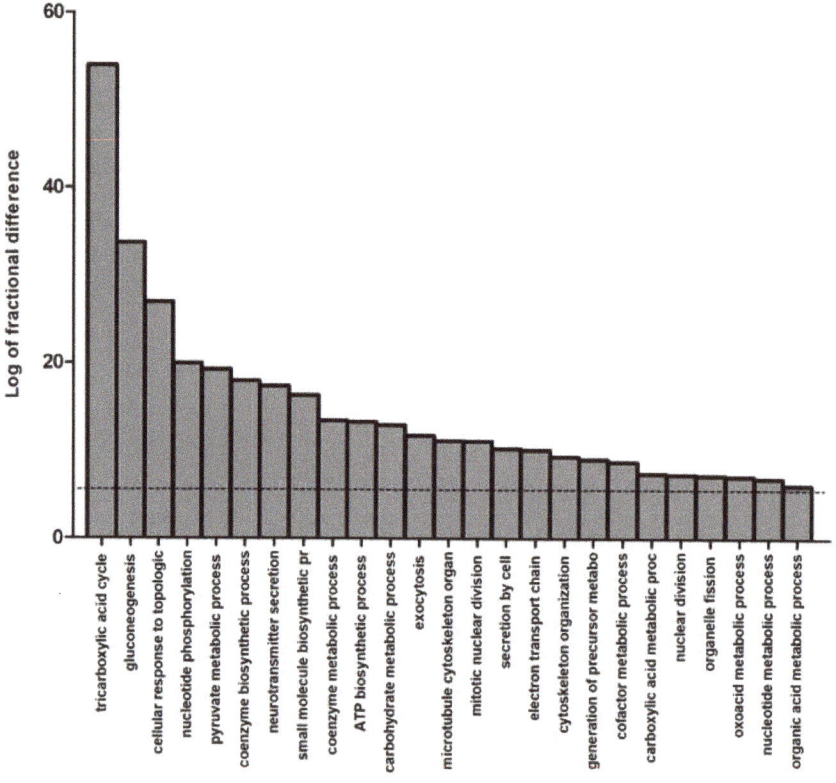

Figure 3. Biological process classification of murine NAGLU$^{-/-}$ brain tissue proteome. The differentially expressed proteins in NAGLU$^{-/-}$ brain versus murine WT brain proteomes were clustered according to their gene ontology (GO) biological process using PANTHER software. The most significant biological processes are listed according to their enriched values, expressed as the log of fractional difference (observed vs. expected): (number of genes for the category − number of genes expected) / (number of genes expected).

In order to obtain additional information from our dataset, the NAGLU$^{-/-}$ differentially abundant proteins were also analyzed using REACTOME and the MetaCore functional ontology enrichment tools.

The REACTOME clustering (Table 2) shows three major significant clusters: "Microtubule-dependent trafficking of connexons from Golgi to the plasma membrane" (R-MMU-190840; $p\ 1.45 \times 10^{-11}$), "Transport of connexons to the plasma membrane" (R-MMU-190872, $p\ 2.12 \times 10^{-11}$) and "Citric acid cycle (TCA cycle)" (R-MMU-71403, $p\ 3.68 \times 10^{-12}$). REACTOME and PANTHER analyses indeed suggest that altered protein trafficking and cellular metabolism play a crucial role in the neuropathology of MPS IIIB disease.

Table 2. REACTOME pathway classification of murine NAGLU$^{-/-}$ brain tissue proteome.

REACTOME Pathways	Mus musculus REFLIST	Client Input	Client Input (Raw p-Value)
Microtubule-dependent trafficking of connexons from Golgi to the plasma membrane (R-MMU-190840)	14	7	1.45×10^{-11}
Citric acid cycle (TCA cycle) (R-MMU-71403)	22	8	3.68×10^{-12}
RHO GTPases activate IQGAPs (R-MMU-5626467)	25	8	8.61×10^{-12}
Carboxyterminal post-translational modifications of tubulin (R-MMU-8955332)	25	7	4.00×10^{-10}
Recycling pathway of L1 (R-MMU-437239)	34	9	1.74×10^{-12}
Lysine catabolism (R-MMU-71064)	12	3	7.16×10^{-05}
HSP90 chaperone cycle for steroid hormone receptors (SHR) (R-MMU-3371497)	51	12	1.00×10^{-15}
COPI-independent Golgi-to-ER retrograde traffic (R-MMU-6811436)	47	10	6.42×10^{-13}
Gluconeogenesis (R-MMU-70263)	35	7	3.07×10^{-09}
Serotonin Neurotransmitter Release Cycle (R-MMU-181429)	17	3	1.76×10^{-04}
Pyruvate metabolism and Citric Acid (TCA) cycle (R-MMU-71406)	51	9	4.21×10^{-11}
GABA synthesis, release, reuptake and degradation (R-MMU-888590)	19	3	2.35×10^{-04}
Dopamine Neurotransmitter Release Cycle (R-MMU-212676)	22	3	3.47×10^{-04}
Glyoxylate metabolism and glycine degradation (R-MMU-389661)	30	4	3.64×10^{-05}
Kinesins (R-MMU-983189)	54	7	4.54×10^{-08}
Intraflagellar transport (R-MMU-5620924)	54	7	4.54×10^{-08}
Recruitment of NuMA to mitotic centrosomes (R-MMU-380320)	86	11	6.28×10^{-12}
RAF activation (R-MMU-5673000)	25	3	4.89×10^{-04}
COPI-mediated anterograde transport (R-MMU-6807878)	98	11	2.29×10^{-11}
The role of GTSE1 in G2/M progression after G2 checkpoint (R-MMU-8852276)	72	8	1.45×10^{-08}
Loss of Nlp from mitotic centrosomes (R-MMU-380259)	67	7	1.77×10^{-07}
AURKA Activation by TPX2 (R-MMU-8854518)	70	7	2.33×10^{-07}
MHC class II antigen presentation (R-MMU-2132295)	120	12	9.50×10^{-12}
Recruitment of mitotic centrosome proteins and complexes (R-MMU-380270)	76	7	3.91×10^{-07}
Regulation of PLK1 Activity at G2/M Transition (R-MMU-2565942)	85	7	7.92×10^{-07}
Hedgehog "on" state (R-MMU-5632684)	103	8	1.91×10^{-07}
ER to Golgi Anterograde Transport (R-MMU-199977)	155	12	1.52×10^{-10}
COPI-dependent Golgi-to-ER retrograde traffic (R-MMU-6811434)	92	7	1.30×10^{-06}
Anchoring of the basal body to the plasma membrane (R-MMU-5620912)	93	7	1.40×10^{-06}
RHO GTPases Activate Formins (R-MMU-5663220)	133	10	7.13×10^{-09}
Resolution of Sister Chromatid Cohesion (R-MMU-2500257)	121	9	4.53×10^{-08}
Hedgehog "off" state (R-MMU-5610787)	109	8	2.87×10^{-07}
Glycolysis (R-MMU-70171)	63	4	5.22×10^{-04}
Separation of Sister Chromatids (R-MMU-2467813)	185	10	1.36×10^{-07}
Mitotic Anaphase (R-MMU-68882)	188	10	1.57×10^{-07}
Neutrophil degranulation (R-MMU-6798695)	553	14	3.17×10^{-06}
Microtubule-dependent trafficking of connexons from Golgi to the plasma membrane (R-MMU-190840)	14	7	1.45×10^{-11}
Citric acid cycle (TCA cycle) (R-MMU-71403)	22	8	3.68×10^{-12}
RHO GTPases activate IQGAPs (R-MMU-5626467)	25	8	8.61×10^{-12}
Carboxyterminal post-translational modifications of tubulin (R-MMU-8955332)	25	7	4.00×10^{-10}
Recycling pathway of L1 (R-MMU-437239)	34	9	1.74×10^{-12}
Lysine catabolism (R-MMU-71064)	12	3	7.16×10^{-05}
Fatty Acids bound to GPR40 (FFAR1) regulate insulin secretion (R-MMU-434316)	8	2	1.33×10^{-03}
HSP90 chaperone cycle for steroid hormone receptors (SHR) (R-MMU-3371497)	51	12	1.00×10^{-15}
COPI-independent Golgi-to-ER retrograde traffic (R-MMU-6811436)	47	10	6.42×10^{-13}
Gluconeogenesis (R-MMU-70263)	35	7	3.07×10^{-09}
Serotonin Neurotransmitter Release Cycle (R-MMU-181429)	17	3	1.76×10^{-04}
Pyruvate metabolism and Citric Acid (TCA) cycle (R-MMU-71406)	51	9	4.21×10^{-11}
GABA synthesis, release, reuptake and degradation (R-MMU-888590)	19	3	2.35×10^{-04}
Dopamine Neurotransmitter Release Cycle (R-MMU-212676)	22	3	3.47×10^{-04}
Glyoxylate metabolism and glycine degradation (R-MMU-389661)	30	4	3.64×10^{-05}
Kinesins (R-MMU-983189)	54	7	4.54×10^{-08}
Intraflagellar transport (R-MMU-5620924)	54	7	4.54×10^{-08}
Recruitment of NuMA to mitotic centrosomes (R-MMU-380320)	86	11	6.28×10^{-12}
RAF activation (R-MMU-5673000)	25	3	4.89×10^{-04}

On the other hand, the MetaCore functional ontology enrichment tool was applied to map identified proteins into two MetaCore ontologies: "diseases by biomarkers" and "process networks". The 20 most significant enriched terms are reported in Figure 4, where the −log(pValue)s of the mapping of the experimental protein set to the ontology terms "diseases by biomarkers" (Figure 4a; FDR

$\leq 2.5 \times 10^{-11}$) and "process networks" (Figure 4b; FDR $\leq 2.8 \times 10^{-3}$) are represented by histograms. The former enrichment highlighted the tight correlation existing between identified differentially abundant proteins and CNS affections. As expected, a number of differences were annotated as biomarkers in (i) CNS diseases, e.g., in some heredodegenerative disorders, prion diseases, tauopathies, and Alzheimer disease; (ii) dementia, epilepsy, and neurocognitive impairments; and iii) mental disorders, as schizophrenia and other psychotic disorders (Table S4).

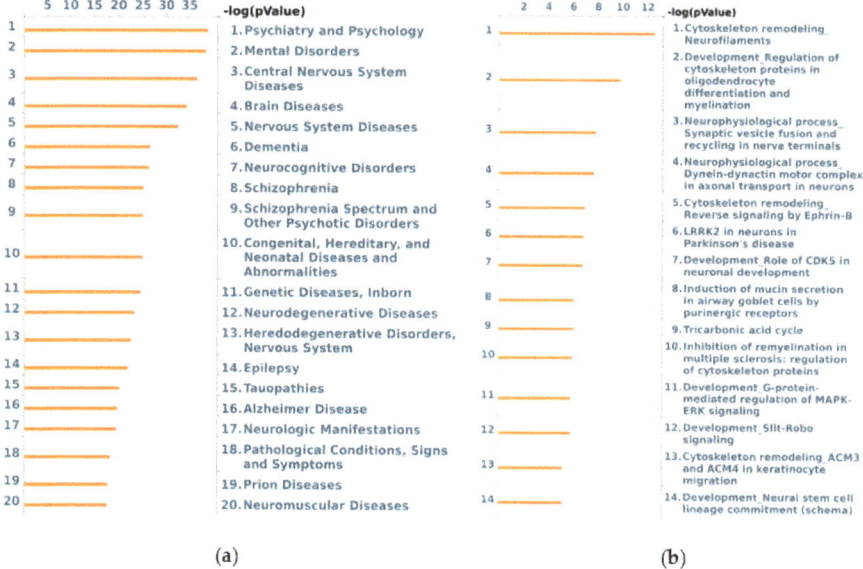

(a)   (b)

Figure 4. MetaCore "diseases by biomarkers" (**a**) and "process networks" (**b**) enrichment analysis of murine NAGLU$^{-/-}$ brain tissues proteome. The MetaCore enriched analysis provides a statistically supported list of (a) diseases in which identified proteins have been previously described as biomarkers; and (b) process networks more represented in identified proteins dataset.

According to "process networks" ontologies, and in line with PANTHER and REACTOME results, cytoskeleton dynamics were suggested as the most representative cellular process affected in NAGLU$^{-/-}$ mouse brains. Spanning from microtubule and microfilaments to intermediate filaments, the three main structural and functional components of cytoskeleton seem actually altered by MPS IIIB. Related to cytoskeleton dysregulation, we also observed a highly significant enrichment of gene ontology (GO) terms concerning cell adhesion, by both integrins and cell junctions, and to neurogenesis (axonal guidance and synaptogenesis) and neurotransmission (GABAergic transmission).

Finally, to functionally correlate the differentially abundant detected proteins, pathway analyses were attempted by applying the STRING and MetaCore resources.

Noteworthy, the STRING protein–protein interaction (PPI) network showed the identified differences clustering in three main paths, that are all related to the above described enrichment analyses: cytoskeletal regulation, metabolism, and synaptic vesicle trafficking (Figure 5). These functional clusters highlight the fundamental role that defects in cytoskeletal organization, synaptic transmission, and energy balance act in MPS IIIB neuropathogenesis.

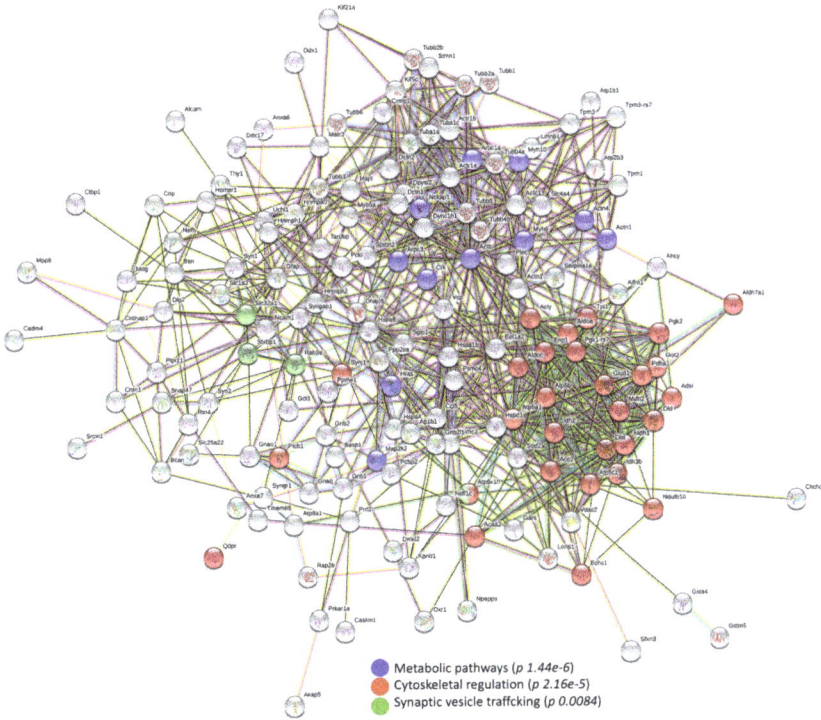

Figure 5. Protein–protein interaction (PPI) in murine NAGLU$^{-/-}$ brain tissue proteome. The PPI network was explored by STRING (Search Tool for the Retrieval of Interacting Genes) software. The cluster analysis shows "Metabolic Pathways" ($p\ 1.44 \times 10^{-6}$), "Cytoskeletal Regulation" ($p\ 2.16 \times 10^{-5}$) and "Synaptic vesicle trafficking" ($p\ 8.40 \times 10^{-3}$) as significant pathways according to KEGG (Kyoto Encyclopedia of Genes and Genomes) database.

The involvement of neuronal plasticity and signal transduction affections, along with an evident dysfunction in cytoskeleton, and even nucleoskeleton organization, with known degenerative consequences for the CNS, are definitively indicated by the MetaCore shortest path analysis as key processes in the neurological manifestations of MPS IIIB. According to the selected parameters, the built net resulted from the tight functional correlation existing among the processed EntrezGene-list corresponding proteins. Of relevance, about 80% of the processed differences entered into the net, thus proving the significance of the obtained data and the biological relevance of their deregulated abundance. Five main central hubs in the net (Figure 6, red circles) resulted: serine/threonine protein phosphatase 2A, catalytic subunit, alpha isoform (collapsed in PP2A catalytic in the MetaCore net; P63330; Fold$_{NSAF}$ = 1.4), receptor for activated protein C kinase 1 (RACK1; P68040; Fold$_{NSAF}$ = −1), C-terminal-binding protein 1 (collapsed in CtBP1 in the MetaCore net; O88712; Fold$_{NSAF}$ = 0.6), GTPase HRas (collapsed in RAS in the MetaCore net; Q61411; Fold$_{NSAF}$ = −2.2), HSC70 (collapsed in HSP70 in the MetaCore net—the protein difference heat shock cognate 71 kDa protein (hspa8; P63017; Fold$_{NSAF}$ = 0.4) also functionally collapsed in this central hub). Despite that they were not designed among the above central hubs, tubulin (in microtubules), actin, and stathmin (Figure 6, green circles) act in key roles for the network by assuming central positions and interacting with several other proteins.

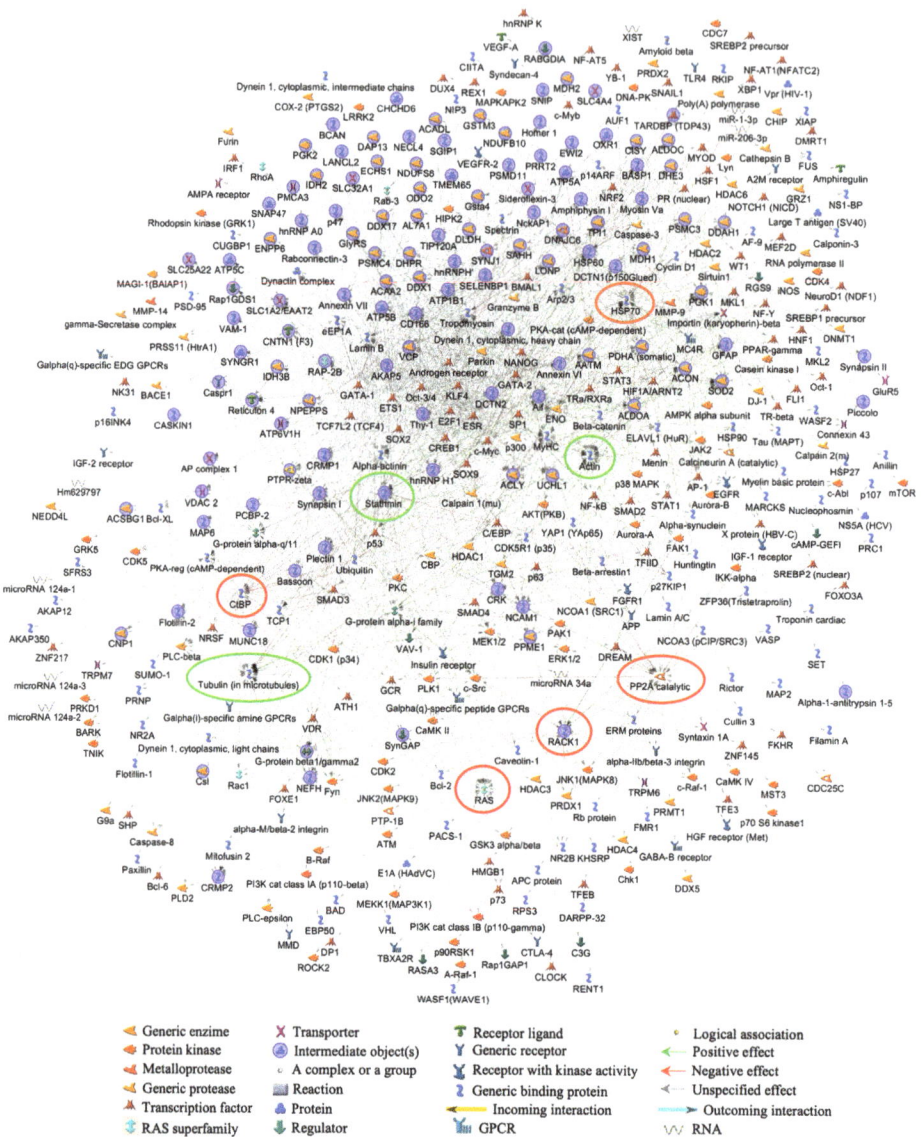

Figure 6. MetaCore protein network of murine NAGLU$^{-/-}$ brain proteome. The protein–protein interactions characterizing the murine NAGLU$^{-/-}$ brain proteome, were explored by MetaCore tools. The experimental proteins (blue circles) were processed according to known protein–protein interactions and other features established in the literature. The relationships existing between individual proteins and their directions were represented by arrows and lines. The following line colors designate the nature of the interaction: red = negative effect, green = positive effect, gray = unspecified effect.

4. Discussion

A label-free quantitative proteomic approach was employed to identify 204 proteins whose expression was found deregulated in NAGLU knockout murine brain tissues versus WT mice. Multiple bioinformatic analyses allowed us to classify these proteins into three major groups of biological processes: regulation of cytoskeleton organization, synaptic vesicle trafficking, and energy metabolism. Here we discuss the proteins that we identified as deregulated in NAGLU$^{-/-}$ brains (Figure 7) within these biological processes and their involvement in the neuropathogenesis of MPS IIIB disease.

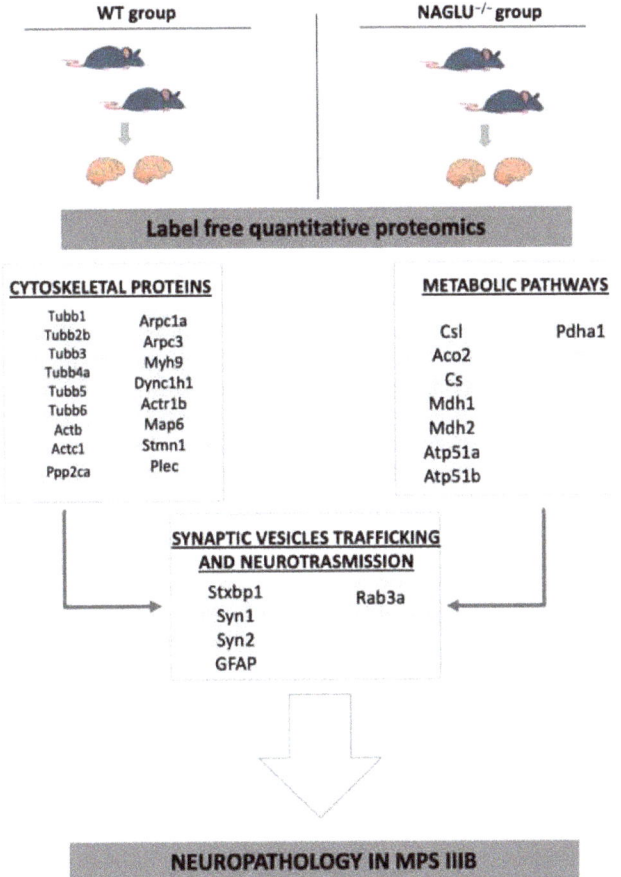

Figure 7. Representation of the main proteomic modifications induced by NAGLU deletion in murine brains. Dysregulation of cytoskeleton associated proteins and the energy metabolism-involved proteins may contribute to impair the lysosomal membrane trafficking pathway linked to the pathogenesis of neuropathy in MPS IIIB disease. Both altered pathways are relevant to preserve brain homeostasis and could be responsible for an impairment of synaptic vesicle formation and activity in the MPS IIIB mouse brain.

4.1. Deregulated Proteins Involved in Cytoskeleton Organization

The major group of dysregulated proteins in MPS IIIB mouse brain is made by cytoskeletal proteins. We found altered levels of a cluster of proteins involved in the cytoskeletal organization composed by Tubb (tubulin beta) 1, Tubb2b, Tubb3, Tubb4a, Tubb5, Tubb6, Actb (actin beta), Actc1 (actin alpha cardiac muscle 1), Arpc1a (actin-related protein 2/3 complex subunit 1a), Arpc3 (actin-related protein 2/3 complex subunit 3), and Myh9 (myosin-9). Furthermore, the cytoskeletal proteins dynein, Actr, Map6, Stmn1, plectin, and Ppp2cA were also found to be deregulated in MPS IIIB mouse brains.

In the developing brain, a large number of tubulin isoforms are expressed in neurons during neuronal migration and differentiation. They are globular proteins forming heterodimers that coassemble into microtubules, important cytoskeletal polymers that are involved in fundamental cellular processes such as cell division, motility, differentiation, intracellular cargo transport, and communications [44,45]. Distinct alpha- and beta-tubulin isoforms are required for the positioning, differentiation, and survival of neurons [46,47]. Mutations in genes encoding for alpha-tubulin (Tuba1a) and beta-tubulin (Tubb2a, Tubb3, Tubb4a) have been associated with a variety of brain malformations, including different types of cortical phenotypes [48]. As the deregulation of the tubulin isotype, Tubb4b was also found in the brain of MPS I mice [49]; the deregulation of tubulin isoforms Tubb1, Tubb2a, Tubb3, Tubb4a, Tubb5, and Tubb6 found in the MPS IIIB mouse brain strongly suggests that microtubule dysfunction may underlie the pathogenic mechanisms of neurological disorders in specific MPS subtypes.

Indeed, microtubule involvement in the MPS neurological component is supported by our results where we found altered expression levels of proteins such as Stathmin (Stmn1) and microtubule-associated protein 6 (Map6) detected in MPS IIIB mouse brain. Stmn1 has been shown to act as a key mediator in neuronal transduction pathways, and it is involved in the physiological regulation of microtubule destabilization. Moreover, it plays a critical role in the pathology of neurodegeneration such as Alzheimer's disease (AD) [50]. Finally, Stmn1 regulates physiological development of Purkinje cell dendrites, controls the microtubule polymerization, and mediates the development of dendritic arbors in neuronal cells [51,52]. Map6 is deputed to stabilize neuronal microtubules and plays an important role in establishing axon–dendrite polarity [53]. Interestingly, we observed also the increased levels of Serine/threonine-protein phosphatase 2A catalytic subunit alpha isoform (Ppp2ca), described as the major phosphatase for microtubule-associated proteins (MAPs). Ppp2ca is the central factor in the NAGLU$^{-/-}$ proteome, given that it establishes the greatest number of functional connections with the other proteins in the dataset hubs as shown in the net. Furthermore, the interaction of Map6 with the lysosomal protein TMEM 106B is crucial for controlling lysosomal trafficking by acting as a molecular brake for retrograde transport [54]. Indeed, lysosomes receive inputs from both endocytic and autophagic pathways, and release degraded products to Golgi apparatus through retrograde trafficking or to the extracellular space through exocytosis [55,56]. Thus, lysosomal misrouting may be responsible for neurodegeneration in MPS diseases. Consistently, in MPS IIIB mouse brains, we also found altered expression levels of the motor protein dynein complex which mediates lysosome movement towards the microtubule-minus ends (retrograde transport). The lysosome retrograde transport mediated by dynein requires the simultaneous binding of the protein to its adaptor dynactyn [57]. An impairment of dynein-mediated retrograde transport and clearance of autophagic vacuoles has been found in several neurodegenerative disorders [58].

Notably, in MPS IIIB mouse brains, we found also the deregulation of plectin, a protein that acts as the main linker of the intermediate filaments with microtubules and microfilaments. Plectin is a member of a structural family of proteins able to interlink different cytoskeletal elements. It might be involved not only in the cross-linking and stabilization of cytoskeletal intermediate filaments network, but also in the dynamic regulation of the cytoskeleton [59,60].

Overall, these findings suggest that the impairment of the lysosomal membrane trafficking pathway due to a deregulation of cytoskeleton-associated proteins may contribute to the pathogenesis of neuropathy in MPS IIIB disease.

4.2. Deregulated Proteins Involved in Metabolic Pathways

A group of proteins deregulated in murine NAGLU knockout brain tissue clustered as "TCA cycle" (Csl, Aco2, Pdha1, Cs, Mdh1), "Pyruvate metabolism" (Csl, Pdha1, Cs, Mdh2), and ATP Synthesis (Atp51a, Atp51b). These alterations strictly correlate with the deregulation of the lysosomal–autophagy pathway. Pharmacological inhibition of this pathway in cultured primary rat cortical neurons showed alterations in TCA cycle intermediates, particularly those downstream of citrate synthase and those linked to glutaminolysis [61]. Furthermore, autophagy impairment affects the quality and activity of mitochondria, including its electron transport chain function [61]. It has been shown that neurons of the mouse model of MPS IIIB accumulate the subunit c of mitochondrial ATP synthase (SCMAS) [62]. On the other hand, mitochondria engulf lysosomes by autophagy [63], a process that is critical for neuronal survival [64]. Suppression of autophagy in neural cells causes neurodegeneration in mice [64,65]. An aberrant lysosomal–autophagy pathway associated with neurodegeneration has been ascertained in various lysosomal storage diseases, including MPSs [31,66,67].

The mechanistic target of rapamycin complex 1 (mTORC1) plays a key role in maintaining cellular homeostasis by regulating metabolic processes [68]. Indeed, in nutrient-rich conditions, mTORC1 stimulates biosynthetic pathways (anabolic metabolism) and inhibits catabolic pathways. Acting in concert with the energy sensor AMP-activated protein kinase (AMPK) [58], mTORC1 drives anabolic or catabolic processes. Lysosomes, among their functions, serve also as platforms for both anabolic or catabolic signaling mediated by mTORC1 and AMPK [69]. These pathways are particularly relevant for maintaining brain homeostasis, and increasing evidence suggests that metabolic alterations strongly influence the initiation and progression of neurodegenerative disorders [70,71].

Our results, that identify dysregulated proteins involved in energy metabolism in MPS IIIB mouse brain, strongly suggest the involvement of metabolic pathway alterations in the development of neurological phenotypes in the MPS IIIB disease.

4.3. Deregulated Proteins Involved in Synaptic Vesicle Trafficking and Neurotransmission

Energy metabolism is relevant for neuronal plasticity, axonal transport, synaptic vesicle trafficking and docking, and thereby neurotransmitter release [72]. In our study, dysregulation of the expression levels of proteins involved in "Synaptic vesicle trafficking" and in "neurotransmitter release" pathways, including the syntaxin-binding protein 1 (Stxbp1), synapsin 1 and 2 (Syn1, Syn2), and Rab3a, was observed in the brain of MPS IIIB mice.

The brain membrane transport protein Stxbp1, also known as Munc18-1, is a key component of synaptic vesicle-fusion machinery, thus playing an important role in neurotransmitter secretion [73]. Heterozygous de novo mutations in the neuronal protein Munc18-1 are associated with epilepsies, movement disorders, intellectual disability, and neurodegeneration [74].

Synapsins (Syns) are the most abundant protein family present on synaptic vesicles and are phosphorylated at multiple sites by various protein kinases [75]. When dephosphorylated Syns are associated with the synaptic vesicle membrane, while when phosphorylated they dissociate from the synaptic vesicles thus stimulating the exocytosis [76,77]. Three isoforms of Syns, namely Syn 1, Syn 2, and Syn 3, are highly expressed in nerve cells, but Syn 1 and Syn 2 are the major isoforms in neurons. They are involved in the elongation of axons, formation of presynaptic terminals, regulation of the vesicle reserve pool at presynaptic terminals, synaptogenesis, and synaptic vesicle docking [78,79]. These proteins display a highly conserved ATP binding site in the central C-domain, and this binding modulates synaptic vesicle clustering and plasticity of inhibitory synapses [80]. The Syn-dependent cluster of synaptic vesicles plays a key role in sustaining the release of neurotransmitter in response to high levels of neuronal activity [75]. Indeed, Syn1 null mice exhibit altered synaptic vesicle organization at presynaptic terminals coupled to a reduced neurotransmitter release, and delayed recovery of synaptic transmission after neurotransmitter depletion [76]. Abnormal expression/activity of Syns has been associated with several neurological disorders including epilepsy, schizophrenia, Huntington's disease, Alzheimer's disease, multiple sclerosis (MS), and autism [78,79].

Finally, in MPS IIIB mouse brain, we found altered expression levels of Rab3a, a GTPase protein which localizes to the synaptosomes and secretory granules. This protein is a critical player in the regulation of secretion and neurotransmitter release [81]. In general, Rab GTPases are involved in the control of vesicular traffic by recruiting effector proteins that bind exclusively to the GTP-bound, active form of the GTPase [82]. Several evidences demonstrate that Rab3a interacts with the cortical actin cytoskeleton via its effector, the nonmuscle myosin heavy chain IIA (NMHC IIA), an actin-dependent motor adaptor responsible for the positioning of the lysosomes at the periphery of the cell [83].

Previous studies in the mouse model of the Gaucher lysosomal storage disease have shown a deregulation of dopamine neurotransmission indicative of synaptic dysfunction [84]. Altered dopamine transport system imaging resulted to be pathologic in Niemann-Pick type C-case reports [85,86]. These findings together with our observations of a deregulation of proteins involved in synaptic vesicle formation and activity in the MPS IIIB mouse brain strongly suggest the involvement of synaptic dysfunction and impaired neurotransmission in the pathogenesis of the neurological disorders associated with some MPS subtypes and other lysosomal storage diseases as well.

4.4. Other Proteins

Altered expression levels of Glial fibrillary acidic protein (GFAP) were found in the MPS IIIB mouse brain. This finding is consistent with previous studies that highlighted a deregulation of GFAP in several lysosomal storage diseases, including MPS IIIB [18,87–95]. The protein GFAP is a molecular marker of astrocytes that are fundamental for the neuronal microenvironment in order to control the metabolism of glucose, neurotransmitters re-uptake, and the formation and maturation of the synapses. Moreover, astrocytes play a crucial role in inflammation and neurodegeneration in the brain. Indeed, they are the source and the target of inflammatory cytokines together with the microglia and oligodendrocytes. Elevated levels of proinflammatory cytokines such as IL-1, TNF-α, MCP-1, and MIP-1α have been found in the CNS of MPS murine models [20,90,96,97] as well as in the mouse models of Gaucher disease and Krabbe [98]. Although most of these cytokines might be released by the activated microglia, activated astrocytes and neurons are also capable to diffuse proinflammatory cytokine signaling. Significant increased levels of MCP-1, MIP-1α, and IL-1α were observed in MPS I and MPS III mouse brains [90,99,100]. Upregulation of TNF-α and TNFR1 gene expression was detected in MPS IIIB mouse brain [96,101]. Serum and synovial fluid levels of TNF-α were found increased in MPS VII mice and dogs, respectively [93,94]. These findings suggest the activation of signaling from the TLRs and IL-1 receptors, which together would contribute to TNF-α production. IL-1β levels were found upregulated in both MPS IIIA and MPS IIIB brains [20,96], in MPS VII dogs synovial fluid, and MPS VI rat fibroblast-like synoviocytes [102–104]. Innate immunity appears to have a dominating role in MPSs by controlling lipid metabolism, glycosaminoglycan degradation, autophagy, and regulation of the cytokines release by the inflammasome [95]. Moreover, the relationship between inflammation and autophagy has been recently linked to the release of the specific IL-1β by the inflammasome [104]. In our study, we also found proteins involved in inflammation dysregulated in the MPS IIIB mouse brains.

5. Conclusions

In this work we analyze for the first time the differences in the proteome profiles between brains from MPS IIIB vs. WT mice and we highlight that alterations in metabolic pathways, organelle homeostasis, and cytoskeletal system may play a fundamental role in the neuropathology of MPS IIIB. Deregulation of cytoskeleton and energy metabolism-associated proteins may contribute to impair the lysosomal membrane trafficking pathway linked to the pathogenesis of neuropathy in MPS IIIB disease. Both altered pathways are relevant to preserve brain homeostasis and could be responsible for the impairment of synaptic vesicle formation and activity in the MPS IIIB mouse brain. We believe that an in depth shotgun proteomic analysis would be required to validate this first study on protein abundance quantifications in the MPS IIIB mouse model. In addition, future studies will be necessary to evaluate the involvement of specific pathways which could be the molecular basis of the neuropathology seen in MPS IIIB patients and animal models. Furthermore, it would be of great interest to investigate the proteomic profiles of brains from other lysosomal diseases and compare them together in order to find common hallmarks of these neurological diseases.

Supplementary Materials: The following are available online at http://www.mdpi.com/2218-273X/10/3/355/s1, Supplemental Table S1: Details of mass spectrometry identifications; Supplemental Table S2: PANTHER Cellular Pathways of murine NAGLU$^{-/-}$ brain tissue proteome; Supplemental Table S3: PANTHER GO-Biological Process of murine NAGLU$^{-/-}$ brain tissue proteome; Supplemental Table S4: Protein distribution in Diseases by biomarkers enrichment. Supplemental Figure S1: Reproducibility of the abundance parameter NSAF; Supplemental Figure S2: Normal distribution, Principal Component Analysis (PCA) and correlation matrix for WT and NAGLU$^{-/-}$ protein dataset. Supplemental Figure S3: Volcano plot analysis of global proteome comparison between NAGLU$^{-/-}$ and WT. Supplemental Figure S4: Western blotting of GFAP protein levels in NAGLU$^{-/-}$ and WT brain.

Author Contributions: Conceptualization, V.D.P., M.C.(Michele Costanzo), M.R., L.M.P. and M.C. (Marianna Caterino); Data curation, R.A.S., M.F.M., L.B. and M.C. (Marianna Caterino); Formal analysis, M.F.M., V.P., L.B. and M.C. (Marianna Caterino); Funding acquisition, M.R.; Investigation, V.D.P., M.C. (Michele Costanzo) and M.C. (Marianna Caterino); Methodology, V.D.P., M.C. (Michele Costanzo), R.A.S., M.F.M., V.P., L.B., E.M. and M.C. (Marianna Caterino); Resources, R.A.S.; Supervision, M.R. and L.M.P.; Validation, R.A.S.; Writing—original draft, V.D.P., M.R., L.M.P. and M.C. (Marianna Caterino) All authors have read and agreed to the published version of the manuscript.

Funding: This research was funded by PRIN (Progetti di Ricerca di Rilevante Interesse Nazionale—grant number Prot. 2017SNRXH3) to M.R.

Acknowledgments: Associazione Culturale DiSciMuS RFC.

Conflicts of Interest: The authors declare no conflict of interest.

References

1. Neufeld, E.F.; Muenzer, J. The mucopolysaccharidoses. In *The Metabolic and Molecular Bases of Inherited Disease*, 8th ed.; Scriver, C.R., Beaudet, A.L., Sly, W.S., Valle, D., Eds.; McGraw-Hill: New York, NY, USA, 2001; pp. 3421–3452.
2. De Pasquale, V.; Pavone, L.M. Heparan sulfate proteoglycans: The sweet side of development turns sour in mucopolysaccharidoses. *Biochim. Biophys. Acta Mol. Basis Dis.* **2019**, *1865*, 165539. [CrossRef] [PubMed]
3. Gilkes, J.A.; Heldermon, C.D. Mucopolysaccharidosis III (Sanfilippo Syndrome) disease presentation and experimental therapies. *Pediatr. Endocrinol. Rev.* **2014**, *12*, 133–140. [PubMed]
4. De Pasquale, V.; Sarogni, P.; Pistorio, V.; Cerulo, G.; Paladino, S.; Pavone, L.M. Targeting Heparan Sulfate Proteoglycans as a Novel Therapeutic Strategy for Mucopolysaccharidoses. *Mol. Ther. Methods Clin. Dev.* **2018**, *10*, 8–16. [CrossRef] [PubMed]
5. De Pasquale, V.; Pezone, A.; Sarogni, P.; Tramontano, A.; Schiattarella, G.G.; Avvedimento, V.E.; Paladino, S.; Pavone, L.M. EGFR activation triggers cellular hypertrophy and lysosomal disease in NAGLU-depleted cardiomyoblasts; mimicking the hallmarks of mucopolysaccharidosis IIIB. *Cell Death Dis.* **2018**, *9*, 40. [CrossRef]
6. Shapiro, E.G.; Jones, S.A.; Escolar, M.L. Developmental and behavioral aspects of mucopolysaccharidoses with brain manifestations—Neurological signs and symptoms. *Mol. Genet. Metab.* **2017**, *122*, 1–7. [CrossRef]
7. Whitley, C.B.; Cleary, M.; Eugen Mengel, K.; Harmatz, P.; Shapiro, E.; Nestrasil, I.; Haslett, P.; Whiteman, D.; Alexanderian, D. Observational prospective natural history of patients with Sanfilippo syndrome type B. *J. Pediatr.* **2018**, *197*, 198–206. [CrossRef]
8. Heldermon, C.D.; Hennig, A.K.; Ohlemiller, K.K.; Ogilvie, J.M.; Herzog, E.D.; Breidenbach, A.; Vogler, C.; Wozniak, D.F.; Sands, M.S. Development of sensory, motor and behavioral deficits in the murine model of Sanfilippo syndrome type B. *PLoS ONE* **2007**, *2*, 772. [CrossRef]
9. Bigger, B.W.; Begley, D.J.; Virgintino, D.; Pshezhetsky, A.V. Anatomical changes and pathophysiology of the brain in mucopolysaccharidosis disorders. *Mol. Genet. Metab.* **2018**, *125*, 322–331. [CrossRef]
10. Zafeiriou, D.I.; Savvopoulou-Augoustidou, P.A.; Sewell, A.; Papadopoulou, F.; Badouraki, M.; Vargiami, E.; Gombakis, N.P.; Katzos, G.S. Serial magnetic resonance imaging findings in mucopolysaccharidosis IIIB (Sanfilippo's syndrome B). *Brain Dev.* **2001**, *23*, 385–389. [CrossRef]
11. Barone, R.; Nigro, F.; Triulzi, F.; Musumeci, S.; Fiumara, A.; Pavone, L. Clinical and neuroradiological follow-up in mucopolysaccharidosis type III (Sanfilippo syndrome). *Neuropediatrics* **1999**, *30*, 270–274. [CrossRef] [PubMed]
12. Ferrer, I.; Cusi, V.; Pineda, M.; Galofre, E.; Vila, J. Focal dendritic swellings in Purkinje cells in mucopolysaccharidoses types I, II and III. A Golgi and ultrastructural study. *Neuropathol. Appl. Neurobiol.* **1988**, *14*, 315–323. [CrossRef]

13. Ellinwood, N.M.; Wang, P.; Skeen, T.; Sharp, N.J.; Cesta, M.; Decker, S.; Edwards, N.J.; Bublot, I.; Thompson, J.N.; Bush, W.; et al. A model of mucopolysaccharidosis IIIB (Sanfilippo syndrome type IIIB): N-acetyl-alpha-D-glucosaminidase deficiency in Schipperke dogs. *J. Inherit. Metab. Dis.* **2003**, *26*, 489–504. [CrossRef] [PubMed]
14. Lavery, M.A.; Green, W.R.; Jabs, E.W.; Luckenbach, M.W.; Cox, J.L. Ocular histopathology and ultrastructure of Sanfilippo's syndrome, type III-B. *Arch. Ophthalmol.* **1983**, *101*, 1263–1274. [CrossRef] [PubMed]
15. McCarty, D.M.; DiRosario, J.; Gulaid, K.; Killedar, S.; Oosterhof, A.; van Kuppevelt, T.H.; Martin, P.T.; Fu, H. Differential distribution of heparan sulfate glycoforms and elevated expression of heparan sulfate biosynthetic enzyme genes in the brain of mucopolysaccharidosis IIIB mice. *Metab. Brain Dis.* **2011**, *26*, 9–19. [CrossRef] [PubMed]
16. McGlynn, R.; Dobrenis, K.; Walkley, S.U. Differential subcellular localization of cholesterol, gangliosides, and glycosaminoglycans in murine models of mucopolysaccharide storage disorders. *J. Comp. Neurol.* **2004**, *480*, 415–426. [CrossRef]
17. Hara, A.; Kitazawa, N.; Taketomi, T. Abnormalities of glycosphingolipids in mucopolysaccharidosis type III B. *J. Lipid Res.* **1984**, *25*, 175–184.
18. Ohmi, K.; Greenberg, D.S.; Rajavel, K.S.; Ryazantsev, S.; Li, H.H.; Neufeld, E.F. Activated microglia in cortex of mouse models of mucopolysaccharidoses I and IIIB. *Proc. Natl. Acad. Sci. USA* **2003**, *100*, 1902–1907. [CrossRef]
19. Fu, H.; Bartz, J.D.; Stephens, R.L., Jr.; McCarty, D.M. Peripheral nervous system neuropathology and progressive sensory impairments in a mouse model of Mucopolysaccharidosis IIIB. *PLoS ONE* **2012**, *7*, 45992. [CrossRef]
20. Ausseil, J.; Desmaris, N.; Bigou, S.; Attali, R.; Corbineau, S.; Vitry, S.; Parent, M.; Cheillan, D.; Fuller, M.; Maire, I.; et al. Early neurodegeneration progresses independently of microglial activation by heparan sulfate in the brain of mucopolysaccharidosis IIIB mice. *PLoS ONE* **2008**, *3*, 2296. [CrossRef]
21. Li, H.H.; Zhao, H.Z.; Neufeld, E.F.; Cai, Y.; Gómez-Pinilla, F. Attenuated plasticity in neurons and astrocytes in the mouse model of Sanfilippo syndrome type B. *J. Neurosci. Res.* **2002**, *69*, 30–38. [CrossRef]
22. Caterino, M.; Corbo, C.; Imperlini, E.; Armiraglio, M.; Pavesi, E.; Aspesi, A.; Loreni, F.; Dianzani, I.; Ruoppolo, M. Differential proteomic analysis in human cells subjected to ribosomal stress. *Proteomics* **2013**, *13*, 1220–1227. [CrossRef]
23. Imperlini, E.; Santorelli, L.; Orrù, S.; Scolamiero, E.; Ruoppolo, M.; Caterino, M. Mass spectrometry-based metabolomic and proteomic strategies in organic acidemias. *BioMed Res. Int.* **2016**, *2016*, 9210408. [CrossRef] [PubMed]
24. Barbarani, G.; Ronchi, A.; Ruoppolo, M.; Santorelli, L.; Steinfelder, R.; Elangovan, S.; Fugazza, C.; Caterino, M. Unravelling pathways downstream Sox6 induction in K562 erythroid cells by proteomic analysis. *Sci. Rep.* **2017**, *7*, 14088. [CrossRef] [PubMed]
25. Costanzo, M.; Cevenini, A.; Marchese, E.; Imperlini, E.; Raia, M.; Del Vecchio, L.; Caterino, M.; Ruoppolo, M. Label-free quantitative proteomics in a methylmalonyl-CoA mutase-silenced neuroblastoma cell line. *Int. J. Mol. Sci.* **2018**, *19*, 3580. [CrossRef] [PubMed]
26. Mi, H.; Muruganujan, A.; Casagrande, J.T.; Thomas, P.D. Large-scale gene function analysis with the PANTHER classification system. *Nat. Protoc.* **2013**, *8*, 1551–1566. [CrossRef] [PubMed]
27. Mi, H.; Huang, X.; Muruganujan, A.; Tang, H.; Mills, C.; Kang, D.; Thomas, P.D. PANTHER version 11: Expanded annotation data from Gene Ontology and Reactome pathways, and data analysis tool enhancements. *Nucleic Acids Res.* **2017**, *45*, 183–189. [CrossRef]
28. Armentano, M.F.; Caterino, M.; Miglionico, R.; Ostuni, A.; Pace, M.C.; Cozzolino, F.; Monti, M.; Milella, L.; Carmosino, M.; Pucci, P.; et al. New insights on the functional role of URG7 in the cellular response to ER stress. *Biol. Cell* **2018**, *110*, 147–158. [CrossRef]
29. Bianchi, L.; Gagliardi, A.; Landi, C.; Focarelli, R.; De Leo, V.; Luddi, A.; Bini, L.; Piomboni, P. Protein pathways working in human follicular fluid: The future for tailored IVF? *Expert Rev. Mol. Med.* **2016**, *8*, 9. [CrossRef]
30. Li, H.H.; Yu, W.H.; Rozengurt, N.; Zhao, H.Z.; Lyons, K.M.; Anagnostaras, S.; Fanselow, M.S.; Suzuki, K.; Vanier, M.T.; Neufeld, E.F. Mouse model of Sanfilippo syndrome type B produced by targeted disruption of the gene encoding alpha-N-acetylglucosaminidase. *Proc. Natl. Acad. Sci. USA* **1999**, *96*, 14505–14510. [CrossRef]

31. Schiattarella, G.G.; Cerulo, G.; De Pasquale, V.; Cocchiaro, P.; Paciello, O.; Avallone, L.; Belfiore, M.P.; Iacobellis, F.; Di Napoli, D.; Magliulo, F.; et al. The Murine Model of Mucopolysaccharidosis IIIB Develops Cardiopathies over Time Leading to Heart Failure. *PLoS ONE* **2015**, *10*, e0131662. [CrossRef]
32. Pavone, L.M.; Rea, S.; Trapani, F.; De Pasquale, V.; Tafuri, S.; Papparella, S.; Paciello, O. Role of serotonergic system in the pathogenesis of fibrosis in canine idiopathic inflammatory myopathies. *Neuromuscul. Disord.* **2012**, *22*, 549–557. [CrossRef] [PubMed]
33. Spina, A.; Rea, S.; De Pasquale, V.; Mastellone, V.; Avallone, L.; Pavone, L.M. Fate map of serotonin transporter-expressing cells in developing mouse thyroid. *Anat. Rec. (Hoboken)* **2011**, *294*, 384–390. [CrossRef] [PubMed]
34. Cerulo, G.; Tafuri, S.; De Pasquale, V.; Rea, S.; Romano, S.; Costagliola, A.; Della Morte, R.; Avallone, L.; Pavone, L.M. Serotonin activates cell survival and apoptotic death responses in cultured epithelial thyroid cells. *Biochimie* **2014**, *105*, 211–215. [CrossRef] [PubMed]
35. Colavita, I.; Esposito, N.; Martinelli, R.; Catanzano, F.; Melo, J.V.; Pane, F.; Ruoppolo, M.; Salvatore, F. Gaining insights into the Bcr-Abl activity-independent mechanisms of resistance to imatinib mesylate in KCL22 cells: A comparative proteomic approach. *Biochim. Biophys. Acta* **2010**, *1804*, 1974–1987. [CrossRef]
36. Caterino, M.; Chandler, R.J.; Sloan, J.L.; Dorko, K.; Cusmano-Ozog, K.; Ingenito, L.; Strom, S.C.; Imperlini, E.; Scolamiero, E.; Venditti, C.P.; et al. The proteome of methylmalonic acidemia (MMA): The elucidation of altered pathways in patient livers. *Mol. Biosyst.* **2016**, *12*, 566–574. [CrossRef]
37. Caterino, M.; Pastore, A.; Strozziero, M.G.; Di Giovamberardino, G.; Imperlini, E.; Scolamiero, E.; Ingenito, L.; Boenzi, S.; Ceravolo, F.; Martinelli, D.; et al. The proteome of cblC defect: In vivo elucidation of altered cellular pathways in humans. *J. Inherit. Metab. Dis.* **2015**, *38*, 969–979. [CrossRef]
38. Caterino, M.; Zacchia, M.; Costanzo, M.; Bruno, G.; Arcaniolo, D.; Trepiccione, F.; Siciliano, R.A.; Mazzeo, M.F.; Ruoppolo, M.; Capasso, G. Urine proteomics revealed a significant correlation between urine-fibronectin abundance and estimated-GFR decline in patients with Bardet-Biedl Syndrome. *Kidney Blood Press. Res.* **2018**, *43*, 389–405. [CrossRef]
39. Alberio, T.; Pieroni, L.; Ronci, M.; Banfi, C.; Bongarzone, I.; Bottoni, P.; Brioschi, M.; Caterino, M.; Chinello, C.; Cormio, A.; et al. Toward the Standardization of Mitochondrial Proteomics: The Italian Mitochondrial Human Proteome Project Initiative. *J. Proteome Res.* **2017**, *16*, 4319–4329. [CrossRef]
40. Caterino, M.; Aspesi, A.; Pavesi, E.; Imperlini, E.; Pagnozzi, D.; Ingenito, L.; Santoro, C.; Dianzani, I.; Ruoppolo, M. Analysis of the interactome of ribosomal protein S19 mutants. *Proteomics* **2014**, *14*, 2286–2296. [CrossRef]
41. Capobianco, V.; Caterino, M.; Iaffaldano, L.; Nardelli, C.; Sirico, A.; Del Vecchio, L.; Martinelli, P.; Pastore, L.; Pucci, P.; Sacchetti, L. Proteome analysis of human amniotic mesenchymal stem cells (hA-MSCs) reveals impaired antioxidant ability, cytoskeleton and metabolic functionality in maternal obesity. *Sci. Rep.* **2016**, *6*, 25270. [CrossRef]
42. Di Pasquale, P.; Caterino, M.; Di Somma, A.; Squillace, M.; Rossi, E.; Landini, P.; Iebba, V.; Schippa, S.; Papa, R.; Selan, L.; et al. Exposure of E. coli to DNA-methylating agents impairs biofilm formation and invasion of eukaryotic cells via down regulation of the N-Acetylneuraminate Lyase NanA. *Front. Microbiol.* **2016**, *7*, 147. [CrossRef] [PubMed]
43. Corbo, C.; Cevenini, A.; Salvatore, F. Biomarker discovery by proteomics-based approaches for early detection and personalized medicine in colorectal cancer. *Proteom. Clin. Appl.* **2017**, *11*, 5–6.
44. Croisé, P.; Estay-Ahumada, C.; Gasman, S.; Ory, S. Rho GTPases; phosphoinositides, and actin: A tripartite framework for efficient vesicular trafficking. *Small GTPases* **2014**, *5*, 29469. [CrossRef] [PubMed]
45. Vemu, A.; Atherton, J.; Spector, J.O.; Moores, C.A.; Roll-Mecak, A. Tubulin isoform composition tunes microtubule dynamics. *Mol. Biol. Cell* **2017**, *28*, 3564–3572. [CrossRef] [PubMed]
46. Tischfield, M.A.; Engle, E.C. Distinct alpha- and beta-tubulin isotypes are required for the positioning, differentiation and survival of neurons: New support for the 'multi-tubulin' hypothesis. *Biosci. Rep.* **2010**, *30*, 319–330. [CrossRef] [PubMed]
47. Engle, E.C. Human genetic disorders of axon guidance. *Cold Spring Harb. Perspect. Biol.* **2010**, *2*, a001784. [CrossRef]
48. Romaniello, R.; Arrigoni, F.; Fry, A.E.; Bassi, M.T.; Rees, M.I.; Borgatti, R.; Pilz, D.T.; Cushion, T.D. Tubulin genes and malformations of cortical development. *Eur. J. Med. Genet.* **2018**, *61*, 744–754. [CrossRef] [PubMed]

49. Ou, L.; Przybilla, M.J.; Whitley, C.B. Proteomic analysis of mucopolysaccharidosis I mouse brain with two-dimensional polyacrylamide gel electrophoresis. *Mol. Genet. Metab.* **2017**, *120*, 101–110. [CrossRef]
50. Cheon, M.S.; Fountoulakis, M.; Cairns, N.J.; Dierssen, M.; Herkner, K.; Lubec, G. Decreased protein levels of stathmin in adult brains with Down syndrome and Alzheimer's disease. *J. Neural Transm. Suppl.* **2001**, *61*, 281–288.
51. Howell, B.; Larsson, N.; Gullberg, M.; Cassimeris, L. Dissociation of the tubulin-sequestering and microtubule catastrophe-promoting activities of oncoprotein 18/stathmin. *Mol. Biol. Cell* **1999**, *10*, 105–118. [CrossRef]
52. Ohkawa, N.; Fujitani, K.; Tokunaga, E.; Furuya, S.; Inokuchi, K. The microtubule destabilizer stathmin mediates the development of dendritic arbors in neuronal cells. *J. Cell Sci.* **2007**, *120*, 1447–1456. [CrossRef] [PubMed]
53. Tortosa, E.; Adolfs, Y.; Fukata, M.; Pasterkamp, R.J.; Kapitein, L.C.; Hoogenraad, C.C. Dynamic Palmitoylation Targets MAP6 to the Axon to Promote Microtubule Stabilization during Neuronal Polarization. *Neuron* **2017**, *17*, 809–825. [CrossRef]
54. Schwenk, B.M.; Lang, C.M.; Hogl, S.; Tahirovic, S.; Orozco, D.; Rentzsch, K.; Lichtenthaler, S.F.; Hoogenraad, C.C.; Capell, A.; Haass, C.; et al. The FTLD risk factor TMEM106B and MAP6 control dendritic trafficking of lysosomes. *EMBO J.* **2014**, *33*, 450–467. [CrossRef]
55. Pu, J.; Guardia, C.M.; Keren-Kaplan, T.; Bonifacino, J.S. Mechanisms and functions of lysosome positioning. *J. Cell Sci.* **2016**, *129*, 4329–4339. [CrossRef]
56. Overly, C.C.; Hollenbeck, P.J. Dynamic organization of endocytic pathways in axons of cultured sympathetic neurons. *J. Neurosci.* **1996**, *16*, 6056–6064. [CrossRef] [PubMed]
57. McKenney, R.J.; Huynh, W.; Tanenbaum, M.E.; Bhabha, G.; Vale, R.D. Activation of cytoplasmic dynein motility by dynactin-cargo adapter complexes. *Science* **2014**, *354*, 337–341. [CrossRef]
58. Lie, P.P.Y.; Nixon, R.A. Lysosome trafficking and signaling in health and neurodegenerative diseases. *Neurobiol. Dis.* **2019**, *122*, 94–105. [CrossRef] [PubMed]
59. Wiche, G. Role of plectin in cytoskeleton organization and dynamics. *J. Cell Sci.* **1998**, *111*, 2477–2486. [PubMed]
60. Leung, C.L.; Green, K.J.; Liem, R.K. Plakins: A family of versatile cytolinker proteins. *Trends Cell Biol.* **2002**, *12*, 37–45. [CrossRef]
61. Redmann, M.; Benavides, G.A.; Berryhill, T.F.; Wani, W.Y.; Ouyang, X.; Johnson, M.S.; Ravi, S.; Barnes, S.; Darley-Usmar, V.M.; Zhang, J. Inhibition of autophagy with bafilomycin and chloroquine decreases mitochondrial quality and bioenergetic function in primary neurons. *Redox Biol.* **2017**, *11*, 73–81. [CrossRef]
62. Ryazantsev, S.; Yu, W.H.; Zhao, H.Z.; Neufeld, E.F.; Ohmi, K. Lysosomal accumulation of SCMAS (subunit c of mitochondrial ATP synthase) in neurons of the mouse model of mucopolysaccharidosis III B. *Mol. Genet. Metab.* **2007**, *90*, 393–401. [CrossRef] [PubMed]
63. Knecht, E.; Martinez-Ramón, A.; Grisolia, S. Autophagy of mitochondria in rat liver assessed by immunogold procedures. *J. Histoch. Cytochem.* **1988**, *36*, 1433–1440. [CrossRef] [PubMed]
64. Komatsu, M.; Waguri, S.; Chiba, T.; Murata, S.; Iwata, J.; Tanida, I.; Ueno, T.; Koike, M.; Uchiyama, Y.; Kominami, E.; et al. Loss of autophagy in the central nervous system causes neurodegeneration in mice. *Nature* **2006**, *441*, 880–884. [CrossRef] [PubMed]
65. Hara, T.; Nakamura, K.; Matsui, M.; Yamamoto, A.; Nakahara, Y.; Suzuki-Migishima, R.; Yokoyama, M.; Mishima, K.; Saito, I.; Okano, H.; et al. Suppression of basal autophagy in neural cells causes neurodegenerative disease in mice. *Nature* **2006**, *441*, 885–889. [CrossRef]
66. Di Malta, C.; Fryer, J.D.; Settembre, C.; Ballabio, A. Autophagy in astrocytes: A novel culprit in lysosomal storage disorders. *Autophagy* **2012**, *8*, 1871–1872. [CrossRef]
67. Fraldi, A.; Klein, A.D.; Medina, D.L.; Settembre, C. Brain disorders due to lysosomal dysfunction. *Ann. Rev. Neurosci.* **2016**, *39*, 277–295. [CrossRef]
68. Kim, S.G.; Hoffman, G.R.; Poulogiannis, G.; Buel, G.R.; Jang, Y.J.; Lee, K.W.; Kim, B.Y.; Erikson, R.L.; Cantley, L.C.; Choo, A.Y.; et al. Metabolic stress controls mTORC1 lysosomal localization and dimerization by regulating the TTT-RUVBL1/2 complex. *Mol. Cell* **2013**, *49*, 172–185. [CrossRef]
69. Napolitano, G.; Ballabio, A. TFEB at a glance. *J. Cell Sci.* **2016**, *129*, 2475–2481. [CrossRef]
70. Camandola, S.; Mattson, M.P. Brain metabolism in health, aging, and neurodegeneration. *EMBO J.* **2017**, *36*, 1474–1492. [CrossRef]

71. García-Cazorla, À.; Saudubray, J.M. Cellular neurometabolism: A tentative to connect cell biology and metabolism in neurology. *J. Inherit. Metab. Dis.* **2018**, *41*, 1043–1054. [CrossRef]
72. Oyarzabal, A.; Marin-Valencia, I. Synaptic energy metabolism and neuronal excitability, in sickness and health. *J. Inherit. Metab. Dis.* **2019**, *42*, 220–236. [CrossRef] [PubMed]
73. Rizo, J. Mechanism of neurotransmitter release coming into focus. *Protein Sci.* **2018**, *27*, 1364–1391. [CrossRef] [PubMed]
74. Guiberson, N.G.L.; Pineda, A.; Abramov, D.; Kharel, P.; Carnazza, K.E.; Wragg, R.T.; Dittman, J.S.; Burré, J. Mechanism-based rescue of Munc18-1 dysfunction in varied encephalopathies by chemical chaperones. *Nat. Commun.* **2018**, *9*, 3986. [CrossRef] [PubMed]
75. Hilfiker, S.; Pieribone, V.A.; Czernik, A.J.; Kao, H.T.; Augustine, G.J.; Greengard, P. Synapsins as regulators of neurotransmitter release. *Philos. Trans. R. Soc. Lond. B Biol. Sci.* **1999**, *354*, 269–279. [CrossRef]
76. Hosaka, M.; Hammer, R.E.; Südhof, T.C. A phospho-switch controls the dynamic association of synapsins with synaptic vesicles. *Neuron* **1999**, *24*, 377–387. [CrossRef]
77. Shin, O.H. Exocytosis and synaptic vesicle function. *Compr. Physiol.* **2014**, *4*, 149–175. [CrossRef]
78. Mirza, F.J.; Zahid, S. The Role of Synapsins in Neurological Disorders. *Neurosci. Bull.* **2018**, *34*, 349–358. [CrossRef]
79. Zahid, S.; Oellerich, M.; Asif, A.R.; Ahmed, N. Differential expression of proteins in brain regions of Alzheimer's disease patients. *Neurochem. Res.* **2014**, *39*, 208–215. [CrossRef]
80. Orlando, M.; Lignani, G.; Maragliano, L.; Fassio, A.; Onofri, F.; Baldelli, P.; Giovedí, S.; Benfenati, F. Functional role of ATP binding to synapsin I in synaptic vesicle trafficking and release dynamics. *J. Neurosci.* **2014**, *34*, 14752–14768. [CrossRef]
81. Vieira, O.V. Rab3a and Rab10 are regulators of lysosome exocytosis and plasma membrane repair. *Small GTPases* **2018**, *9*, 349–351. [CrossRef]
82. Zhen, Y.; Stenmark, H. Cellular functions of Rab GTPases at a glance. *J. Cell Sci.* **2015**, *128*, 3171–3176. [CrossRef] [PubMed]
83. Encarnacao, M.; Espada, L.; Escrevente, C.; Mateus, D.; Ramalho, J.; Michelet, X.; Santarino, I.; Hsu, V.W.; Brenner, M.B.; Barral, D. A Rab3a-dependent complex essential for lysosome positioning and plasma membrane repair. *J. Cell Biol.* **2016**, *213*, 631–640. [CrossRef] [PubMed]
84. Ginns, E.I.; Mak, S.K.; Ko, N.; Karlgren, J.; Akbarian, S.; Chou, V.P.; Guo, Y.; Lim, A.; Samuelsson, S.; LaMarca, M.L.; et al. Neuroinflammation and α-synuclein accumulation in response to glucocerebrosidase deficiency are accompanied by synaptic dysfunction. *Mol. Genet. Metab.* **2014**, *111*, 152–162. [CrossRef] [PubMed]
85. Tomic, S. Dopamine transport system imaging is pathologic in Niemann-Pick type C-case report. *Neurol. Sci.* **2018**, *39*, 1139–1140. [CrossRef]
86. Terbeek, J.; Latour, P.; Van Laere, K.; Vandenberghe, W. Abnormal dopamine transporter imaging in adult-onset Niemann-Pick disease type C. *Park. Relat. Disord.* **2017**, *36*, 107–108. [CrossRef]
87. Xu, S.; Sleat, D.E.; Jadot, M.; Lobel, P. Glial fibrillary acidic protein is elevated in the lysosomal storage disease classical late-infantile neuronal ceroid lipofuscinosis, but is not a component of the storage material. *Biochem. J.* **2010**, *428*, 355–362. [CrossRef]
88. Baldo, G.; Mayer, F.Q.; Martinelli, B.; Dilda, A.; Meyer, F.; Ponder, K.P.; Giugliani, R.; Matte, U. Evidence of a progressive motor dysfunction in Mucopolysaccharidosis type I mice. *Behav. Brain Res.* **2012**, *233*, 169–175. [CrossRef]
89. Pressey, S.N.; Smith, D.A.; Wong, A.M.; Platt, F.M.; Cooper, J.D. Early glial activation, synaptic changes and axonal pathology in the thalamocortical system of Niemann-Pick type C1 mice. *Neurobiol. Dis.* **2012**, *45*, 1086–1100. [CrossRef]
90. Wilkinson, F.L.; Holley, R.J.; Langford-Smith, K.J.; Badrinath, S.; Liao, A.; Langford-Smith, A.; Cooper, J.D.; Jones, S.A.; Wraith, J.E.; Wynn, R.F.; et al. Neuropathology in mouse models of mucopolysaccharidosis type I, IIIA and IIIB. *PLoS ONE* **2012**, *7*, e35787. [CrossRef]
91. Vitner, E.B.; Futerman, A.H. Neuronal forms of Gaucher disease. *Handb. Exp. Pharmacol.* **2013**, *216*, 405–419. [CrossRef]
92. Tsuji, D. Molecular pathogenesis and therapeutic approach of GM2 gangliosidosis. *Yakugaku Zasshi* **2013**, *133*, 269–274. [CrossRef] [PubMed]

93. Hordeaux, J.; Dubreil, L.; Robveille, C.; Deniaud, J.; Pascal, Q.; Dequéant, B.; Pailloux, J.; Lagalice, L.; Ledevin, M.; Babarit, C.; et al. Long-term neurologic and cardiac correction by intrathecal gene therapy in Pompe disease. *Acta Neuropathol. Commun.* **2017**, *5*, 1–66. [CrossRef] [PubMed]
94. Lotfi, P.; Tse, D.Y.; Di Ronza, A.; Seymour, M.L.; Martano, G.; Cooper, J.D.; Pereira, F.A.; Passafaro, M.; Wu, S.M.; Sardiello, M. Trehalose reduces retinal degeneration, neuroinflammation and storage burden caused by a lysosomal hydrolase deficiency. *Autophagy* **2018**, *14*, 1419–1434. [CrossRef] [PubMed]
95. Parker, H.; Bigger, B.W. The role of innate immunity in mucopolysaccharide diseases. *J. Neurochem.* **2019**, *148*, 639–651. [CrossRef]
96. Arfi, A.; Richard, M.; Gandolphe, C.; Bonnefont-Rousselot, D.; Therond, P.; Scherman, D. Neuroinflammatory and oxidative stress phenomena in MPS IIIA mouse model: The positive effect of long-term aspirin treatment. *Mol. Genet. Metab.* **2011**, *103*, 18–25. [CrossRef]
97. Martins, C.; Hůlková, H.; Dridi, L.; Dormoy-Raclet, V.; Grigoryeva, L.; Choi, Y.; Langford-Smith, A.; Wilkinson, F.L.; Ohmi, K.; DiCristo, G.; et al. Neuroinflammation, mitochondrial defects and neurodegeneration in mucopolysaccharidosis III type C mouse model. *Brain* **2015**, *138*, 336–355. [CrossRef]
98. Vitner, E.B.; Farfel-Becker, T.; Ferreira, N.S.; Leshkowitz, D.; Sharma, P.; Lang, K.S.; Futerman, A.H. Induction of the type I interferon response in neurological forms of Gaucher disease. *J. Neuroinflamm.* **2016**, *13*, 104. [CrossRef]
99. Guo, H.; Callaway, J.B.; Ting, J.P. Inflammasomes: Mechanism of action, role in disease, and therapeutics. *Nat. Med.* **2015**, *21*, 677–687. [CrossRef]
100. Holley, R.J.; Ellison, S.M.; Fil, D.; O'Leary, C.; McDermott, J.; Senthivel, N.; Langford-Smith, A.W.W.; Wilkinson, F.L.; D'Souza, Z.; Parker, H.; et al. Macrophage enzyme and reduced inflammation drive brain correction of mucopolysaccharidosis IIIB by stem cell gene therapy. *Brain* **2018**, *141*, 99–116. [CrossRef]
101. Trudel, S.; Trecherel, E.; Gomila, C.; Peltier, M.; Aubignat, M.; Gubler, B.; Morliere, P.; Heard, J.M.; Ausseil, J. Oxidative stress is independent of inflammation in the neurodegenerative Sanfilippo syndrome type B. *J. Neurosci. Res.* **2015**, *93*, 424–432. [CrossRef]
102. Simonaro, C.M.; Ge, Y.; Eliyahu, E.; He, X.; Jepsen, K.J.; Schuchman, E.H. Involvement of the Toll-like receptor 4 pathway and use of TNF-alpha antagonists for treatment of the mucopolysaccharidoses. *Proc. Natl. Acad. Sci. USA* **2010**, *107*, 222–227. [CrossRef] [PubMed]
103. Simonaro, C.M.; D'Angelo, M.; He, X.; Eliyahu, E.; Shtraizent, N.; Haskins, M.E.; Schuchman, E.H. Mechanism of glycosaminoglycan-mediated bone and joint disease: Implications for the mucopolysaccharidoses and other connective tissue diseases. *Am. J. Pathol.* **2008**, *172*, 112–122. [CrossRef] [PubMed]
104. Simonaro, C.M.; Haskins, M.E.; Schuchman, E.H. Articular chondrocytes from animals with a dermatan sulfate storage disease undergo a high rate of apoptosis and release nitric oxide and inflammatory cytokines: A possible mechanism underlying degenerative joint disease in the mucopolysaccharidoses. *Lab. Investig.* **2001**, *81*, 1319–1328. [CrossRef]

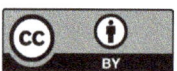

© 2020 by the authors. Licensee MDPI, Basel, Switzerland. This article is an open access article distributed under the terms and conditions of the Creative Commons Attribution (CC BY) license (http://creativecommons.org/licenses/by/4.0/).

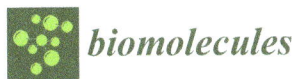

Article

Upregulation of Sortilin, a Lysosomal Sorting Receptor, Corresponds with Reduced Bioavailability of Latent TGFβ in Mucolipidosis II Cells

Jarrod W. Barnes [1], Megan Aarnio-Peterson [2,†], Joy Norris [2], Mark Haskins [3], Heather Flanagan-Steet [2] and Richard Steet [2,*]

1. Division of Pulmonary, Allergy and Critical Care Medicine, University of Alabama at Birmingham, Birmingham, AL 35294, USA; barnesj5@uab.edu
2. Greenwood Genetic Center, Greenwood, SC 29646, USA; mcaarnio@gmail.com (M.A.-P.); jwnorris@ggc.org (J.N.); heatherfs@ggc.org (H.F.-S.)
3. Emeritus Professor, Pathology and Medical Genetics, School of Veterinary Medicine, University of Pennsylvania, Philadelphia, PA 19104-6051, USA; mhaskins@vet.upenn.edu
* Correspondence: rsteet@ggc.org; Fax: +(864)-388-1707
† Current address: Sangamo Therapeutics, Brisbane, CA 94005, USA.

Received: 17 February 2020; Accepted: 20 April 2020; Published: 26 April 2020

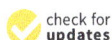

Abstract: Mucolipidosis II (ML-II) is a lysosomal disease caused by defects in the carbohydrate-dependent sorting of soluble hydrolases to lysosomes. Altered growth factor signaling has been identified as a contributor to the phenotypes associated with ML-II and other lysosomal disorders but an understanding of how these signaling pathways are affected is still emerging. Here, we investigated transforming growth factor beta 1 (TGFβ1) signaling in the context of ML-II patient fibroblasts, observing decreased TGFβ1 signaling that was accompanied by impaired TGFβ1-dependent wound closure. We found increased intracellular latent TGFβ1 complexes, caused by reduced secretion and stable localization in detergent-resistant lysosomes. Sortilin, a sorting receptor for hydrolases and TGFβ-related cytokines, was upregulated in ML-II fibroblasts as well as *GNPTAB*-null HeLa cells, suggesting a mechanism for inappropriate lysosomal targeting of TGFβ. Co-expression of sortilin and TGFβ in HeLa cells resulted in reduced TGFβ1 secretion. Elevated sortilin levels correlated with normal levels of cathepsin D in ML-II cells, consistent with a compensatory role for this receptor in lysosomal hydrolase targeting. Collectively, these data support a model whereby sortilin upregulation in cells with lysosomal storage maintains hydrolase sorting but suppresses TGFβ1 secretion through increased lysosomal delivery. These findings highlight an unexpected link between impaired lysosomal sorting and altered growth factor bioavailability.

Keywords: mucolipidosis II; sortilin; TGF-beta; lysosomes; cathepsin D

1. Introduction

The lysosomal disease mucolipidosis type II (ML-II) is caused by a defect in the biosynthesis of mannose 6-phosphate (Man-6-P) residues, the carbohydrate-based tag responsible for lysosomal targeting of acid hydrolases [1,2]. Loss of this residue results in hypersecretion of several enzymes into the extracellular space and hydrolase-deficient lysosomes. Mutations in the *GNPTAB* gene, which encodes two of the three subunits of the GlcNAc-1-phosphotransferase enzyme, lead to ML-II. The severe, multisystem manifestations of this disorder include pronounced cartilage and bone defects, many of which are noted at birth [3–5]. Patients with ML-II exhibit short stature, craniofacial defects and osteoporosis, which have been attributed to impaired development and function of mesenchymal cell types. An attenuated form of ML-II, referred to as ML-IIIα/β, is characterized by partial loss of mannose phosphorylation, later onset of disease symptoms and clinically distinct skeletal phenotypes [4,6,7]. The bone and cartilage findings in ML-II and ML-IIIα/β human patients are mirrored, albeit with notable differences in severity, within animal models of the disease. Phenotypic analysis of both feline and murine ML-II models has revealed changes in the cellular organization of growth plates, abnormal chondrocyte morphology and reduced endochondral ossification [8–13]. Moreover, defective chondrocyte development and excessive deposition of type II collagen were observed in a zebrafish model for ML-II [14]. These phenotypes were subsequently linked to an imbalance in TGFβ/BMP signaling caused by the inappropriate activity of the cysteine protease cathepsin K [15–17]. Notably, these phenotypes occur in the absence of any detectable lysosomal storage in the developing embryos [14].

Collectively, the complex nature of ML-II patient phenotypes suggests that the alterations in cell behavior and development of different tissues likely involve the dysregulation of multiple growth factor signaling pathways. Indeed, the clinical manifestations of ML-II resemble many conditions with documented growth factor dysregulation, including arthritis, osteoporosis and the congenital skeletal disorders such as Camurati-Engelmann, Marfan's disease and geleophysic dysplasia [18–24]. The relevance of storage-independent alterations in growth factor signaling during early development in the context of MPSII has been documented by recent studies [25–27]. Despite these advances, the mechanisms whereby lysosomal dysfunction impacts the key growth factor signaling pathways implicated in aberrant bone and cartilage development and homeostasis remain largely unknown.

Transforming growth factor beta 1 (TGFβ1) mediates a broad spectrum of biological processes including wound repair, angiogenesis and immunity and plays specific roles in the development of cartilage, connective tissue and bone [28–35]. TGFβ1 and its related isoforms are initially synthesized as pre-proproteins consisting of a signal peptide, the latency-associated peptide (LAP) and the mature TGFβ1 ligand [36,37]. Prior to secretion, the TGFβ1 precursor undergoes proteolytic and post-translational modification. During this processing, the LAP portion is cleaved from the TGFβ1 ligand and non-covalently re-associates with it to form the small latent complex (SLC) [38]. In some cases, the SLC also covalently attaches to one of four latent TGFβ1 binding proteins (LTBPs), generating the large latent complex (LLC) [39]. Association with LTBPs has been shown to both facilitate rapid secretion of latent TGFβ1 and target it for storage within the extracellular matrix (ECM) [40,41]. Direct interaction between the LLC and several matrix components, such as fibrillins, fibronectin and heparan sulfate mediate growth factor latency [42–46]. In vivo activation of ECM-stored latent TGFβ1 can occur by various mechanisms, including those governed by integrins and thrombospondin-1 [47–49]. Mannose phosphorylation of latent TGFβ1 has been proposed to mediate its proteolytic activation at the cell surface [50,51]. Thus, loss of this modification could directly inhibit activation. This idea has, however, been challenged by the demonstration that latent TGFβ1 is very poorly modified with Man-6-P under physiological conditions [52].

In this study, to further address the involvement of TGFβ1 signaling in ML-II pathogenesis, the biosynthesis and regulation of this growth factor was analyzed in cultured dermal fibroblasts. One of the few available human cell culture systems for this disease, these cells exhibit the classic biochemical hallmarks of ML-II (hypersecretion of hydrolases and lysosomal storage) and are able to synthesize, secrete and respond to TGFβ1. ML-II-specific decreases in TGFβ1 signaling were noted and found to be associated with impaired wound closure and accumulation of latent complexes within the lysosomal compartment. Sortilin-1, a multifunctional lysosomal sorting receptor that has been shown to mediate lysosomal delivery of TGFβ-related cytokines, was shown to be upregulated in multiple ML-II cell models. The results of this study support two distinct molecular outcomes governed by sortilin upregulation in ML-II: (i) compensatory, carbohydrate-independent lysosomal sorting of the protease cathepsin D and (ii) impaired secretion and bioavailability of latent TGFβ1 complexes due to inappropriate delivery to this same compartment. To our knowledge, this discovery represents the first example of increased sortilin expression in the context of an inherited lysosomal storage disorder.

Implications for the impaired bioavailability of latent TGFβ1 and other sortilin ligands towards ML-II pathogenesis are discussed.

2. Materials and Methods

Cell lines and reagents—Human control fibroblasts (CRL-1509), ML-III (GM-03391) and ML-II (GM-01586) skin fibroblasts were obtained from Coriell (Camden, NJ) and cultured in Dulbecco's modified Eagle's medium (DMEM) containing 18% fetal bovine serum (FBS) supplemented with 100 μg/mL penicillin in addition to streptomycin and maintained in a humidified 5% CO2 atmosphere. GM-01586 is homozygous for a 2-bp deletion in exon 19 of the GNPTAB gene [3665_3666delTC] resulting in a frameshift and truncation of the protein in the beta subunit [L1168fsX1172]. This cell line has been shown to have < 0.1% residual GlcNAc-1-phosphotransferase activity. GM-03391 is homozygous for a 1-bp deletion at nucleotide 445 of the GNPTG gene [445delG]. Synovial membranes were taken from unaffected and ML-II feline littermates raised at the School of Veterinary Medicine at the University of Pennsylvania, under NIH and USDA guidelines for the care and use of animals in research. Fibroblast-like synoviocytes were isolated from the membranes using collagenase 1A (Sigma St. Louis, MO, USA) digestion. All primary cell lines were grown in RPMI media supplemented with 10% FBS with the addition of 100 μg/mL streptomycin and penicillin and maintained in humidified 5% CO_2 atmosphere. HeLa cells were maintained in DMEM containing 10% FBS supplemented with penicillin and streptomycin and maintained as described above. Goat antisera against human LAP and monoclonal antibody against human LTBP was purchased from R & D systems (USA), while the monoclonal antibody γ-tubulin was obtained from Sigma. The anti-human LT-1 (LAP) rabbit polyclonal antibody was a generous gift from Dr. Kohei Miyazono (University of Tokyo, Tokyo, Japan). Rabbit antisera against human phospho-Smad 2 and monoclonal anti-human Smad 2/3 were purchased from Millipore (Billirica, MA, USA), whereas mouse anti-human sortilin-1 and GS28 were obtained from BD Transduction Labs (San Jose, CA, USA). Rabbit anti-human ERp29 and the protease inhibitor cocktail were obtained from Thermo Scientific (Rockford, IL) and Sigma (St. Louis, MO), respectively. The LAMP-2 mouse monoclonal antibody was obtained from the Developmental Studies Hybridoma Bank (Iowa City, IA). Rabbit anti-human cathepsin D antibody was a kind gift from Dr. Stuart Kornfeld (Washington University in Saint Louis). Recombinant TGFβ1 ligand was purchased from PeproTech Inc (Rocky Hill, NJ). TGFβ1 mink lung epithelial cells (T-MLECs) stably transfected with a luciferase gene driven by a TGFβ-responsive plasminogen activator inhibitor-1 promoter sequence was a kind gift from D. Rifkin (New York University Langone Medical Center, New York, NY).

Plasmids and constructs—Human latent TGFβ1 was synthesized from GeneArt (Invitrogen, Carlsbad, CA, USA). The cysteine at position 33 within the TGFβ1 sequence was mutated to a serine to prevent to formation of the LLC in transfected HeLa cells to ensure the sortilin-1 was interacting with the SLC [53]. Human sortilin-1 I.M.A.G.E. clone (clone I.D. 4123836) was obtained from Open Biosystems (Thermo Scientific, Waltham, MA) and was subcloned with the addition of flanking restriction digest sites (5'- Xho1 and 3'- Xba1) and ligated into pcDNA 3.1 expression vector as previously described. The glycopepsinogen in pcDNA 3.1 was kindly provided by Dr. Stuart Kornfeld (Washington University in St. Louis).

RT-PCR analysis of transcript abundance—RNA was extracted from pellets of ~10^6 trypsinized control and ML-II cells using Trizol reagent (Life Technologies, Grand Island, NY). RNA (500 ng) was reverse transcribed using the iScript cDNA synthesis kit (BioRad, Hercules, CA). Primers used for PCR amplification (35 cycles; melting temperature: 98 °C, annealing temperature: 59 °C, extension temperature: 72 °C) were as follows—human sortilin-1 5' TGGGTTTGGCACAATCTTTACC 3'; 5'CCACAATGATGCCTCCAGAATC 3' and RPL4 5' CAGAGCTGTGGCTCGAATTCC 3'; 5' AGTTACTCTTGAGGGAAGCGGC 3'. To ensure resulting PCR products represented RNA and were not due to genomic DNA contamination, all primers were designed to exon sequences flanking an intron. RPL4 was used as a normalizing control.

Preparation of SDS whole cell lysates, DOC (deoxycholate)-soluble, DOC-insoluble fractions and media collection—In preparation for western blot analysis, human and feline fibroblasts were plated at equal density (2.5×10^5 cells/mL), cultured for times indicated and collected by scraping with rubber policeman. For SDS whole cell lysate preparations, cell pellets were treated with 1% SDS in PBS 7.4, plus protease inhibitors followed by brief sonication and centrifugation. These cell preparations result in full solubility of cellular components. DOC-soluble and insoluble fractions were prepared as described [40]. The insoluble fraction was solubilized in SDS containing buffer (3 % SDS, 15% glycerol and 75 mM Tris pH 6.5). Both SDS whole cell and DOC preparations were normalized to total protein using micro BCA protein assay (Pierce/Thermo Scientific, Rockford, IL) and prepared for SDS-PAGE and Western blot analysis as described [54]. As a loading control for SDS whole cell preps, nitrocellulose membranes were lightly stripped and re-probed for γ-tubulin. For the additional collection of conditioned media, cells were washed twice with PBS and incubated in 1 mL of serum free DMEM overnight, 24 h before collection. Media was then concentrated from 1 mL to 100 µL, in the presence of protease inhibitors, using Centricon 10 tubes (Milllipore, Billirica, MA) and was assayed for equivalent loading concentration using microBCA protein assay kit (Pierce, Rockford, IL).

Wound healing assays—Control and ML-II cells were plated and grown to confluency followed by washing with PBS and culturing cells overnight in 0.1% FBS supplement DMEM. After serum starvation, cells were scratched with a pipette tip and washed extensively to remove cell debris. Fresh culture media containing 2% FBS was added to cultures and incubated for 24 h in the presence or absence of TGFβ1 ligand (10 ng/mL). Images were prepared at 0 and 24 h post scarring using a 10x Plan C objective attached to an Olympus CX41 compound light microscope and pictures of wound closure fields were taken with a Retiga 2000R Fast 1394 camera equipped with Qcapture software v2.8.1. Measurement of wound closure was determined within several fields by defining an initial wound boundary and counting cells that migrated into the wound at the times indicated.

Metabolic ^{35}S labeling—Pulse-chase analysis of latent TGFβ1 was performed as described [54] with modifications. Fibroblast cultures were metabolically labeled with TRAN^{35}S-label (MP Biomedicals, Solon, OH) in methionine- and cysteine-free DMEM (Invitrogen, USA). The media was removed and the cells were methionine deprived for 30 minutes in met/cys free media and subsequently labeled with ^{35}S methionine (0.75 mCi/mL) in met/cys free media with 10% dialyzed FBS for 1 hr. Media was change to DMEM supplemented with 20% FBS to initiate the chase for times indicated in each experiment. Samples were Immunoprecipitated overnight with anti-LAP antibody, incubated with protein A sepharose beads at 4 °C for 1h, washed extensively and prepared for SDS-PAGE and autoradiography detection.

TGFβ1 mink lung luciferase activity assay—WT and ML-II human skin fibroblasts were cultured for 3-4 days in a 60 mm dish and scraped with a rubber policeman in PBS. Cells were then pelleted by centrifugation and subsequently lysed with 1% DOC and prepared as described above. For the TGFβ1 reporter experiments, DOC-insoluble pellets were washed and broken apart using a pipette in 200 µL of DMEM (serum free). Homogenized samples were split into two 100 µL aliquots. One set was subjected to 80 °C heat activation for 10 minutes, while to other sample was not heated. After a final spin to pellet the insoluble material, media from both samples was added directly to previously plated mink lung reporter cells (1.6×10^5 cells/mL) and incubated for 16 h at 37 °C. Media was then removed and cells were lysed and assayed for luciferase activity using a Luciferase Assay Kit (Promega, Madison, WI).

Percoll gradient fractionation—Percoll gradient fractionation was performed as previously described with minor modifications [55]. After gradient formation, nine 1 mL fractions were collected from the bottom of the centrifuge tube and assayed for β-hexosaminidase activity to determine the distribution of the dense lysosomes within the collected fractions. Fractions were combined as follows—fractions 1–3 (pool I; Dense Lysosomes), fractions 4–6 (pool II; intermediate density organelles) and fractions 7–9 (pool III; Golgi, ER, endosomes and plasma membrane) based on the β-Hexosaminidase activity assays and the organelle distribution within collected Percoll gradient fractions that has been previously described [56]. Pooled fractions were precipitated with cold ethanol (100%) precipitation and subjected to SDS-PAGE and Western blot analysis.

Co-immunoprecipitation experiments in ML-II fibroblasts—ML-II fibroblasts were grown in a 10cm cell culture dish to confluency. Cells were washed and collected in cold PBS followed by lysis of cells using RIPA buffer containing a protease inhibitor cocktail (Sigma, St. Louis, MO) and sonication. Cell lysates were subjected to 4 °C post-nuclear centrifugation using a tabletop centrifuge. To pre-clear cell lysates, 50 μL of unblocked protein A sepharose (Pierce, Rockford, IL) was added and rotated at 4 °C for 4 h. Protein A sepharose beads were removed from pre-cleared cell lysates and either antisera against sortilin-1 or LAP (LT-1) was used for the 4 °C overnight immunoprecipitation. Protein-antibody complexes were purified from cell lysates using blocked protein A sepharose followed by six washes using RIPA buffer and 2 washes with a final wash buffer containing 20 mM Tris-HCl pH 6.8. Purified protein complexes were eluded from the protein A beads by boiling in a 3% SDS buffer containing 75 mM Tris pH 6.8 and 15% glycerol and subjected to SDS-PAGE (under non-reducing conditions) and Western blot analysis. In all cases, 5% of the whole cell lysate was set aside as a Western blot input control.

Transient transfection and latent TGFβ1 secretion assays—HeLa cells were transfected with latent TGFβ1, glycopepsinogen, and/or sortilin-1 in Opti-MEM using Lipofectamine PLUS reagents as previously described [52]. In all co-transfection experiments, 2.5 μg of sortilin-1 and 0.3 μg of latent TGFβ1 or glycopepsinogen DNA were used. For secretion assays, transfection medium was removed after overnight incubation and cells were washed once with sterile PBS and assays were initialized by the addition of fresh Opti-MEM and incubated overnight. Media from each experiment was subjected to cold ethanol precipitation, while cells were trypsinized, collected and lysed in RIPA buffer containing a protease inhibitor cocktail followed by SDS-PAGE and Western blot analysis. To ensure equal sample loading, media aliquots were normalized total cellular protein from whole cell lysates determined by BCA protein assay (Pierce, Rockford, IL). In addition, membranes were stained with Ponceau S azo dye after protein transfer or were lightly stripped and re-probed for cellular γ-tubulin to further demonstrate equal loading of media or cell samples, respectively.

Inhibition of lysosomal function in HeLa cells with bafilomycin A1—Latent TGFβ1 was co-transfected with sortilin-1 in HeLa cells as described above. Following the removal of the transfection medium, fresh Opti-MEM was added to the transfected cells and incubated in the presence or absence of bafilomycin A1 (10 nM) for 24 h. Cells were collected and subjected to BCA protein assay, SDS-PAGE and Western blot analysis as described above.

3. Results

ML-II fibroblasts exhibit reduced TGFβ1 signaling accompanied by impaired TGFβ1-dependent wound closure—To explore whether TGFβ1 signaling is sensitive in ML-II, the level of phosphorylated Smad2 (p-Smad2), a downstream effector of TGFβ1 signaling, was investigated in control and ML-II human skin fibroblasts. The levels of p-Smad2, relative to total Smad2/3, were decreased two-fold in ML-II fibroblasts, indicating a possible reduction in canonical TGFβ1-mediated signaling (Figure 1A,B). To determine whether the decrease in phosphorylation was functionally relevant and could impact the behavior of ML-II fibroblasts, wound closure assays were performed. Wound closure following mechanical scarring is a well-established TGFβ1-dependent process, requiring the biosynthesis and remodeling of the extracellular matrix [57]. For these experiments, confluent cultures of control and ML-II fibroblasts were "wounded" and subsequently incubated in the presence or absence of TGFβ1 ligand. The extent of wound closure was assessed as the number of individual cells within the wound 24 h post-scarring (Figure 1C,D). Using this parameter, wound repair was significantly reduced in ML-II fibroblasts (63.1 ± 6.8% fewer than control fibroblasts). While addition of purified TGFβ1 did not affect this process in control cultures, it partially ameliorated the wound closure defect noted in ML-II cells. This is evidenced by an increase in the number of cells present within

TGFβ1 treated ML-II wounds compared to untreated wounds (39.3 ± 13.5% fewer than control cells). These data indicate that the delayed wound closure in ML-II is at least partially TGFβ1 dependent.

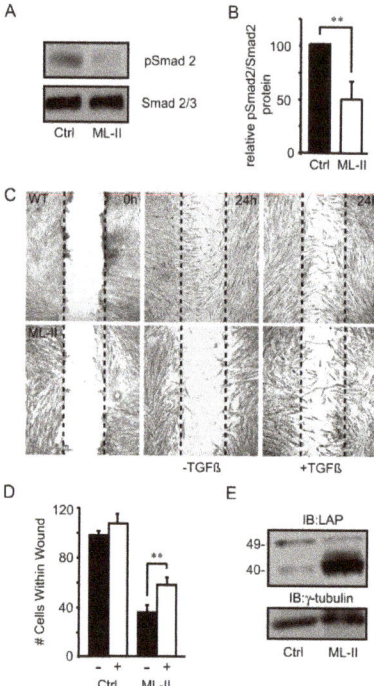

Figure 1. ML-II fibroblasts exhibit reduced transforming growth factor beta 1 (TGFβ1) signaling accompanied by impaired TGFβ1-dependent wound closure. (**A**) Western blot analysis of control and ML-II human fibroblast lysates using antibodies against human Smad 2/3 and phosphorylated Smad 2. (**B**) Quantification of the relative intensity of phosphorylated Smad 2 vs. Smad 2/3 protein in control and ML-II cells (n = 3), ** $p \leq 0.01$. (**C**) Representative images of wound healing assays using control and ML-II fibroblasts in the presence and absence of 10 ng/mL TGFβ1 ligand. (**D**) Quantification of the number of cells migrating into the wounded area after 24 h (n = 3), ** $p \leq 0.01$. (**E**) Western blot analysis of latent TGFβ1 in whole SDS lysates using an antibody against LAP. Note the pronounced increase in the level of the 40kDa LAP band in ML-II fibroblasts.

In light of the positive effect that TGFβ1 addition had on ML-II wound closure, one explanation for its decreased signaling is reduced expression of the TGFβ1 precursor. Transcript analysis did not reveal any differences in TGFβ1 expression between control and ML-II samples. In contrast, Western blot analysis revealed a robust increase in steady state levels of latent TGFβ1 protein present within ML-II fibroblasts. As shown in Figure 1E, the 40-kDa band corresponding to the LAP portion of the latent complex is dramatically increased in cellular lysates derived from trypsinized ML-II cultures. These data demonstrate that the decrease in TGFβ1 signaling noted in ML-II is associated with intracellular accumulation of latent growth factor.

The secretion of newly synthesized latent TGF-beta is decreased in ML-II fibroblasts—To ask whether the accumulation of latent TGFβ1 within ML-II cells results from its impaired secretion, the processing and trafficking of newly synthesized growth factor was monitored using metabolic labeling experiments. As shown in Figure 2, after a 1 h pulse, ^{35}S-labeled TGFβ1 precursor (49-kD) was detected within both control and ML-II fibroblasts. Analysis of media fractions (Figure 2A,B; right panel), however, revealed significant reductions in the amount of both the small latent complex (SLC) and large latent complex (LLC) secreted from ML-II cells. Increased levels of an unidentified 65-kD LAP-reactive band were also noted in the media from ML-II cultures. This 65-kDa band, along with low levels of LLC, were the only TGFβ1 related species detected within the media of ML-II cultures (Figure 2B, right panel). The identity of this band is not known but may represent a biosynthetic intermediate of latent TGFβ1. Although roughly corresponding to the molecular size expected for dimerized LAP, this protein species was completely insensitive to chemical reduction, which has been described previously [58]. Together, these data clearly show that the secretion of latent TGFβ1 is reduced in ML-II, providing a biochemical mechanism to explain the impaired signaling in these cells.

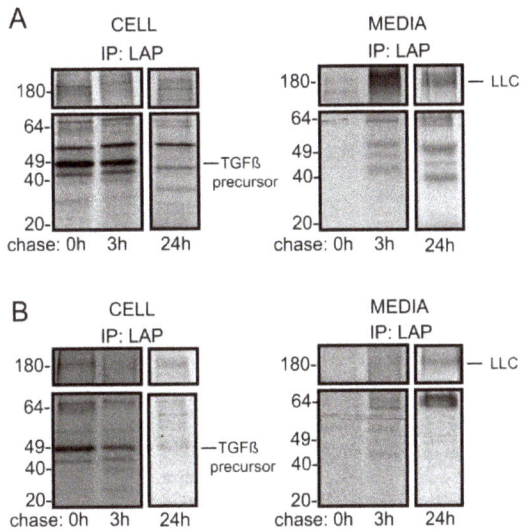

Figure 2. Accumulation of latent TGFβ1 in ML-II fibroblasts is associated with impaired secretion. Representative autoradiographs of ^{35}S-labeled latent TGFβ1 complexes Immunoprecipitated from control (**A**) and ML-II (**B**) human fibroblast lysates and media samples at times indicated and resolved by sodium dodecyl sulfate polyacrylamide gel electrophoresis (SDS-PAGE) (n = 4). The expected migration of the TGFβ1 precursor and the large latent complex (LLC) is shown.

Increased intracellular latent TGF-beta is localized within dense, detergent-insoluble fractions—To identify the intracellular location of accumulating latent TGFβ1, control and ML-II cellular homogenates were fractionated using Percoll gradients and the presence of latent TGFβ1 complexes probed by Western blot (Figure 3A). Percoll gradient fractionation separates dense lysosomes and intermediate density organelles from other cellular organelles, including the endoplasmic reticulum and Golgi, providing a means to determine where intracellular latent TGFβ1 has accumulated within the secretory pathway [55,59]. The identity of individual fractions was confirmed with organelle–specific markers, including the lysosomal membrane protein LAMP-2, the ER protein ERp29 and the Golgi-associated protein GS-28. While most of the latent TGFβ1 detected in control homogenates was found in the lighter ER- and Golgi-containing pool (III), the majority of protein in ML-II homogenates was recovered in the density pool (I), which corresponds to lysosomes. Moreover, several additional high molecular weight LAP-reactive species were detected in this pool, consistent with aggregate forms of latent TGFβ1. To address whether the appearance of these higher molecular weight forms corresponds to decreased solubility of latent TGFβ1, lysates from control and ML-II fibroblast cultures grown in serum free media were treated with sodium deoxycholate (DOC) and the soluble and insoluble fractions resolved by SDS-PAGE prior to Western blot analysis. The serum free media was also collected from these cultures and analyzed. Using antisera against LAP and LTBP, the majority of latent TGFβ1 (both LLC and SLC) isolated from control fibroblasts was detected in either the media or DOC-soluble cell-associated pools (Figure 3B). In contrast, these complexes were highly enriched within both the DOC-soluble and DOC-insoluble fractions of ML-II cells, demonstrating that the increased levels of latent TGFβ1 correlate with enhanced insolubility (Figure 3B). Further, the presence of reactive bands migrating at 40 kDa, 80 kDa and 160 kDa is highly suggestive of LAP aggregation. In line with the pulse-chase analyses, ML-II media fractions were essentially devoid of both SLC and LLC. In contrast, free LTBP (~180kDa) was detected within ML-II media fractions, further suggesting that LAP is not secreted from the ML-II fibroblasts, instead leaving the free LTBP to be released from the cell alone. (Figure 3B). In the pulse/chase experiments, the use of the mild detergent to solubilize these cells, which kept any aggregated LAP insoluble, likely accounts for the absence of intracellular LAP accumulation. It is equally feasible that the pool detected in the whole SDS lysates represents protein that has stably accumulated in the lysosome with extended culture time.

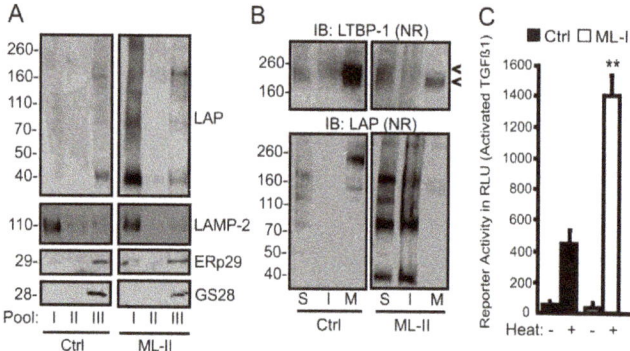

Figure 3. Increased intracellular latent TGFβ1 in ML-II fibroblasts is localized within dense, detergent-insoluble lysosomal fractions. (**A**) Western blot analysis of pooled Percoll gradient fractions from control and ML-II cellular lysates (n = 4). SDS-PAGE-resolved fractions were subjected to analysis using antibodies against markers for lysosomes (LAMP-2), Golgi (GS28) and ER (ERp29) as well as LAP. Pool I, dense membranes (lysosomes); pool II, intermediate density organelles; pool III, ER and Golgi membranes. (**B**) Western blots of human control and ML-II cells fractionated into deoxycholate (DOC)-soluble (S) and –insoluble (I) fractions (n = 4). Along with concentrated media (M) fractions, these pools were resolved by non-reducing (NR) SDS-PAGE and immunoblotted with antibodies against human LAP or LTBP-1. The upper and lower arrowheads indicate the position of the LLC and free LTBP-1, respectively (**C**) Luciferase assays (n = 3) of heat-treated deoxycholate-insoluble fractions that were applied to mink lung TGFβ1 reporter cells; luciferase activity was measured in relative luminescence units, ** $p \leq 0.01$.

Insoluble aggregates of latent TGFβ1 in ML-II cells are capable of ligand activation—Since SDS-PAGE conditions liberate the active ligand from latent complexes, it was not clear from the previous experiments whether the forms of LAP detected represented latent growth factor complexes yet to be "activated," residual LAP monomers or LAP-aggregates generated following release of the active ligand. To distinguish between these possibilities, DOC-insoluble pellets from 4-day control and ML-II cultures were heat-treated to release any latent ligand and TGFβ1 activity tested using a luciferase reporter assay. A three-fold increase in TGFβ1 activity was detected in the insoluble fractions of ML-II cells following heat treatment, indicating that the accumulating latent TGFβ1 represents latent TGFβ1 complexes that are still capable of releasing active ligand (Figure 3C). Collectively, these results demonstrate that latent TGFβ1 is subject to accumulation within lysosomes in a form that is capable of activation. Furthermore, these accumulating latent complexes appear to be prone to aggregation.

Impaired secretion and increased insolubility of latent TGFβ1 are also observed in feline fibroblast-like synoviocytes—To establish whether this unusual biochemical profile for latent TGFβ1 is a general feature of ML-II, the localization, solubility and activity of this growth factor was investigated in feline fibroblast-like synoviocytes isolated from the synovial membranes of control and ML-II kittens. The same properties noted in human dermal fibroblasts, including reduced secretion, increased insolubility and decreased activity were observed in these cells (Figure 4). These data demonstrate that this biochemical profile is a general feature of ML-II. Interestingly, the same pattern of growth factor aggregation was not observed in the feline cells, possibly indicating that certain aspects of latent TGFβ1 processing within the secretory pathway differ between cell types or species.

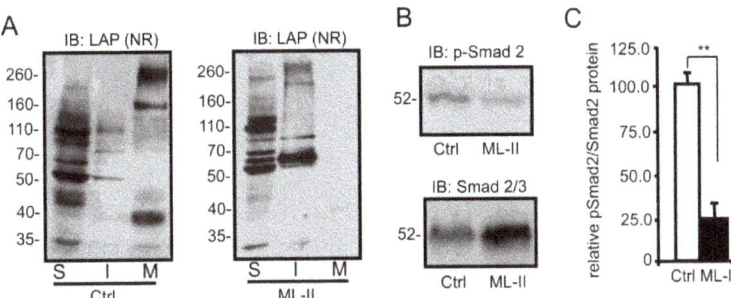

Figure 4. Impaired secretion and increased insolubility and of latent TGFβ1 and reduced TGFβ1 signaling, are also noted in feline ML-II fibroblast-like synoviocytes. (**A**) Western blots of feline control and ML-II cells fractionated into deoxycholate-soluble (S) and –insoluble (I) fractions (n = 3). These fractions and concentrated media (M) from cultures, were resolved by non-reducing (NR) SDS-PAGE and immunoblotted with an antibody against human LAP. (**B**) Western blot analysis of control and ML-II feline fibroblast lysates using antibodies against Smad 2/3 and phosphorylated Smad 2. (**C**) Quantification of the relative intensity of phosphorylated Smad 2 vs. Smad 2/3 protein in control and ML-II cells (n = 3), ** p ≤ 0.01.

Sortilin-1 protein and transcript levels are increased in ML-II cells—Having established that latent TGFβ1 is subject to lysosomal accumulation in ML-II cells, the mechanism of its delivery to this compartment was investigated. In addition to its role as a carbohydrate-independent sorting receptor for certain lysosomal hydrolases, namely cathepsins D and H and acid sphingomyelinase, sortilin has also been shown to regulate the extracellular level and lysosomal targeting of a diverse set of substrates including the TGFβ superfamily member, BMP4, BDNF, alpha-1-antitrypsin and APOB [60–62]. In light of this, we hypothesized that this receptor might also play a role in limiting TGFβ secretion in ML-II cells. Western blot analysis of sortilin was performed on control and ML-II fibroblast lysates. These results demonstrated that sortilin levels were substantially increased in ML-II cells relative to control cells (Figure 5A). A similar elevation in sortilin levels was also noted in the feline ML-II synoviocytes, demonstrating that higher sortilin levels are a common feature of primary ML-II cells (Figure 5B). We also demonstrated that sortilin steady-state levels were increased in CRISPR-Cas9 generated *GNPTAB*-null HeLa cells (Figure 5C), indicating that augmented sortilin expression also occurs in cells engineered to have impaired lysosomal targeting. In the human fibroblasts, elevated protein levels within DOC-soluble pools accounted for much of this increase but a detectable elevation in sortilin levels was also seen within the insoluble pool (Figure 5D).

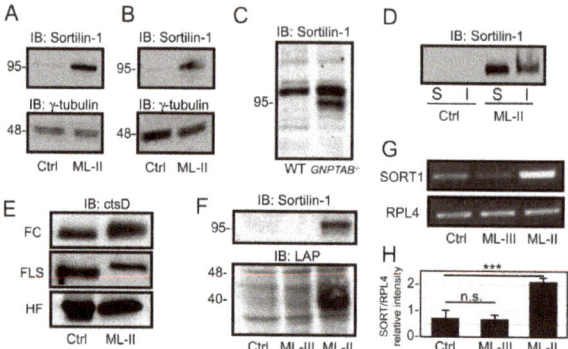

Figure 5. Sortilin-1 protein and transcript levels are elevated in ML-II but not ML-III, fibroblasts. Western blots for sortilin-1 in control and ML-II human fibroblasts (**A**) and feline fibroblast-like synoviocytes (**B**) using a mouse monoclonal antibody against human sortilin-1 (n = 3). (**C**) Sortilin-1 Western blot in WT and GNPTAB-/- (KO) HeLa cells (n = 2). (**D**) Sortilin-1 Western blot of DOC-soluble and –insoluble fractions of human control and ML-II fibroblasts (n = 3). (**E**) Western blot of control and ML-II feline chondrocytes (FC) and fibroblast-like synoviocytes (FLS) as well as control and ML-II human fibroblasts (HF) using a polyclonal antibody against human cathepsin D (n = 2). (**F**) Immunoblots for sortilin-1 and LAP in control, ML-III and ML-II human fibroblasts. Note the correlation of increased sortilin levels and accumulation of LAP in ML-II but not ML-III cells. (**G**) Representative reverse transcription-polymerase chain reaction (RT-PCR) analysis of sortilin-1 transcripts. Ribosomal Protein L4 (RPL4) transcript abundance is shown as a loading control. (**H**) Quantification of the intensity of SORT1 relative to RPL4 (n = 3), *** $p \leq 0.001$.

Since sortilin has been shown to bind and play a partial role in the lysosomal delivery of cathepsin D, the possibility that ML-II cells maintain normal levels of this protease was also investigated. As shown in Figure 5E, the steady state level of cathepsin D is largely unchanged within both ML-II human fibroblasts and two different feline cell lines. Consistent with earlier reports the differences in mobility in control and ML-II cells reflect changes in glycan processing (to primarily complex-type N-glycans) that occur upon loss of mannose phosphorylation [8,63]. These findings strongly support the conclusion that this protease is capable of being retained to some extent despite the absence of Man-6-P residues and that increased sortilin-1 levels correspond to its active role in lysosomal trafficking.

Since the increased expression of this receptor may be a response to the loss of Man-6-P dependent targeting in ML-II cells, the possibility that sortilin levels were also increased in human ML-III fibroblasts was investigated. While catalytically compromised, GlcNAc-1-phosphotransferase is still expressed in ML-III; therefore, these cells retain the ability to synthesize low levels of Man-6-P residues and do not exhibit the same visible lysosomal storage and proliferation as their ML-II counterparts. The presence of residual enzyme activity in ML-III is in contrast to ML-II, where frameshift mutations yield non-functional null alleles. Interestingly, sortilin is not detectably increased in ML-III fibroblasts, suggesting a relationship between the degree of residual mannose phosphorylation and the steady state level of this alternate sorting receptor (Figure 5F). Lastly, we determined whether an increase in sortilin-1 transcripts in ML cells was associated with the elevated levels of this protein (Figure 5G). Sortilin transcripts were indeed increased in ML-II more than two-fold but not ML-III cells, indicating that these cells either actively stimulate transcription or stabilize sortilin transcripts (Figure 5H). Although some of the increase in sortilin protein levels may be a function of slower turnover or its detergent insolubility, the robust increase in sortilin-1 transcript abundance points instead to upregulation of sortilin gene expression.

Co-expression of latent TGFβ1 and sortilin in HeLa cells reduced latent TGFβ1 secretion—To address the link between sortilin expression and cytokine sorting, sortilin was overexpressed to determine if it could alter the secretion of latent TGFβ1 when cDNA encoding the two proteins was introduced into HeLa cells. Endogenous sortilin levels were low in HeLa cells but could be increased following transfection with sortilin cDNA, analogous to what was observed in *GNPTAB*-null HeLa cells (Figure 6A). Upon co-expression of both proteins, increased sortilin expression reduced the amount of both intracellular and extracellular latent TGFβ1, suggesting a reduction in growth factor secretion. The extent of these reductions was quantified and the results shown in Figure 6B. As a control, sortilin and glycopepsinogen, a glycosylated form of the protease pepsinogen [64], were co-expressed in HeLa cells and analyzed as before. In contrast to latent TGFβ1, neither the intracellular nor the secreted level of glycopepsinogen was sensitive to sortilin overexpression (Figure 6C,D), consistent with the ability of this sorting receptor to specifically associate with TGFβ1 and target them to the lysosome. To determine whether the decrease in intracellular levels of latent TGFβ1 (and its subsequent impaired secretion) were due to lysosomal degradation, HeLa cells co-expressing latent TGFβ1 and sortilin were treated with balifomycin, which disrupts lysosomal function and lysates from trypsinized cells were analyzed by Western blot (Figure 6E). Treatment with bafilomycin resulted in a modest increase in intracellular latent TGFβ1 levels (Figure 6F), providing further evidence that this growth factor was targeted to lysosomes and subsequently degraded when sortilin levels are increased.

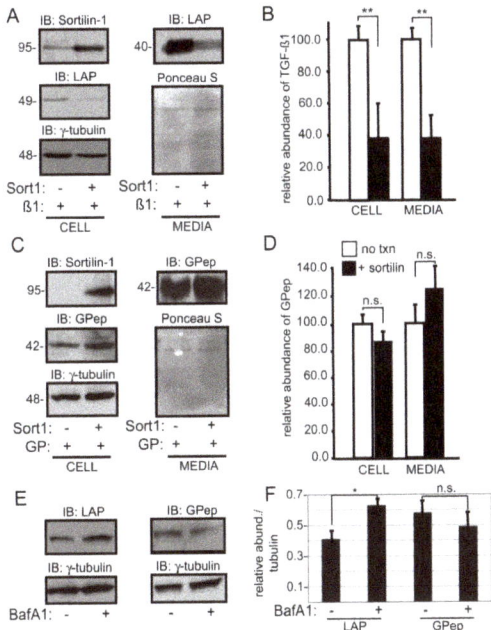

Figure 6. Co-expression of latent TGFβ1 and sortilin in HeLa cells reduced latent TGFβ1 secretion. (**A**) HeLa cells were transfected with DNA encoding sortilin-1 and the TGFβ1 precursor and Western blot analysis performed on cell lysates or media. Immunoblots were subsequently reprobed with antibodies specific for γ-tubulin (cell) or were stained with Ponceau S (media) as a loading control. (**B**) Relative levels of TGFβ1 in the presence and absence of exogenously expressed sortilin were quantified based on band intensity on Western blots from three separate experiments. Average intensity in cells not transfected with sortilin-1 were set to 100. (**C,D**) Parallel experiments and quantification in HeLa cells transfected with DNA encoding sortilin-1 and human glycopepsinogen. (**E**) HeLa cells transfected with sortilin-1 and either TGFβ1 precursor or glycopepsinogen were treated with bafilomycin A1 (BafA1) to disrupt lysosomal function and subjected to SDS-PAGE and Western blot analysis; representative images are shown. (**F**) Quantification of the intensity of LAP or glycopepsinogen relative to γ-tubulin (n = 3), * $p \leq 0.05$, ** $p \leq 0.01$.

Lastly, we assessed whether introduction of cDNA for TGFβ1 protein into the *GNPTAB*-null HeLa cells resulted in its reduced secretion. While these cells did not transfect as well as WT HeLa cells, we demonstrated that TGFβ1 secretion was lower in the *GNPTAB*-null HeLa cells (Figure 7A). Unlike the WT HeLa cells, we did not observe an increase in intracellular TGFβ1 following bafilomycin treatment in the knockout cells (Figure 7B). Rather, there was a slight reduction in the steady-state level that can be interpreted to either reflect a lack of responsiveness to the drug or that these cells lack the proteolytic capacity in their lysosomes to degrade the growth factor.

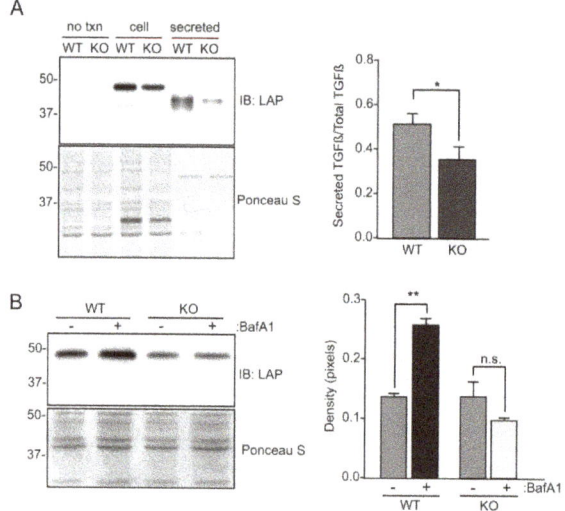

Figure 7. Expression of latent TGFβ1 in GNPTAB[-/-] HeLa cells modestly lowers latent TGFβ1 secretion. (**A**) WT and GNPTAB[-/-] HeLa cells were transfected with DNA encoding the TGFβ1 precursor and Western blot analysis performed on cell lysates or media. Immunoblots were subsequently stained with Ponceau S as a loading control. The relative amount of latent TGFβ1 to total TGFβ1 in the cell lysates and media (secreted) fractions was quantified (n = 3), * p ≤ 0.05. (**B**) WT and GNPTAB[-/-] HeLa cells transfected with TGFβ1 precursor cDNA were treated with or without bafilomycin A1 and cell lysates subjected to SDS-PAGE and Western blot analysis. The abundance of latent TGFβ1 protein in cell lysates is plotted (n = 3), ** p ≤ 0.01.

4. Discussion

In addition to demonstrated roles for sortilin in controlling extracellular levels of several different factors [65–69], numerous studies have also indicated a role for sortilin in the progression of human disorders [70–72]. Loss-of-function or underexpression of sortilin and its related family members has been shown to impact the pathogenic process in Alzheimer's disease by increasing production of the Aβ peptide [73–75]. On the other hand, increased hepatic sortilin expression has been shown to reduce hepatic APOB secretion and increases LDL catabolism, providing a molecular basis for reduced plasma LDL-C levels and lower cardiovascular risk in humans with variations at the SORT1 locus [62,76]. The present results support a unique effect for sortilin in the context of ML-II, where the increased levels of this receptor negatively impact TGFβ1 secretion despite potential positive benefits toward hydrolase sorting. Although we did not perform experiments to directly test whether a reduction in sortilin levels in ML-II fibroblasts could reverse this phenomenon, the reciprocal relationship between its upregulation and the inappropriate lysosomal delivery of latent TGFβ1 to the lysosome is clearly reflected by the co-existence of these phenotypes in ML-II but not the closely related ML-III, fibroblasts. This hypothesis is further supported by observations that sortilin and intracellular latent TGFβ1 are present at very low levels within control fibroblasts and HeLa cells. The observation that these biochemical phenotypes are largely reproduced within early passage feline ML-II cultures is significant in that it further reinforces the disease specificity and eliminates the possibility that sortilin upregulation is simply a byproduct of fibroblasts approaching senescence. Lastly, we acknowledge the limitations in our study of only using a single control fibroblast line but note that the processing and secretion of latent TGFβ1 is highly consistent with metabolic labeling experiments from prior studies [40,41].

Latent TGFβ1 complexes accumulate in dense, detergent-resistant compartments corresponding to dense lysosomes in ML-II fibroblasts. The accumulating complexes do not appear to be subject to intracellular activation since the active TGFβ1 ligand is still capable of being released following heat treatment. Several mechanisms can be envisioned to account for this lack of activation. First, the aggregation of latent TGFβ1 complexes within detergent-resistant compartments in the ML-II cells alone likely contributes to their stability. In light of the abundant storage in ML-II cells, the aggregation and insolubility may reflect still other compensatory mechanisms utilized in these cells to manage the accumulation of storage material. Sortilin has been shown to sort prosaposin and other proteins to detergent-resistant membranes, which may explain the relative insolubility of both the receptor and ligand [77]. Second, the lysosomes in ML-II fibroblasts are generally deficient in protease activity due to the loss of Man-6-P-dependent sorting. This loss of proteolytic capacity is evidenced by the altered conversion of intermediate forms of cathepsin D to its heavy and light chain fragments within ML-II fibroblasts [63]. Since proteases are known activators of latent TGFβ1 [78], their deficiency in this compartment may spare it from efficient degradation.

Although it is unclear at this time whether increased sortilin expression is directly stimulated by the loss of Man-6-P dependent lysosomal targeting or another secondary mechanism, several observations support a direct relationship between impaired mannose phosphorylation and increased sortilin levels. First, sortilin protein and transcript levels are not increased in ML-III fibroblasts, which exhibit only partial loss of mannose phosphorylation capacity. Second, increased sortilin expression was not detected in either mucopolysaccharidosis-I or mucolipidosis-IV (mucolipin deficiency) human fibroblasts (data not shown), suggesting that elevation of this receptor is not a feature of all lysosomal storage disorders and may therefore be specific to ML-II. Sortilin has not been identified as a gene that is regulated by the transcription factor TFEB, a recently defined master regulator of lysosomal biogenesis [79,80]. This observation suggests that additional mechanisms are capable of sensing the need for Man-6-P-independent lysosomal targeting in ML-II cells. The possibility that upregulation of sortilin arises in response to either altered growth factor signaling or increased secretion of other non-lysosomal sortilin ligands also cannot be ruled out. Further analyses of the tissue-specific mechanisms that regulate sortilin expression should provide insight into these unresolved issues.

Sortilin-mediated decreases in the signaling of TGFβ1 (or any other molecules known to bind this receptor) may be relevant to the pathogenesis of ML-II and provide a novel mechanism to explain the surprising clinical distinction between the ML-II and ML-III skeletal phenotypes. The complex skeletal manifestations associated with ML-II suggest that the normal programs by which osteoblasts and chondrocytes mature are disrupted. These processes are tightly linked to the presentation and activation of TGFβ superfamily members. Our prior work in a zebrafish model for ML-II showed that increased TGFβ signaling played a central role in cartilage phenotypes associated with impaired lysosomal targeting. While this finding is seemingly contradictory to what we observed in ML-II fibroblasts, the zebrafish model lacks any signs of lysosomal storage at early developmental stages [14]. Instead the TGFβ-related phenotypes are driven by the extracellular action of cathepsin K [15–17]. This highlights the need to consider whether lysosomal storage is present in a particular cell type and whether sortilin expression is increased, in order to comprehensively assess any effects on TGFβ signaling. Although we did not directly assess BMP activation in the fibroblasts, a sortilin-mediated decrease in the activity of several of these growth factors in cell types that exhibit storage may contribute to the altered skeletal formation in ML-II. Indeed, sortilin upregulation occurs during osteoblast differentiation of mesenchymal stem cells, suggesting that this receptor may have a normal physiological function in bone development [81]. We have shown that another cytokine relevant to bone formation, leukemia inhibitory factor, is subject to higher extracellular levels when mannose phosphorylation and subsequent lysosomal degradation, is decreased [54].

Thus, there appear to be multiple mechanisms whereby decreased mannose phosphorylation and subsequent adaptations are capable of impacting the growth factor and cytokine signaling pathways that control bone and cartilage homeostasis. The tissue- or species-specific manner by which these factors are balanced may account for the variable nature of the phenotypes associated with the human disease as well as those defects noted within animal models of ML-II. In summary, the present findings provide a new prospective on the pathogenesis of ML-II by suggesting that increased expression of alternate hydrolase sorting receptors can negatively impact growth factor signaling in the context of impaired mannose phosphorylation.

5. Conclusions

The sorting receptor sortilin is specifically upregulated in ML-II cells with storage in order to compensate for the loss of carbohydrate-dependent targeting of hydrolases. This increase in sortilin expression, however, reduces the secretion of latent TGFβ by instead directing it to detergent-resistant lysosomes. These findings suggest that the enhanced expression of alternate sorting receptors can have unintended consequences on the availability and activity of growth factors and cytokines.

Author Contributions: Conceptualization, J.W.B., H.F.-S. and R.S.; methodology, J.W.B. and R.S.; validation, J.W.B. and J.N.; formal analysis, J.W.B., H.F.-S. and R.S; investigation, J.W.B., M.A.-P. and J.N; resources, M.H.; writing—original draft preparation, J.W.B. and R.S.; writing—review and editing, J.W.B. and R.S.; supervision and project administration, J.W.B., H.F.-S. and R.S.; funding acquisition, J.W.B., M.H. and R.S. All authors have read and agreed to the published version of the manuscript.

Funding: This work was supported by grants from the NIH (R00HL131866 to J.W.B., P40OD012095 to M.H. and R01GM086524 to R.S.).

Acknowledgments: We are grateful to Daniel Rifkin (NYU Langone Medical Center) for providing the mink lung reporter cells and to Carl-Henrik Heldin (Uppsala University, Sweden) and Kohei Miyazono (University of Tokyo, Tokyo, Japan) for agreeing to provide the LT-1 antibody. We also thank Stuart Kornfeld (Washington University in Saint Louis, USA) for sharing the GNPTAB$^{-/-}$ HeLa cells [82].

Conflicts of Interest: The authors declare no conflict of interest.

Abbreviations

Man-6-P	mannose 6-phosphate;
ML-II	mucolipidosis II;
TGFβ	transforming growth factor beta;
LAP	latency-associated peptide;
SLC	small latent complex;
LLC	large latent complex;
LTBP	latent TGFβ binding protein;
LAMP	lysosomal associated membrane protein;
DOC	deoxycholate;
LDL	low density lipoprotein;
APOB	apolipoprotein B;
BDNF	brain-derived neurotrophic factor;
RPL4	ribosomal protein L4.

References

1. Reitman, M.L.; Varki, A.; Kornfeld, S. Fibroblasts from patients with I-cell disease and pseudo-Hurler polydystrophy are deficient in uridine 5′-diphosphate-N-acetylglucosamine: Glycoprotein N-acetylglucosaminylphosphotransferase activity. *J. Clin. Investig.* **1981**, *67*, 1574–1579. [CrossRef] [PubMed]

2. Tiede, S.; Storch, S.; Lubke, T.; Henrissat, B.; Bargal, R.; Raas-Rothschild, A.; Braulke, T. Mucolipidosis II is caused by mutations in GNPTA encoding the alpha/beta GlcNAc-1-phosphotransferase. *Nat. Med.* **2005**, *11*, 1109–1112. [CrossRef] [PubMed]
3. David-Vizcarra, G.; Briody, J.; Ault, J.; Fietz, M.; Fletcher, J.; Savarirayan, R.; Wilson, M.; McGill, J.; Edwards, M.; Munns, C.; et al. The natural history and osteodystrophy of mucolipidosis types II and III. *J. Paediatr. Child Health* **2010**, *46*, 316–322. [CrossRef] [PubMed]
4. Cathey, S.S.; Leroy, J.G.; Wood, T.; Eaves, K.; Simensen, R.J.; Kudo, M.; Stevenson, R.E.; Friez, M.J. Phenotype and genotype in mucolipidoses II and III alpha/beta: A study of 61 probands. *J. Med. Genet.* **2010**, *47*, 38–48. [CrossRef] [PubMed]
5. Saul, R.A.; Proud, V.; Taylor, H.A.; Leroy, J.G.; Spranger, J. Prenatal mucolipidosis type II (I-cell disease) can present as Pacman dysplasia. *Am. J. Med. Genet. A* **2005**, *135*, 328–332. [CrossRef] [PubMed]
6. Cathey, S.S.; Kudo, M.; Tiede, S.; Raas-Rothschild, A.; Braulke, T.; Beck, M.; Taylor, H.A.; Canfield, W.M.; Leroy, J.G.; Neufeld, E.F.; et al. Molecular order in mucolipidosis II and III nomenclature. *Am. J. Med. Genet. A* **2008**, *146*, 512–513. [CrossRef]
7. Qian, Y.; van Meel, E.; Flanagan-Steet, H.; Yox, A.; Steet, R.; Kornfeld, S. Analysis of mucolipidosis II/III GNPTAB missense mutations identifies domains of UDP-GlcNAc:Lysosomal enzyme GlcNAc-1-phosphotransferase involved in catalytic function and lysosomal enzyme recognition. *J. Biol. Chem.* **2015**, *290*, 3045–3056. [CrossRef]
8. Gelfman, C.M.; Vogel, P.; Issa, T.M.; Turner, C.A.; Lee, W.S.; Kornfeld, S.; Rice, D.S. Mice lacking alpha/beta subunits of GlcNAc-1-phosphotransferase exhibit growth retardation, retinal degeneration and secretory cell lesions. *Investig. Ophthalmol. Vis. Sci.* **2007**, *48*, 5221–5228. [CrossRef]
9. Boonen, M.; van Meel, E.; Oorschot, V.; Klumperman, J.; Kornfeld, S. Vacuolization of mucolipidosis type II mouse exocrine gland cells represents accumulation of autolysosomes. *Mol. Biol. Cell* **2011**, *22*, 1135–1147. [CrossRef]
10. Vogel, P.; Payne, B.J.; Read, R.; Lee, W.S.; Gelfman, C.M.; Kornfeld, S. Comparative pathology of murine mucolipidosis types II and IIIC. *Vet. Pathol.* **2009**, *46*, 313–324. [CrossRef] [PubMed]
11. Kollmann, K.; Damme, M.; Markmann, S.; Morelle, W.; Schweizer, M.; Hermans-Borgmeyer, I.; Rochert, A.K.; Pohl, S.; Lubke, T.; Michalski, J.C.; et al. Lysosomal dysfunction causes neurodegeneration in mucolipidosis II 'knock-in' mice. *Brain* **2012**, *135*, 2661–2675. [CrossRef] [PubMed]
12. Marschner, K.; Kollmann, K.; Schweizer, M.; Braulke, T.; Pohl, S. A key enzyme in the biogenesis of lysosomes is a protease that regulates cholesterol metabolism. *Science* **2011**, *333*, 87–90. [CrossRef] [PubMed]
13. Mazrier, H.; Van Hoeven, M.; Wang, P.; Knox, V.W.; Aguirre, G.D.; Holt, E.; Wiemelt, S.P.; Sleeper, M.M.; Hubler, M.; Haskins, M.E.; et al. Inheritance, biochemical abnormalities and clinical features of feline mucolipidosis II: The first animal model of human I-cell disease. *J. Hered.* **2003**, *94*, 363–373. [CrossRef]
14. Flanagan-Steet, H.; Sias, C.; Steet, R. Altered chondrocyte differentiation and extracellular matrix homeostasis in a zebrafish model for mucolipidosis II. *Am. J. Pathol.* **2009**, *175*, 2063–2075. [CrossRef] [PubMed]
15. Petrey, A.C.; Flanagan-Steet, H.; Johnson, S.; Fan, X.; De la Rosa, M.; Haskins, M.E.; Nairn, A.V.; Moremen, K.W.; Steet, R. Excessive activity of cathepsin K is associated with cartilage defects in a zebrafish model of mucolipidosis II. *Dis. Models Mech.* **2012**, *5*, 177–190. [CrossRef]
16. Flanagan-Steet, H.; Aarnio, M.; Kwan, B.; Guihard, P.; Petrey, A.; Haskins, M.; Blanchard, F.; Steet, R. Cathepsin-mediated alterations in TGFbeta-related signaling underlie disrupted cartilage and bone maturation associated with impaired lysosomal targeting. *J. Bone Miner. Res.* **2016**, *31*, 535–548. [CrossRef]
17. Flanagan-Steet, H.; Christian, C.; Lu, P.N.; Aarnio-Peterson, M.; Sanman, L.; Archer-Hartmann, S.; Azadi, P.; Bogyo, M.; Steet, R.A. TGF-beta regulates cathepsin activation during normal and pathogenic development. *Cell Rep.* **2018**, *22*, 2964–2977. [CrossRef]
18. Saito, T.; Kinoshita, A.; Yoshiura, K.; Makita, Y.; Wakui, K.; Honke, K.; NIIkawa, N.; Taniguchi, N. Domain-specific mutations of a transforming growth factor (TGF)-beta 1 latency-associated peptide cause Camurati-Engelmann disease because of the formation of a constitutively active form of TGF-beta 1. *J. Biol. Chem.* **2001**, *276*, 11469–11472. [CrossRef]
19. Janssens, K.; Gershoni-Baruch, R.; Guanabens, N.; Migone, N.; Ralston, S.; Bonduelle, M.; Lissens, W.; Van Maldergem, L.; Vanhoenacker, F.; Verbruggen, L.; et al. Mutations in the gene encoding the latency-associated peptide of TGF-beta 1 cause Camurati-Engelmann disease. *Nat. Genet.* **2000**, *26*, 273–275. [CrossRef]

20. Neptune, E.R.; Frischmeyer, P.A.; Arking, D.E.; Myers, L.; Bunton, T.E.; Gayraud, B.; Ramirez, F.; Sakai, L.Y.; Dietz, H.C. Dysregulation of TGF-beta activation contributes to pathogenesis in Marfan syndrome. *Nat. Genet.* **2003**, *33*, 407–411. [CrossRef]
21. Nistala, H.; Lee-Arteaga, S.; Siciliano, G.; Smaldone, S.; Ramirez, F. Extracellular regulation of transforming growth factor beta and bone morphogenetic protein signaling in bone. *Ann. N. Y. Acad. Sci.* **2010**, *1192*, 253–256. [CrossRef] [PubMed]
22. Cohen, M.M., Jr. The new bone biology: Pathologic, molecular and clinical correlates. *Am. J. Med. Genet. A* **2006**, *140*, 2646–2706. [CrossRef] [PubMed]
23. Le Goff, C.; Cormier-Daire, V. From tall to short: The role of TGFbeta signaling in growth and its disorders. *Am. J. Med. Genet. C Semin. Med. Genet.* **2012**, *160*, 145–153. [CrossRef] [PubMed]
24. Le Goff, C.; Morice-Picard, F.; Dagoneau, N.; Wang, L.W.; Perrot, C.; Crow, Y.J.; Bauer, F.; Flori, E.; Prost-Squarcioni, C.; Krakow, D.; et al. ADAMTSL2 mutations in geleophysic dysplasia demonstrate a role for ADAMTS-like proteins in TGF-beta bioavailability regulation. *Nat. Genet.* **2008**, *40*, 1119–1123. [CrossRef]
25. Bellesso, S.; Salvalaio, M.; Lualdi, S.; Tognon, E.; Costa, R.; Braghetta, P.; Giraudo, C.; Stramare, R.; Rigon, L.; Filocamo, M.; et al. FGF signaling deregulation is associated with early developmental skeletal defects in animal models for mucopolysaccharidosis type II (MPSII). *Hum. Mol. Genet.* **2018**, *27*, 2262–2275. [CrossRef]
26. Costa, R.; Urbani, A.; Salvalaio, M.; Bellesso, S.; Cieri, D.; Zancan, I.; Filocamo, M.; Bonaldo, P.; Szabo, I.; Tomanin, R.; et al. Perturbations in cell signaling elicit early cardiac defects in mucopolysaccharidosis type II. *Hum. Mol. Genet.* **2017**, *26*, 1643–1655. [CrossRef] [PubMed]
27. Moro, E.; Tomanin, R.; Friso, A.; Modena, N.; Tiso, N.; Scarpa, M.; Argenton, F. A novel functional role of iduronate-2-sulfatase in zebrafish early development. *Matrix Biol.* **2010**, *29*, 43–50. [CrossRef] [PubMed]
28. Massague, J.; Blain, S.W.; Lo, R.S. TGFbeta signaling in growth control, cancer and heritable disorders. *Cell* **2000**, *103*, 295–309. [CrossRef]
29. Massague, J.; Chen, Y.G. Controlling TGF-beta signaling. *Genes Dev.* **2000**, *14*, 627–644. [PubMed]
30. Taylor, A.W. Review of the activation of TGF-beta in immunity. *J. Leukoc. Biol.* **2009**, *85*, 29–33. [CrossRef]
31. Chen, G.; Deng, C.; Li, Y.P. TGF-beta and bmp signaling in osteoblast differentiation and bone formation. *Int. J. Biol. Sci.* **2012**, *8*, 272–288. [CrossRef] [PubMed]
32. Kitisin, K.; Saha, T.; Blake, T.; Golestaneh, N.; Deng, M.; Kim, C.; Tang, Y.; Shetty, K.; Mishra, B.; Mishra, L. TGF-beta signaling in development. *Sci. STKE* **2007**, *2007*. [CrossRef] [PubMed]
33. Serra, R.; Chang, C. TGF-beta signaling in human skeletal and patterning disorders. *Birth Defects Res. C Embryo Today* **2003**, *69*, 333–351. [CrossRef]
34. Janssens, K.; ten Dijke, P.; Janssens, S.; Van Hul, W. Transforming growth factor-beta1 to the bone. *Endocr. Rev.* **2005**, *26*, 743–774. [CrossRef] [PubMed]
35. Moustakas, A.; Pardali, K.; Gaal, A.; Heldin, C.H. Mechanisms of TGF-beta signaling in regulation of cell growth and differentiation. *Immunol. Lett.* **2002**, *82*, 85–91. [CrossRef]
36. Gentry, L.E.; Webb, N.R.; Lim, G.J.; Brunner, A.M.; Ranchalis, J.E.; Twardzik, D.R.; Lioubin, M.N.; Marquardt, H.; Purchio, A.F. Type 1 transforming growth factor beta: Amplified expression and secretion of mature and precursor polypeptides in Chinese hamster ovary cells. *Mol. Cell Biol.* **1987**, *7*, 3418–3427. [CrossRef]
37. Gentry, L.E.; Lioubin, M.N.; Purchio, A.F.; Marquardt, H. Molecular events in the processing of recombinant type 1 pre-pro-transforming growth factor beta to the mature polypeptide. *Mol. Cell Biol.* **1988**, *8*, 4162–4168. [CrossRef]
38. Rifkin, D.B.; Kojima, S.; Abe, M.; Harpel, J.G. TGF-beta: Structure, function and formation. *Thromb. Haemost.* **1993**, *70*, 177–179.
39. Rifkin, D.B. Latent transforming growth factor-beta (TGF-beta) binding proteins: Orchestrators of TGF-beta availability. *J. Biol. Chem.* **2005**, *280*, 7409–7412. [CrossRef]
40. Taipale, J.; Miyazono, K.; Heldin, C.H.; Keski-Oja, J. Latent transforming growth factor-beta 1 associates to fibroblast extracellular matrix via latent TGF-beta binding protein. *J. Cell Biol.* **1994**, *124*, 171–181. [CrossRef]
41. Miyazono, K.; Olofsson, A.; Colosetti, P.; Heldin, C.H. A role of the latent TGF-beta 1-binding protein in the assembly and secretion of TGF-beta 1. *EMBO J.* **1991**, *10*, 1091–1101. [CrossRef]
42. Chen, Q.; Sivakumar, P.; Barley, C.; Peters, D.M.; Gomes, R.R.; Farach-Carson, M.C.; Dallas, S.L. Potential role for heparan sulfate proteoglycans in regulation of transforming growth factor-beta (TGF-beta) by modulating assembly of latent TGF-beta-binding protein-1. *J. Biol. Chem.* **2007**, *282*, 26418–26430. [CrossRef] [PubMed]

43. Dallas, S.L.; Sivakumar, P.; Jones, C.J.; Chen, Q.; Peters, D.M.; Mosher, D.F.; Humphries, M.J.; Kielty, C.M. Fibronectin regulates latent transforming growth factor-beta (TGF beta) by controlling matrix assembly of latent TGF beta-binding protein-1. *J. Biol. Chem.* **2005**, *280*, 18871–18880. [CrossRef] [PubMed]
44. Ramirez, F.; Rifkin, D.B. Extracellular microfibrils: Contextual platforms for TGFbeta and BMP signaling. *Curr. Opin. Cell Biol.* **2009**, *21*, 616–622. [CrossRef] [PubMed]
45. Zhou, Y.; Koli, K.; Hagood, J.S.; Miao, M.; Mavalli, M.; Rifkin, D.B.; Murphy-Ullrich, J.E. Latent transforming growth factor-beta-binding protein-4 regulates transforming growth factor-beta1 bioavailability for activation by fibrogenic lung fibroblasts in response to bleomycin. *Am. J. Pathol.* **2009**, *174*, 21–33. [CrossRef]
46. Isogai, Z.; Ono, R.N.; Ushiro, S.; Keene, D.R.; Chen, Y.; Mazzieri, R.; Charbonneau, N.L.; Reinhardt, D.P.; Rifkin, D.B.; Sakai, L.Y. Latent transforming growth factor beta-binding protein 1 interacts with fibrillin and is a microfibril-associated protein. *J. Biol. Chem.* **2003**, *278*, 2750–2757. [CrossRef] [PubMed]
47. Horiguchi, M.; Ota, M.; Rifkin, D.B. Matrix control of transforming growth factor-beta function. *J. Biochem.* **2012**, *152*, 321–329. [CrossRef]
48. Munger, J.S.; Huang, X.; Kawakatsu, H.; Griffiths, M.J.; Dalton, S.L.; Wu, J.; Pittet, J.F.; Kaminski, N.; Garat, C.; Matthay, M.A.; et al. The integrin alpha V beta 6 binds and activates latent TGF beta 1: A mechanism for regulating pulmonary inflammation and fibrosis. *Cell* **1999**, *96*, 319–328. [CrossRef]
49. Crawford, S.E.; Stellmach, V.; Murphy-Ullrich, J.E.; Ribeiro, S.M.; Lawler, J.; Hynes, R.O.; Boivin, G.P.; Bouck, N. Thrombospondin-1 is a major activator of TGF-beta1 in vivo. *Cell* **1998**, *93*, 1159–1170. [CrossRef]
50. Godar, S.; Horejsi, V.; Weidle, U.H.; Binder, B.R.; Hansmann, C.; Stockinger, H. M6P/IGFII-receptor complexes urokinase receptor and plasminogen for activation of transforming growth factor-beta1. *Eur. J. Immunol.* **1999**, *29*, 1004–1013. [CrossRef]
51. Dennis, P.A.; Rifkin, D.B. Cellular activation of latent transforming growth factor beta requires binding to the cation-independent mannose 6-phosphate/insulin-like growth factor type II receptor. *Proc. Natl. Acad. Sci. USA* **1991**, *88*, 580–584. [CrossRef] [PubMed]
52. Barnes, J.; Warejcka, D.; Simpliciano, J.; Twining, S.; Steet, R. Latency-associated peptide of transforming growth factor-beta1 is not subject to physiological mannose phosphorylation. *J. Biol. Chem.* **2012**, *287*, 7526–7534. [CrossRef] [PubMed]
53. Chen, Y.; Dabovic, B.; Annes, J.P.; Rifkin, D.B. Latent TGF-beta binding protein-3 (LTBP-3) requires binding to TGF-beta for secretion. *FEBS Lett.* **2002**, *517*, 277–280. [CrossRef]
54. Barnes, J.; Lim, J.M.; Godard, A.; Blanchard, F.; Wells, L.; Steet, R. Extensive mannose phosphorylation on leukemia inhibitory factor (LIF) controls its extracellular levels by multiple mechanisms. *J. Biol. Chem.* **2011**, *286*, 24855–24864. [CrossRef] [PubMed]
55. Rohrer, J.; Schweizer, A.; Johnson, K.F.; Kornfeld, S. A determinant in the cytoplasmic tail of the cation-dependent mannose 6-phosphate receptor prevents trafficking to lysosomes. *J. Cell Biol.* **1995**, *130*, 1297–1306. [CrossRef]
56. Steet, R.A.; Chung, S.; Wustman, B.; Powe, A.; Do, H.; Kornfeld, S.A. The iminosugar isofagomine increases the activity of N370S mutant acid beta-glucosidase in Gaucher fibroblasts by several mechanisms. *Proc. Natl. Acad. Sci. USA* **2006**, *103*, 13813–13818. [CrossRef]
57. Barrientos, S.; Stojadinovic, O.; Golinko, M.S.; Brem, H.; Tomic-Canic, M. Growth factors and cytokines in wound healing. *Wound Repair Regen.* **2008**, *16*, 585–601. [CrossRef]
58. Miyazono, K.; Thyberg, J.; Heldin, C.H. Retention of the transforming growth factor-beta 1 precursor in the golgi complex in a latent endoglycosidase H-sensitive form. *J. Biol. Chem.* **1992**, *267*, 5668–5675.
59. Schaub, B.E.; Nair, P.; Rohrer, J. Analysis of protein transport to lysosomes. *Curr. Protoc. Cell Biol.* **2005**, *27*, 15–18. [CrossRef]
60. Canuel, M.; Korkidakis, A.; Konnyu, K.; Morales, C.R. Sortilin mediates the lysosomal targeting of cathepsins d and h. *Biochem. Biophys. Res. Commun.* **2008**, *373*, 292–297. [CrossRef]
61. Nykjaer, A.; Willnow, T.E. Sortilin: A receptor to regulate neuronal viability and function. *Trends Neurosci.* **2012**, *35*, 261–270. [CrossRef] [PubMed]
62. Strong, A.; Ding, Q.; Edmondson, A.C.; Millar, J.S.; Sachs, K.V.; Li, X.; Kumaravel, A.; Wang, M.Y.; Ai, D.; Guo, L.; et al. Hepatic sortilin regulates both apolipoprotein B secretion and ldl catabolism. *J. Clin. Investig.* **2012**, *122*, 2807–2816. [CrossRef] [PubMed]

63. Steet, R.A.; Hullin, R.; Kudo, M.; Martinelli, M.; Bosshard, N.U.; Schaffner, T.; Kornfeld, S.; Steinmann, B. A splicing mutation in the alpha/beta GlcNAc-1-phosphotransferase gene results in an adult onset form of mucolipidosis III associated with sensory neuropathy and cardiomyopathy. *Am. J. Med. Genet. A* **2005**, *132*, 369–375. [CrossRef] [PubMed]
64. Steet, R.; Lee, W.S.; Kornfeld, S. Identification of the minimal lysosomal enzyme recognition domain in cathepsin D. *J. Biol. Chem.* **2005**, *280*, 33318–33323. [CrossRef]
65. Evans, S.F.; Irmady, K.; Ostrow, K.; Kim, T.; Nykjaer, A.; Saftig, P.; Blobel, C.; Hempstead, B.L. Neuronal brain-derived neurotrophic factor is synthesized in excess, with levels regulated by sortilin-mediated trafficking and lysosomal degradation. *J. Biol. Chem.* **2011**, *286*, 29556–29567. [CrossRef]
66. Kwon, S.; Christian, J.L. Sortilin associates with transforming growth factor-beta family proteins to enhance lysosome-mediated degradation. *J. Biol. Chem.* **2011**, *286*, 21876–21885. [CrossRef]
67. Chen, Z.Y.; Ieraci, A.; Teng, H.; Dall, H.; Meng, C.X.; Herrera, D.G.; Nykjaer, A.; Hempstead, B.L.; Lee, F.S. Sortilin controls intracellular sorting of brain-derived neurotrophic factor to the regulated secretory pathway. *J. Neurosci.* **2005**, *25*, 6156–6166. [CrossRef]
68. Gelling, C.L.; Dawes, I.W.; Perlmutter, D.H.; Fisher, E.A.; Brodsky, J.L. The endosomal protein-sorting receptor sortilin has a role in trafficking alpha-1 antitrypsin. *Genetics* **2012**, *192*, 889–903. [CrossRef]
69. Strong, A.; Rader, D.J. Sortilin as a regulator of lipoprotein metabolism. *Curr. Atheroscler. Rep.* **2012**, *14*, 211–218. [CrossRef]
70. Calkin, A.C.; Tontonoz, P. Genome-wide association studies identify new targets in cardiovascular disease. *Sci. Transl. Med.* **2010**, *2*, 48ps46. [CrossRef]
71. Rogaeva, E.; Meng, Y.; Lee, J.H.; Gu, Y.; Kawarai, T.; Zou, F.; Katayama, T.; Baldwin, C.T.; Cheng, R.; Hasegawa, H.; et al. The neuronal sortilin-related receptor SORL1 is genetically associated with Alzheimer disease. *Nat. Genet.* **2007**, *39*, 168–177. [CrossRef] [PubMed]
72. Conlon, D.M. Role of sortilin in lipid metabolism. *Curr. Opin. Lipidol.* **2019**, *30*, 198–204. [CrossRef] [PubMed]
73. Ciarlo, E.; Massone, S.; Penna, I.; Nizzari, M.; Gigoni, A.; Dieci, G.; Russo, C.; Florio, T.; Cancedda, R.; Pagano, A. An intronic ncRNA-dependent regulation of SORL1 expression affecting abeta formation is upregulated in post-mortem Alzheimer's disease brain samples. *Dis. Models Mech.* **2012**, *6*, 424–433. [CrossRef] [PubMed]
74. Lane, R.F.; Raines, S.M.; Steele, J.W.; Ehrlich, M.E.; Lah, J.A.; Small, S.A.; Tanzi, R.E.; Attie, A.D.; Gandy, S. Diabetes-associated SorCS1 regulates Alzheimer's amyloid-beta metabolism: Evidence for involvement of SORL1 and the retromer complex. *J. Neurosci.* **2010**, *30*, 13110–13115. [CrossRef] [PubMed]
75. Rohe, M.; Carlo, A.S.; Breyhan, H.; Sporbert, A.; Militz, D.; Schmidt, V.; Wozny, C.; Harmeier, A.; Erdmann, B.; Bales, K.R.; et al. Sortilin-related receptor with a-type repeats (SORLA) affects the amyloid precursor protein-dependent stimulation of ERK signaling and adult neurogenesis. *J. Biol. Chem.* **2008**, *283*, 14826–14834. [CrossRef]
76. Musunuru, K.; Strong, A.; Frank-Kamenetsky, M.; Lee, N.E.; Ahfeldt, T.; Sachs, K.V.; Li, X.; Li, H.; Kuperwasser, N.; Ruda, V.M.; et al. From noncoding variant to phenotype via SORT1 at the 1p13 cholesterol locus. *Nature* **2010**, *466*, 714–719. [CrossRef]
77. Canuel, M.; Bhattacharyya, N.; Balbis, A.; Yuan, L.; Morales, C.R. Sortilin and prosaposin localize to detergent-resistant membrane microdomains. *Exp. Cell Res.* **2009**, *315*, 240–247. [CrossRef]
78. Lyons, R.M.; Keski-Oja, J.; Moses, H.L. Proteolytic activation of latent transforming growth factor-beta from fibroblast-conditioned medium. *J. Cell Biol.* **1988**, *106*, 1659–1665. [CrossRef]
79. Palmieri, M.; Impey, S.; Kang, H.; di Ronza, A.; Pelz, C.; Sardiello, M.; Ballabio, A. Characterization of the clear network reveals an integrated control of cellular clearance pathways. *Hum. Mol. Genet.* **2011**, *20*, 3852–3866. [CrossRef]
80. Sardiello, M.; Palmieri, M.; di Ronza, A.; Medina, D.L.; Valenza, M.; Gennarino, V.A.; Di Malta, C.; Donaudy, F.; Embrione, V.; Polishchuk, R.S.; et al. A gene network regulating lysosomal biogenesis and function. *Science* **2009**, *325*, 473–477. [CrossRef]

81. Maeda, S.; Nobukuni, T.; Shimo-Onoda, K.; Hayashi, K.; Yone, K.; Komiya, S.; Inoue, I. Sortilin is upregulated during osteoblastic differentiation of mesenchymal stem cells and promotes extracellular matrix mineralization. *J. Cell Physiol.* **2002**, *193*, 73–79. [CrossRef] [PubMed]
82. van Meel, E.; Lee, W.S.; Liu, L.; Qian, Y.; Doray, B.; Kornfeld, S. Multiple Domains of GlcNAc-1-phosphotransferase Mediate Recognition of Lysosomal Enzymes. *J. Biol. Chem.* **2016**, *291*, 8295–8307. [CrossRef] [PubMed]

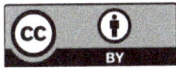

© 2020 by the authors. Licensee MDPI, Basel, Switzerland. This article is an open access article distributed under the terms and conditions of the Creative Commons Attribution (CC BY) license (http://creativecommons.org/licenses/by/4.0/).

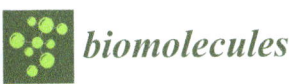 *biomolecules*

Review

Gene Therapy for Lysosomal Storage Disorders: Ongoing Studies and Clinical Development

Giulia Massaro [1,*], Amy F. Geard [1,2], Wenfei Liu [1], Oliver Coombe-Tennant [1], Simon N. Waddington [2,3], Julien Baruteau [4,5], Paul Gissen [5] and Ahad A. Rahim [1]

1. UCL School of Pharmacy, University College London, London WC1N 1AX, UK; amy.geard.16@ucl.ac.uk (A.F.G.); wenfei.liu.10@ucl.ac.uk (W.L.); o.coombe-tennant@ucl.ac.uk (O.C.-T.); a.rahim@ucl.ac.uk (A.A.R.)
2. Wits/SAMRC Antiviral Gene Therapy Research Unit, Faculty of Health Sciences, University of the Witwatersrand, Johannesburg 2193, South Africa; s.waddington@ucl.ac.uk
3. Gene Transfer Technology Group, EGA Institute for Women's Health, University College London, London WC1E 6HX, UK
4. Metabolic Medicine Department, Great Ormond Street Hospital for Children NHS Foundation Trust, London WC1N 1EH, UK; j.baruteau@ucl.ac.uk
5. Great Ormond Street Hospital Biomedical Research Centre, Great Ormond Street Institute of Child Health, National Institute of Health Research, University College London, London WC1N 1EH, UK; p.gissen@ucl.ac.uk
* Correspondence: giulia.massaro.13@ucl.ac.uk

Abstract: Rare monogenic disorders such as lysosomal diseases have been at the forefront in the development of novel treatments where therapeutic options are either limited or unavailable. The increasing number of successful pre-clinical and clinical studies in the last decade demonstrates that gene therapy represents a feasible option to address the unmet medical need of these patients. This article provides a comprehensive overview of the current state of the field, reviewing the most used viral gene delivery vectors in the context of lysosomal storage disorders, a selection of relevant pre-clinical studies and ongoing clinical trials within recent years.

Keywords: lysosomal diseases; gene therapy; viral vectors

1. Introduction

Lysosomal storage disorders (LSDs) form a group of genetic errors of metabolism, comprising more than 70 different diseases [1]. These monogenic disorders result from defects in proteins crucial for lysosomal function, such as lysosomal hydrolases, as well as transporters, integral membrane proteins, co-factors and enzyme modifiers or activators [2]. Moreover, mutations in non-lysosomal proteins that play a role in lysosome-related processes can also cause LSDs. The lysosome is a complex organelle, involved in several cellular processes such as autophagy, signalling cascades, lipid and calcium homeostasis, exocytosis, membrane repair and cell viability [3,4]. As a consequence of genetic defects, these cellular functions and mechanisms are disrupted, leading to inflammatory responses and ultimately cell death. Typical LSDs involve accumulation of undegraded substrates in the lysosome due to defective hydrolase enzymes, and classification of the disorder can be based on the nature of the accumulated substrate. However, the identification of additional defects in integral proteins for which the function is not fully understood has broadened the traditional classification of LSDs [5]. The disease can also be classified by the causative underlying defect. Although LSDs are individually considered rare diseases, some populations have a higher carrier frequency, and the collective prevalence as a group is relatively common, with an estimated incidence of 1 in 5000 live births [1].

Specific treatments that aim to correct the metabolic defect have been developed for many LSDs. These include haematopoietic stem cell transplantation (HSCT), enzyme replacement therapy (ERT), pharmacological chaperone therapy (PCT) and substrate reduction therapy (SRT). HSCT involves the transplantation of haematopoietic stem cells, usually derived from bone marrow. The rationale relies on transplanted stem cells engrafting in the bone marrow and differentiating into various cells of the haematopoietic lineage; some of the cells then cross the blood brain barrier (BBB) and potentially may differentiate into resident microglia of the central nervous system that can secrete functioning lysosomal enzymes [6,7]. HSCT is considered the standard or optional therapy for some LSDs such as mucopolysaccharidosis type I (MPS I), when diagnosed before 2.5 years of age [8], alpha mannosidosis and globoid cell leukodystrophy, where early-stage treatment correlates with better clinical outcomes, and it could be indicated for other inherited metabolic disorders [9]. However, this approach is not feasible in disorders such as the late infantile form of metachromatic leukodystrophy, where engraftment and expansion of donor-derived cells are significantly slower than the rapid progression of the disease, and the treatment is not able to prevent the development of neuropathology [10].

ERT is based on the premise that LSDs could be treated by administering the recombinant functional enzyme to patients to compensate for their abnormal or defective protein. The concept was originally suggested by Christian de Duve in 1964 [11] and is supported by the discovery that many lysosomal proteins are targeted via the mannose-6-phosphate (M6P) receptor pathway [12]. According to the mechanism of 'cross-correction', the addition of a mannose group to the recombinant enzyme facilitates interaction with the mannose receptor on the surface of macrophages, allowing uptake by neighbouring cells and facilitating its transport to the lysosomes [13]. Alglucerase was the first recombinant enzyme approved for use in humans for the treatment of type 1 Gaucher disease in 1991 [14]. The enzyme was originally harvested from human placental tissue; however, subsequent therapies producing recombinant enzyme using gene activation technology in Chinese hamster ovary cells (Imiglucerase, Genzyme), human fibrosarcoma cells (Velaglucerase alfa, Takeda) or a carrot cell line (Taliglucerase alfa, Pfizer) are equally efficacious [15–17]. ERT is now considered the standard of care for many LSDs and is currently approved for the treatment of Fabry, Gaucher and Pompe diseases, alpha-mannosidosis, acid lipase deficiency, late infantile neuronal ceroid lipofuscinosis type 2 (CLN2) and mucopolysaccharidoses type I, II, IVA, VI and VII [18,19]. ERT is typically given by repeated intravenous (IV) administrations, but despite being effective, the regular nature of administration affects the quality of life of patients, as well as having a considerable economic impact on the health system [20]. In addition, repeated infusions of high concentrations of the recombinant enzyme can lead to the development of immune reactions to the protein requiring complex management [21,22]. Another drawback of this therapy is that it is unable to cross the BBB, therefore preventing treatment of the neurological phenotypes of some LSDs [19]. To overcome the limitations of using ERT to treat neuropathology, direct administration to the cerebral ventricles is successfully used to deliver the tripeptidyl peptidase 1 enzyme (cerliponase alfa, Brineura®) to CLN2 patients [23]. The nature of the affected tissue limits the use of ERT for certain LSDs, as some tissues can be refractive to penetration by most molecules [19], such as skeletal manifestations of Gaucher disease, cardiac valves in MPS or the neurological phenotype of many LSDs.

PCT involves the use of molecular chaperones that may stabilise conformation of unstable or misfolded proteins due to mutations that cause LSDs. This prevents rapid degradation of proteins and allows them to perform their enzymatic function [24]. The only approved therapy is Migalastat for the treatment of Fabry disease [25,26]; however, Ambroxol is currently in a phase 2 clinical trial (NCT03950050) as a potential therapeutic for type 1 Gaucher disease. The PCT approach shows promise, but its use is limited to mutations that affect only the stability of the mutant enzyme and may not be effective in those cases where the mutation affects the catalytic site of the protein. Endogenous molecular chaperone proteins can be activated in response to the heat shock response (HSR) following cellular stress or damage [27]. Heat Shock Protein 70 (HSP70) activators, such as the small molecule Arimoclomol (Orphazyme), can induce the chaperone response, promoting correct protein folding or clearance of damaged proteins in the cytosol. Arimoclomol is currently being investigated for the treatment of Niemann-Pick type C (NCT02612129) and Gaucher patients (NCT03746587).

SRT has been investigated as a potential therapy to treat neurological phenotypes. These small molecules aim to reduce accumulation of undegraded substrate by limiting its synthesis or the synthesis of its precursors [28,29]. Miglustat (Zavesca, Actelion Pharmaceuticals) and Eliglustat (Cerdelga, Sanofi Genzyme) have been approved for the treatment of type 1 Gaucher disease as second- and first-line therapies, respectively [30,31]. However, Miglustat has not been proven to be more efficacious than ERT [32]. Eliglustat is unable to cross the BBB and therefore cannot be used to treat neuronopathic forms of the disease. Miglustat has also been approved by the European Medicines Agency for the treatment of Niemann-Pick type C (NPC) as it showed a significant reduction in neurological disease progression [33].

Gene therapy is the delivery of nucleic acids to cells for patient benefit using viral or non-viral derived vectors. In the context of LSDs, this is usually delivery of a functional copy of the defective gene. LSDs are an ideal candidate disease group for gene therapy because they are typically well-characterised monogenic disorders for which the defective gene has been identified and animal models have been developed that allow for preclinical testing. For some disorders, the newly synthesized enzyme is secreted into systemic circulation for recapture and use by non-neighbouring cells. This 'cross-correction' process allows certain organs, such as the liver, to act as an enzyme factory where the protein is produced and delivered to other organs via blood circulation. Moreover, the amount of enzyme correction required to sufficiently clear the accumulating substrate is estimated to be between 1 and 10% of normal concentrations, although this will vary by disease [34]. Thus, a complete recovery of the physiological enzyme activity might not be needed to ameliorate disease phenotypes. However, those LSDs that are caused by defective membrane bound proteins that are not secreted are more challenging since there is no cross-correction. Ideal viral vector systems exploit the efficient ability of viruses to infect cells while preventing the expression of viral genes that can lead to replication and subsequent toxicity. Importantly, genes encoding replication and capsid or envelope functions are removed from the viral genome and provided in trans during the vector production process. Viral genes are replaced with the expression cassette sequences encoding the transgene of interest, promoter of choice and other regulatory elements. Great focus has been placed on vectors that avoid activation of oncogenes if nearby vector integration occurs and can control gene expression to target cells in order to prevent toxicity and the efficient gene transfer into these target cells, whether ex vivo or in vivo [35]. The most common viral vector systems used include retroviruses, lentiviruses, adenoviruses and adeno-associated viruses. Each of the different viral vector systems possesses certain characteristics that determine its suitability for specific applications (Table 1, Figure 1).

Table 1. Characteristics of the most used viral vectors in gene therapy for LSDs.

Vector	Size (nm)	Genome	Packaging Capacity (Kb)	Cell Type	Integration Profile
Retroviral	100	RNA	8	Dividing	Integrating
Lentiviral	100	RNA	14	Dividing and non-dividing	Integrating
Adenoviral	70–100	dsDNA	8–10	Dividing and non-dividing	Non-integrating
AAV	25–20	ssDNA	4.7	Dividing and non-dividing	Non-integrating

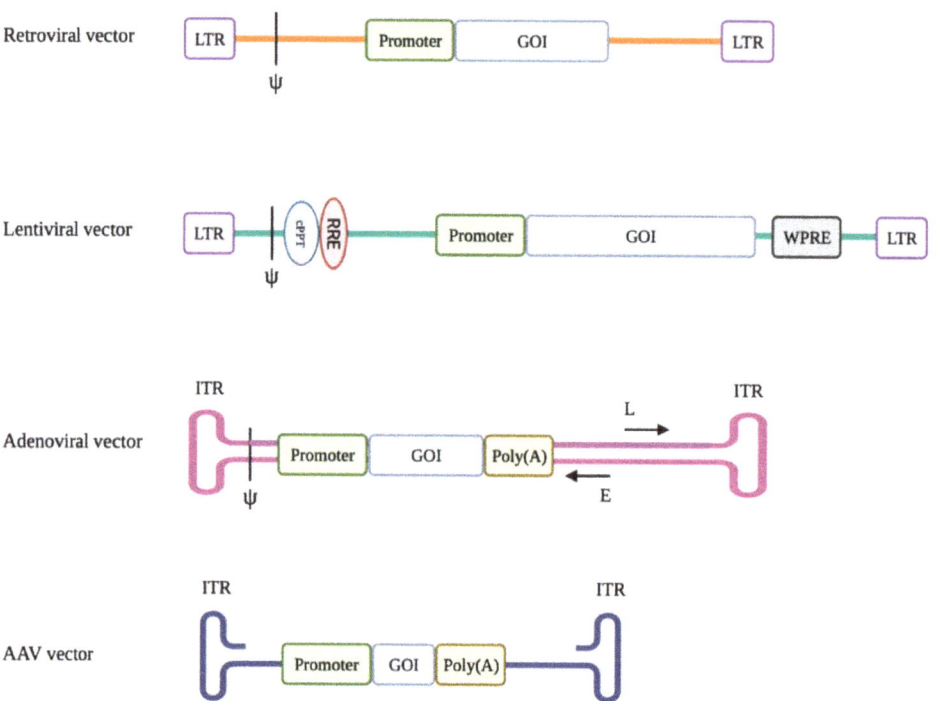

Figure 1. Schematic representation of the vector genomes (LTR: Long Terminal Repeat; Ψ: packaging signal; GOI: Gene of Interest; cPPT: central Polypurine Tract; RRE: rev-binding element; WPRE: Woodchuck Post-transcriptional Regulatory Element; ITR: Inverted Terminal Repeat; L: Late adenoviral genes; E: Early adenoviral genes).

1.1. Retroviral Vectors

Retroviruses are lipid-enveloped particles that contain a RNA genome. The viral envelope glycoprotein is responsible for interaction of the retroviral particles with receptors on target cells, thus controlling the host tropism and biodistribution [36]. Substitution of the receptor-binding proteins on the viral envelope with those from other, unrelated viral strains is known as pseudotyping [37]. This engineering strategy has been successfully used to expand the target range of retroviral vectors. Following entry into target cells, the RNA genome is retrotranscribed by reverse transcriptase into double-stranded linear DNA strands that then randomly integrate into the host genome [36]. While integration into the host genome enables long-term gene expression in dividing cells, possible insertion of genetic material near oncogenes could cause disease [38]. Moreover, further undesirable traits of retroviral vectors include their highly immunogenic nature and their ability to only transduce dividing cells [37]. Therefore, they are most commonly used for ex vivo applications.

1.2. Lentiviral Vectors

Lentiviruses are a genus of the retrovirus family. Lentivirus-based vectors mediate more stable transgene expression and efficient gene transfer than previous retroviral vectors [35]. The lentiviral genome has been engineered to contain self-inactivating long terminal repeats (LTRs), and the vectors have been shown to significantly reduce insertional genotoxicity [39–41]. The current generation of lentiviral vectors is based on the HIV type 1 virus, elements of which integrate into the host cell genome, posing a risk for clinical translation. Recently Vink and colleagues [42] described a novel lentiviral vector with reduced packaging of HIV-1 sequences within the LTRs. LTR1 vectors showed increased safety profile, titre and transgene expression. These vectors are widely used in the context of ex vivo gene therapy but have also been recently employed in in vivo trials where, when administered to the patient, they are able to give rise to robust and stable transgene expression [43,44]. Unlike retroviral vectors, such as gammaretroviral vectors, lentiviral vectors are able to transduce non-dividing cells by nuclear targeting using the nuclear import machinery of the host cell [45]. Moreover, these vectors do not usually induce a severe immune response upon administration. However, it is possible for T-cell responses to be activated against the transgene delivered by the vector. Lentiviral vectors pseudotyped with the G glycoprotein of the vesicular stomatitis virus (VSV-G) exhibit expanded tropism compared with the original HIV1-derived lentivirus [46]. Pseudotyping involves substituting the receptors of the original envelope with those from VSV-G, which may also improve the stability of the vector [46]. This vector has been successfully used, preclinically, in both in vivo and ex vivo applications. Lentivirus vectors have been used with resounding success clinically in ex vivo gene therapy, for example, in the treatment of primary immune deficiencies [47] and as an anti-cancer therapy in the generation of CAR T-cells [48].

1.3. Adenoviral Vectors

Adenoviruses are non-enveloped viruses with an icosahedral capsid containing a double-stranded DNA (dsDNA) genome [37]. More than 50 adenoviral serotypes derived from human and other species have been identified, and while the natural viruses cause disease in humans, they can be engineered and exploited to safely and efficiently deliver genes to a variety of cell types [36]. Unlike with retroviral vectors, a packaging cell line has not been engineered. To increase the carrying capacity of the vector, a helper-dependent vector system was developed [49], where a helper virus contains the genes needed for replication, thus allowing 28–32 kb of packaging capacity contained between two inverted terminal repeat sequences (ITRs) in a second vector. ITRs play a role in adenoviral DNA replication and transcriptional activity. This second vector also contains the normal packaging recognition signal, allowing its packaging and release from cells. Adenoviral vectors are considered to be among the most immunogenic of the viral vector groups, which limits their use for treatment of monogenic disease for in vivo gene therapy [50]. However, this makes them an excellent choice for use in oncolytic virotherapy [51] and as a vaccine against, for example, Severe Acute Respiratory Syndrome Coronavirus 2 SARS-Cov2 [52].

1.4. Adeno-Associated Viral Vectors

Adeno-associated viruses (AAVs) are part of the Parvoviridae family and are replication-deficient non-enveloped viruses. AAVs typically require a helper virus, such as the adenovirus, to facilitate infection. In the absence of a helper virus, the AAV genome remains latent in the host cell [53] in an episomal state. AAVs are not known to cause disease in humans, with 11 known human viral serotypes presenting wide and differential cellular tropism [54]. AAV2 is the most well-known serotype, and current AAV vectors are based on its genome. The wild-type AAV genome contains rep and cap genes that encode proteins involved in DNA replication [55] and capsid formation [56], respectively. The genome is flanked by 145-bp inverted terminal repeats (ITRs) which function in cis as packaging signals, denoting the coding region that will be packaged into the capsid and inserted into the host cell [57]. In recombinant AAV (rAAV) vectors, the rep and cap genes are provided in trans and are replaced with the transgene cassette that is flanked by the ITRs. Using this method, the recombinant AAV2 genome has successfully been packaged into various capsids of other serotypes, thus enhancing the tropism of this vector [58,59]. The rAAV system is the most promising for low-immunogenic [60], long-term gene expression [61,62] and is able to transduce a wide range of tissues. Similar to the lentivirus, wild-type AAV serotypes are not highly immunogenic. However, T-cell responses to the transgene may arise after administration of the AAV-based vector, particularly if the vector transduces cells that are involved in antigen presentation, such as dendritic cells [37,63]. It is important to note that majority of the human population has been exposed to wild-type AAV serotypes, and the prevalence of neutralizing anti-capsid antibodies is high [64,65]. Moreover, the development of neutralizing antibodies after the first administration in patients may hinder vector re-administration [66].

2. In Vitro Haematopoietic Stem Cell Gene Therapy

The theoretical basis of haematopoietic stem cell transplantation for LSDs lies in (1) identification of the M6P receptor pathway [67], through which lysosomal enzymes secreted by a cell can bind to the M6P receptor on the cell membrane of surrounding cells with subsequent uptake and transport to the lysosome and (2) transplanted haematopoietic stem cells (HSCs) or their progeny can settle in various tissues to contribute to the local macrophage populations and thus become sources of the required lysosomal enzyme.

The history of HSCT for LSDs started from conventional allogeneic HSCT, which employs HSCs from a healthy person to supply the lysosomal enzyme deficient in the transplant recipient. In the field of LSDs, conventional allogeneic HSCT has performed well in treating MPS I-H, which is caused by *IDUA* mutations resulting in alpha-L-iduronidase deficiency and affects multiple tissues including the central nervous system (CNS). The first trial was reported in 1981, which described biochemical and clinical improvements of an MPS I-H patient that received allogeneic HSCT at one year of age [68]. Since then, more HSCT has been performed for the treatment of MPS I-H, but the clinical outcomes are highly variable among patients as well as among different tissues, as reviewed by Aldenhoven et al. in 2008 [69]. More recently, a long-term longitudinal study including 217 patients from multiple clinical centres was reported to provide more information on the efficacy of allogeneic HSCT for treating MPS I-H [70]. Encouragingly, dramatic improvement of clinical course and lifespan was observed. However, a significant residual disease burden remained, and as lifespan was increased, various clinical manifestations emerged during long-term follow-up. In general, the outcomes of HSCT are affected by various aspects of the transplant such as haploidentity between the donor and recipient, severity of myeloablative conditioning, phenotypic severity at the age of HSCT, degree and persistence of donor chimerism and post-transplant complications [71,72]. A critical predictor for better outcome is sufficient circulating enzyme concentrations obtained post-HSCT, which could be affected by the degree of donor chimerism. This is particularly challenging in the CNS, and limited therapeutic benefits for the CNS are a relatively common finding from LSD treatment with HSCT.

Haematopoietic stem cell gene therapy (HSC-GT) holds great potential. An advantage of HSC-GT is the ability to perform autologous transplantation, which bypasses the difficulty in donor selection for allogeneic HSCT and avoids the risk of graft-versus-host disease. Addition of gene therapy to HSCT using viral vectors may provide supraphysiological expression of the required lysosomal enzymes as with other gene therapies. This is of particular interest for LSDs, as secretion of the therapeutic protein is enhanced due to gene overexpression in the transplanted cells, resulting in a higher degree of cross-correction. Considering the heredity of all LSDs, matched sibling donors (commonly employed in allogeneic HSCT) may also bear the disease mutation and thus cannot provide HSCs of sufficient therapeutic efficacy. The general approach of HSC-GT proceeds as follows: (1) autologous HSCs are collected from the patient, (2) collected HSCs are genetically corrected by transduction with a viral vector harbouring the therapeutic gene and (3) the transduced HSCs are transplanted back into the patient following transplant conditioning treatment similar to that required for HSCT. The most commonly used vectors for HSC-GT are lentiviral and gammaretroviral vectors. Both are able to transduce HSCs as well as to integrate into the host genome, allowing permanent target gene expression by transduced cells and, more importantly, by their progeny in the context of HSCT. However, genome integration is always a double-edged sword with risk of oncogenesis and mutagenesis over time, as discussed above. Thus, gene therapy employing these integrating vectors requires careful safety studies, preferentially with large-scale analysis and long-term follow-up. To date, clinical trials of HSC-GT have been initiated for treatment of various LSDs, including metachromatic leukodystrophy (MLD), MPS IIIA, MPS I-H, cystinosis, Gaucher disease and Fabry disease (Table 2).

Table 2. HSC-GT clinical trials recruiting LSDs patients or currently active (LV: lentiviral vector).

Disease	NCT Ref.	Intervention	Status	Est. Participants
MLD	NCT01560182	OTL-200 (autologous CD34$^+$ enriched cell fraction transduced with human ARSA LV)	Phase 1/2; Active, not recruiting	20
MLD	NCT03392987	OTL-200	Phase 2; Active, not recruiting	10
MLD	NCT04283227	OTL-200	Phase 3; Recruiting	6
MLD	NCT02559830	Transduced CD34$^+$ autologous HSCs	Phase 1/2; Recruiting	50
MPS IIIA	NCT04201405	Autologous CD34$^+$ cells transduced with the human SGSH LV	Phase 1/2; Recruiting	5
MPS I-H	NCT03488394	Autologous CD34$^+$ cells transduced with human IDUA LV	Phase 1/2; Recruiting	8
Cystinosis	NCT03897361	CTNS-RD-04 (autologous CD34$^+$ enriched cells transduced with human CTNS LV)	Phase 1/2; Recruiting	6
Fabry	NCT03454893	AVR-RD-01 (autologous CD34$^+$ cell-enriched fraction transduced with human AGA LV)	Phase 1/2; Recruiting	12
Gaucher	NCT04145037	AVR-RD-02 (autologous CD34$^+$ enriched HSCs transduced with human GBA gene LV)	Phase 1/2; Recruiting	16

2.1. Metachromatic Leukodystrophy (MLD)

One of the best examples of HSC-GT for treating LSDs, to date, is for metachromatic leukodystrophy. MLD is caused by a deficiency of arylsulfatase A (ARSA) due to mutations in the ARSA gene. ARSA is a soluble lysosomal enzyme with its lysosomal targeting dependent on the M6P receptor pathway. The physiological properties of ARSA, together with the extensive neurological involvement of MLD, offer hope for the disease to be a potential candidate for HSC-GT. Preclinical HSC-GT studies provided supportive data for clinical trials. Initially, Matzner et al. investigated HSC-GT using a mouse model of MLD and bone-marrow-derived HSCs transduced with a retroviral vector (murine stem cell virus, MSCV) harbouring the human ARSA gene [73–75]. Significant correction of lysosomal storage was observed in visceral organs such as the liver and kidney. However, improvement of CNS pathology and behavioural performance was only minor, despite the forebrain ARSA concentration in the treated MLD mice being increased to 10–33% of that of the wild-type. This may suggest that, for MLD, a better therapeutic outcome in the CNS may require even higher expression of the therapeutic enzyme and/or more extensive CNS microglia/macrophage reconstitution by progeny of the transduced HSCs allowing for broader cross correction. Furthermore, the authors found that although a long-term high bone marrow engraftment rate was obtained, the transduction efficiency and the quantity of transgene expression in the HSCs were highly variable and thus hampered consistency of the enzymatic correction, which could be at least partially due to the integration patterns of retroviral vectors. A few years later, Biffi et al. tested advanced-generation lentiviral vector-mediated HSC-GT in MLD mice [76,77] and achieved strikingly enhanced outcomes. They showed that both neurological pathology and behavioural performance were vastly improved, whether transplanted at the pre-symptomatic [76] or early-symptomatic [77] stage. Such corrections were not achieved by using conventional HSCT from wild-type donors without transduction, suggesting the importance of overexpressing the therapeutic gene to boost efficacy. Additionally, using the HSC-GT expressing HA-tagged ARSA gene, they detected ARSA in both microglia/macrophages in the CNS (representing transduced mononuclear cells engrafted into the CNS) and neurons plus other cell types (providing evidence for cross correction), whereas HSC-GT expressing *EGFP* resulted in GFP detection only in microglia/macrophages in the CNS [77]. Compared with previous studies, the therapeutic success of this work, as suggested by the authors, may lie in the more efficient HSC transduction and transgene overexpression by advanced-generation lentiviral vectors to reach the threshold enzyme concentrations required for a good therapeutic effect. This threshold could vary between different LSDs and thus should be investigated on a case-to-case basis.

Based on these preclinical studies, clinical trials have been performed to treat MLD patients. Promising outcomes have been reported from a phase 1/2 clinical trial of HSC-GT in MLD children (NCT01560182) [78,79]. MLD patients with mutations associated with early-onset MLD received HSC-GT transduced with lentiviral vectors harbouring human *ARSA* at pre-symptomatic or very early symptomatic stages, with myeloablative busulfan pre-transplant conditioning. The patients were then followed up for 18–54 months post transplantation. Stable engraftment of transduced HSCs was observed during follow-up, and ARSA activity was reconstituted to physiological or supra-physiological concentrations in haematopoietic cells and in the cerebrospinal fluid (CSF). The therapeutic efficacy was promising. Eight of nine patients showed prevention of disease onset or arrest of progression in accordance with clinical and instrumental assessment. In addition, skin biopsy exhibited occurrence of peripheral nerve remyelination in some of the patients. No serious adverse effects due to the medicinal product were reported during follow-up, and no haematopoietic malignancy was observed. The most frequent adverse events were cytopenia and mucositis, which are common complications of the chemotherapy conditioning for HSCT. A recent case report by Calbi et al. showed post-HSCT endothelial injury could be prevented by using Defibrotide and adjusting busulfan exposure to a lower but still myeloablative area under the curve (AUC) [80], as shown for other HSCT indications. To date, HSC-GT has shown exciting outcomes for MLD, which offers hope and valuable information for development of HSC-GT for other LSDs. In late 2020, the European Commission granted full market authorisation for Libmeldy (Orchard Therapeutics) for the treatment of MLD patients.

2.2. Mucopolysaccharidosis Type IIIA (MPS IIIA)

Recently, a phase 1/2 clinical trial was initiated (NCT04201405) for treatment of mucopolysaccharidosis type IIIA (MPS IIIA) [81]. MPS IIIA is a neurodegenerative LSD, caused by deficiency in the lysosomal enzyme *N*-sulfoglucosamine sulfohydrolase (SGSH) due to mutations in the *SGSH* gene. Patients usually have onset of disease in their first decade of life and present with heparan sulphate accumulation, progressive neurodegeneration and behavioural abnormalities, leading to death in their second decade. Currently most therapies for MPS IIIA are supportive treatments directed towards multisystem complications, whereas no effective disease-modifying therapy is available to prevent disease progression [81]. HSC-GT was initially investigated in an MPS IIIA mouse model but did not display dramatic therapeutic benefits [82]. The authors compared HSC-GT using wild-type donor cells transduced ex vivo with lentiviral vectors expressing SGSH (LV-WT-HSCT) or MPS IIIA deficient cells transduced ex vivo with lentiviral vectors expressing SGSH (LV-IIIA-HSCT) versus conventional wild-type donor cell transplant (WT-HSCT). Among these three strategies, the LV-IIIA-HSCT is apparently the best representative of autologous HSC-GT in humans which, however, showed no significant effect on behavioural performance, despite high bone marrow engraftment and the brain enzymatic activity correction to 7% of wild-type concentrations. The same research group then hypothesized that specifically enhancing the transgene expression in the myeloid lineage could make autologous HSC-GT more efficient in the myeloid precursors that can engraft in the brain, thus achieving better therapeutic benefits. Therefore, they optimised the vector by transducing MPS IIIA HSCs with a novel lentiviral vector containing a codon-optimized SGSH gene under the myeloid-specific CD11b promoter (instead of the ubiquitous phosphoglycerate kinase (PGK) promoter) [83]. While it was not clear whether engrafting cells would retain microglia characteristics (e.g., at the transcriptional level), the outcomes were promising; brain lysosomal storage accumulation, neuroinflammation and abnormal open-field behaviour of the MPS IIIA mice were all corrected. In preparations for clinical trials, the authors performed a further study to evaluate the efficiency of the CD11b vector in transducing human HSCs, as well as a safety study [84]. The authors showed that the clinical grade Good Manufacturing Practice (GMP) lentiviral vector expressing *SGHG* under the CD11b promoter could effectively transduce human HSCs, which could also be effectively scaled up for a sufficient dose necessary for the clinic. HSC-GT with this vector in a humanised mouse model resulted in effective engraftment and biodistribution, with no vector shedding or transmission to germline cells. The vector genotoxicity assay showed low transformation potential, which was comparable to other lentiviral vectors currently used in the clinic. Orchard Therapeutics has initiated a phase 1/2 clinical trial for autologous HSC-GT in MPS IIIA patients using this vector (ClinicalTrials.gov Identifier: NCT04201405). In summary, compared with other HSC-GT using ubiquitous promoters, this example offers evidence for a strategy using a myeloid-specific promoter to drive transgene expression as an alternative option of (1) boosting expression of the transgene in myeloid cells that engraft and differentiate into microglia-like cells in the CNS, which would be especially useful for LSDs with extensive CNS involvement and (2) preventing potential toxicity associated with supraphysiological enzyme concentrations in the general circulation.

2.3. Mucopolysacchridosis Type I, Hurler Variant (MPS I-H)

Although allogeneic HSCT has been used as a treatment, HSC-GT has also been studied for MPS I-H. The importance of studying HSC-GT in MPS I-H is to eliminate the problem of histocompatibility in allogeneic HSCT and to potentially provide higher concentrations of the therapeutic enzyme by overexpression for this most severe type of MPS I. An early study using an MPS I-H mouse model firstly evaluated potential therapeutic effects of HSC-GT mediated by an MND retroviral vector expressing the human *IDUA* gene [85]. The tissue concentrations of alpha-L-iduronidase activity achieved by *IDUA*-transduced HSCs were variable between experiments, but a significant reduction of glycosaminoglycan accumulation and histological improvement were consistently observed in visceral organs, with the exception of the brain. A few years later, a study led by Biffi et al. tested HSC-GT mediated by lentiviral vectors and showed complete therapeutic correction in a mouse model [86]. In particular, neurological and skeletal impairments, a challenge to conventional HSCT and other therapies, were successfully corrected. This example, as well as the HSC-GT studies in MLD, suggests that second-generation lentiviral vectors perhaps represent a more efficacious strategy than RVs in HSC-GT, especially for LSDs with CNS involvement. Additionally, with regard to the safety issue, lentiviral vectors show a lower risk of genotoxicity than retroviral vectors when used to transduce HSCs [39,87,88]. A phase 1/2 clinical trial was started in 2018 to evaluate the efficacy and safety of lentiviral vector-mediated autologous HSC-GT in the treatment of MPS I-H patients (ClinicalTrials.gov Identifier: NCT03488394). In early 2021, Orchard Therapeutics shared the first encouraging preliminary clinical data from the follow up of the initial proof-of concept study, showing sustained IDUA expression in the CSF and normalization of pathology biomarkers in all treated patients [89].

2.4. Gaucher Disease

Numerous and successful results in preclinical studies using a type 1 mouse model [90–92] demonstrated the feasibility and safety of HSC-GT for Gaucher patients. Gene therapy not only prevented disease development but resulted also in long-term amelioration of hepatosplenomegaly and blood parameters, correcting the already established phenotypes. Avrobio has initiated a phase 1/2 HSC-GT clinical trial (NCT04145037) where autologous CD34+ enriched HSCs are modified with a lentiviral vector and administered in conjunction with a conditioning regime to type 1 Gaucher subjects. The self-inactivating vector expresses a codon-optimised *GBA* sequence under the control of the elongation factor 1α short (EFS) promoter. The data on the first treated patient reported a significant decrease in the toxic metabolite Lyso-Gb1 and in the biomarker chitotriosidase, with consequent interruption of ERT [93]. Importantly this approach has the potential to improve bone mass and density; in fact, the skeletal system is usually not targeted by ERT, and bone crises are a common feature in the lives of Gaucher patients.

2.5. Cystinosis

Although the mechanism of 'cross-correction' is applicable for soluble enzymes, diseases caused by defects in transmembrane proteins can also be targeted with an ex vivo gene therapy approach. This is the case for cystinosis, a disease caused by mutations in the *CTNS* gene encoding the lysosomal membrane-specific transporter for cystine. Cystine accumulation appears in all tissues, and the major cause of death is severe renal damage. A preclinical study by Harrison et al. demonstrated in a *Ctns* deficient mouse model that HSCs transduced with a lentiviral vector expressing human *CTNS* were capable of achieving engraftment and expressing transgene in all tissues tested [94]. Cystine accumulation in tissues was largely reduced, including in the kidney. Renal function was assessed eight months post-transplantation, and in the treated *Ctns* deficient mice, serum creatinine, urine phosphate and urine volume were significantly decreased compared with non-treated *Ctns* deficient mice. To date, a phase 1/2 clinical trial has been initiated to evaluate the efficacy and safety of HSC-GT in cystinosis patients (ClinicalTrials.gov Identifier: NCT03897361).

2.6. Other Pre-Clinical Studies

In addition to MPS IIIA and I-H discussed above, HSC-GT has been studied in animal models for treating other MPS types such as MPS II [95–97], MPS IIIB [98,99] and MPS VII [100,101]. All these disorders involve the CNS, which likely makes them better candidates for HSC-GT because of the CNS engraftment of the enzyme-proficient donor HSCs. Although it has been revealed that the renewal and maintenance of microglia and other CNS myeloid cells are independent of circulating monocytes under physiological conditions [102], use of a myeloablating conditioning regimen prior to transplantation allows re-population of CNS myeloid cells with the donor immigrants [103], which then becomes the local source for the CNS enzyme correction. The majority of these studies utilised lentiviral vectors to transduce HSCs and showed therapeutic benefits, suggesting that HSC-GT appears to be a promising approach to treat LSDs with CNS involvement.

Numerous pre-clinical studies of HSC-GT have been performed in Pompe disease [104–107]. Pompe disease is caused by a deficiency of the acid alpha-glucosidase (GAA) enzyme due to mutations in the *GAA* gene, resulting in the accumulation of lysosomal glycogen in a variety of cell types. The typical cause of death in this disease is cardio-respiratory failure which results from hypertrophic cardiomyopathy and skeletal muscle weakness. An early study in the Netherlands [107] using a Pompe mouse model showed that HSC-GT with a lentiviral vector expressing *GAA* reversed cardiac remodelling and improved disease manifestations, without obvious toxicity caused by *GAA* overexpression. However, complete correction of lysosomal glycogen accumulation in the skeletal muscle and the CNS cells was not achieved, and motor performance was only partially improved. Recently, the same research group conducted an HSC-GT study for Pompe mice using a novel lentiviral vector expressing codon-optimised *GAA*, which resulted in significantly higher GAA activity in peripheral blood [106]. The treatment led to almost complete correction of glycogen accumulation in the heart, skeletal muscles, brain and other organs, as well as restoration of locomotor functions tested at 10–12 months post-transplantation. Furthermore, vector integration site analysis was performed and confirmed that none of the genes near common integration sites was an oncogene. These promising results appear to pave the way for clinical trials using this vector to treat Pompe disease.

2.7. Innovative Techniques

One of the major advantages of HSC-GT for LSDs compared to conventional HSCT is the ability to overexpress the therapeutic gene in the HSCs and their progeny. This results in higher enzyme concentrations and better cross-correction once the transgene-expressing cells repopulate various tissue compartments. HSC-GT is attractive for treating the neurological manifestation of the diseases compared to other therapies such as ERT that cannot cross the BBB and conventional HSCT which produces relatively lower enzyme levels in the CNS. As discussed above, obtaining sufficient tissue enzyme activity for clinical benefits is an important issue for some LSDs. This has been studied with various optimisiation methods, such as the careful selection of vectors and promoters and codon-optimisation of the gene sequence. There are also alternative approaches that have been studied in the field of LSDs. Gleitz et al. [95] investigated a lentiviral vector expressing the target gene fused with *ApoEII* for treating MPS II in animal models, which resulted in the human IDS protein fused to a receptor-binding domain of human ApoE. The theoretical basis of this experiment was the ability of the receptor-binding portion of ApoE to form a high-affinity binding complex with heparan sulphate, which could potentially promote cross-correction in addition to uptake via the M6P-R pathway. The plasma enzyme concentration and uptake across the BBB were elevated, whereas the enzymatic activity was not affected by this modification. When compared to HSCT without vector transduction and HSC-GT with a lentiviral vector expressing normal IDS in an MPS II mouse model, this IDS/ApoEII approach produced significantly enhanced therapeutic effects, resulting in complete correction of brain pathology and behaviour.

Gene editing techniques such as CRISPR-Cas have also been introduced to HSC-GT as an alternative to traditional viral vector-based gene augmentation. With this approach, the addition of the therapeutic gene is achieved by delivering the Cas9 nuclease and a short guide RNA (sgRNA) targeting a nonessential genomic sequence (a "safe harbour"), where an expression cassette (the therapeutic gene with a promoter) will be inserted. In vitro studies have already provided evidence for successful genetic modification of HSCs using CRISPR-Cas9 [108,109]. Very recently, two studies reported pre-clinical utilisation of CRISPR-Cas9 HSC-GT for MPS I [110] and Gaucher disease [111], which will be further discussed in the Gene Editing section of this review. These two studies have established a novel approach for HSC-GT, which is highly flexible and could serve as a platform to obtain supraphysiological expression of a therapeutic protein. Moreover, compared with HSC-GT driven by RV/LV vectors, it reduces the potential risk of toxic random genome integration, and the amount of transgene expression is more predictable and consistent because of limited insertion sites. However, off-target editing remains a concern.

In summary, HSC-GT is a valuable gene therapy approach for LSDs. Gene therapy overcomes limitations of allogeneic transplantation and allows amplified expression of the therapeutic gene. Cross-correction via the M6P-R-pathway which is used by many lysosomal proteins, makes it possible to treat disease by correcting a proportion of deficient cells, especially when the therapeutic protein is overexpressed in those cells via gene therapy. In the CNS, HSC-GT is a potentially good option compared to ERT since the recombinant enzyme does not cross the BBB, and to conventional HSCT which shows limited efficacy in the CNS. HSC-GT research is particularly important for LSDs involving extensive pathologies in both the CNS and the periphery, whereas for disease predominantly affecting the brain rather than other organs, direct gene therapy targeting the brain might be more beneficial. Several attempts have been made to improve HSC-GT, as discussed above, and promising results have emerged and paved the way. In the future, several uncertainties or limitations will need to be better addressed: long-term efficacy follow-up and safety analysis, particularly with regard to viral genome integration and transgene overexpression, optimisation of current approaches and technology to better regulate the transgene expression and improve therapeutic effects and reducing complications related to pre-conditioning for transplantation.

3. In Vivo Gene Therapy

In vivo gene transfer therapies are based on the ability to introduce the therapeutic genetic material into affected tissues by direct administration into the patient (Figure 2). While ex vivo gene therapy represents a feasible therapeutic approach mostly for secreted enzyme deficiencies, direct administration of gene therapy vectors has now been successfully applied in many pre-clinical and clinical studies. Notably, with significant advances in vector technology and production, in vivo gene transfer has emerged as a safe and efficient technique to target the nervous system.

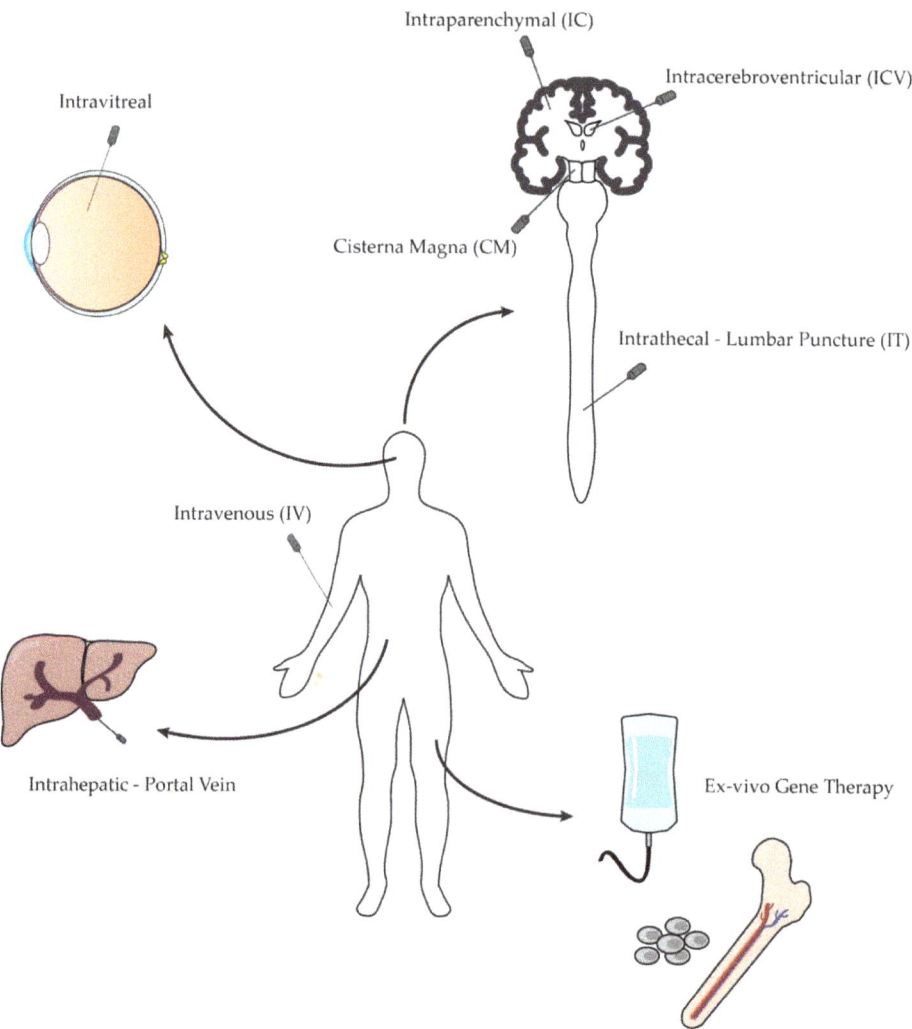

Figure 2. Main routes of administration for in vivo gene delivery to LSDs patients.

3.1. Systemic Administration

While enzyme replacement therapy is an effective treatment option, systemic gene delivery offers the opportunity for a sustained therapeutic effect comparable to long-term effects of ERT, with a single or limited number of administrations and the additional prospect of treating the CNS. The earliest vectors used for systemic delivery were based on or derived from the retroviral Moloney murine leukaemia virus. These vectors have been used to deliver the *IDUA* gene to MPS I mice [112,113] via injection into the temporal vein of neonates. Although the visceral pathology was partially rescued, a high dose was required to achieve sufficient expression, particularly in the brain. The ability of retroviral vectors to transduce only dividing cells limits their possible application for the treatment of the CNS. Similar effects were achieved when neonatal MPS VII mice were administered a high dose vector expressing the *GUSB* gene [114,115]. Similarly, neonatal MPS VII dogs injected systemically with a retroviral vector expressing the canine β-glucuronidase gene showed significant improvement in body weight, bone and joint abnormalities, motor coordination and visual impairment [116]. While neonatal gene therapy can lead to improvements in the viscera and brain, adult systemic administration of retroviral vectors can cause extensive cytotoxic T lymphocyte immune response if not combined with immunosuppressant treatment [117].

Gammaretroviral vectors have been succeeded by lentiviral vectors based on immunodeficiency viruses and have the ability to also transduce non-dividing cells. Lentiviruses show the ability to efficiently transduce hepatocytes following systemic administration. In fact, gene therapy targeted to the growing liver exploits clonal expansion of the transduced hepatocytes, resulting in high gene expression in the liver. A lentiviral vector based on the feline immunodeficiency virus FIV was first used to deliver the β-glucuronidase gene to MPS VII adult mice with the aim of providing sustained therapeutic enzyme following liver transduction [118]. Further optimisation led to the development of lentiviral vectors based on the human HIV-1 virus and their application for in vivo pre-clinical studies. A Pompe disease mouse model was treated intravenously on the day of birth with an HIV-1 based lentiviral vector expressing human *GAA* [119]. Then, 24 weeks after administration, glycogen accumulation was partially cleared in cardiac and skeletal muscles. Importantly, neonatal gene transfer elicited only a minimal antibody response despite expressing the GAA enzyme at supraphysiological concentrations. Systemic administration of lentiviral vectors expressing the IDUA gene to both neonatal [120] and adult [121] MPS I knock-out mice resulted in decreased GAG storage and improved survival. In treated animals, 1% of physiological enzymatic activity was sufficient to normalise substrate concentrations in the urine, liver and spleen. However, six months after adult injections, enzyme-specific antibodies were found to be present, causing loss of therapeutic protein expression in evaluated tissues. Conversely, seven months post-administration, long-term expression was detected in the visceral organs of adult MPS IIIB [122] and IIIA mice injected with a lentiviral vector expressing the murine sulphamidase gene [123,124]. Interestingly, these two studies from the same research group reported contrasting results regarding the effects of the therapy on the central nervous system pathology. Partial correction of the brain pathology following systemic gene therapy was achieved when the murine β-glucuronidase gene was delivered to adult MPS VII mice up to seven months after gene transfer [125]. The authors suggested that the enzyme is mainly produced in the viscera and transferred across the BBB via the mannose-6-phosphate/insulin-like growth factor 2 receptor. In addition, the expression of enzymes from transduced cells of haematopoietic origin might have further contributed to improve CNS pathology.

Adenoviral vectors have also been employed to deliver the β-glucuronidase gene to MPS VII mice [126,127], with resulting elevation of enzymatic activity in the liver and spleen. However, systemic administration of the vector failed to improve pathology within the brain. Preferential liver transduction following IV injections of the adenoviral vector was also reported in Tay-Sachs adult mice co-administered with vectors coding for both α- and β-subunits [128]. Similarly, hepatomegaly was rescued by adenoviral vector-mediated delivery of the human *LIPA* gene in a mouse model of lysosomal acid lipase (LAL) deficiency [129]. A single intravenous injection of an adenoviral vector allowed for *GAA* expression in multiple muscle groups in a quail model of Pompe disease [130] and *GAA*-knock-out mice [131,132]. In these studies, the efficient hepatic transduction following systemic gene delivery led to secretion of the enzyme at high concentrations into the plasma of treated animals, with uptake into both skeletal and cardiac muscle.

With their wide cellular tropism, low toxicity and sustained gene-expression, recombinant AAV vectors represent a compelling candidate for systemic (IV) gene delivery. Although capsids such as AAV8 and AAV9 preferentially transduce liver and muscle [133], a more modest increase in enzyme concentrations in other tissues can also contribute to reducing the amount of accumulating substrates and treating the visceral component of the diseases in different models (Table 3). Efficient and widespread visceral expression following systemic administration is achieved in a dose-dependent manner. Recent advances in the ability to produce recombinant AAV vectors at a fairly large scale has resulted in the translation of many pre-clinical studies to clinical trials. The use of AAV systemic gene therapy in paediatric patients is possibly the first step in applying this approach for LSDs within the clinic. Sio Gene Therapies in collaboration with the National Human Genome Research Institute is investigating the efficacy of intravenous high-dose (1.5×10^{13} to 4.5×10^{13} vg/kg) AAV9 gene therapy in infantile (6–12 months) type I and young (2–12 years) type II GM1 gangliosidosis patients (NCT03952637). Despite the challenges associated with manufacturing of the ever larger batches of the viral vector required for intravenous delivery in the clinic, several clinical trials involving adult patients are currently on-going. Adult Fabry disease patients have received AAV6 (NCT04046224) or other engineered capsids (NCT04040049, NCT04519749) with the aim to test safety and tolerability of the treatment following a single intravenous injection. Similarly, two phase I/II clinical trials delivering AAV8 to adults with late onset Pompe disease (NCT04093349, NCT04174105), and a self-complementary AAV9 vector to MPSIIA patients (NCT04088734 and long-term follow up NCT02716246) are now active and remain ongoing.

Table 3. Overview of some AAV pre-clinical studies using systemic gene delivery to treat various animal models of LSDs (vg: vector genomes; gc: genome content, equivalent of vg; iu: infective units; P: Post-natal day).

Delivery Route	Disease	Species	Model	Vector	Dose	Time of injection	Ref.
Tail Vein	Gaucher	Mouse	UBC-creERT2-Gba$^{flox/flox}$	AAV9-CMV-Gba or AAV9-SYN-Gba	3–5×10^{11} vg	4 weeks	[134]
	GM1	Mouse	C57BL/6J-$\beta gal^{-/-}$	AAV9-CAG-βgal	1×10^{11} or 3×10^{11} vg	6 weeks	[135]
	GM2 (Sandhoff)	Mouse	C57BL/6C129-Hexb$^{-/-}$	AAV9-CMV-HEXB	2.5×10^{14} or 3.5×10^{13} vg/kg	P1 or 6 weeks	[136]
	GM2 (Sandhoff)	Mouse	Hexb$^{-/-}$	AAV9 or PHP.B-BiCBA-mHEXA/mHEXB, AAV9 or PHP.B-P2-HEX	AAV9: 1×10^{12}–4×10^{12} vg; PHP.B: 3×10^{11}–1×10^{12} vg	4 weeks	[137]
	Krabbe	Mouse	C57BL-twi/twi	AAVhr10-CAG-mGALC	2×10^{11} vg	P10–12	[138]
	MPS I	Mouse	C57BL/6-Idua$^{-/-}$	AAV9-CAG-IDUA or AAVh10-CAG-IDUA	1×10^{12} vg	8–21 weeks	[139]
	MPS II	Mouse	ids$^{y/-}$	AAV8-EF1α-IDS	1×10^{11} vg	NA	[140]
	MPS IIIA	Mouse	C57BL/6-Sgsh$^{-/-}$	scAAVh74-U1a-hSGSH	5×10^{12} vg/kg	4–6 weeks	[141]
	MPS IIIA	Mouse	C57BL/6-Sgsh^{G91A}	AAV9-CAG-mSGSH	1×10^{12} vg/kg	2 months	[142]
	MPS IIIB	Mouse	C57BL/6-Naglu$^{-/-}$	AAV9-CAG-hNAGLU	1×10^{13} vg/kg	4–6 weeks	[143]
	MPS IIIB	Mouse	C57BL/6-Naglu$^{-/-}$	AAV2-CMV-hNAGLU	4×10^{11} vg	4–6 weeks	[144]
	MPS VII	Mouse	b6.C-H-abm1/byBir-gus$^{mps/mps}$	AAV9-βGluc	1×10^{12} vg	6 weeks	[145]
Temporal/Cephalic Vein	Gaucher	Mouse	CD1-K14-ln/ln	AAV9-GUSB-hGBA1	4×10^{11} gc	P0–P1	[146]
	Gaucher	Mouse	CD1-K14-ln/ln	AAV9-SYN-hGBA1	2.4×10^{12} vg	P0–P1	[147]
	MPS I	Mouse	Idua$^{-/-}$	AAV2-CAG-hIDUA	10^{10} vp	P1–P2	[148]
	MPS II	Mouse	ids$^{y/-}$	AAV5-CMV-hIDS	1×10^{11} vg	P2	[149]
	MPS VII	Mouse	B6.C-H-2bm1/ByBir-gus$^{mps/mps}$	AAV-CAG-hGUSB	5×10^{9} iu/kg	P2	[150]
	MPS VII	Mouse	B6.C-H-2bm1/ByBir-gus$^{mps/mps}$	AAV-CAG-hGUSB	8×10^{10} iu/kg	P2	[151]
	MSD	Mouse	C57B6/S129J-Sgsh$^{-/-}$	AAV9-CMV-hSUMF1	2×10^{11} vg	P1	[152]
Jugular Vein	MLD	Mouse	C57BL/6-ASA$^{-/-}$	AAV9-CAG-hARSA	2×10^{12} vg	P1–2	[153]
Retro-orbital Sinus	Pompe	Mouse	C57BL/6J-GAA$^{-/-}$	AAV-PHP.B-CAG-hGAA	5×10^{12} vg/kg	2 weeks	[154]
Combination							
IV + ICV	MSD	Mouse	C57B6/S129J-Sgsh$^{-/-}$	AAV9-CMV-hSUMF1	IV: 2×10^{11} vg; ICV: 6×10^{9} vg	P1	[152]
IV + IT	MPS VII	Mouse	C57BL6/J-Gus$^{b/b}$	AAV2-CMV-GUSB	IV: 4.1×10^{11} vg; IT: 3×10^{10} vg	P3–P4	[155]
IV + CM	MPS IIIB	Mouse	C57BL/6-Naglu$^{-/-}$	AAV2-CMV-hNAGLU	IV: 4×10^{11} vg; CM: 5×10^{10} vg	4–8 weeks	[156]

The ability of AAV vectors, particularly AAV9, to transduce neurons following systemic administration to animal models [157] and the recent commercialisation of Zolgensma for spinal muscular atrophy in paediatric patients have provided significant evidence to justify the use of AAV vectors as a therapeutic option for LSDs with neuropathology. However, the dose required to achieve sufficient and extensive CNS expression via intravenous administration is high and raises concerns around toxicity [158]. Severe adverse events have been reported in different clinical trials where relatively high doses of the vector (6.7×10^{13}–3×10^{14} vg/kg) were administered to neonates and children, ranging from elevated serum transaminase in the SMA1 Novartis trial (NCT03306277), complement activation and acute kidney injury in the Duchenne Muscular Dystrophy trial (NCT03362502) to death from sepsis [159] in the recent ASPIRO trial (NCT03199469). As a result of a T cell-mediated immune response to high amounts of capsid antigen, hepatotoxicity is the most common adverse effect in systemic gene therapy trials [160]. This immune response is not always evident in animal models; therefore, pre-clinical studies might fail to predict the adverse effects developed by patients during trials.

Although systemic administration is arguably the most feasible approach to target diseases caused by deficiencies in secreted enzymes, gene delivery has also been used to successfully treat lysosomal defects involving membrane-bound proteins. Neonatal NPC mice received a retro-orbital injection of AAV9 vectors expressing the human NPC1 gene [161]. Treatment with vectors containing both the neuronal-specific and the ubiquitous promoter vector resulted in increased life span, reduction in cholesterol storage in the liver and a variable degree of cholesterol reduction in the brain.

3.2. Organs as Enzyme Factories for Systemic Expression
3.2.1. Liver

The selective targeting of organs in order to produce and secrete therapeutic proteins into the bloodstream is an attractive approach to treat systemic diseases such as LSDs. Highly vascularised organs, such as the liver or the lungs, are prime candidates for this gene transfer modality. The development of a successful gene therapy for haemophilia A [62] and B [162] demonstrated that hepatocytes can be easily transduced following intravenous injection, ensuring safe and long-term transgene expression. Systemic delivery has proved to be a non-invasive delivery route, which provides the same liver transduction efficiency as direct intrahepatic administration [163]. In addition, the intravenous route allows the delivery of high doses of vectors, therefore achieving widespread and efficient transduction. However, this can come at the cost of a possible immune reaction [164,165].

While the initial choice of serotype was the early characterised AAV2, other capsids such as AAV8, AAV3B and novel engineered vectors including LK03 [166] or NP59 [167] have recently shown superior transduction efficiency in mouse and human hepatocytes. This approach was successful in rescuing a mouse model of Pompe disease following systemic delivery of an AAV8 vector that expressed an engineered acid-α-glucosidase protein secreted by hepatocytes [168]. Freeline Therapeutics has recently used both AAV8 and novel capsid AAVS3 to deliver a *GBA* vector to cells and mice in a proof-of-concept study, supporting the development of a liver-directed therapy for Gaucher disease [169]. In addition, liver-specific promoters have been designed to further improve efficacy and safety, as demonstrated in pre-clinical studies in Fabry disease [170,171], Gaucher disease [172] and Pompe disease [173,174] mouse models. Notably, systemic administration of low-dose AAV8 containing a liver-specific promoter did not result in a detectable immune response in Pompe mice, in contrast with the elevated rate of anti-GAA antibody formation following ERT administration [175]. The safety and bioactivity of an AAV8 vector expressing the human *GAA* gene under control of a liver-specific promoter are currently being assessed in a clinical trial on late-onset Pompe patients (NCT03533673). A similar approach has been tested in MPS I cats [176], and MPS VI mice [177] and cats [178] where gene expression was controlled by the thyroxine binding globulin (TBG) liver promoter. Gene therapy reduced GAG accumulation and corrected the aortic valve lesions in treated cats. The authors briefly addressed the possible effects of AAV8-mediated liver-directed gene therapy in the CNS of MPS I cats. Interestingly, although GAG storage was substantially improved in the meninges, there was no detectable improvement in the brain parenchyma and corneas of injected animals. This AAV8-based vector has been administered to MPS IV patients in a multi-centre phase I/II clinical trial (NCT03173521).

Intraparenchymal administration of an AAV2 vector expressing the murine β-glucuronidase gene to MPS VII mice resulted in increased quantities of enzyme in the viscera as a consequence of both direct transduction of extrahepatic organs and circulation of the enzyme produced in the liver through the bloodstream [179]. Interestingly, a high dose of vector partially improved the pathology in some brain regions, reducing storage accumulation in the cortex, corpus callosum and striatum.

For devastating diseases with rapid progression such as most acute forms of LSDs, early intervention is essential to prevent the development of severe pathology and ultimately early death. As already mentioned, viral gene delivery to paediatric patients presents the advantage of preventing or slowing the accumulation of macromolecules at an early stage, when the pathology is not extensive and the progression might still be reversible. Additionally, neonates are more likely to have not yet developed antibodies [180] or T cell immunity to the viruses, allowing safe and efficient administration of high doses of the vector. Liver-directed gene delivery to neonatal MPS I mice using retroviral vectors has been attempted in the past [113]. The early intervention led to high *IDUA* expression in the plasma, completely correcting cardiac, bone, eye and ear manifestations eight months post-administration. Rucker and colleagues raised the idea of early intervention by delivering an AAV vector expressing the human *GAA* gene to the liver of fetal Pompe mice [181].

Although prenatal and neonatal/paediatric application is an attractive prospect for liver-targeted gene therapy, one has to consider that the fast cell proliferation rate and turnover of hepatocytes can lead to a loss of vector genomes when using vectors considered to be non-integrating such as AAVs [182]. There are also safety concerns around the possible genotoxic effects of AAV-mediated gene therapy and its potential connection with hepatocellular carcinoma [183,184].

3.2.2. Lungs

The lung can also be used as a metabolic factory for targeting systemic diseases, exploiting its large surface and extensive vascularisation. In fact, nasal delivery is a non-invasive technique that results in systemic gene expression and might offer the possibility of safe re-administration [185]. An adenoviral vector expressing α-galactosidase A was delivered via inhalation to a Fabry mouse model, resulting in increased enzymatic concentrations in some visceral organs, including the heart, liver and spleen [186]. Interestingly, no viral DNA was detected in the viscera, confirming the enzyme was produced and secreted from the lung and then taken up by other organs.

3.2.3. Muscle

Skeletal muscle has also been considered a potential organ factory to produce lysosomal enzymes, especially as certain AAV serotypes are particularly efficient in transducing myofibers [187]. Intramuscular injections of AAV vectors have been used to deliver recombinant enzyme to the systemic circulation in murine models of MPS VII [188] and Pompe disease [189]. Overall, gene transfer resulted in strong expression in the muscle and increased amounts of enzyme in some visceral organs. However, the therapeutic efficacy was not always sufficient for reversing the pathology in organs distant from the site of injection. On the other hand, muscle-directed gene transfer resulted in long-term expression of circulating enzyme in a Fabry mouse model [190], proving that intramuscular administration might be effective for certain lysosomal disorders.

3.3. CNS-Directed Gene Therapy

While different gene therapy strategies have been effective in improving the majority of visceral manifestations, the severe neuropathology that characterises many LSDs remains a significant issue for the treatment of these patients. Drug delivery to the central nervous system, particularly to the brain, is challenging because of its unique complexity and limited access through physical barriers such as the skull and the BBB. In the last two decades, AAVs have been the vectors of choice for most of the CNS-directed gene therapy studies (Table 4).

Table 4. Selection of the most relevant pre-clinical studies on CNS-directed gene therapy in animal models of LSDs using AAV vectors (vg: vector genomes; gc: genome content, equivalent of vg; vp: viral particles; iu: infective units; pu: purified units; P: Post-natal day; E: Embryonic day; NHP: non-human primate).

Delivery Route	Disease	Species	Model	Vector	Dose	Time of injection	Ref.
Intraparenchymal (IC)							
	CLN1 Batten	Mouse	C57BL/6-Ppt1$^{-/-}$	AAV9-CAG-hPPT1	1×10^{12} vg/mL	P1	[191]
	CLN2 Batten	Mouse	C57BL/6-CLN2$^{-/-}$	AAV2 or AAV5-CAG-hCLN2	3.6×10^9 gc	6 or 10 weeks	[192]
	CLN2 Batten	Mouse	C57BL/6:129Sv-TPP1$^{-/-}$	AAV2 or AAV5-CAG-hCLN2	1.2–3.6×10^9 gc	6 or 10 weeks	[192]
	CLN3 Batten	Mouse	C57BL/6N-Cln3$^{\Delta ex7/8}$	AAVrh10-CAG-hCLN3	3×10^{10} gc	P2	[193]
	Gaucher	Mouse	GBA$^{L444P/L444P}$	AVV5-CAG-hGBA	3.5×10^{13} vg/mL	8 months	[194]
	GM1	Mouse	C57BL/6-βgal$^{-/-}$	AAV1-CAG-mβgal	4×10^{10} gc	6–8 weeks	[195]
	GM2 (Sandhoff)	Mouse	C57BL/6-Hexb$^{-/-}$	AAV1-HEXA and AAV1-HEXB	9.9×10^9 and 1.4×10^{10} gc	1 month	[196]
	Krabbe	Mouse	C57BL/6-twi^{W339X} or C57BL/129SVJ/FVB/N-twi-trs	AAV1-CMV-mGALC	3×10^{10} vp	P0–P1	[197]
	Krabbe	Mouse	B6.CE-Galc^{twi}/J	AAV2 or AAV5-CAG-GALC	5.5×10^6 iu	P3	[198]
	MLD	Mouse	C57BL/6J-ASA$^{-/-}$	AAVrh10-CAG-hARSA or AAV5-PGK-hARSA	2.3×10^9 vg	8 and 16 months	[199]
	MPS I	Mouse	C57BL/6-Idua$^{-/-}$	AAV2 or AAV5-PGK-hIDUA	10^9 vg	6–7 weeks	[200]
	MPS I	Mouse	C57BL/6-Idua$^{-/-}$	AAV2 or AVA5-mPGK-hIDUA	10^9 vg	6–7 weeks	[200]
	MPS IIIA	Mouse	C57BL/6-Sgsh$^{-/-}$	AAVrh10-PGK-SGSH-IRES-SUMF1	7.5×10^9 gc	5 weeks	[201]
	MPS IIIA	Mouse	C57BL/6-Sgsh$^{-/-}$	AAVrh10-CMV-SGSH-IRES-SUMF1	7.5×10^9 gc	5 weeks	[201]
	MPS IIIA	Mouse	C57BL/6-Sgsh$^{-/-}$	AAVrh10-CAG-hSGSH	$8.4 \times 10^8, 4.1 \times 10^{10}, 9 \times 10^{10}$ vg	5–6 weeks	[202]
	MPS IIIB	Mouse	C57BL/6-Naglu$^{-/-}$	AAV2 or AAV5-mPGK-hNAGLU	10^9 vg	6 weeks	[203]
	MPS IIIB	Mouse	C57BL/6-Naglu$^{-/-}$	AAV5-CAG-hNAGLU	1.8×10^{10} vp	P2–4	[204]
	MPS IIIC	Mouse	Hgsnat$^{-/-}$	AAV2TT-CAG-hcoHGSNAT	5.2×10^9 vg	8 weeks	[205]
	MPS VII	Mouse	B6.C-H-2^{bm1}/byBirgus^{mps}/+	AAV5-RSV-GUSB	3×10^9 vg	6–8 weeks	[206]
	MPS VII	Mouse	C3H/HeOuJ-Gusb^{mps-2J}	AAV1, AAV9 or AAVrh10-GUSB-hGUSB	1.2–1.3×10^{10} vg	>2 months	[207]
	NP-A	Mouse	C57BL/6-ASMKO$^{-/-}$	AVV2-CMV-hASM	1.86×10^{10} gc	10 weeks	[208]
	GM1	Cat	fGM1	AAV1 or AAVrh8-CAG-fβgal	$3 \times 10^{11}, 4 \times 10^{12}$ or 1.2×10^{13} vg	1.3–3 months	[209]
	GM2 (Sandhoff)	Cat	fG$_{M2}$	AAV1-CAG-fHEXA/B or AAV8-DC172-HEXA/B	3×10^{11}– 3.2×10^{12} vg	0.9–2.6 months	[210]
	GM2 (Sandhoff)	Cat	fG$_{M2}$	AAVrh8-CAG-HEXA, AAVrh8-CAG-HEXB	1.6–4.5×10^{11} vg	1 month	[211]
	MPS I	Dog	IDUA$^{-/-}$	AAV5-PGK-hIDUA	5×10^{11}– 2.1×10^{12} vg	18–30 months	[212]
	MPS IIIB	Dog	Schipperke Naglu$^{-/-}$	AAV5-PGK-hNAGLU	5×10^{11}– 2.1×10^{12} vg	18–30 months	[212]
	CLN2 Batten	Rat	Fisher 344	AAV2-CAG-TPP1	10^9–10^{10} pu	NA	[213]
	CLN2 Batten	NHP	C. sabaeus	AAV2-CAG-TPP1	3.6×10^{11} pu	5–10 years	[213]
Intrathecal (IT)							
	Krabbe	Mouse	B6.CE-Galc^{twi}/J	AAV9, AAVrh10 or AAVOlig001-CAGGS-mβgal	2×10^{11} vg	P10–11	[214]
	MPS I	Mouse	C57BL/6-IDUA$^{-/-}$	AAV2-CMV-hIDUA	2×10^9–4×10^{10} vp	2–4 months	[215]

Table 4. Cont.

Delivery Route	Disease	Species	Model	Vector	Dose	Time of injection	Ref.
	MPS VII	Mouse	$Gusb^{-/-}$	AAV2-CMV-mGUSB	1×10^{11} and 5×10^{11} vp	P3 and 7–13 weeks	[216]
	GM1	Cat	$\beta gal^{-/-}$	AAVrh10-βgal	1×10^{12} vg/kg	NA	[217]
	MPS I	Cat	$IDUA^{-/-}$	AVV9-IDUA	1×10^{12} gc/kg	NA	[218]
Cisterna Magna (CM)							
	MPS IIIA	Mouse	C57BL/6-$SGSH^{D31N}$	AAV9-CAG-mSgsh	5×10^9–5×10^{10} vg	2 months	[219]
	MPS IIIB	Mouse	C57BL/6-$Naglu^{-/-}$	AVV9-CAG-mNaglu	3×10^{10} vg	2 months	[220]
	MPS IIID	Mouse	C57BL/6NTac-$Gns^{tm1e(EUCOMM)Hmgu}$	AAV9-CAG-mGns	5×10^{10} vg	2 months	[221]
	Pompe	Mouse	6neo/6neo	AAV9 or AAVrh10-CAG-hGAA	10^{11} vg	1 month	[222]
	AMD	Cat	$MANB^{-/-}$	AAV1-GUSB-fMANB	1×10^{13} gc	4–6 weeks	[223]
	GM1	Cat	$\beta gal^{-/-}$	AAVrh10-βgal	1×10^{12} vg/kg	NA	[217]
	MPS I	Cat	$IDUA^{-/-}$	AAV9-CB-fIDUA, AAV9-CMV-fIDUA	10^{12} gc/kg	4–7 months	[224]
	MPS I	Dog	$IDUA^{-/-}$	AAV9-CAG-IDUA	10^{12} gc/kg	1 month	[225]
	MPS I	Dog	$IDUA^{-/-}$	AAV9-CAG-IDUA	10^{11}–10^{12} gc/kg	1 month	[226]
	MPS VII	Dog	$GUSB^{-/-}$	AAV9 or AAVrh10-CAG-caGUSB	5×10^{12} gc/kg	3 weeks	[227]
Intracerebroventricular (ICV)							
	CLN6 Batten	Mouse	$Cln6^{nclf}$	AAV9-CMV-hCLN6	5×10^{10}–5×10^{11} vg	P0	[228]
	CLN8 Batten	Mouse	C57BL/6J-$Cln8^{mnd}$	AAV9.pT-MecP2.CLN8	5×10^{10} vg	P0–P1	[229]
	Gaucher	Mouse	CD1-K14-ln/ln	AAV9-GUSB-hGBA1	5×10^{10} gc	E16 and P0	[146]
	GM1	Mouse	$\beta gal^{-/-}$	AAV1-CAG-mβgal	3.2×10^9 vg	P0	[230]
	Krabbe	Mouse	C57BL/6-twi^{W339X} or C57BL/129SVJ/FVB/N-twi-trs	AAV1-CMV-mGALC	3×10^{10} vp	P0–P1	[197]
	MLD	Mouse	C57BL/6J-$Asra^{tm1Gie}$	AAV1-CAG-ARSA	2×10^{11} vg	8–12 weeks	[231]
	MLD	Mouse	C57BL/6J-$Asra^{tm1Gie}$	AAV1, 9-CAG-ARSA	1.1×10^{11}–2.3×10^{11} vg	8 and 18 weeks	[232]
	MPS I	Mouse	C57BL/6-$IDUA^{-/-}$	AAV8-CAG-hIDUA	2×10^{10} vg	P4-P6	[233]
	MPS I	Mouse	C57BL/6-$IDUA^{null}$	AAV5-CBA-hIDUA	1×10^{11} vp	8–11 weeks	[234]
	MPS IIIA	Mouse	B6Cg-$Sgsh^{(mps3/Pstl)}$	AAV5-CMV-SGSH-IRES-SUMF1	6×10^9–3×10^{10} vp	P0	[235]
	MPS III A	Mouse	B6Cg-$Sgsh^{(mps3a/Pstl)}$	AAV9-CMV-IDSspSGSH-IRES-SUMF1	5.4×10^{12} gc/kg	P60	[236]
	MPS VII	Mouse	C3H/HeOuJ-$Gusb^{mps-2J}$	AVV1, 2, 5-GUSB-GUSB	1.8×10^{10} vg	P0	[237]
	MPS VII	Mouse	B6.C-H-2^{bm1}/byBirgus^{mps}/+	AAV4-RSV-hGUSB	1×10^{10} vg	6–8 weeks	[238]
	MSD	Mouse	C57B6/S129J-$Sumf^{-/-}$	AAV4, 9-CMV-SUMF1	1.2×10^{10} vg	P1	[152]
	NP-C	Mouse	BALB/cNctr-$Npc1^{m1N}$/J	AAV9-hSYN-hNPC1	4.6×10^9 vg	P0	[239]
	GM1	Cat	$\beta gal^{-/-}$	AAVrh10-βgal	1×10^{12} vg/kg	NA	[217]
	CLN2 Batten	Dog	Dachshunds $TPP1^{null}$	AAV2-CAG-caTPP1	1.6×10^7 vg	3 months	[240]
	CLN5 Batten	Sheep	$CLN5^{-/-}$	AAV9-CBh-CLN5	4×10^{12} vg	2–3 months	[241]
Combination							
IC + IT	CLN1 Batten	Mouse	C57BL/6-$Ptt1^{-/-}$	AAV9-CAG-hPTT1	1×10^{12} vg/ml	P1	[191]
IC + ICV	GM2 (Sandhoff)	Cat	fG_{M2}	AAVrh8-CAG-HEXA/B	1.1×10^{12} vg	1.1–1.6 months	[242]
IC + ICV	GM2 (Sandhoff)	Cat	fG_{M2}	AAVrh8-CAG-HEXA, AAVrh8-CAG-HEXB	IC: 1.6–4.5 $\times 10^{11}$ vg; ICV: 6.4 $\times 10^{11}$ vg	1 month	[211]
CM + ICV	CLN2 Batten	Dog	Dachshunds $TPP1^{null}$	AAV2-CAG-caTPP1	1.6×10^{12} vg	3 months	[240]
IC + ICV	CLN5 Batten	Sheep	$CLN5^{-/-}$	AAV9-CBh-CLN5	3.1×10^{12} vg	2–3 months	[241]
IC + ICV	GM2 (Tay-Sachs)	Sheep	TSD	AAVrh8-CAG-HEXA, AAVrh8-CAG-HEXA/B	6.3×10^{12} vg, 4.2×10^{12}–1.3×10^{13} vg	2–4 months	[243]

The first approaches were mainly based on the direct infusion of the product into the brain parenchyma. Intraparenchymal (IC) injections have the advantage of providing targeted administration to the affected area and can overcome the challenge of the vector permeating efficiently through the BBB. On the other hand, the limited spread of the vector might not be efficient in treating disorders where the neuropathology is extensive and high concentrations of therapeutic protein expression are required in multiple brain areas. However, this drawback could be overcome by administering the therapy to multiple injection sites in the brain parenchyma, ensuring widespread expression in different regions. This method has been applied in clinical trials for MPS IIIA (NCT01474343), MPS IIIB

(ISRCTN19853672), early onset MLD (NCT01801709) and late infantile NCL (NCT01161576, NCT01414985), where the intervention consisted of six or 12 vector deposits to different brain regions during a single neurosurgical session.

Delivery to the cerebrospinal fluid is an alternative approach to achieve widespread gene expression in the CNS. Intrathecal (IT) administration into the lumbar cistern has proven particularly efficient when using AAV9-based vectors [244]. While gene expression following IT injection in mice is restricted to the lower segments of the spinal cord, delivery to larger animals such as pigs [245] and NHPs [246] results in more diffuse transduction of the spinal cord and brain. However, studies conducted by Hinderer and colleagues showed that intrathecal delivery resulted in lower gene expression in the cervical section of the spinal cord and in the brain compared to other CSF delivery methods [247,248], even when the animals were placed in the Trendelenburg position after injection [249]. Nevertheless, the lumbar puncture procedure is widely used in the clinic. Due to its feasibility and reduced invasiveness, IT delivery was chosen as the route of administration in a phase I/II safety study where an AAV9-based vector expressing the *CLN6* gene was administered via lumbar puncture to patients with CLN6 type late infantile NCL (NCT02725580), following positive results in NHPs experimentation [250].

An extensive study conducted by Ohno et al. compared the kinetics of vector clearance from the CSF following infusion of AAV vectors to the lumbar cistern and the cerebromedullary cistern, or cisterna magna (CM) in NHPs [251]. This and other studies demonstrated that administration via suboccipital puncture to the cisterna magna is remarkably efficient in widely transducing the brain and spinal cord in NHPs [252,253]. In addition, the pattern of transduction in the brain of NHPs infused with an AAV9 vector via CM was identical to the one produced by systemic administration to the carotid artery, with particularly high gene expression in the brain [254]. CM and IV routes of administration have also been compared in an MPS VII dog model [227]. The CNS-directed treatment resulted in higher expression levels of GUSB following injection of both AAV9 and AAVrh10 vectors. MPS I dogs were also injected with an AAV9 vector into the cisterna magna, one month after preventive immune tolerization via systemic administration during the perinatal period [225]. The tolerised animals did not develop antibodies against the *IDUA* enzyme in the brain, allowing a safe and effective re-administration to the CSF. Together, these studies suggest that CM gene delivery can be a feasible approach for treating the neuropathology in many LSDs, with the advantage of a lower vector dose requirement and reduced exposure of the vector to the peripheral organs compared to systemic administration. In 2020, Prevail Therapeutics started recruiting type II Gaucher patients to enrol in the PROVIDE clinical study (NCT04411654), where infants diagnosed with the acute form of nGD will receive a CM injection of an AAV9 vector. However, it has been shown that CM delivery is not easily translatable to the clinic, as this technique might be associated with risks related to high vascularisation of the tissue in human patients [253,255]. In addition, there are reports of dorsal root ganglia (DRG) sensory neuron degeneration and secondary axonopathy following CM administration of AAV9 delivering human iduronidase to NHPs [252]. The possible mechanisms responsible for this reaction currently remain undefined. Hordeaux et al. down-regulated transgene expression in the DRG neurons of NHP by incorporating into the vector genome sequence targets for the microRNA miR183, which is present almost exclusively in the DRG, into the vector genome [256]. This modification resulted in reduced toxicity in the DRG, while gene expression was not affected in the rest of the CNS. Recently, Taghian and colleagues developed a novel delivery technique using a microcatheter inserted in the lumbar region that reaches the cisterna magna in the suboccipital space through the spinal canal [257]. The safety and biodistribution of this delivery approach were first evaluated in sheep. Extensive transduction of brain cortical regions and the spinal cord and modest biodistribution in the peripheral organs were detected in the animals three weeks following administration. Two infant Tay-Sachs patients were also dosed using a spinal canal microcatheter, with no reported adverse effects during the infusion or post-treatment. In 2019, Regenxbio Inc.

commenced a phase I/II clinical trial (NCT03566043), where three infant MPS II patients received an AAV9 vector via CM infusion. The first results showed that the treatment was well tolerated and caused a sustained reduction of heparan sulphate in the CNS [258].

Extensive transduction of the CNS is also achieved via intracerebroventricular (ICV) administration. ICV delivery to NHPs results in larger cortical distribution of the vector compared to the intrathecal route, with substantial transduction of the cerebellum [251] and a comparable distribution throughout the brain and spinal cord to CM administration [249]. ICV administration is a relatively common technique compared to CM and it has proven particularly effective in neonatal animals, where it mediates extensive vector distribution in the parenchyma with widespread neuronal transduction and partial transduction of some peripheral organs in animal models of severe neuro-metabolic diseases [146,239]. In addition, delivery to the lateral ventricles can be efficiently combined with systemic AAV administration, resulting in further improvement of the treatment as demonstrated in a pre-clinical study developing gene therapy for multiple sulfatase deficiency [152].

A self-inactivating HIV-based lentivirus vector expressing the human arylsulfatase A *ARSA* gene was used in a pre-clinical study in metachromatic leukodystrophy [259]: 10-month-old knock-out mice received unilateral injection into the right fimbria in the hippocampus under stereotactic guidance and were examined one, three and five months later. Extensive transduction of neurons and astrocytes was detected in different areas of the hippocampus, with no major adverse effects. The treatment resulted in reduced neuronal loss and lipid deposition, increased enzyme expression and activity in both the treated and the contralateral uninjected hemisphere; and rescued short-term and long-term spatial memory. Although lentivirus-mediated transduction spread is usually limited to the focal administration area, the authors speculated that the widespread enzymatic activity was caused by the mechanism of cross-correction. Therefore, lentiviral vector-based gene therapy could be an effective therapeutic option for MLD, as less than 5% of wild-type enzymatic activity would be required to prevent the neurological symptoms [260]. This approach has been recently translated to the clinic, where a phase I/II clinical trial (NCT03725670) is currently exploring the safety and efficacy of brain-direct gene therapy using a self-inactivating lentiviral vector in MLD patients.

The characteristic temporal and spatial expression patterns can limit the applicability of lentiviral vectors for those disorders where widespread transgene expression might not be required or might cause brain toxicity. Widespread gene delivery to the brain has been achieved using a recombinant adenoviral vector expressing the human β-glucuronidase gene to the striatum of MPS VII mice [261]. Increased enzymatic activity was detected not only in many regions of the ipsilateral hemisphere but also in the liver of treated mice up to 16 weeks post-injection when administered in combination with a systemic injection [126]. However, because of the acute immune response associated with adenoviral vectors, the animals were transiently treated with the immunosuppressant MR-1. To avoid loss of transgene expression due to the immune response, researchers developed a new generation of helper-dependent vectors based on the canine adenovirus type 2 (CAV-2) [262]. These vectors do not induce adaptive cell-mediated immune response and therefore mediate long-term gene expression with limited need for immunosuppression. A CAV-2 vector was used to deliver the β-glucuronidase gene to the brain of MPS VII mice via bilateral striatal injections [263]; 16 weeks post-administration, enzymatic activity was detected in several areas of the forebrain and midbrain, with significant correction of pathology in neurons and glial cells. Preferential neuronal transduction and correction of brain pathology were also achieved in the MPS VII dog model, following brain-direct administration of the same vector [264].

A similar approach was developed for the treatment of MPS IIIA mice, where 6–18-week-old adult mice received bilateral injections into the thalamus with a CAV-2 vector expressing the *SGSH* gene [265]. However, transgene expression was dose-dependent and enzymatic activity was already undetectable two weeks post-injection. On the contrary, long-lasting expression was achieved following neonatal administration via bilateral injections into the lateral ventricles. Enzymatic activity was elevated 20 weeks post-treatment with a significant reduction in lysosomal storage and a lack of neutralising antibody formation.

Despite CAV-2 vectors having proven effectiveness in transducing neurons following brain-directed administration and their ability to promote widespread gene expression following retrograde axonal transportation [266], their application has currently not been translated to the clinic. The ability of CAV-2 to transduce neuronal cells depends on the expression of the CAR receptor, which is restricted to neurons in the mouse brain [267]. However, CAR expression varies considerably in different species and neuronal types [266]; therefore, CAV-2 vectors might not be able to efficiently transduce CAR-negative neurons in the human brain.

3.4. Other Organ-Targeted Gene Therapy Approaches

3.4.1. Eye

While brain-directed gene therapy showed promising results for the treatment of the neurological manifestations in many LSDs, correction of the disease is usually limited to the brain. However, other structures of the CNS might be affected by substrate accumulation and cell loss. Batten disease, for example, is characterised by severe and progressive degeneration of the retina [268]. As of today, correction of retinal atrophy and consequent visual loss have not been achieved following brain-directed gene therapy. However, focal intravitreal administration of an AAV2/7m8 vector prevented loss of photoreceptor cells in the retina of a CLN6 mouse model [269]. Interestingly, direct transduction of photoreceptors did not result in any therapeutic effect, while overexpression of the CLN6 gene in the bipolar cell layer significantly slowed retinal degeneration and loss of photoreceptor functionality. This study showed that bipolar cells could be a therapeutic target for several Batten disorders, although transduction efficiency of the AAV7m8 vector in human bipolar cells has not yet been assessed. Sub-retinal injections of another novel AAV capsid (AAV-TT) resulted in higher transduction of photoreceptor cells compared to standard AAV2 [205]. A similar approach was previously adopted in pre-clinical studies with the aim of treating the progressive retinal degeneration and photoreceptor cell loss characteristic of MPS VII, using AAV-mediated intravitreal gene delivery [270,271].

3.4.2. Muscle

Localised administration to the muscle has been widely used to treat skeletal myopathy caused by glycogen accumulation in Pompe disease. Several studies have shown that injection of AAV2 [189], AAV6 [272] and AAV9 [273] vectors to the tibialis anterior or the gastrocnemius muscle of *Gaa* knock-out mice led to glycogen clearance and amelioration of the neuromuscular phenotype. However, prolonged overexpression of *GAA* is associated with transgene immunogenicity. The immune reaction was successfully attenuated using immune deficient *Gaa*-KO/SCID mice [272]. A similar approach was adopted in a current clinical trial (NCT02240407), assessing the safety of two consecutive administrations of an AAV9 vector to both legs of Pompe patients under a regime of immunosuppressive drugs.

Pompe disease is characterised by weakening of the diaphragm and other respiratory skeletal muscles, resulting in ventilatory insufficiency [274]. Although direct gene delivery was efficient in increasing GAA enzymatic activity in the leg muscle, intramuscular injections did not produce any effect in the diaphragm of treated animals. An interesting gene delivery method that combines an AAV2 vector and glycerin-based gel has been successfully used to transduce the diaphragm of *Gaa* knock-out mice [275]. Topical delivery of the vector resulted in substantially increased enzymatic activity in the diaphragm of treated animals and improved ventilatory function. However, as with the intramuscular injections, early intervention in young mice was more efficient in normalising the pathology compared to the treatment of older animals. The safety of intramuscular administration to the diaphragm of Pompe patients was also investigated in a phase I/II clinical study (NCT00976352) using an AAV1 vector to deliver the therapeutic gene to late infantile/juvenile subjects.

In addition, Pompe patients often present with tongue weakness and typically develop pharyngeal dysphagia due to hypoglossal XII motor neuron dysfunction [276]. In an attempt to target the TXII motor neurons, ElMallah and colleagues delivered AAV1 and AAV9 vectors to the tongue of *Gaa* knock-out mice [277]. Exploiting the retrograde axonal transport to the neurons, gene therapy resulted in overexpression of *GAA* and the clearance of glycogen storage in XII motor neurons, with consequent improvement in the upper airway motor function of treated mice.

Further research supported the contribution of the CNS to the respiratory muscle impairment in Pompe disease [278]. With the aim of targeting the respiratory and cardiac dysfunctions, while potentially delivering the functional enzyme to the phrenic and intercostal motor neurons via retrograde transportation, the authors administered an AAV9 vector intrapleurally to adult *Gaa* knock-out mice. Six months post-injection, enzymatic activity was significantly improved in the lungs and myocardium of treated mice, with consequent clearance of glycogen storage. Interestingly, vector genome copies were also detected in the diaphragm and spinal cord, supporting the hypothesis that transduction of respiratory motor neurons can be beneficial in improving respiratory function in Pompe disease.

4. Gene Editing

The gene therapy approaches mentioned so far in this review rely on gene augmentation, rather than correction of the detrimental mutations in the patients' genome. Genome editing aims to manipulate the patient's genome in a controlled manner. For example, it may allow insertion of the desired gene at a specific site within the host genome. When targeting actively dividing cells, this would overcome the problems of dilution of a non-integrating vector and the potential genotoxic effects of uncontrolled insertion [160]. The ultimate goal of gene editing is to be able to selectively correct a harmful mutation in the patient's own genome to the correct nucleotide base sequences.

4.1. Double-Strand Breaks (DSBs)

Gene editing involves the manipulation of the cell system for repairing double-strand breaks in the genome. Two of the most common methods are non-homologous end joining (NHEJ) and homology directed repair (HDR). The NHEJ repair mechanism mediates the direct re-ligation of the broken DNA without the need of a homologous template to guide repair. The NHEJ mechanism is the quickest at restoring the DNA strand; however, the repair mechanism is highly error prone and sequence independent, frequently leading to small insertions and deletions (indels) [279]. This can be beneficial when trying to create a knock-out model, as it can lead to a reading frame shift and the formation of an early stop codon. However, NHEJ is unsuitable in the therapeutic setting, as the random nature of the system means that the end population of cells could exhibit a diverse array of mutations [280–282].

HDR is a naturally occurring system which can repair DNA DSBs with high efficiency. HDR requires a homologous DNA repair template, which contains the desired edit within stretches of the homologous sequence both immediately upstream and downstream of the target site. These are typically ~1.2 kb in length for mammalian cells [279,283,284]. A Holliday junction is created when there is sufficient homology for the template strand to displace the host strand and form a single strand cross over [285]. This is then cleaved by endonuclease GEN1 and the strands are fused together by a ligase. This method of repair only occurs during the S and G2 phases of the cell cycle, thus limiting this mechanism to actively replicating cells [286].

4.2. Zinc Finger Nucleases (ZFNs)

Zinc finger nucleases (ZFNs) are synthetic, engineered proteins consisting of the non-specific cleavage domain of FokI endonuclease and zinc finger proteins [287]. These motifs are able to bind to DNA by inserting into the major groove of the double helix and recognising specific base triplets [288]. When ZFNs bind to unique sequences within the genome, the FokI nucleases create a double-strand break at the target site allowing for local homologous recombination and consequent targeted delivery of a therapeutic gene [289].

In the LSD field, approaches with ZFNs have been explored for Gaucher disease [290], Fabry disease [290], MPS I [290,291] and MPS II [290,292]. Wild-type mice were treated with 3×10^{11} vg of both AAV8-ZFNs and 1.5×10^{12} vg AAV8-donors which contained either acid-β-glucosidase (Gaucher), α-galactosidase A (Fabry), α-L-iduronidase (MPS I) or iduronate-2 sulfatase (MPS II). The ZFNs were designed to induce a double-strand break in the albumin gene, while the donor genes were flanked by homologous repeats and a splice acceptor sequence. Four weeks post-administration, supraphysiological concentrations of enzymes were detected in the liver, while a 3-fold increase in enzymatic activity persisted for eight weeks post injection. Sequencing analysis of the genomic DNA showed a 31.4% modification at the intended target with less than 2% at queried off target loci.

α-L-iduronidase *IDUA* knockout mouse models, aged 4 to 10 weeks old, were intravenously injected with 1.5×10^{11} vg of each AAV8-ZFN targeted at intron 1 of the albumin locus and 1.2×10^{12} vg AAV8-IDUA donor [291]. This approach led to 34–47% insertions by one month post-injection. The *IDUA* activity in the liver was 10- to 16-fold higher compared to wild-type controls, and enzyme activity in the plasma was 7- to 9-fold higher compared to the control mice at 28 days post injection. Secondary tissues including the spleen, heart, lungs and muscle also showed an increase in *IDUA* activity one month post-administration; however, no significant increase was observed in the brain. This suggested that uptake by the M6P-R pathway allowed for a degree of cross correction to occur, as confirmed by the reduction of the glycosaminoglycan concentrations in the liver and all peripheral tissues at the four-month time point.

Similar experiments were also performed on a mouse model of MPS II [292]. Male mice between six and nine weeks old were intravenously injected with AAV8 ZFN vectors and the AAV8 IDS donor at three doses, with the highest being 1.5×10^{11} vg AAV-ZFN and 1.2×10^{12} vg AAV-donor. The enzyme concentration in the liver was 207-fold higher compared to the wild-type mice at four months post-injection, with the GAG concentration restored to wild-type levels.

In a clinical trial for the treatment of MPS I (NCT02702115), three participants were enrolled in a phase 1/2 trial to receive ascending single doses of SB-318 (a three-component therapeutic of AAV6-ZFN1, AAV6-ZFN2 and AAV6-IDAU donor) administered by intravenous infusion. The purpose of this study was to assess the safety and tolerability of the agent, with the secondary outcomes being measured including the change in *IDUA* activity, the change of urine GAG levels and AAV6 clearance. The trial sponsored by Sangamo Therapeutics has been terminated as the study did not demonstrate a clear clinical benefit.

4.3. Transcription Activator-Like Effector Nucleases (TALENs)

The transcription activator-like effector (TALE) protein is derived from the pathogenic plant bacteria *Xanthomonas* [283,293]. The protein has repeats of a DNA binding module, consisting of 34 amino acids that allow specific single DNA base recognition. These DNA binding domains are able to be synthesized in tandem to form an array that can recognise a specific target sequence with more flexibility than ZFNs due to single base pair reading compared to triplets. TALE proteins are fused with FokI nucleases. This allows FokI to dimerise upon binding to the target DNA and create a double-strand break at a targeted location within the genome [294,295]. Exogenous DNA can be inserted at the DSB site via a non-homologous end-joining repair mechanism, using transfected dsDNA sequences as a template for the repair. The use of TALENs with regards to LSDs has been limited so far, having only been used to produce models of Gaucher disease in human-induced pluripotent stem cells and zebrafish [282,296].

4.4. Clustered Regularly Interspaced Short Palindromic Repeats (CRISPR)

A Nobel Prize winning advancement in the field of gene editing was the discovery of the CRISPR system [297]. Bacteria have an RNA-mediated adaptive immune system based on clustered regularly interspaced short palindromic repeats (CRISPR). When foreign pathogenic DNA is detected within the cell, short strands of the invading DNA are incorporated into the bacterial genome between CRISPR repeat sequences [298]. The CRISPR-associated protein 9 (Cas9) is an endonuclease that recognises CRISPR repeats and cleaves specific complementary DNA sequences. By complexing Cas9 with a synthetic guide RNA sequence (gRNA), which targets a specific genomic sequence and forms a scaffold for the Cas9 enzyme, the CRISPR technology can be used to modify, remove or add genes in vivo.

The use of CRISPR in the field of LSDs has been explored for the creation of novel disease models [282] and the development of potential therapeutic strategies, where a therapeutic cDNA sequence is inserted at different loci within the genome, such as the albumin locus, acting as a safe harbour. One of these strategies, for the treatment of MPS I, follows on from previous work using ZFNs to try and insert the *IDUA* gene into the albumin locus [291]. A system was designed using CRISPR technology to create a DSB in the albumin gene, allowing for insertion of the *IDUA* cDNA [299]. Neonatal MPS I mice were injected intravenously with two AAV-based vectors, one carrying the CRISPR/Cas9 system and the other the donor *IDUA* sequence. At 11 months post-administration, a significant increase in *IDUA* activity was observed in the liver, heart, spleen and brain tissue of the animals treated with the highest dose; 3×10^{14} vg/kg AAV-IDUA and 5×10^{13} vg/kg AAV-Cas9. These encouraging results were also reflected in the GAG concentrations with a significant decrease in the treated mice compared to the untreated controls. Examination of the tissue by light microscopy revealed a reduced incidence of foam cells in the liver and decreased vacuolation of Purkinje cells in the brain of treated mice. Noticeable behavioural improvement was observed, with treated mice showing restored memory and learning ability.

Another similar approach using the albumin locus as a safe harbour has also been investigated for the treatment of Tay-Sachs and Sandhoff diseases [300]. The inserted gene was a modified human Hex hybrid μ-subunit (*HEXM*), which incorporates the active site of subunit-α and stable subunit-β interface along with areas from each subunit required to interact with the GM2 activator protein. Together, these subunits form a homodimer capable of degrading GM2 gangliosides [210,301,302]. Neonatal Sandhoff mice were injected with a dual AAV system consisting of AAV8-SaCas9 (5×10^9 vg/g) and AAV8-HEXM-sgRNA (3×10^{10} vg/g) via the temporal facial vein. One month post administration, the plasma 4-methylumbelliferyl-β-N-acetylglucosamine-6-sulphate (MUGS) and 4-methylumbelliferyl-β-N-acetylglucosamine (MUG) activity increased 144-fold and 17-fold, respectively, when compared to the wild-type. The tissues were harvested following euthanasia at four months of age and assessed for enzymatic activity. There was a 7-fold increase in the liver of treated mice compared to the wild-type, and a significant increase in the brain, heart and spleen compared to the untreated group. The rotarod results showed that there was also a significant locomotor improvement in the treated mice.

A frequent mutation in South American MPS I patients is a 1205G>A mutation which leads to the formation of a premature stop codon [282,303]. The use of the CRISPR/Cas9 technology was combined with the provision of a single strand of wild-type donor sequence for *IDUA* to allow for HDR. The agents were first delivered to human fibroblasts using a non-viral nano-emulsion system, and then to new-born MPS I mice via systemic administration. The serum *IDUA* activity was restored to around 6% of normal, and the enzymatic activity in the peripheral organs examined showed a significant increase compared to the untreated controls.

Ex vivo gene editing has also been evaluated for the treatment of MPS I [110,304]. In order to generate human CD34+ haematopoietic stem cells, sgRNA for the *CCR5* gene and Cas9 protein were electroporated into HPSCs followed by AAV6-mediated transduction for delivery of the homologous templates [110]. The *CCR5* site was chosen as the safe harbour, because it is a non-essential gene which poses no detrimental effect at deficiency. The frequency of modification was reported as 54 ± 10% for cord blood-derived HSPCs, and 44 ± 7% for peripheral blood-derived HSPCs. The *IDUA* gene was placed under the control of the spleen focus forming virus (SFFV) or phosphoglycerate kinase promoters, which led to a 250-fold and 50-fold increase in enzymatic activity, respectively. Upon co-culture with MPS I patient-derived fibroblasts, the modified HSPCs led to a decrease in lysosomal compartment size by means of cross correction. Subsequently, homozygous NOD-scid-gamma (NSD)-IDUA$^{X/X}$ mice were created by CRISPR-Cas9 as a model of MPS I. At 18 weeks post-engraftment, the GAG concentrations in urine had reduced by 65% compared to the sham-treated mice.

The research group then established this approach for potential treatment of another LSD; Gaucher disease [111]. Again, the *CCR5* gene was selected as the safe harbour, and the glucocerebrosidase expression cassette was inserted at the targeted site. The modified HSCs were confirmed for their capacity for long-term engraftment and multi-lineage differentiation in the injected mice, as well as confined glucocerebrosidase overexpression specific to the monocyte/macrophage lineage.

4.5. Base Editing

A further iteration of the CRISPR/Cas9 system has been the development of base editors, which come in two classes: cytosine base editors (CBEs) [305], which are capable of converting C•G base pairs to T•A, and adenine base editors (ABEs) [306], which convert the base pair A•T to C•G. These proteins have been engineered to perform transition mutations without the formation of a DSB [279].

One of the factors which has limited the use of base editors for in vivo work so far, has been the size of the DNA strand encoding the editor [307]. At 5.2 kb for the editor alone without any of the regulatory elements or gRNA, this exceeds the carrying capacity of AAV capsids. A method to overcome this limitation has been developed where the editor is split in half and fused to a fast-splicing split intein. Inteins are segments of a protein sequence located at a splicing site, which are removed from the precursor peptide allowing for ligation of the remaining adjacent regions [308]. The two halves can then be delivered by a dual AAV vector system. Following transduction of a single cell by both AAV vectors and expression of the complementary gene sequences, protein splicing occurs and all exogenous sequences are removed, leaving the base editor in its original form.

This system was then explored for its therapeutic potential for the treatment of Niemann-Pick type C disease [307]. The T3182C mutation was selected as the target, and P0 pups of a NPC1 mouse model were injected retro-orbitally with the dual AAV system at two distinct doses, with the highest being 5×10^{10} vg of each AAV. The treatment led to a 9.2% increase in lifespan compared to the untreated mice. At around 100 days post-injection, the number of surviving Purkinje neurons was found to have modestly increased in the treated mice to 38% of wild-type levels. In order to examine the extent of editing efficiency, the brain tissue was also examined, with nearly 50% of the cortical neurons been edited.

4.6. Prime Editing

Base editors are a powerful tool in the genome editing toolkit; however, they are limited to transition purine-to-purine or pyrimidine-to-pyrimidine mutations. Prime editing is a novel technology capable of making a wider range of changes to the genome such as targeted insertions, targeted deletions, all four transition mutations and all eight transversion mutations, either alone or in combination [309]. Prime editors consist of a reverse transcriptase fused to an RNA-programmable nickase, which functions with a prime editing guide RNA (pegRNA). The pegRNA acts in a manner similar to that of the guide RNA in the CRISPR/Cas9 system, where the sequence hybridizes to the target DNA and act as the template strand for the reverse transcriptase component of the prime editor.

With regards to LSDs, the most common mutation which causes Tay-Sachs disease is a TATC insertion into the *HEXA* gene at the 1278 position [309]. Anzalone et al. initially used the third-generation prime editor (PE3) to install the 4-bp insertion into the *HEXA* gene of HEK293T cells, with a 31% efficiency and 0.8% indel rate. The authors then isolated two cell lines that were homologous for the mutated gene and attempted to rectify the mutation. The most successful correction to wild-type *HEXA* had 33% efficiency and 0.32% indel formation [309]. These results supported the possible use of prime editing to correct pathogenic genetic variants; however, strategies to improve delivery to the target cells and an increase the editing efficiency will have to be further investigated before translating this technology to a clinical setting.

5. Conclusions

Lysosomal diseases have proven to be fertile ground for the development of gene therapy. This is understandable given the number of conditions, knowledge of the defective gene, the availability of animal models for pre-clinical studies and the frequent absence of effective treatments. Some of these conditions may be considered 'lower hanging fruit', where the gene therapy approach would benefit from secretion of the protein or enzyme from transduced cells and uptake by other untransduced cells. However, improvement in the viral vector technology and a better understanding of the appropriate route of administration now permit targeting of more difficult conditions. These involve non-secreted or membrane-bound proteins where efficacy is more dependent on the transduction efficiency of the viral vector in the relevant organs. Engineering of the vector and expression cassette can improve transduction efficiency and penetration into specific tissues. This is particularly important for LSDs with a neurological component, where efficient administration of the vector to the CNS is essential and may also require supplementation via other routes of delivery.

While gene therapy is an attractive therapeutic option, ethical concerns related to the possible risk profile require careful consideration. The absence of alternative treatments is clearly a strong argument in favour of gene therapy; however, the risk of extending the life span of the patient while only partially restoring their pathology without significant improvements in their quality of life, is still a critical concern. Therefore, scientists and clinicians should be mindful and carefully evaluate suitability of the therapy to protect both patients and caregivers' interests.

Although LSDs are rare disorders, the large number of gene therapy companies invested in the LSD field is encouraging and also gives a sense of the optimism for future licensed therapies for conditions with unmet medical needs. In addition, progress in developing novel therapies proceeds in parallel with the assessment of new biomarkers necessary to diagnose new patients earlier and more efficiently and to monitor the course of the treatments over time. Overall, this advancement means that the outcome of the ongoing and soon to be initiated clinical trials is of vital importance, first to the patients and their families, but also for future development of novel advanced therapy medicinal products in other fields other than gene augmentation therapy for LSDs.

Author Contributions: Conceptualization, G.M.; writing—original draft preparation, G.M., A.F.G., W.L., O.C.-T.; writing—review, G.M., A.F.G., W.L., O.C.-T., S.N.W., J.B., P.G., A.A.R. All authors have read and agreed to the published version of the manuscript.

Funding: G.M. is supported by the NIHR Great Ormond Street Hospital Biomedical Research Centre (562868), and the Wellcome Trust (562646); W.L. is supported by the UK Medical Research Council (MR/R025134/1); J.B. is a recipient of a UK Medical Research Council Clinician Scientist Fellowship (MR/T008024/1), Innovate UK Biomedical Catalyst award 14720, NIHR Great Ormond Street Hospital Biomedical Research Centre, Nutricia Metabolic Research Grant, and London Advanced Therapy/Confidence in Collaboration Award (2CiC017); S.W. is supported by Wellbeing of Women, LifeArc, GOSH/SPARKS and Dravet Syndrome UK, UK Biomedical Catalyst Early stage award No 14720; P.G. is supported by the NIHR Great Ormond Street Hospital Biomedical Research Centre (562868), UK Medical Research Council (MR/S019111/1); A.R. is supported by UK Medical Research

Council Grants (MR/R025134/1, MR/S009434/1, MR/S036784/1, MR/T044853/1), the Wellcome Trust Institutional Strategic Support Fund/UCL Therapeutic Acceleration Support (TAS) Fund (204841/Z/16/Z), Action Medical Research (GN2485), Asociación Niemann Pick de Fuenlabrada, The Sigrid Rausing Trust/UCL Neurogenetic Therapies Programme and funded by the NIHR GOSH BRC. The views expressed are those of the authors and not necessarily those of the NHS, the NIHR or the Department of Health.

Institutional Review Board Statement: Not applicable.

Informed Consent Statement: Not applicable.

Data Availability Statement: Not applicable.

Conflicts of Interest: The authors declare no conflict of interest.

References

1. Platt, F.M.; D'Azzo, A.; Davidson, B.L.; Neufeld, E.F.; Tifft, C.J. Lysosomal storage diseases. *Nat. Rev. Dis. Prim.* **2018**, *4*, 27. [CrossRef] [PubMed]
2. Parenti, G.; Andria, G.; Ballabio, A. Lysosomal Storage Diseases: From Pathophysiology to Therapy. *Annu. Rev. Med.* **2015**, *66*, 471–486. [CrossRef] [PubMed]
3. Marques, A.R.A.; Saftig, P. Lysosomal storage disorders—Challenges, concepts and avenues for therapy: Beyond rare diseases. *J. Cell Sci.* **2019**, *132*, jcs221739. [CrossRef] [PubMed]
4. Xu, H.; Martinoia, E.; Szabo, I. Organellar channels and transporters. *Cell Calcium* **2015**, *58*, 1–10. [CrossRef] [PubMed]
5. Boustany, R.-M.N. Lysosomal storage diseases—the horizon expands. *Nat. Rev. Neurol.* **2013**, *9*, 583–598. [CrossRef] [PubMed]
6. Krivit, W. Microglia: The effector cell for reconstitution of the central nervous system following bone marrow transplantation for lysosomal and peroxisomal storage diseases. *Cell Transplant.* **1995**, *4*, 385–392. [CrossRef] [PubMed]
7. Kierdorf, K.; Katzmarski, N.; Haas, C.A.; Prinz, M. Bone Marrow Cell Recruitment to the Brain in the Absence of Irradiation or Parabiosis Bias. *PLoS ONE* **2013**, *8*, e58544. [CrossRef]
8. De Ru, M.H.; Boelens, J.J.; Das, A.M.; Jones, S.A.; Van Der Lee, J.H.; Mahlaoui, N.; Mengel, E.; Offringa, M.; O'Meara, A.; Parini, R.; et al. Enzyme Replacement Therapy and/or Hematopoietic Stem Cell Transplantation at diagnosis in patients with Mucopolysaccharidosis type I: Results of a European consensus procedure. *Orphanet J. Rare Dis.* **2011**, *6*, 55. [CrossRef]
9. Tan, E.Y.; Boelens, J.J.; Jones, S.A.; Wynn, R.F. Hematopoietic Stem Cell Transplantation in Inborn Errors of Metabolism. *Front. Pediatr.* **2019**, *7*, 433. [CrossRef]
10. Welling, L.; Marchal, J.P.; Van Hasselt, P.; Van Der Ploeg, A.T.; Wijburg, F.A.; Boelens, J.J.; Zschocke, J.; Baumgartner, M.; Gibson, K.M.; Patterson, M.; et al. Early Umbilical Cord Blood-Derived Stem Cell Transplantation Does Not Prevent Neurological Deterioration in Mucopolysaccharidosis Type III. *JIMD Rep.* **2014**, *18*, 63–68. [CrossRef]
11. Deduve, C. From Cytases to Lysosomes. *Fed. Proc.* **1964**, *23*, 1045–1049.
12. Platt, F.M.; Lachmann, R.H. Treating lysosomal storage disorders: Current practice and future prospects. *Biochim. Biophys. Acta (BBA) Bioenerg.* **2009**, *1793*, 737–745. [CrossRef]
13. Cox, T.M.; Cachón-González, M.B. The cellular pathology of lysosomal diseases. *J. Pathol.* **2011**, *226*, 241–254. [CrossRef]
14. Barton, N.W.; Brady, R.O.; Dambrosia, J.M.; Di Bisceglie, A.M.; Doppelt, S.H.; Hill, S.C.; Mankin, H.J.; Murray, G.J.; Parker, R.I.; Argoff, C.E.; et al. Replacement Therapy for Inherited Enzyme Deficiency—Macrophage-Targeted Glucocerebrosidase for Gaucher's Disease. *N. Engl. J. Med.* **1991**, *324*, 1464–1470. [CrossRef]
15. Aviezer, D.; Brill-Almon, E.; Shaaltiel, Y.; Hashmueli, S.; Bartfeld, D.; Mizrachi, S.; Liberman, Y.; Freeman, A.; Zimran, A.; Galun, E. A Plant-Derived Recombinant Human Glucocerebrosidase Enzyme—A Preclinical and Phase I Investigation. *PLoS ONE* **2009**, *4*, e4792. [CrossRef] [PubMed]
16. Grabowski, G.A.; Golembo, M.; Shaaltiel, Y. Taliglucerase alfa: An enzyme replacement therapy using plant cell expression technology. *Mol. Genet. Metab.* **2014**, *112*, 1–8. [CrossRef]
17. Zimran, A.; Altarescu, G.; Philips, M.; Attias, D.; Jmoudiak, M.; Deeb, M.; Wang, N.; Bhirangi, K.; Cohn, G.M.; Elstein, D. Phase 1/2 and extension study of velaglucerase alfa replacement therapy in adults with type 1 Gaucher disease: 48-month experience. *Blood* **2010**, *115*, 4651–4656. [CrossRef]
18. Sun, A. Lysosomal storage disease overview. *Ann. Transl. Med.* **2018**, *6*, 476. [CrossRef]
19. Desnick, R.; Schuchman, E. Enzyme Replacement Therapy for Lysosomal Diseases: Lessons from 20 Years of Experience and Remaining Challenges. *Annu. Rev. Genom. Hum. Genet.* **2012**, *13*, 307–335. [CrossRef]
20. Rombach, S.M.; Hollak, C.E.M.; Linthorst, G.E.; Dijkgraaf, M.G.W. Cost-effectiveness of enzyme replacement therapy for Fabry disease. *Orphanet J. Rare Dis.* **2013**, *8*, 29. [CrossRef]
21. Baruteau, J.; Broomfield, A.; Crook, V.; Finnegan, N.; Harvey, K.; Burke, D.; Burch, M.; Shepherd, G.; Vellodi, A. Successful Desensitisation in a Patient with CRIM-Positive Infantile-Onset Pompe Disease. *JIMD Rep.* **2013**, *12*, 99–102. [CrossRef] [PubMed]
22. Broomfield, A.; Jones, S.A.; Hughes, S.M.; Bigger, B.W. The impact of the immune system on the safety and efficiency of enzyme replacement therapy in lysosomal storage disorders. *J. Inherit. Metab. Dis.* **2016**, *39*, 499–512. [CrossRef] [PubMed]

23. Mole, S.E.; Anderson, G.; Band, H.A.; Berkovic, S.F.; Cooper, J.D.; Holthaus, S.-M.K.; McKay, T.R.; Medina, D.L.; Rahim, A.A.; Schulz, A.; et al. Clinical challenges and future therapeutic approaches for neuronal ceroid lipofuscinosis. *Lancet Neurol.* **2019**, *18*, 107–116. [CrossRef]
24. Parenti, G.; Andria, G.; Valenzano, K.J. Pharmacological Chaperone Therapy: Preclinical Development, Clinical Translation, and Prospects for the Treatment of Lysosomal Storage Disorders. *Mol. Ther.* **2015**, *23*, 1138–1148. [CrossRef]
25. Markham, A. Migalastat: First Global Approval. *Drugs* **2016**, *76*, 1147–1152. [CrossRef]
26. Hughes, D.A.; Nicholls, K.; Shankar, S.P.; Sunder-Plassmann, G.; Koeller, D.; Nedd, K.; Vockley, G.; Hamazaki, T.; Lachmann, R.; Ohashi, T.; et al. Oral pharmacological chaperone migalastat compared with enzyme replacement therapy in Fabry disease: 18-month results from the randomised phase III ATTRACT study. *J. Med. Genet.* **2017**, *54*, 288–296. [CrossRef]
27. Liu, Y.; Chang, A. Heat shock response relieves ER stress. *EMBO J.* **2008**, *27*, 1049–1059. [CrossRef]
28. Platt, F.M.; Neises, G.R.; Reinkensmeier, G.; Townsend, M.J.; Perry, V.H.; Proia, R.L.; Winchester, B.; Dwek, R.A.; Butters, T.D. Prevention of Lysosomal Storage in Tay-Sachs Mice Treated with N-Butyldeoxynojirimycin. *Science* **1997**, *276*, 428–431. [CrossRef]
29. Platt, F.M.; Jeyakumar, M. Substrate reduction therapy. *Acta Paediatr.* **2008**, *97*, 88–93. [CrossRef]
30. Balwani, M.; Burrow, T.A.; Charrow, J.; Goker-Alpan, O.; Kaplan, P.; Kishnani, P.S.; Mistry, P.; Ruskin, J.; Weinreb, N. Recommendations for the use of eliglustat in the treatment of adults with Gaucher disease type 1 in the United States. *Mol. Genet. Metab.* **2016**, *117*, 95–103. [CrossRef]
31. Belmatoug, N.; Di Rocco, M.; Fraga, C.; Giraldo, P.; Hughes, D.; Lukina, E.; Maison-Blanche, P.; Merkel, M.; Niederau, C.; Plöckinger, U.; et al. Management and monitoring recommendations for the use of eliglustat in adults with type 1 Gaucher disease in Europe. *Eur. J. Intern. Med.* **2017**, *37*, 25–32. [CrossRef]
32. Elstein, D.; Dweck, A.; Attias, D.; Hadas-Halpern, I.; Zevin, S.; Altarescu, G.; Aerts, J.F.M.G.; Van Weely, S.; Zimran, A. Oral maintenance clinical trial with miglustat for type I Gaucher disease: Switch from or combination with intravenous enzyme replacement. *Blood* **2007**, *110*, 2296–2301. [CrossRef] [PubMed]
33. Fecarotta, S.; Romano, A.; Della Casa, R.; Del Giudice, E.; Bruschini, D.; Mansi, G.; Bembi, B.; Dardis, A.; Fiumara, A.; Di Rocco, M.; et al. Long term follow-up to evaluate the efficacy of miglustat treatment in Italian patients with Niemann-Pick disease type C. *Orphanet J. Rare Dis.* **2015**, *10*, 22. [CrossRef]
34. Cheng, S.H.; Smith, A.E. Gene therapy progress and prospects: Gene therapy of lysosomal storage disorders. *Gene Ther.* **2003**, *10*, 1275–1281. [CrossRef]
35. Naldini, L. Ex vivo gene transfer and correction for cell-based therapies. *Nat. Rev. Genet.* **2011**, *12*, 301–315. [CrossRef]
36. Kay, M.A.; Glorioso, J.C.; Naldini, L. Viral vectors for gene therapy: The art of turning infectious agents into vehicles of therapeutics. *Nat. Med.* **2001**, *7*, 33–40. [CrossRef]
37. Thomas, C.E.; Ehrhardt, A.; Kay, M.A. Progress and problems with the use of viral vectors for gene therapy. *Nat. Rev. Genet.* **2003**, *4*, 346–358. [CrossRef]
38. Neil, J.C. Safety of Retroviral Vectors in Clinical Applications: Lessons from Retroviral Biology and Pathogenesis. *eLS* **2017**, 1–10. [CrossRef]
39. Montini, E.; Cesana, D.; Schmidt, M.; Sanvito, F.; Ponzoni, M.; Bartholomae, C.; Sergi, L.S.; Benedicenti, F.; Ambrosi, A.; Di Serio, C.; et al. Hematopoietic stem cell gene transfer in a tumor-prone mouse model uncovers low genotoxicity of lentiviral vector integration. *Nat. Biotechnol.* **2006**, *24*, 687–696. [CrossRef] [PubMed]
40. Montini, E.; Cesana, D.; Schmidt, M.; Sanvito, F.; Bartholomae, C.C.; Ranzani, M.; Benedicenti, F.; Sergi, L.S.; Ambrosi, A.; Ponzoni, M.; et al. The genotoxic potential of retroviral vectors is strongly modulated by vector design and integration site selection in a mouse model of HSC gene therapy. *J. Clin. Investig.* **2009**, *119*, 964–975. [CrossRef] [PubMed]
41. Zhou, S.; Mody, D.; DeRavin, S.S.; Hauer, J.; Lu, T.; Ma, Z.; Abina, S.H.-B.; Gray, J.T.; Greene, M.R.; Cavazzana-Calvo, M.; et al. A self-inactivating lentiviral vector for SCID-X1 gene therapy that does not activate LMO2 expression in human T cells. *Blood* **2010**, *116*, 900–908. [CrossRef]
42. Vink, C.A.; Counsell, J.R.; Perocheau, D.P.; Karda, R.; Buckley, S.M.; Brugman, M.H.; Galla, M.; Schambach, A.; McKay, T.R.; Waddington, S.N.; et al. Eliminating HIV-1 Packaging Sequences from Lentiviral Vector Proviruses Enhances Safety and Expedites Gene Transfer for Gene Therapy. *Mol. Ther.* **2017**, *25*, 1790–1804. [CrossRef] [PubMed]
43. Maus, M.V.; Fraietta, J.A.; Levine, B.L.; Kalos, M.; Zhao, Y.; June, C.H. Adoptive Immunotherapy for Cancer or Viruses. *Annu. Rev. Immunol.* **2014**, *32*, 189–225. [CrossRef]
44. Rosenberg, S.A.; Restifo, N.P. Adoptive cell transfer as personalized immunotherapy for human cancer. *Science* **2015**, *348*, 62–68. [CrossRef]
45. Michael, I.B. HIV-1 nuclear import: In search of a leader; update 1999. *Front. Biosci.* **1999**, *4*, d772-81. [CrossRef]
46. Naldini, L.; Blömer, U.; Gallay, P.; Ory, D.; Mulligan, R.; Gage, F.H.; Verma, I.M.; Trono, D. In Vivo Gene Delivery and Stable Transduction of Nondividing Cells by a Lentiviral Vector. *Science* **1996**, *272*, 263–267. [CrossRef]
47. Mamcarz, E.; Zhou, S.; Lockey, T.; Abdelsamed, H.; Cross, S.J.; Kang, G.; Ma, Z.; Condori, J.; Dowdy, J.; Triplett, B.; et al. Lentiviral Gene Therapy Combined with Low-Dose Busulfan in Infants with SCID-X1. *N. Engl. J. Med.* **2019**, *380*, 1525–1534. [CrossRef]
48. Maude, S.L.; Laetsch, T.W.; Buechner, J.; Rives, S.; Boyer, M.; Bittencourt, H.; Bader, P.; Verneris, M.R.; Stefanski, H.E.; Myers, G.D.; et al. Tisagenlecleucel in Children and Young Adults with B-Cell Lymphoblastic Leukemia. *N. Engl. J. Med.* **2018**, *378*, 439–448. [CrossRef]

49. Morsy, M.A.; Caskey, C. Expanded-capacity adenoviral vectors—the helper-dependent vectors. *Mol. Med. Today* **1999**, *5*, 18–24. [CrossRef]
50. Lee, C.S.; Bishop, E.S.; Zhang, R.; Yu, X.; Farina, E.M.; Yan, S.; Zhao, C.; Zeng, Z.; Shu, Y.; Wu, X.; et al. Adenovirus-mediated gene delivery: Potential applications for gene and cell-based therapies in the new era of personalized medicine. *Genes Dis.* **2017**, *4*, 43–63. [CrossRef]
51. Cunliffe, T.G.; Bates, E.A.; Parker, A.L. Hitting the Target but Missing the Point: Recent Progress towards Adenovirus-Based Precision Virotherapies. *Cancers* **2020**, *12*, 3327. [CrossRef] [PubMed]
52. Logunov, D.Y.; Dolzhikova, I.V.; Shcheblyakov, D.V.; Tukhvatulin, A.I.; Zubkova, O.V.; Dzharullaeva, A.S.; Kovyrshina, A.V.; Lubenets, N.L.; Grousova, D.M.; Erokhova, A.S.; et al. Safety and efficacy of an rAd26 and rAd5 vector-based heterologous prime-boost COVID-19 vaccine: An interim analysis of a randomised controlled phase 3 trial in Russia. *Lancet* **2021**, *397*, 671–681. [CrossRef]
53. Yakobson, B.; Koch, T.; Winocour, E. Replication of adeno-associated virus in synchronized cells without the addition of a helper virus. *J. Virol.* **1987**, *61*, 972–981. [CrossRef] [PubMed]
54. Balakrishnan, B.; Jayandharan, G.R. Basic Biology of Adeno-Associated Virus (AAV) Vectors Used in Gene Therapy. *Curr. Gene Ther.* **2014**, *14*, 86–100. [CrossRef]
55. Pereira, D.J.; Mccarty, D.M.; Muzyczka, N. The adeno-associated virus (AAV) Rep protein acts as both a repressor and an activator to regulate AAV transcription during a productive infection. *J. Virol.* **1997**, *71*, 1079–1088. [CrossRef]
56. Daya, S.; Berns, K.I. Gene Therapy Using Adeno-Associated Virus Vectors. *Clin. Microbiol. Rev.* **2008**, *21*, 583–593. [CrossRef]
57. Calos, M.P.; Miller, J.H. Transposable elements. *Cell* **1980**, *20*, 579–595. [CrossRef]
58. Rabinowitz, J.E.; Rolling, F.; Li, C.; Conrath, H.; Xiao, W.; Xiao, X.; Samulski, R.J. Cross-Packaging of a Single Adeno-Associated Virus (AAV) Type 2 Vector Genome into Multiple AAV Serotypes Enables Transduction with Broad Specificity. *J. Virol.* **2002**, *76*, 791–801. [CrossRef]
59. Gao, G.-P.; Alvira, M.R.; Wang, L.; Calcedo, R.; Johnston, J.; Wilson, J.M. Novel adeno-associated viruses from rhesus monkeys as vectors for human gene therapy. *Proc. Natl. Acad. Sci. USA* **2002**, *99*, 11854–11859. [CrossRef]
60. Somanathan, S.; Breous, E.; Bell, P.; Wilson, J.M. AAV Vectors Avoid Inflammatory Signals Necessary to Render Transduced Hepatocyte Targets for Destructive T Cells. *Mol. Ther.* **2010**, *18*, 977–982. [CrossRef]
61. Buchlis, G.; Podsakoff, G.M.; Radu, A.; Hawk, S.M.; Flake, A.W.; Mingozzi, F.; High, K.A. Factor IX expression in skeletal muscle of a severe hemophilia B patient 10 years after AAV-mediated gene transfer. *Blood* **2012**, *119*, 3038–3041. [CrossRef] [PubMed]
62. Nathwani, A.C.; Reiss, U.M.; Tuddenham, E.G.; Rosales, C.; Chowdary, P.; McIntosh, J.; Della Peruta, M.; Lheriteau, E.; Patel, N.; Raj, D.; et al. Long-Term Safety and Efficacy of Factor IX Gene Therapy in Hemophilia B. *N. Engl. J. Med.* **2014**, *371*, 1994–2004. [CrossRef] [PubMed]
63. Rossi, A.; Dupaty, L.; Aillot, L.; Zhang, L.; Gallien, C.; Hallek, M.; Odenthal, M.; Adriouch, S.; Salvetti, A.; Büning, H. Vector uncoating limits adeno-associated viral vector-mediated transduction of human dendritic cells and vector immunogenicity. *Sci. Rep.* **2019**, *9*, 3631. [CrossRef] [PubMed]
64. Gao, G.; Vandenberghe, L.H.; Alvira, M.R.; Lu, Y.; Calcedo, R.; Zhou, X.; Wilson, J.M. Clades of Adeno-Associated Viruses Are Widely Disseminated in Human Tissues. *J. Virol.* **2004**, *78*, 6381–6388. [CrossRef]
65. Boutin, S.; Monteilhet, V.; Veron, P.; Leborgne, C.; Benveniste, O.; Montus, M.F.; Masurier, C. Prevalence of Serum IgG and Neutralizing Factors Against Adeno-Associated Virus (AAV) Types 1, 2, 5, 6, 8, and 9 in the Healthy Population: Implications for Gene Therapy Using AAV Vectors. *Hum. Gene Ther.* **2010**, *21*, 704–712. [CrossRef]
66. Verdera, H.C.; Kuranda, K.; Mingozzi, F. AAV Vector Immunogenicity in Humans: A Long Journey to Successful Gene Transfer. *Mol. Ther.* **2020**, *28*, 723–746. [CrossRef]
67. Hasilik, A.; Klein, U.; Waheed, A.; Strecker, G.; Von Figura, K. Phosphorylated oligosaccharides in lysosomal enzymes: Identification of alpha-N-acetylglucosamine(1)phospho(6)mannose diester groups. *Proc. Natl. Acad. Sci. USA* **1980**, *77*, 7074–7078. [CrossRef]
68. Hobbs, J. Reversal of Clinical Features of Hurler's Disease and Biochemical Improvement after Treatment by Bone-Marrow Transplantation. *Lancet* **1981**, *318*, 709–712. [CrossRef]
69. Aldenhoven, M.; Boelens, J.J.; De Koning, T.J. The Clinical Outcome of Hurler Syndrome after Stem Cell Transplantation. *Biol. Blood Marrow Transplant.* **2008**, *14*, 485–498. [CrossRef]
70. Aldenhoven, M.; Wynn, R.F.; Orchard, P.J.; O'Meara, A.; Veys, P.; Fischer, A.; Valayannopoulos, V.; Neven, B.; Rovelli, A.; Prasad, V.K.; et al. Long-term outcome of Hurler syndrome patients after hematopoietic cell transplantation: An international multicenter study. *Blood* **2015**, *125*, 2164–2172. [CrossRef]
71. Peters, C.A.; Nmdp, I.O.B.O.T.; Steward, C.G. Hematopoietic cell transplantation for inherited metabolic diseases: An overview of outcomes and practice guidelines. *Bone Marrow Transplant.* **2003**, *31*, 229–239. [CrossRef] [PubMed]
72. Steward, C.G. Haemopoietic stem cell transplantation for genetic disorders. *Arch. Dis. Child.* **2005**, *90*, 1259–1263. [CrossRef]
73. Matzner, U.; Harzer, K.; Learish, R.; Barranger, J.; Gieselmann, V. Long-term expression and transfer of arylsulfatase A into brain of arylsulfatase A-deficient mice transplanted with bone marrow expressing the arylsulfatase A cDNA from a retroviral vector. *Gene Ther.* **2000**, *7*, 1250–1257. [CrossRef]

74. Matzner, U.; Schestag, F.; Hartmann, D.; Lüllmann-Rauch, R.; D'Hooge, R.; De Deyn, P.P.; Gieselmann, V. Bone Marrow Stem Cell Gene Therapy of Arylsulfatase A-Deficient Mice, Using an Arylsulfatase A Mutant That Is Hypersecreted from Retrovirally Transduced Donor-Type Cells. *Hum. Gene Ther.* **2001**, *12*, 1021–1033. [CrossRef]
75. Matzner, U.; Hartmann, D.; Lüllmann-Rauch, R.; Coenen, R.; Rothert, F.; Månsson, J.-E.; Fredman, P.; Hooge, R.D.; De Deyn, P.; Gieselmann, V. Bone marrow stem cell-based gene transfer in a mouse model for metachromatic leukodystrophy: Effects on visceral and nervous system disease manifestations. *Gene Ther.* **2002**, *9*, 53–63. [CrossRef]
76. Biffi, A.; De Palma, M.; Quattrini, A.; Del Carro, U.; Amadio, S.; Visigalli, I.; Sessa, M.; Fasano, S.; Brambilla, R.; Marchesini, S.; et al. Correction of metachromatic leukodystrophy in the mouse model by transplantation of genetically modified hematopoietic stem cells. *J. Clin. Investig.* **2004**, *113*, 1118–1129. [CrossRef]
77. Biffi, A.; Capotondo, A.; Fasano, S.; Del Carro, U.; Marchesini, S.; Azuma, H.; Malaguti, M.C.; Amadio, S.; Brambilla, R.; Grompe, M.; et al. Gene therapy of metachromatic leukodystrophy reverses neurological damage and deficits in mice. *J. Clin. Investig.* **2006**, *116*, 3070–3082. [CrossRef]
78. Biffi, A.; Montini, E.; Lorioli, L.; Cesani, M.; Fumagalli, F.; Plati, T.; Baldoli, C.; Martino, S.; Calabria, A.; Canale, S.; et al. Lentiviral Hematopoietic Stem Cell Gene Therapy Benefits Metachromatic Leukodystrophy. *Science* **2013**, *341*, 1233158. [CrossRef]
79. Sessa, M.; Lorioli, L.; Fumagalli, F.; Acquati, S.; Redaelli, D.; Baldoli, C.; Canale, S.; Lopez, I.D.; Morena, F.; Calabria, A.; et al. Lentiviral haemopoietic stem-cell gene therapy in early-onset metachromatic leukodystrophy: An ad-hoc analysis of a non-randomised, open-label, phase 1/2 trial. *Lancet* **2016**, *388*, 476–487. [CrossRef]
80. Calbi, V.; Fumagalli, F.; Consiglieri, G.; Penati, R.; Acquati, S.; Redaelli, D.; Attanasio, V.; Marcella, F.; Cicalese, M.P.; Migliavacca, M.; et al. Use of Defibrotide to help prevent post-transplant endothelial injury in a genetically predisposed infant with metachromatic leukodystrophy undergoing hematopoietic stem cell gene therapy. *Bone Marrow Transplant.* **2018**, *53*, 913–917. [CrossRef]
81. Yilmaz, B.S.; Davison, J.; Jones, S.A.; Baruteau, J. Novel therapies for mucopolysaccharidosis type III. *J. Inherit. Metab. Dis.* **2021**, *44*, 129–147. [CrossRef] [PubMed]
82. Langford-Smith, A.; Wilkinson, F.L.; Langford-Smith, K.J.; Holley, R.J.; Sergijenko, A.; Howe, S.J.; Bennett, W.R.; Jones, S.A.; Wraith, J.; Merry, C.L.; et al. Hematopoietic Stem Cell and Gene Therapy Corrects Primary Neuropathology and Behavior in Mucopolysaccharidosis IIIA Mice. *Mol. Ther.* **2012**, *20*, 1610–1621. [CrossRef] [PubMed]
83. Sergijenko, A.; Langford-Smith, A.; Liao, A.Y.; Pickford, C.E.; McDermott, J.C.; Nowinski, G.; Langford-Smith, K.J.; Merry, C.L.R.; Jones, S.A.; Wraith, J.E.; et al. Myeloid/Microglial Driven Autologous Hematopoietic Stem Cell Gene Therapy Corrects a Neuronopathic Lysosomal Disease. *Mol. Ther.* **2013**, *21*, 1938–1949. [CrossRef] [PubMed]
84. Ellison, S.M.; Liao, A.; Wood, S.; Taylor, J.; Youshani, A.S.; Rowlston, S.; Parker, H.; Armant, M.; Biffi, A.; Chan, L.; et al. Pre-clinical Safety and Efficacy of Lentiviral Vector-Mediated Ex Vivo Stem Cell Gene Therapy for the Treatment of Mucopolysaccharidosis IIIA. *Mol. Ther. Methods Clin. Dev.* **2019**, *13*, 399–413. [CrossRef]
85. Zheng, Y.; Rozengurt, N.; Ryazantsev, S.; Kohn, D.B.; Satake, N.; Neufeld, E.F. Treatment of the mouse model of mucopolysaccharidosis I with retrovirally transduced bone marrow. *Mol. Genet. Metab.* **2003**, *79*, 233–244. [CrossRef]
86. Visigalli, I.; Delai, S.; Politi, L.S.; Di Domenico, C.; Cerri, F.; Mrak, E.; D'Isa, R.; Ungaro, D.; Stok, M.; Sanvito, F.; et al. Gene therapy augments the efficacy of hematopoietic cell transplantation and fully corrects mucopolysaccharidosis type I phenotype in the mouse model. *Blood* **2010**, *116*, 5130–5139. [CrossRef]
87. Cattoglio, C.; Facchini, G.; Sartori, D.; Antonelli, A.; Miccio, A.; Cassani, B.; Schmidt, M.; Von Kalle, C.; Howe, S.; Thrasher, A.J.; et al. Hot spots of retroviral integration in human CD34+ hematopoietic cells. *Blood* **2007**, *110*, 1770–1778. [CrossRef]
88. De Palma, M.; Montini, E.; De Sio, F.R.S.; Benedicenti, F.; Gentile, A.; Medico, E.; Naldini, L. Promoter trapping reveals significant differences in integration site selection between MLV and HIV vectors in primary hematopoietic cells. *Blood* **2005**, *105*, 2307–2315. [CrossRef]
89. Orchard Therapeutics Outlines Comprehensive Presence at 2021 WORLDSymposium™. Orchard Therapeutics. Available online: https://ir.orchard-tx.com/news-releases/news-release-details/orchard-therapeutics-outlines-comprehensive-presence-2021 (accessed on 8 March 2021).
90. Enquist, I.B.; Nilsson, E.C.; Ooka, A.; Månsson, J.-E.; Olsson, K.; Ehinger, M.; Brady, R.O.; Richter, J.; Karlsson, S. Effective cell and gene therapy in a murine model of Gaucher disease. *Proc. Natl. Acad. Sci. USA* **2006**, *103*, 13819–13824. [CrossRef]
91. Enquist, I.B.; Nilsson, E.; Månsson, J.-E.; Ehinger, M.; Richter, J.; Karlsson, S. Successful Low-Risk Hematopoietic Cell Therapy in a Mouse Model of Type 1 Gaucher Disease. *STEM CELLS* **2009**, *27*, 744–752. [CrossRef]
92. Dahl, M.; Smith, E.M.; Warsi, S.; Rothe, M.; Ferraz, M.J.; Aerts, J.M.; Golipour, A.; Harper, C.; Pfeifer, R.; Pizzurro, D.; et al. Correction of pathology in mice displaying Gaucher disease type 1 by a clinically-applicable lentiviral vector. *Mol. Ther. Methods Clin. Dev.* **2021**, *20*, 312–323. [CrossRef]
93. Jacobsen, L. The GuardOne Clinical Trial: A First-in-Human, Open-Label, Multinational Phase 1/2 Study of AVR-RD-02 Ex Vivo Lentiviral Vector, Autologous Gene Therapy for Gaucher Disease. In Proceedings of the WORLDSymposium, Manchester Grand Hyatt, San Diego, CA, USA, 8–12 February 2021.
94. Harrison, F.; Yeagy, B.A.; Rocca, C.J.; Kohn, D.B.; Salomon, D.R.; Cherqui, S. Hematopoietic Stem Cell Gene Therapy for the Multisystemic Lysosomal Storage Disorder Cystinosis. *Mol. Ther.* **2013**, *21*, 433–444. [CrossRef]

95. Gleitz, H.F.; Liao, A.Y.; Cook, J.R.; Rowlston, S.F.; Forte, G.M.; D'Souza, Z.; O'Leary, C.; Holley, R.J.; Bigger, B.W. Brain-targeted stem cell gene therapy corrects mucopolysaccharidosis type II via multiple mechanisms. *EMBO Mol. Med.* **2018**, *10*, e8730. [CrossRef]
96. Miwa, S.; Watabe, A.M.; Shimada, Y.; Higuchi, T.; Kobayashi, H.; Fukuda, T.; Kato, F.; Ida, H.; Ohashi, T. Efficient engraftment of genetically modified cells is necessary to ameliorate central nervous system involvement of murine model of mucopolysaccharidosis type II by hematopoietic stem cell targeted gene therapy. *Mol. Genet. Metab.* **2020**, *130*, 262–273. [CrossRef] [PubMed]
97. Wakabayashi, T.; Shimada, Y.; Akiyama, K.; Higuchi, T.; Fukuda, T.; Kobayashi, H.; Eto, Y.; Ida, H.; Ohashi, T. Hematopoietic Stem Cell Gene Therapy Corrects Neuropathic Phenotype in Murine Model of Mucopolysaccharidosis Type II. *Hum. Gene Ther.* **2015**, *26*, 357–366. [CrossRef]
98. Holley, R.J.; Ellison, S.M.; Fil, D.; O'Leary, C.; McDermott, J.; Senthivel, N.; Langford-Smith, A.W.W.; Wilkinson, F.L.; D'Souza, Z.; Parker, H.; et al. Macrophage enzyme and reduced inflammation drive brain correction of mucopolysaccharidosis IIIB by stem cell gene therapy. *Brain* **2017**, *141*, 99–116. [CrossRef]
99. Zheng, Y.; Ryazantsev, S.; Ohmi, K.; Zhao, H.-Z.; Rozengurt, N.; Kohn, D.B.; Neufeld, E.F. Retrovirally transduced bone marrow has a therapeutic effect on brain in the mouse model of mucopolysaccharidosis IIIB. *Mol. Genet. Metab.* **2004**, *82*, 286–295. [CrossRef]
100. Hofling, A.A.; Devine, S.; Vogler, C.; Sands, M.S. Human CD34+ hematopoietic progenitor cell-directed lentiviral-mediated gene therapy in a xenotransplantation model of lysosomal storage disease. *Mol. Ther.* **2004**, *9*, 856–865. [CrossRef]
101. Sakurai, K.; Iizuka, S.; Shen, J.-S.; Meng, X.-L.; Mori, T.; Umezawa, A.; Ohashi, T.; Eto, Y. Brain transplantation of genetically modified bone marrow stromal cells corrects CNS pathology and cognitive function in MPS VII mice. *Gene Ther.* **2004**, *11*, 1475–1481. [CrossRef]
102. Goldmann, T.; Wieghofer, P.; Jordão, M.J.C.; Prutek, F.; Hagemeyer, N.; Frenzel, K.; Amann, L.; Staszewski, O.; Kierdorf, K.; Krueger, M.; et al. Origin, fate and dynamics of macrophages at central nervous system interfaces. *Nat. Immunol.* **2016**, *17*, 797–805. [CrossRef]
103. Capotondo, A.; Milazzo, R.; Politi, L.S.; Quattrini, A.; Palini, A.; Plati, T.; Merella, S.; Nonis, A.; Di Serio, C.; Montini, E.; et al. Brain conditioning is instrumental for successful microglia reconstitution following hematopoietic stem cell transplantation. *Proc. Natl. Acad. Sci. USA* **2012**, *109*, 15018–15023. [CrossRef]
104. Douillard-Guilloux, G.; Richard, E.; Batista, L.; Caillaud, C. Partial phenotypic correction and immune tolerance induction to enzyme replacement therapy after hematopoietic stem cell gene transfer of α-glucosidase in Pompe disease. *J. Gene Med.* **2009**, *11*, 279–287. [CrossRef]
105. Piras, G.; Montiel-Equihua, C.; Chan, Y.-K.A.; Wantuch, S.; Stuckey, D.; Burke, D.; Prunty, H.; Phadke, R.; Chambers, D.; Partida-Gaytan, A.; et al. Lentiviral Hematopoietic Stem Cell Gene Therapy Rescues Clinical Phenotypes in a Murine Model of Pompe Disease. *Mol. Ther. Methods Clin. Dev.* **2020**, *18*, 558–570. [CrossRef] [PubMed]
106. Stok, M.; De Boer, H.; Huston, M.W.; Jacobs, E.H.; Roovers, O.; Visser, T.P.; Jahr, H.; Duncker, D.J.; Van Deel, E.D.; Reuser, A.J.; et al. Lentiviral Hematopoietic Stem Cell Gene Therapy Corrects Murine Pompe Disease. *Mol. Ther. Methods Clin. Dev.* **2020**, *17*, 1014–1025. [CrossRef] [PubMed]
107. Van Til, N.P.; Stok, M.; Kaya, F.S.F.A.; De Waard, M.C.; Farahbakhshian, E.; Visser, T.P.; Kroos, M.A.; Jacobs, E.H.; Willart, M.A.; Van Der Wegen, P.; et al. Lentiviral gene therapy of murine hematopoietic stem cells ameliorates the Pompe disease phenotype. *Blood* **2010**, *115*, 5329–5337. [CrossRef] [PubMed]
108. Dever, D.P.; Bak, R.O.; Reinisch, A.; Camarena, J.; Washington, G.; Nicolas, C.E.; Pavel-Dinu, M.; Saxena, N.; Wilkens, A.B.; Mantri, S.; et al. CRISPR/Cas9 β-globin gene targeting in human haematopoietic stem cells. *Nat. Cell Biol.* **2016**, *539*, 384–389. [CrossRef] [PubMed]
109. Schiroli, G.; Ferrari, S.; Conway, A.; Jacob, A.; Capo, V.; Albano, L.; Plati, T.; Castiello, M.C.; Sanvito, F.; Gennery, A.R.; et al. Preclinical modeling highlights the therapeutic potential of hematopoietic stem cell gene editing for correction of SCID-X1. *Sci. Transl. Med.* **2017**, *9*, eaan0820. [CrossRef]
110. Gomez-Ospina, N.; Scharenberg, S.G.; Mostrel, N.; Bak, R.O.; Mantri, S.; Quadros, R.M.; Gurumurthy, C.B.; Lee, C.; Bao, G.; Suarez, C.J.; et al. Human genome-edited hematopoietic stem cells phenotypically correct Mucopolysaccharidosis type I. *Nat. Commun.* **2019**, *10*, 1–14. [CrossRef]
111. Scharenberg, S.G.; Poletto, E.; Lucot, K.L.; Colella, P.; Sheikali, A.; Montine, T.J.; Porteus, M.H.; Gomez-Ospina, N. Engineering monocyte/macrophage–specific glucocerebrosidase expression in human hematopoietic stem cells using genome editing. *Nat. Commun.* **2020**, *11*, 11. [CrossRef]
112. Chung, S.; Ma, X.; Liu, Y.; Lee, D.; Tittiger, M.; Ponder, K.P. Effect of neonatal administration of a retroviral vector expressing α-l-iduronidase upon lysosomal storage in brain and other organs in mucopolysaccharidosis I mice. *Mol. Genet. Metab.* **2007**, *90*, 181–192. [CrossRef]
113. Liu, Y.; Xu, L.; Hennig, A.K.; Kovács, A.; Fu, A.; Chung, S.; Lee, D.; Wang, B.; Herati, R.S.; Ogilvie, J.M.; et al. Liver-directed neonatal gene therapy prevents cardiac, bone, ear, and eye disease in mucopolysaccharidosis I mice. *Mol. Ther.* **2005**, *11*, 35–47. [CrossRef] [PubMed]
114. Mango, R.L. Neonatal retroviral vector-mediated hepatic gene therapy reduces bone, joint, and cartilage disease in mucopolysaccharidosis VII mice and dogs. *Mol. Genet. Metab.* **2004**, *82*, 4–19. [CrossRef] [PubMed]

115. Xu, L.; Mango, R.L.; Sands, M.S.; Haskins, M.E.; Ellinwood, N.M.; Ponder, K.P. Evaluation of Pathological Manifestations of Disease in Mucopolysaccharidosis VII Mice after Neonatal Hepatic Gene Therapy. *Mol. Ther.* **2002**, *6*, 745–758. [CrossRef]
116. Ponder, K.P.; Melniczek, J.R.; Xu, L.; Weil, M.A.; O'Malley, T.M.; O'Donnell, P.A.; Knox, V.W.; Aguirre, G.D.; Mazrier, H.; Ellinwood, N.M.; et al. Therapeutic neonatal hepatic gene therapy in mucopolysaccharidosis VII dogs. *Proc. Natl. Acad. Sci. USA* **2002**, *99*, 13102–13107. [CrossRef]
117. Ma, X.; Liu, Y.; Tittiger, M.; Hennig, A.; Kovacs, A.; Popelka, S.; Wang, B.; Herati, R.S.; Bigg, M.; Ponder, K.P.; et al. Improvements in Mucopolysaccharidosis I Mice After Adult Retroviral Vector–mediated Gene Therapy with Immunomodulation. *Mol. Ther.* **2007**, *15*, 889–902. [CrossRef] [PubMed]
118. Stein, C.S.; Kang, Y.; Sauter, S.L.; Townsend, K.; Staber, P.; Derksen, T.A.; Martins, I.; Qian, J.; Davidson, B.L.; McCray, P.B.; et al. In Vivo Treatment of Hemophilia A and Mucopolysaccharidosis Type VII Using Nonprimate Lentiviral Vectors. *Mol. Ther.* **2001**, *3*, 850–856. [CrossRef]
119. Kyosen, S.; Iizuka, S.; Kobayashi, H.; Kimura, T.; Fukuda, T.; Shen, J.; Shimada, Y.; Ida, H.; Eto, Y.; Ohashi, T. Neonatal gene transfer using lentiviral vector for murine Pompe disease: Long-term expression and glycogen reduction. *Gene Ther.* **2009**, *17*, 521–530. [CrossRef] [PubMed]
120. Kobayashi, H.; Carbonaro, D.; Pepper, K.; Petersen, D.; Ge, S.; Jackson, H.; Shimada, H.; Moats, R.; Kohn, D.B. Neonatal Gene Therapy of MPS I Mice by Intravenous Injection of a Lentiviral Vector. *Mol. Ther.* **2005**, *11*, 776–789. [CrossRef]
121. Di Domenico, C.; Villani, G.R.; Di Napoli, D.; Reyero, E.G.Y.; Lombardo, A.; Naldini, L.; Di Natale, P. Gene Therapy for a Mucopolysaccharidosis Type I Murine Model with Lentiviral-IDUA Vector. *Hum. Gene Ther.* **2005**, *16*, 81–90. [CrossRef]
122. Di Natale, P.; Di Domenico, C.; Gargiulo, N.; Castaldo, S.; Reyero, E.G.Y.; Mithbaokar, P.; De Felice, M.; Follenzi, A.; Naldini, L.; Villani, G.R.D. Treatment of the mouse model of mucopolysaccharidosis type IIIB with lentiviral-NAGLU vector. *Biochem. J.* **2005**, *388*, 639–646. [CrossRef]
123. McIntyre, C.; Roberts, A.L.D.; Ranieri, E.; Clements, P.R.; Byers, S.; Anson, D.S. Lentiviral-mediated gene therapy for murine mucopolysaccharidosis type IIIA. *Mol. Genet. Metab.* **2008**, *93*, 411–418. [CrossRef] [PubMed]
124. McIntyre, C.; Byers, S.; Anson, D.S. Correction of mucopolysaccharidosis type IIIA somatic and central nervous system pathology by lentiviral-mediated gene transfer. *J. Gene Med.* **2010**, *12*, 717–728. [CrossRef] [PubMed]
125. Bielicki, J.; McIntyre, C.; Anson, D.S. Comparison of ventricular and intravenous lentiviral-mediated gene therapy for murine MPS VII. *Mol. Genet. Metab.* **2010**, *101*, 370–382. [CrossRef] [PubMed]
126. Stein, C.S.; Ghodsi, A.; Derksen, T.; Davidson, B.L. Systemic and Central Nervous System Correction of Lysosomal Storage in Mucopolysaccharidosis Type VII Mice. *J. Virol.* **1999**, *73*, 3424–3429. [CrossRef] [PubMed]
127. Ohashi, T.; Watabe, K.; Uehara, K.; Sly, W.S.; Vogler, C.; Eto, Y. Adenovirus-mediated gene transfer and expression of human -glucuronidase gene in the liver, spleen, and central nervous system in mucopolysaccharidosis type VII mice. *Proc. Natl. Acad. Sci. USA* **1997**, *94*, 1287–1292. [CrossRef]
128. Guidotti, J.E.; Mignon, A.; Haase, G.; Caillaud, C.; McDonell, N.; Kahn, A.; Poenaru, L. Adenoviral gene therapy of the Tay-Sachs disease in hexosaminidase A-deficient knock-out mice. *Hum. Mol. Genet.* **1999**, *8*, 831–838. [CrossRef]
129. Du, H.; Heur, M.; Witte, D.P.; Ameis, D.; Grabowski, G.A. Lysosomal Acid Lipase Deficiency: Correction of Lipid Storage by Adenovirus-Mediated Gene Transfer in Mice. *Hum. Gene Ther.* **2002**, *13*, 1361–1372. [CrossRef]
130. McVie-Wylie, A.J.; Ding, E.Y.; Lawson, T.; Serra, D.; Migone, F.K.; Pressley, D.; Mizutani, M.; Kikuchi, T.; Chen, Y.T.; Amalfitano, A. Multiple muscles in the AMD quail can be "cross-corrected" of pathologic glycogen accumulation after intravenous injection of an [E1-, polymerase-] adenovirus vector encoding human acid-α-glucosidase. *J. Gene Med.* **2002**, *5*, 399–406. [CrossRef]
131. Amalfitano, A.; McVie-Wylie, A.J.; Hu, H.; Dawson, T.L.; Raben, N.; Plotz, P.; Chen, Y.T. Systemic correction of the muscle disorder glycogen storage disease type II after hepatic targeting of a modified adenovirus vector encoding human acid- -glucosidase. *Proc. Natl. Acad. Sci. USA* **1999**, *96*, 8861–8866. [CrossRef]
132. Pauly, D.F.; Fraites, T.J.; Toma, C.; Bayes, H.S.; Huie, M.L.; Hirschhorn, R.; Plotz, P.H.; Raben, N.; Kessler, P.D.; Byrne, B.J. Intercellular Transfer of the Virally Derived Precursor Form of Acid α-Glucosidase Corrects the Enzyme Deficiency in Inherited Cardioskeletal Myopathy Pompe Disease. *Hum. Gene Ther.* **2001**, *12*, 527–538. [CrossRef]
133. Asokan, A.; Schaffer, D.V.; Samulski, R.J. The AAV Vector Toolkit: Poised at the Clinical Crossroads. *Mol. Ther.* **2012**, *20*, 699–708. [CrossRef]
134. Du, S.; Ou, H.; Cui, M.R.; Jiang, M.N.; Zhang, M.M.; Li, M.X.; Ma, J.; Zhang, J.; Ma, D. Delivery of Glucosylceramidase Beta Gene Using AAV9 Vector Therapy as a Treatment Strategy in Mouse Models of Gaucher Disease. *Hum. Gene Ther.* **2019**, *30*, 155–167. [CrossRef]
135. Weismann, C.M.; Ferreira, J.; Keeler, A.M.; Su, Q.; Qui, L.; Shaffer, S.A.; Xu, Z.; Gao, G.; Sena-Esteves, M. Systemic AAV9 gene transfer in adult GM1 gangliosidosis mice reduces lysosomal storage in CNS and extends lifespan. *Hum. Mol. Genet.* **2015**, *24*, 4353–4364. [CrossRef]
136. Walia, J.S.; Altaleb, N.; Bello, A.; Kruck, C.; LaFave, M.C.; Varshney, G.K.; Burgess, S.M.; Chowdhury, B.; Hurlbut, D.; Hemming, R.; et al. Long-Term Correction of Sandhoff Disease Following Intravenous Delivery of rAAV9 to Mouse Neonates. *Mol. Ther.* **2015**, *23*, 414–422. [CrossRef]
137. Lahey, H.G.; Webber, C.J.; Golebiowski, D.; Izzo, C.M.; Horn, E.; Taghian, T.; Rodriguez, P.; Batista, A.R.; Ellis, L.E.; Hwang, M.; et al. Pronounced Therapeutic Benefit of a Single Bidirectional AAV Vector Administered Systemically in Sandhoff Mice. *Mol. Ther.* **2020**, *28*, 2150–2160. [CrossRef]

138. Rafi, M.A.; Rao, H.Z.; Luzi, P.; Luddi, A.; Curtis, M.T.; Wenger, D.A. Intravenous injection of AAVrh10-GALC after the neonatal period in twitcher mice results in significant expression in the central and peripheral nervous systems and improvement of clinical features. *Mol. Genet. Metab.* **2015**, *114*, 459–466. [CrossRef]
139. Belur, L.R.; Podetz-Pedersen, K.M.; Tran, T.A.; Mesick, J.A.; Singh, N.M.; Riedl, M.; Vulchanova, L.; Kozarsky, K.F.; McIvor, R.S. Intravenous delivery for treatment of mucopolysaccharidosis type I: A comparison of AAV serotypes 9 and rh10. *Mol. Genet. Metab. Rep.* **2020**, *24*, 100604. [CrossRef]
140. Jung, S.-C.; Park, E.-S.; Choi, E.N.; Kim, C.H.; Kim, S.J.; Jin, D.-K. Characterization of a novel mucopolysaccharidosis type II mouse model and recombinant AAV2/8 vector-mediated gene therapy. *Mol. Cells* **2010**, *30*, 13–18. [CrossRef]
141. Duncan, F.J.; Naughton, B.J.; Zaraspe, K.; Murrey, D.A.; Meadows, A.S.; Clark, K.R.; Newsome, D.E.; White, P.; Fu, H.; Mccarty, D.M. Broad Functional Correction of Molecular Impairments by Systemic Delivery of scAAVrh74-hSGSH Gene Delivery in MPS IIIA Mice. *Mol. Ther.* **2015**, *23*, 638–647. [CrossRef]
142. Ruzo, A.; Marcó, S.; Garcia, M.; Villacampa, P.; Ribera, A.; Ayuso, E.; Maggioni, L.; Mingozzi, F.; Haurigot, V.A.; Bosch, F. Correction of Pathological Accumulation of Glycosaminoglycans in Central Nervous System and Peripheral Tissues of MPSIIIA Mice Through Systemic AAV9 Gene Transfer. *Hum. Gene Ther.* **2012**, *23*, 1237–1246. [CrossRef]
143. Naughton, B.J.; Duncan, F.J.; Murrey, D.; Ware, T.; Meadows, A.; Mccarty, D.M.; Fu, H. Amyloidosis, Synucleinopathy, and Prion Encephalopathy in a Neuropathic Lysosomal Storage Disease: The CNS-Biomarker Potential of Peripheral Blood. *PLoS ONE* **2013**, *8*, e80142. [CrossRef]
144. Mccarty, D.M.; DiRosario, J.; Gulaid, K.; Muenzer, J.; Fu, H. Mannitol-facilitated CNS entry of rAAV2 vector significantly delayed the neurological disease progression in MPS IIIB mice. *Gene Ther.* **2009**, *16*, 1340–1352. [CrossRef] [PubMed]
145. Chen, Y.H.; Claflin, K.; Geoghegan, J.C.; Davidson, B.L. Sialic Acid Deposition Impairs the Utility of AAV9, but Not Peptide-modified AAVs for Brain Gene Therapy in a Mouse Model of Lysosomal Storage Disease. *Mol. Ther.* **2012**, *20*, 1393–1399. [CrossRef] [PubMed]
146. Massaro, G.; Mattar, C.N.Z.; Wong, A.M.S.; Sirka, E.; Buckley, S.M.K.; Herbert, B.R.; Karlsson, S.; Perocheau, D.P.; Burke, D.; Heales, S.; et al. Fetal gene therapy for neurodegenerative disease of infants. *Nat. Med.* **2018**, *24*, 1317–1323. [CrossRef] [PubMed]
147. Massaro, G.; Hughes, M.P.; Whaler, S.M.; Wallom, K.-L.; Priestman, D.A.; Platt, F.M.; Waddington, S.N.; Rahim, A.A. Systemic AAV9 gene therapy using the synapsin I promoter rescues a mouse model of neuronopathic Gaucher disease but with limited cross-correction potential to astrocytes. *Hum. Mol. Genet.* **2020**, *29*, 1933–1949. [CrossRef] [PubMed]
148. Hartung, S.D.; Frandsen, J.L.; Pan, D.; Koniar, B.L.; Graupman, P.; Gunther, R.; Low, W.C.; Whitley, C.B.; McIvor, R.S. Correction of metabolic, craniofacial, and neurologic abnormalities in MPS I mice treated at birth with adeno-associated virus vector transducing the human α-l-iduronidase gene. *Mol. Ther.* **2004**, *9*, 866–875. [CrossRef] [PubMed]
149. Polito, V.A.; Cosma, M.P. IDS Crossing of the Blood-Brain Barrier Corrects CNS Defects in MPSII Mice. Expanding the Spectrum of BAF-Related Disorders: De Novo Variants in SMARCC2 Cause a Syndrome with Intellectual Disability and Developmental Delay. *AJHG* **2009**, *85*, 296–301. [CrossRef]
150. Daly, T.M.; Vogler, C.; Levy, B.; Haskins, M.E.; Sands, M.S. Neonatal gene transfer leads to widespread correction of pathology in a murine model of lysosomal storage disease. *Proc. Natl. Acad. Sci. USA* **1999**, *96*, 2296–2300. [CrossRef]
151. Daly, T.M.; Ohlemiller, K.K.; Roberts, M.S.; Vogler, C.A.; Sands, M.S. Prevention of systemic clinical disease in MPS VII mice following AAV-mediated neonatal gene transfer. *Gene Ther.* **2001**, *8*, 1291–1298. [CrossRef]
152. Spampanato, C.; De Leonibus, E.; Dama, P.; Gargiulo, A.; Fraldi, A.; Sorrentino, N.C.; Russo, F.; Nusco, E.; Auricchio, A.; Surace, E.M.; et al. Efficacy of a Combined Intracerebral and Systemic Gene Delivery Approach for the Treatment of a Severe Lysosomal Storage Disorder. *Mol. Ther.* **2011**, *19*, 860–869. [CrossRef]
153. Miyake, N.; Miyake, K.; Asakawa, N.; Yamamoto, M.; Shimada, T. Long-term correction of biochemical and neurological abnormalities in MLD mice model by neonatal systemic injection of an AAV serotype 9 vector. *Gene Ther.* **2014**, *21*, 427–433. [CrossRef]
154. Lim, J.-A.; Yi, H.; Gao, F.; Raben, N.; Kishnani, P.S.; Sun, B. Intravenous Injection of an AAV-PHP.B Vector Encoding Human Acid α-Glucosidase Rescues Both Muscle and CNS Defects in Murine Pompe Disease. *Mol. Ther. Methods Clin. Dev.* **2019**, *12*, 233–245. [CrossRef] [PubMed]
155. Elliger, S.S.; Elliger, C.A.; Lang, C.; Watson, G.L. Enhanced Secretion and Uptake of β-Glucuronidase Improves Adeno-associated Viral-Mediated Gene Therapy of Mucopolysaccharidosis Type VII Mice. *Mol. Ther.* **2002**, *5*, 617–626. [CrossRef] [PubMed]
156. Fu, H.; Kang, L.; Jennings, J.S.; Moy, S.S.; Perez, A.; DiRosario, J.; Mccarty, D.M.; Muenzer, J. Significantly increased lifespan and improved behavioral performances by rAAV gene delivery in adult mucopolysaccharidosis IIIB mice. *Gene Ther.* **2007**, *14*, 1065–1077. [CrossRef]
157. Gray, S.J.; Matagne, V.; Bachaboina, L.; Yadav, S.; Ojeda, S.R.; Samulski, R.J. Preclinical Differences of Intravascular AAV9 Delivery to Neurons and Glia: A Comparative Study of Adult Mice and Nonhuman Primates. *Mol. Ther.* **2011**, *19*, 1058–1069. [CrossRef] [PubMed]
158. Hinderer, C.; Katz, N.; Buza, E.L.; Dyer, C.; Goode, T.; Bell, P.; Richman, L.K.; Wilson, J.M. Severe Toxicity in Nonhuman Primates and Piglets Following High-Dose Intravenous Administration of an Adeno-Associated Virus Vector Expressing Human SMN. *Hum. Gene Ther.* **2018**, *29*, 285–298. [CrossRef]
159. Wilson, J.M.; Flotte, T.R. Moving Forward After Two Deaths in a Gene Therapy Trial of Myotubular Myopathy. *Hum. Gene Ther.* **2020**, *31*, 695–696. [CrossRef]

160. Colella, P.; Ronzitti, G.; Mingozzi, F. Emerging Issues in AAV-Mediated In Vivo Gene Therapy. *Mol. Ther. Methods Clin. Dev.* **2018**, *8*, 87–104. [CrossRef]
161. Chandler, R.J.; Williams, I.M.; Gibson, A.L.; Davidson, C.D.; Incao, A.A.; Hubbard, B.T.; Porter, F.D.; Pavan, W.J.; Venditti, C.P. Systemic AAV9 gene therapy improves the lifespan of mice with Niemann-Pick disease, type C1. *Hum. Mol. Genet.* **2016**, *26*, 52–64. [CrossRef]
162. George, L.A.; Sullivan, S.K.; Giermasz, A.; Rasko, J.E.; Samelson-Jones, B.J.; Ducore, J.; Cuker, A.; Sullivan, L.M.; Majumdar, S.; Teitel, J.; et al. Hemophilia B Gene Therapy with a High-Specific-Activity Factor IX Variant. *N. Engl. J. Med.* **2017**, *377*, 2215–2227. [CrossRef]
163. Nathwani, A.C.; Gray, J.T.; McIntosh, J.; Ng, C.Y.C.; Zhou, J.; Spence, Y.; Cochrane, M.; Gray, E.; Tuddenham, E.G.D.; Davidoff, A.M. Safe and efficient transduction of the liver after peripheral vein infusion of self-complementary AAV vector results in stable therapeutic expression of human FIX in nonhuman primates. *Blood* **2006**, *109*, 1414–1421. [CrossRef]
164. Mingozzi, F.; High, K.A. Immune responses to AAV vectors: Overcoming barriers to successful gene therapy. *Blood* **2013**, *122*, 23–36. [CrossRef]
165. Baruteau, J.; Waddington, S.N.; Alexander, I.E.; Gissen, P. Gene therapy for monogenic liver diseases: Clinical successes, current challenges and future prospects. *J. Inherit. Metab. Dis.* **2017**, *40*, 497–517. [CrossRef]
166. Kattenhorn, L.M.; Tipper, C.H.; Stoica, L.; Geraghty, D.S.; Wright, T.L.; Clark, K.R.; Wadsworth, S.C. Adeno-Associated Virus Gene Therapy for Liver Disease. *Hum. Gene Ther.* **2016**, *27*, 947–961. [CrossRef]
167. Paulk, N.K.; Pekrun, K.; Zhu, E.; Nygaard, S.; Li, B.; Xu, J.; Chu, K.; Leborgne, C.; Dane, A.P.; Haft, A.; et al. Bioengineered AAV Capsids with Combined High Human Liver Transduction In Vivo and Unique Humoral Seroreactivity. *Mol. Ther.* **2018**, *26*, 289–303. [CrossRef] [PubMed]
168. Puzzo, F.; Colella, P.; Biferi, M.G.; Bali, D.; Paulk, N.K.; Vidal, P.; Collaud, F.; Simon-Sola, M.; Charles, S.; Hardet, R.; et al. Rescue of Pompe disease in mice by AAV-mediated liver delivery of secretable acid α-glucosidase. *Sci. Transl. Med.* **2017**, *9*, eaam6375. [CrossRef]
169. Miranda, C.J.; Canavese, M.; Chisari, E.; Pandya, J.; Cocita, C.; Portillo, M.; McIntosh, J.; Kia, A.; Foley, J.H.; Dane, A.; et al. Liver-Directed AAV Gene Therapy for Gaucher Disease. *Blood* **2019**, *134*, 3354. [CrossRef]
170. Jung, S.-C.; Han, I.P.; Limaye, A.; Xu, R.; Gelderman, M.P.; Zerfas, P.; Tirumalai, K.; Murray, G.J.; During, M.J.; Brady, R.O.; et al. Adeno-associated viral vector-mediated gene transfer results in long-term enzymatic and functional correction in multiple organs of Fabry mice. *Proc. Natl. Acad. Sci. USA* **2001**, *98*, 2676–2681. [CrossRef]
171. Ziegler, R.J.; Lonning, S.M.; Armentano, D.; Li, C.; Souza, D.W.; Cherry, M.; Ford, C.; Barbon, C.M.; Desnick, R.J.; Gao, G.; et al. AAV2 Vector Harboring a Liver-Restricted Promoter Facilitates Sustained Expression of Therapeutic Levels of α-Galactosidase A and the Induction of Immune Tolerance in Fabry Mice. *Mol. Ther.* **2004**, *9*, 231–240. [CrossRef]
172. McEachern, K.A.; Nietupski, J.B.; Chuang, W.-L.; Armentano, D.; Johnson, J.; Hutto, E.; Grabowski, G.A.; Cheng, S.H.; Marshall, J. AAV8-mediated expression of glucocerebrosidase ameliorates the storage pathology in the visceral organs of a mouse model of Gaucher disease. *J. Gene Med.* **2006**, *8*, 719–729. [CrossRef]
173. Franco, L.M.; Sun, B.; Yang, X.; Bird, A.; Zhang, H.; Schneider, A.; Brown, T.; Young, S.P.; Clay, T.M.; Amalfitano, A.; et al. Evasion of Immune Responses to Introduced Human Acid α-Glucosidase by Liver-Restricted Expression in Glycogen Storage Disease Type II. *Mol. Ther.* **2005**, *12*, 876–884. [CrossRef]
174. Wang, G.; Young, S.P.; Bali, D.; Hutt, J.; Li, S.; Benson, J.; Koeberl, D.D. Assessment of toxicity and biodistribution of recombinant AAV8 vector–mediated immunomodulatory gene therapy in mice with Pompe disease. *Mol. Ther. Methods Clin. Dev.* **2014**, *1*, 14018. [CrossRef] [PubMed]
175. Han, S.-O.; Ronzitti, G.; Arnson, B.; Leborgne, C.; Li, S.; Mingozzi, F.; Koeberl, D. Low-Dose Liver-Targeted Gene Therapy for Pompe Disease Enhances Therapeutic Efficacy of ERT via Immune Tolerance Induction. *Mol. Ther. Methods Clin. Dev.* **2017**, *4*, 126–136. [CrossRef] [PubMed]
176. Hinderer, C.; Bell, P.; Gurda, B.L.; Wang, Q.; Louboutin, J.-P.; Zhu, Y.; Bagel, J.; O'Donnell, P.; Sikora, T.; Ruane, T.; et al. Liver-directed gene therapy corrects cardiovascular lesions in feline mucopolysaccharidosis type I. *Proc. Natl. Acad. Sci. USA* **2014**, *111*, 14894–14899. [CrossRef] [PubMed]
177. Ferla, R.; Alliegro, M.; Marteau, J.-B.; Dell'Anno, M.; Nusco, E.; Pouillot, S.; Galimberti, S.; Valsecchi, M.G.; Zuliani, V.; Auricchio, A. Non-clinical Safety and Efficacy of an AAV2/8 Vector Administered Intravenously for Treatment of Mucopolysaccharidosis Type VI. *Mol. Ther. Methods Clin. Dev.* **2017**, *6*, 143–158. [CrossRef]
178. Cotugno, G.; Annunziata, P.; Tessitore, A.; O'Malley, T.; Capalbo, A.; Faella, A.; Bartolomeo, R.; O'Donnell, P.; Wang, P.; Russo, F.; et al. Long-term Amelioration of Feline Mucopolysaccharidosis VI After AAV-mediated Liver Gene Transfer. *Mol. Ther.* **2011**, *19*, 461–469. [CrossRef]
179. Sferra, T.J.; Backstrom, K.; Wang, C.; Rennard, R.; Miller, M.; Hu, Y. Widespread Correction of Lysosomal Storage Following Intrahepatic Injection of a Recombinant Adeno-associated Virus in the Adult MPS VII Mouse. *Mol. Ther.* **2004**, *10*, 478–491. [CrossRef]
180. Perocheau, D.P.; Cunningham, S.C.; Lee, J.; Diaz, J.A.; Waddington, S.N.; Gilmour, K.; Eaglestone, S.; Lisowski, L.; Thrasher, A.J.; Alexander, I.E.; et al. Age-Related Seroprevalence of Antibodies Against AAV-LK03 in a UK Population Cohort. *Hum. Gene Ther.* **2019**, *30*, 79–87. [CrossRef]

181. Rucker, M.; Fraites, T.J.; Porvasnik, S.L.; Lewis, M.A.; Zolotukhin, I.; Cloutier, D.A.; Byrne, B.J. Rescue of enzyme deficiency in embryonic diaphragm in a mouse model of metabolic myopathy: Pompe disease. *Development* **2004**, *131*, 3007–3019. [CrossRef]
182. Cunningham, S.C.; Dane, A.P.; Spinoulas, A.; Alexander, I.E. Gene Delivery to the Juvenile Mouse Liver Using AAV2/8 Vectors. *Mol. Ther.* **2008**, *16*, 1081–1088. [CrossRef]
183. Chandler, R.J.; LaFave, M.C.; Varshney, G.K.; Trivedi, N.S.; Carrillo-Carrasco, N.; Senac, J.S.; Wu, W.; Hoffmann, V.; Elkahloun, A.G.; Burgess, S.M.; et al. Vector design influences hepatic genotoxicity after adeno-associated virus gene therapy. *J. Clin. Investig.* **2015**, *125*, 870–880. [CrossRef]
184. La Bella, T.; Imbeaud, S.; Peneau, C.; Mami, I.; Datta, S.; Bayard, Q.; Caruso, S.; Hirsch, T.Z.; Calderaro, J.; Morcrette, G.; et al. Adeno-associated virus in the liver: Natural history and consequences in tumour development. *Gut* **2020**, *69*, 737–747. [CrossRef]
185. Auricchio, A.; O'Connor, E.; Weiner, D.; Gao, G.-P.; Hildinger, M.; Wang, L.; Calcedo, R.; Wilson, J.M. Noninvasive gene transfer to the lung for systemic delivery of therapeutic proteins. *J. Clin. Investig.* **2002**, *110*, 499–504. [CrossRef]
186. Li, C.; Ziegler, R.J.; Cherry, M.; Lukason, M.; Desnick, R.J.; Yew, N.S.; Cheng, S.H. Adenovirus-Transduced Lung as a Portal for Delivering α-Galactosidase A into Systemic Circulation for Fabry Disease. *Mol. Ther.* **2002**, *5*, 745–754. [CrossRef]
187. Muraine, M.L.; Bensalah, M.; Dhiab, M.J.; Cordova, G.; Arandel, L.; Marhic, M.A.; Chapart, M.M.; Vasseur, S.; Benkhelifa-Ziyyat, S.; Bigot, A.; et al. Transduction Efficiency of Adeno-Associated Virus Serotypes After Local Injection in Mouse and Human Skeletal Muscle. *Hum. Gene Ther.* **2020**, *31*, 233–240. [CrossRef]
188. Daly, T.M.; Okuyama, T.; Vogler, C.; Haskins, M.E.; Muzyczka, N.; Sands, M.S. Neonatal Intramuscular Injection with Recombinant Adeno-Associated Virus Results in Prolonged beta-Glucuronidase Expression in Situ and Correction of Liver Pathology in Mucopolysaccharidosis Type VII Mice. *Hum. Gene Ther.* **1999**, *10*, 85–94. [CrossRef]
189. Fraites, T.J.; Schleissing, M.R.; Shanely, R.; Walter, G.A.; Cloutier, D.A.; Zolotukhin, I.; Pauly, D.F.; Raben, N.; Plotz, P.H.; Powers, S.K.; et al. Correction of the Enzymatic and Functional Deficits in a Model of Pompe Disease Using Adeno-associated Virus Vectors. *Mol. Ther.* **2002**, *5*, 571–578. [CrossRef]
190. Takahashi, H.; Hirai, Y.; Migita, M.; Seino, Y.; Fukuda, Y.; Sakuraba, H.; Kase, R.; Kobayashi, T.; Hashimoto, Y.; Shimada, T. Long-term systemic therapy of Fabry disease in a knockout mouse by adeno-associated virus-mediated muscle-directed gene transfer. *Proc. Natl. Acad. Sci. USA* **2002**, *99*, 13777–13782. [CrossRef]
191. Shyng, C.; Nelvagal, H.R.; Dearborn, J.T.; Tyynelä, J.; Schmidt, R.E.; Sands, M.S.; Cooper, J.D. Synergistic effects of treating the spinal cord and brain in CLN1 disease. *Proc. Natl. Acad. Sci. USA* **2017**, *114*, E5920–E5929. [CrossRef] [PubMed]
192. Passini, M.A.; Dodge, J.C.; Bu, J.; Yang, W.; Zhao, Q.; Sondhi, L.; Hackett, N.R.; Kaminsky, S.M.; Mao, Q.; Shihabuddin, L.S.; et al. Intracranial Delivery of CLN2 Reduces Brain Pathology in a Mouse Model of Classical Late Infantile Neuronal Ceroid Lipofuscinosis. *J. Neurosci.* **2006**, *26*, 1334–1342. [CrossRef]
193. Sondhi, L.; Scott, E.C.; Chen, A.; Hackett, N.R.; Wong, A.M.; Kubiak, A.; Nelvagal, H.R.; Pearse, Y.; Cotman, S.L.; Cooper, J.D.; et al. Partial Correction of the CNS Lysosomal Storage Defect in a Mouse Model of Juvenile Neuronal Ceroid Lipofuscinosis by Neonatal CNS Administration of an Adeno-Associated Virus Serotype rh.10 Vector Expressing the Human CLN3 Gene. *Hum. Gene Ther.* **2014**, *25*, 223–239. [CrossRef] [PubMed]
194. Yun, S.P.; Kim, D.; Kim, S.; Kim, S.; Karuppagounder, S.S.; Kwon, S.-H.; Lee, S.; Kam, T.-I.; Lee, S.; Ham, S.; et al. α-Synuclein accumulation and GBA deficiency due to L444P GBA mutation contributes to MPTP-induced parkinsonism. *Mol. Neurodegener.* **2018**, *13*, 1–19. [CrossRef]
195. Baek, R.C.; Broekman, M.L.D.; Leroy, S.G.; Tierney, L.A.; Sandberg, M.A.; D'Azzo, A.; Seyfried, T.N.; Sena-Esteves, M. AAV-Mediated Gene Delivery in Adult GM1-Gangliosidosis Mice Corrects Lysosomal Storage in CNS and Improves Survival. *PLoS ONE* **2010**, *5*, e13468. [CrossRef] [PubMed]
196. Sargeant, T.J.; Wang, S.; Bradley, J.; Smith, N.J.; Raha, A.A.; McNair, R.; Ziegler, R.J.; Cheng, S.H.; Cox, T.M.; Cachón-González, M.B. Adeno-associated virus-mediated expression of β-hexosaminidase prevents neuronal loss in the Sandhoff mouse brain. *Hum. Mol. Genet.* **2011**, *20*, 4371–4380. [CrossRef] [PubMed]
197. Rafi, M.A.; Rao, H.Z.; Passini, M.A.; Curtis, M.; Vanier, M.T.; Zaka, M.; Luzi, P.; Wolfe, J.H.; Wenger, D.A. AAV-Mediated expression of galactocerebrosidase in brain results in attenuated symptoms and extended life span in murine models of globoid cell leukodystrophy. *Mol. Ther.* **2005**, *11*, 734–744. [CrossRef]
198. Lin, D.; Fantz, C.R.; Levy, B.; Rafi, M.A.; Vogler, C.; Wenger, D.A.; Sands, M.S. AAV2/5 vector expressing galactocerebrosidase ameliorates CNS disease in the murine model of globoid-cell leukodystrophy more efficiently than AAV2. *Mol. Ther.* **2005**, *12*, 422–430. [CrossRef]
199. Piguet, F.; Sondhi, D.; Piraud, M.; Fouquet, F.; Hackett, N.R.; Ahouansou, O.; Vanier, M.-T.; Bieche, I.; Aubourg, P.; Crystal, R.G.; et al. Correction of Brain Oligodendrocytes by AAVrh.10 Intracerebral Gene Therapy in Metachromatic Leukodystrophy Mice. *Hum. Gene Ther.* **2012**, *23*, 903–914. [CrossRef]
200. Desmaris, N.; Verot, L.; Puech, J.P.; Caillaud, C.; Heard, J.M. Prevention of neuropathology in the mouse model of hurler syndrome. *Ann. Neurol.* **2004**, *56*, 68–76. [CrossRef]
201. Winner, L.K.; Beard, H.; Hassiotis, S.; Lau, A.A.; Luck, A.J.; Hopwood, J.J.; Hemsley, K.M. A Preclinical Study Evaluating AAVrh10-Based Gene Therapy for Sanfilippo Syndrome. *Hum. Gene Ther.* **2016**, *27*, 363–375. [CrossRef]
202. Hocquemiller, M.; Hemsley, K.M.; Douglass, M.L.; Tamang, S.J.; Neumann, D.; King, B.M.; Beard, H.; Trim, P.J.; Winner, L.K.; Lau, A.A.; et al. AAVrh10 Vector Corrects Disease Pathology in MPS IIIA Mice and Achieves Widespread Distribution of SGSH in Large Animal Brains. *Mol. Ther. Methods Clin. Dev.* **2020**, *17*, 174–187. [CrossRef]

203. Cressant, A.; Desmaris, N.; Verot, L.; Bréjot, T.; Froissart, R.; Vanier, M.-T.; Maire, I.; Heard, J.M. Improved Behavior and Neuropathology in the Mouse Model of Sanfilippo Type IIIB Disease after Adeno-Associated Virus-Mediated Gene Transfer in the Striatum. *J. Neurosci.* **2004**, *24*, 10229–10239. [CrossRef] [PubMed]
204. Heldermon, C.D.; Ohlemiller, K.K.; Herzog, E.D.; Vogler, C.; Qin, E.; Wozniak, D.F.; Tan, Y.; Orrock, J.L.; Sands, M.S. Therapeutic Efficacy of Bone Marrow Transplant, Intracranial AAV-mediated Gene Therapy, or Both in the Mouse Model of MPS IIIB. *Mol. Ther.* **2010**, *18*, 873–880. [CrossRef] [PubMed]
205. Tordo, J.; O'Leary, C.; Antunes, A.S.L.M.; Palomar, N.; Aldrin-Kirk, P.; Basche, M.; Bennett, A.; D'Souza, Z.; Gleitz, H.; Godwin, A.; et al. A novel adeno-associated virus capsid with enhanced neurotropism corrects a lysosomal transmembrane enzyme deficiency. *Brain* **2018**, *141*, 2014–2031. [CrossRef]
206. Liu, G.; Chen, Y.H.; He, X.; Martins, I.; Heth, J.A.; Chiorini, J.A.; Davidson, B.L. Adeno-associated Virus Type 5 Reduces Learning Deficits and Restores Glutamate Receptor Subunit Levels in MPS VII Mice CNS. *Mol. Ther.* **2007**, *15*, 242–247. [CrossRef] [PubMed]
207. Cearley, C.N.; Wolfe, J.H. A Single Injection of an Adeno-Associated Virus Vector into Nuclei with Divergent Connections Results in Widespread Vector Distribution in the Brain and Global Correction of a Neurogenetic Disease. *J. Neurosci.* **2007**, *27*, 9928–9940. [CrossRef] [PubMed]
208. Passini, M.A.; Macauley, S.L.; Huff, M.R.; Taksir, A.T.V.; Bu, J.; Wu, I.-H.; Piepenhagen, P.A.; Dodge, J.C.; Shihabuddin, L.S.; O'Riordan, C.R.; et al. AAV Vector-Mediated Correction of Brain Pathology in a Mouse Model of Niemann–Pick A Disease. *Mol. Ther.* **2005**, *11*, 754–762. [CrossRef]
209. McCurdy, V.J.; Johnson, A.K.; Gray-Edwards, H.L.; Randle, A.N.; Brunson, B.L.; Morrison, N.E.; Salibi, N.; Johnson, J.A.; Hwang, M.; Beyers, R.J.; et al. Sustained Normalization of Neurological Disease after Intracranial Gene Therapy in a Feline Model. *Sci. Transl. Med.* **2014**, *6*, 231ra48. [CrossRef] [PubMed]
210. Bradbury, A.M.; Cochran, J.N.; McCurdy, V.J.; Johnson, A.K.; Brunson, B.L.; Gray-Edwards, H.; Leroy, S.G.; Hwang, M.; Randle, A.N.; Jackson, L.S.; et al. Therapeutic Response in Feline Sandhoff Disease Despite Immunity to Intracranial Gene Therapy. *Mol. Ther.* **2013**, *21*, 1306–1315. [CrossRef]
211. Gray-Edwards, H.L.; Brunson, B.L.; Holland, M.; Hespel, A.-M.; Bradbury, A.M.; McCurdy, V.J.; Beadlescomb, P.M.; Randle, A.N.; Salibi, N.; Denney, T.S.; et al. Mucopolysaccharidosis-like phenotype in feline Sandhoff disease and partial correction after AAV gene therapy. *Mol. Genet. Metab.* **2015**, *116*, 80–87. [CrossRef]
212. Ellinwood, N.M.; Ausseil, J.; Desmaris, N.; Bigou, S.; Liu, S.; Jens, J.K.; Snella, E.M.; Mohammed, E.E.A.; Thomson, C.B.; Raoul, S.; et al. Safe, Efficient, and Reproducible Gene Therapy of the Brain in the Dog Models of Sanfilippo and Hurler Syndromes. *Mol. Ther.* **2011**, *19*, 251–259. [CrossRef]
213. Sondhi, D.; Peterson, D.A.; Giannaris, E.L.; Sanders, C.T.; Mendez, B.S.; De, B.; Rostkowski, A.B.; Blanchard, B.; Bjugstad, K.; Sladek, J.R.; et al. AAV2-mediated CLN2 gene transfer to rodent and non-human primate brain results in long-term TPP-I expression compatible with therapy for LINCL. *Gene Ther.* **2005**, *12*, 1618–1632. [CrossRef]
214. Karumuthil-Melethil, S.; Marshall, M.S.; Heindel, C.; Jakubauskas, B.; Bongarzone, E.R.; Gray, S.J. Intrathecal administration of AAV/GALC vectors in 10-11-day-old twitcher mice improves survival and is enhanced by bone marrow transplant. *J. Neurosci. Res.* **2016**, *94*, 1138–1151. [CrossRef] [PubMed]
215. Watson, G.; Bastacky, J.; Belichenko, P.; Buddhikot, M.; Jungles, S.; Vellard, M.; Mobley, W.C.; Kakkis, E. Intrathecal administration of AAV vectors for the treatment of lysosomal storage in the brains of MPS I mice. *Gene Ther.* **2006**, *13*, 917–925. [CrossRef] [PubMed]
216. Elliger, S.S.; Elliger, C.A.; Aguilar, C.P.; Raju, N.R.; Watson, G.L. Elimination of lysosomal storage in brains of MPS VII mice treated by intrathecal administration of an adeno-associated virus vector. *Gene Ther.* **1999**, *6*, 1175–1178. [CrossRef]
217. Gross, A.L.; Gray-Edwards, H.; Murdock, B.; Taylor, A.; Brunson, B.; Randle, A.N.; Stocia, L.; Todessa, S.; Lata, J.; Sena-Esteves, M.; et al. 605. Cerebrospinal Fluid for Delivery of AAV Gene Therapy in GM1 Gangliosidosis. *Mol. Ther.* **2016**, *24*, S240. [CrossRef]
218. 604. Intrathecal AAV9-Mediated Gene Delivery Corrects Lysosomal Storage Throughout the CNS in a Large Animal Model of Mucopolysaccharidosis Type I. *Mol. Ther.* **2014**, *22*, S233–S234. [CrossRef]
219. Haurigot, V.; Marcó, S.; Ribera, A.; Garcia, M.; Ruzo, A.; Villacampa, P.; Ayuso, E.; Añor, S.; Andaluz, A.; Pineda, M.; et al. Whole body correction of mucopolysaccharidosis IIIA by intracerebrospinal fluid gene therapy. *J. Clin. Investig.* **2013**, *123*, 3254–3271. [CrossRef] [PubMed]
220. Ribera, A.; Haurigot, V.; Garcia, M.; Marcó, S.; Motas, S.; Villacampa, P.; Maggioni, L.; León, X.; Molas, M.; Sánchez, V.; et al. Biochemical, histological and functional correction of mucopolysaccharidosis Type IIIB by intra-cerebrospinal fluid gene therapy. *Hum. Mol. Genet.* **2015**, *24*, 2078–2095. [CrossRef]
221. Roca, C.; Motas, S.; Marcó, S.; Ribera, A.; Sánchez, V.; Sánchez, X.; Bertolin, J.; León, X.; Pérez, J.; Garcia, M.; et al. Disease correction by AAV-mediated gene therapy in a new mouse model of mucopolysaccharidosis type IIID. *Hum. Mol. Genet.* **2017**, *26*, 1535–1551. [CrossRef]
222. Hordeaux, J.; Dubreil, L.; Robveille, C.; Deniaud, J.; Pascal, Q.; Dequéant, B.; Pailloux, J.; Lagalice, L.; Ledevin, M.; Babarit, C.; et al. Long-term neurologic and cardiac correction by intrathecal gene therapy in Pompe disease. *Acta Neuropathol. Commun.* **2017**, *5*, 1–19. [CrossRef]
223. Yoon, S.Y.; Bagel, J.H.; O'Donnell, P.A.; Vite, C.H.; Wolfe, J.H. Clinical Improvement of Alpha-mannosidosis Cat Following a Single Cisterna Magna Infusion of AAV1. *Mol. Ther.* **2016**, *24*, 26–33. [CrossRef] [PubMed]

224. Hinderer, C.; Bell, P.; Gurda, B.L.; Wang, Q.; Louboutin, J.-P.; Zhu, Y.; Bagel, J.; O'Donnell, P.; Sikora, T.; Ruane, T.; et al. Intrathecal Gene Therapy Corrects CNS Pathology in a Feline Model of Mucopolysaccharidosis I. *Mol. Ther.* **2014**, *22*, 2018–2027. [CrossRef] [PubMed]
225. Hinderer, C.; Bell, P.; Louboutin, J.-P.; Zhu, Y.; Yu, H.; Lin, G.; Choa, R.; Gurda, B.L.; Bagel, J.; O'Donnell, P.; et al. Neonatal Systemic AAV Induces Tolerance to CNS Gene Therapy in MPS I Dogs and Nonhuman Primates. *Mol. Ther.* **2015**, *23*, 1298–1307. [CrossRef] [PubMed]
226. Hinderer, C.; Bell, P.; Louboutin, J.-P.; Katz, N.; Zhu, Y.; Lin, G.; Choa, R.; Bagel, J.; O'Donnell, P.; Fitzgerald, C.A.; et al. Neonatal tolerance induction enables accurate evaluation of gene therapy for MPS I in a canine model. *Mol. Genet. Metab.* **2016**, *119*, 124–130. [CrossRef]
227. Gurda, B.L.; Lataillade, A.D.G.D.; Bell, P.; Zhu, Y.; Yu, H.; Wang, P.; Bagel, J.; Vite, C.H.; Sikora, T.; Hinderer, C.; et al. Evaluation of AAV-mediated Gene Therapy for Central Nervous System Disease in Canine Mucopolysaccharidosis VII. *Mol. Ther.* **2016**, *24*, 206–216. [CrossRef]
228. Holthaus, S.-M.K.; Herranz-Martin, S.; Massaro, G.; Aristorena, M.; Hoke, J.; Hughes, M.P.; Maswood, R.; Semenyuk, O.; Basche, M.; Shah, A.Z.; et al. Neonatal brain-directed gene therapy rescues a mouse model of neurodegenerative CLN6 Batten disease. *Hum. Mol. Genet.* **2019**, *28*, 3867–3879. [CrossRef]
229. Johnson, T.B.; White, K.A.; Brudvig, J.J.; Cain, J.T.; Langin, L.; Pratt, M.A.; Booth, C.D.; Timm, D.J.; Davis, S.S.; Meyerink, B.; et al. AAV9 Gene Therapy Increases Lifespan and Treats Pathological and Behavioral Abnormalities in a Mouse Model of CLN8-Batten Disease. *Mol. Ther.* **2021**, *29*, 162–175. [CrossRef]
230. Broekman, M.L.D.; Baek, R.C.; Comer, L.A.; Fernandez, J.L.; Seyfried, T.N.; Sena-Esteves, M. Complete Correction of Enzymatic Deficiency and Neurochemistry in the GM1-gangliosidosis Mouse Brain by Neonatal Adeno-associated Virus–mediated Gene Delivery. *Mol. Ther.* **2007**, *15*, 30–37. [CrossRef]
231. Yamazaki, Y.; Hirai, Y.; Miyake, K.; Shimada, T. Targeted gene transfer into ependymal cells through intraventricular injection of AAV1 vector and long-term enzyme replacement via the CSF. *Sci. Rep.* **2014**, *4*, 5506. [CrossRef]
232. Hironaka, K.; Yamazaki, Y.; Hirai, Y.; Yamamoto, M.; Miyake, N.; Miyake, K.; Okada, T.; Morita, A.; Shimada, T. Enzyme replacement in the CSF to treat metachromatic leukodystrophy in mouse model using single intracerebroventricular injection of self-complementary AAV1 vector. *Sci. Rep.* **2015**, *5*, 13104. [CrossRef]
233. Wolf, D.A.; Lenander, A.W.; Nan, Z.; Belur, L.R.; Whitley, C.B.; Gupta, P.; Low, W.C.; McIvor, R.S. Direct gene transfer to the CNS prevents emergence of neurologic disease in a murine model of mucopolysaccharidosis type I. *Neurobiol. Dis.* **2011**, *43*, 123–133. [CrossRef]
234. Janson, C.G.; Romanova, L.G.; Leone, P.; Nan, Z.; Belur, L.; McIvor, R.S.; Low, W.C. Comparison of Endovascular and Intraventricular Gene Therapy With Adeno-Associated Virus–α-L-Iduronidase for Hurler Disease. *Neurosurg.* **2013**, *74*, 99–111. [CrossRef]
235. Fraldi, A.; Hemsley, K.; Crawley, A.; Lombardi, A.; Lau, A.; Sutherland, L.; Auricchio, A.; Ballabio, A.; Hopwood, J.J. Functional correction of CNS lesions in an MPS-IIIA mouse model by intracerebral AAV-mediated delivery of sulfamidase and SUMF1 genes. *Hum. Mol. Genet.* **2007**, *16*, 2693–2702. [CrossRef]
236. Sorrentino, N.C.; Cacace, V.; De Risi, M.; Maffia, V.; Strollo, S.; Tedesco, N.; Nusco, E.; Romagnoli, N.; Ventrella, D.; Huang, Y.; et al. Enhancing the Therapeutic Potential of Sulfamidase for the Treatment of Mucopolysaccharidosis IIIA. *Mol. Ther. Methods Clin. Dev.* **2019**, *15*, 333–342. [CrossRef]
237. Passini, M.A.; Watson, D.J.; Vite, C.H.; Landsburg, D.J.; Feigenbaum, A.L.; Wolfe, J.H. Intraventricular Brain Injection of Adeno-Associated Virus Type 1 (AAV1) in Neonatal Mice Results in Complementary Patterns of Neuronal Transduction to AAV2 and Total Long-Term Correction of Storage Lesions in the Brains of β-Glucuronidase-Deficient Mice. *J. Virol.* **2003**, *77*, 7034–7040. [CrossRef] [PubMed]
238. Liu, G.; Martins, I.; Wemmie, J.A.; Chiorini, J.A.; Davidson, B.L. Functional Correction of CNS Phenotypes in a Lysosomal Storage Disease Model Using Adeno-Associated Virus Type 4 Vectors. *J. Neurosci.* **2005**, *25*, 9321–9327. [CrossRef]
239. Hughes, M.P.; Smith, D.A.; Morris, L.; Fletcher, C.; Colaço, A.; Huebecker, M.; Tordo, J.; Palomar, N.; Massaro, G.; Henckaerts, E.; et al. AAV9 intracerebroventricular gene therapy improves lifespan, locomotor function and pathology in a mouse model of Niemann–Pick type C1 disease. *Hum. Mol. Genet.* **2018**, *27*, 3079–3098. [CrossRef] [PubMed]
240. Katz, M.L.; Tecedor, L.; Chen, Y.; Williamson, B.G.; Lysenko, E.; Wininger, F.A.; Young, W.M.; Johnson, G.C.; Whiting, R.E.H.; Coates, J.R.; et al. AAV gene transfer delays disease onset in a TPP1-deficient canine model of the late infantile form of Batten disease. *Sci. Transl. Med.* **2015**, *7*, 313ra180. [CrossRef]
241. Mitchell, N.L.; Russell, K.N.; Wellby, M.P.; Wicky, H.E.; Schoderboeck, L.; Barrell, G.K.; Melzer, T.R.; Gray, S.J.; Hughes, S.M.; Palmer, D.N. Longitudinal In Vivo Monitoring of the CNS Demonstrates the Efficacy of Gene Therapy in a Sheep Model of CLN5 Batten Disease. *Mol. Ther.* **2018**, *26*, 2366–2378. [CrossRef]
242. Rockwell, H.E.; McCurdy, V.J.; Eaton, S.C.; Wilson, D.U.; Johnson, A.K.; Randle, A.N.; Bradbury, A.M.; Gray-Edwards, H.L.; Baker, H.J.; Hudson, J.A.; et al. AAV-Mediated Gene Delivery in a Feline Model of Sandhoff Disease Corrects Lysosomal Storage in the Central Nervous System. *ASN Neuro* **2015**, *7*. [CrossRef]
243. Gray-Edwards, H.L.; Randle, A.N.; Maitland, S.A.; Benatti, H.R.; Hubbard, S.M.; Canning, P.F.; Vogel, M.B.; Brunson, B.L.; Hwang, M.; Ellis, L.E.; et al. Adeno-Associated Virus Gene Therapy in a Sheep Model of Tay–Sachs Disease. *Hum. Gene Ther.* **2018**, *29*, 312–326. [CrossRef] [PubMed]

244. Snyder, B.R.; Gray, S.J.; Quach, E.T.; Huang, J.W.; Leung, C.H.; Samulski, R.J.; Boulis, N.M.; Federici, T. Comparison of Adeno-Associated Viral Vector Serotypes for Spinal Cord and Motor Neuron Gene Delivery. *Hum. Gene Ther.* **2011**, *22*, 1129–1135. [CrossRef] [PubMed]
245. Federici, T.; Taub, J.S.; Baum, G.R.; Gray, S.J.; Grieger, J.C.; Matthews, K.A.; Handy, C.R.; Passini, M.A.; Samulski, R.J.; Boulis, N.M. Robust spinal motor neuron transduction following intrathecal delivery of AAV9 in pigs. *Gene Ther.* **2011**, *19*, 852–859. [CrossRef] [PubMed]
246. Gray, S.J.; Kalburgi, S.N.; McCown, T.J.; Samulski, R.J. Global CNS gene delivery and evasion of anti-AAV-neutralizing antibodies by intrathecal AAV administration in non-human primates. *Gene Ther.* **2013**, *20*, 450–459. [CrossRef] [PubMed]
247. Hinderer, C.; Bell, P.; Vite, C.H.; Louboutin, J.-P.; Grant, R.; Bote, E.; Yu, H.; Pukenas, B.; Hurst, R.; Wilson, J.M. Widespread gene transfer in the central nervous system of cynomolgus macaques following delivery of AAV9 into the cisterna magna. *Mol. Ther. Methods Clin. Dev.* **2014**, *1*, 14051. [CrossRef] [PubMed]
248. Hinderer, C.; Katz, N.; Dyer, C.; Goode, T.; Johansson, J.; Bell, P.; Richman, L.; Buza, E.; Wilson, J.M. Translational Feasibility of Lumbar Puncture for Intrathecal AAV Administration. *Mol. Ther. Methods Clin. Dev.* **2020**, *17*, 969–974. [CrossRef] [PubMed]
249. Hinderer, C.; Bell, P.; Katz, N.; Vite, C.H.; Louboutin, J.-P.; Bote, E.; Yu, H.; Zhu, Y.; Casal, M.L.; Bagel, J.; et al. Evaluation of Intrathecal Routes of Administration for Adeno-Associated Viral Vectors in Large Animals. *Hum. Gene Ther.* **2018**, *29*, 15–24. [CrossRef]
250. Cain, J.T.; Likhite, S.; White, K.A.; Timm, D.J.; Davis, S.S.; Johnson, T.B.; Dennys-Rivers, C.N.; Rinaldi, F.; Motti, D.; Corcoran, S.; et al. Gene Therapy Corrects Brain and Behavioral Pathologies in CLN6-Batten Disease. *Mol. Ther.* **2019**, *27*, 1836–1847. [CrossRef]
251. Ohno, K.; Samaranch, L.; Hadaczek, P.; Bringas, J.R.; Allen, P.C.; Sudhakar, V.; Stockinger, D.E.; Snieckus, C.; Campagna, M.V.; Sebastian, W.S.; et al. Kinetics and MR-Based Monitoring of AAV9 Vector Delivery into Cerebrospinal Fluid of Nonhuman Primates. *Mol. Ther. Methods Clin. Dev.* **2019**, *13*, 47–54. [CrossRef]
252. Hordeaux, J.; Hinderer, C.; Goode, T.; Katz, N.; Buza, E.L.; Bell, P.; Calcedo, R.; Richman, L.K.; Wilson, J.M. Toxicology Study of Intra-Cisterna Magna Adeno-Associated Virus 9 Expressing Human Alpha-L-Iduronidase in Rhesus Macaques. *Mol. Ther. Methods Clin. Dev.* **2018**, *10*, 79–88. [CrossRef]
253. Katz, N.; Goode, T.; Hinderer, C.; Hordeaux, J.; Wilson, J.M. Standardized Method for Intra-Cisterna Magna Delivery Under Fluoroscopic Guidance in Nonhuman Primates. *Hum. Gene Ther. Methods* **2018**, *29*, 212–219. [CrossRef]
254. Samaranch, L.; Salegio, E.A.; Sebastian, W.S.; Kells, A.P.; Foust, K.D.; Bringas, J.R.; Lamarre, C.; Forsayeth, J.; Kaspar, B.K.; Bankiewicz, K.S. Adeno-Associated Virus Serotype 9 Transduction in the Central Nervous System of Nonhuman Primates. *Hum. Gene Ther.* **2012**, *23*, 382–389. [CrossRef]
255. Samaranch, L.; Bringas, J.; Pivirotto, P.; Sebastian, W.S.; Forsayeth, J.; Bankiewicz, K.S. Cerebellomedullary Cistern Delivery for AAV-Based Gene Therapy: A Technical Note for Nonhuman Primates. *Hum. Gene Ther. Methods* **2016**, *27*, 13–16. [CrossRef]
256. Hordeaux, J.; Buza, E.L.; Jeffrey, B.; Song, C.; Jahan, T.; Yuan, Y.; Zhu, Y.; Bell, P.; Li, M.; Chichester, J.A.; et al. MicroRNA-mediated inhibition of transgene expression reduces dorsal root ganglion toxicity by AAV vectors in primates. *Sci. Transl. Med.* **2020**, *12*, eaba9188. [CrossRef]
257. Taghian, T.; Marosfoi, M.G.; Puri, A.S.; Cataltepe, O.; King, R.M.; Diffie, E.B.; Maguire, A.S.; Martin, D.R.; Fernau, D.; Batista, A.R.; et al. A Safe and Reliable Technique for CNS Delivery of AAV Vectors in the Cisterna Magna. *Mol. Ther.* **2020**, *28*, 411–421. [CrossRef]
258. Nevoret, M.-L. TRGX-121 Gene Therapy for Severe Mucopolysaccharidosis Type II (MPS II): Interim Results of an Ongoing First in Human Trialitle. In Proceedings of the WORLDSymposium, Manchester Grand Hyatt, San Diego, CA, USA, 8–12 February 2021.
259. Consiglio, A.; Quattrini, A.; Martino, S.; Bensadoun, J.C.; Dolcetta, D.; Trojani, A.; Benaglia, G.; Marchesini, S.; Cestari, V.; Oliverio, A.; et al. In vivo gene therapy of metachromatic leukodystrophy by lentiviral vectors: Correction of neuropathology and protection against learning impairments in affected mice. *Nat. Med.* **2001**, *7*, 310–316. [CrossRef]
260. Penzien, J.M.; Kappler, J.; Herschkowitz, N.; Schuknecht, B.; Leinekugel, P.; Propping, P.; Tønnesen, T.; Lou, H.; Moser, H.; Zierz, S.; et al. Compound heterozygosity for metachromatic leukodystrophy and arylsulfatase A pseudodeficiency alleles is not associated with progressive neurological disease. *Am. J. Hum. Genet.* **1993**, *52*, 557–564.
261. Ghodsi, A.; Stein, C.; Derksen, T.; Yang, G.; Anderson, R.D.; Davidson, B.L. Extensiveβ-Glucuronidase Activity in Murine Central Nervous System after Adenovirus-Mediated Gene Transfer to Brain. *Hum. Gene Ther.* **1998**, *9*, 2331–2340. [CrossRef]
262. Bru, T.; Salinas, S.; Kremer, E.J. An Update on Canine Adenovirus Type 2 and Its Vectors. *Viruses* **2010**, *2*, 2134–2153. [CrossRef]
263. Ariza, L.; Giménez-Llort, L.; Cubizolle, A.; Pagès, G.; García-Lareu, B.; Serratrice, N.; Cots, D.; Thwaite, R.; Chillón, M.; Kremer, E.J.; et al. Central Nervous System Delivery of Helper-Dependent Canine Adenovirus Corrects Neuropathology and Behavior in Mucopolysaccharidosis Type VII Mice. *Hum. Gene Ther.* **2014**, *25*, 199–211. [CrossRef]
264. Cubizolle, A.; Serratrice, N.; Skander, N.; Colle, M.-A.; Ibanes, S.; Gennetier, A.; Bayo-Puxan, N.; Mazouni, K.; Mennechet, F.; Joussemet, B.; et al. Corrective GUSB Transfer to the Canine Mucopolysaccharidosis VII Brain. *Mol. Ther.* **2014**, *22*, 762–773. [CrossRef]
265. Lau, A.A.; Hopwood, J.J.; Kremer, E.J.; Hemsley, K.M. SGSH gene transfer in mucopolysaccharidosis type IIIA mice using canine adenovirus vectors. *Mol. Genet. Metab.* **2010**, *100*, 168–175. [CrossRef] [PubMed]
266. Del Rio, D.; Beucher, B.; Lavigne, M.; Wehbi, A.; Dopeso-Reyes, I.G.; Saggio, I.; Kremer, E.J. CAV-2 Vector Development and Gene Transfer in the Central and Peripheral Nervous Systems. *Front. Mol. Neurosci.* **2019**, *12*, 71. [CrossRef] [PubMed]

267. Zussy, C.; Loustalot, F.; Junyent, F.; Gardoni, F.; Bories, C.; Valero, J.; Desarménien, M.G.; Bernex, F.; Henaff, D.; Bayo-Puxan, N.; et al. Coxsackievirus Adenovirus Receptor Loss Impairs Adult Neurogenesis, Synapse Content, and Hippocampus Plasticity. *J. Neurosci.* **2016**, *36*, 9558–9571. [CrossRef] [PubMed]
268. Johnson, T.B.; Cain, J.T.; White, K.A.; Ramirez-Montealegre, D.; Pearce, D.A.; Weimer, J.M. Therapeutic landscape for Batten disease: Current treatments and future prospects. *Nat. Rev. Neurol.* **2019**, *15*, 161–178. [CrossRef]
269. Holthaus, S.-M.K.; Ribeiro, J.; Abelleira-Hervas, L.; Pearson, R.A.; Duran, Y.; Georgiadis, A.; Sampson, R.D.; Rizzi, M.; Hoke, J.; Maswood, R.; et al. Prevention of Photoreceptor Cell Loss in a Cln6 Mouse Model of Batten Disease Requires CLN6 Gene Transfer to Bipolar Cells. *Mol. Ther.* **2018**, *26*, 1343–1353. [CrossRef] [PubMed]
270. Li, T.; Davidson, B.L. Phenotype correction in retinal pigment epithelium in murine mucopolysaccharidosis VII by adenovirus-mediated gene transfer. *Proc. Natl. Acad. Sci. USA* **1995**, *92*, 7700–7704. [CrossRef] [PubMed]
271. Hennig, A.K.; Ogilvie, J.M.; Ohlemiller, K.K.; Timmers, A.M.; Hauswirth, W.W.; Sands, M.S. AAV-mediated intravitreal gene therapy reduces lysosomal storage in the retinal pigmented epithelium and improves retinal function in adult MPS VII mice. *Mol. Ther.* **2004**, *10*, 106–116. [CrossRef]
272. Sun, B.; Zhang, H.; Franco, L.M.; Brown, T.; Bird, A.; Schneider, A.; Koeberl, D.D. Correction of glycogen storage disease type II by an adeno-associated virus vector containing a muscle-specific promoter. *Mol. Ther.* **2005**, *11*, 889–898. [CrossRef]
273. Todd, A.G.; Bsc, J.A.M.; Grange, R.W.; Fuller, D.D.; Walter, G.A.; Byrne, B.J.; Falk, D.J. Correcting Neuromuscular Deficits With Gene Therapy in Pompe Disease. *Ann. Neurol.* **2015**, *78*, 222–234. [CrossRef]
274. Kishnani, P.S.; Steiner, R.D.; Bali, D.; Berger, K.; Byrne, B.J.; Case, L.E.; Crowley, J.F.; Downs, S.; Howell, R.R.; Kravitz, R.M.; et al. Pompe disease diagnosis and management guideline. *Genet. Med.* **2006**, *8*, 267–288. [CrossRef]
275. Mah, C.S.; Falk, D.J.; Germain, S.A.; Kelley, J.S.; Lewis, M.A.; Cloutier, D.A.; DeRuisseau, L.R.; Conlon, T.J.; Cresawn, K.O.; Fraites, T.J.F., Jr.; et al. Gel-mediated Delivery of AAV1 Vectors Corrects Ventilatory Function in Pompe Mice With Established Disease. *Mol. Ther.* **2010**, *18*, 502–510. [CrossRef]
276. McCall, A.L.; ElMallah, M.K. Macroglossia, Motor Neuron Pathology, and Airway Malacia Contribute to Respiratory Insufficiency in Pompe Disease: A Commentary on Molecular Pathways and Respiratory Involvement in Lysosomal Storage Diseases. *Int. J. Mol. Sci.* **2019**, *20*, 751. [CrossRef]
277. ElMallah, M.K.; Falk, D.J.; Nayak, S.; Federico, R.A.; Sandhu, M.S.; Poirier, A.; Byrne, B.J.; Fuller, D.D. Sustained Correction of Motoneuron Histopathology Following Intramuscular Delivery of AAV in Pompe Mice. *Mol. Ther.* **2014**, *22*, 702–712. [CrossRef]
278. Falk, D.J.; Mah, C.S.; Soustek, M.S.; Lee, K.-Z.; Elmallah, M.K.; Cloutier, D.A.; Fuller, D.D.; Byrne, B.J. Intrapleural Administration of AAV9 Improves Neural and Cardiorespiratory Function in Pompe Disease. *Mol. Ther.* **2013**, *21*, 1661–1667. [CrossRef]
279. Rees, H.A.; Liu, D.R. Base editing: Precision chemistry on the genome and transcriptome of living cells. *Nat. Rev. Genet.* **2018**, *19*, 770–788. [CrossRef]
280. Lieber, M.R. The Mechanism of Double-Strand DNA Break Repair by the Nonhomologous DNA End-Joining Pathway. *Annu. Rev. Biochem.* **2010**, *79*, 181–211. [CrossRef]
281. Chang, H.H.Y.; Pannunzio, N.R.; Adachi, N.; Lieber, H.H.Y.C.N.R.P.M.R. Non-homologous DNA end joining and alternative pathways to double-strand break repair. *Nat. Rev. Mol. Cell Biol.* **2017**, *18*, 495–506. [CrossRef]
282. Leal, A.F.; Espejo-Mojica, A.J.; Sánchez, O.F.; Ramírez, R.; Reyes, L.H.; Cruz, J.C.; Alméciga-Díaz, C.J. Lysosomal storage diseases: Current therapies and future alternatives. *J. Mol. Med.* **2020**, *98*, 931–946. [CrossRef]
283. Ho, B.X.; Loh, S.J.H.; Chan, W.K.; Soh, B.S. In Vivo Genome Editing as a Therapeutic Approach. *Int. J. Mol. Sci.* **2018**, *19*, 2721. [CrossRef]
284. Rouet, P.; Smih, F.; Jasin, M. Expression of a site-specific endonuclease stimulates homologous recombination in mammalian cells. *Proc. Natl. Acad. Sci. USA* **1994**, *91*, 6064–6068. [CrossRef] [PubMed]
285. Sung, P.; Klein, H.L. Mechanism of homologous recombination: Mediators and helicases take on regulatory functions. *Nat. Rev. Mol. Cell Biol.* **2006**, *7*, 739–750. [CrossRef] [PubMed]
286. Ranjha, L.; Howard, S.M.; Cejka, P. Main steps in DNA double-strand break repair: An introduction to homologous recombination and related processes. *Chromosoma* **2018**, *127*, 187–214. [CrossRef] [PubMed]
287. Durai, S. Zinc finger nucleases: Custom-designed molecular scissors for genome engineering of plant and mammalian cells. *Nucleic Acids Res.* **2005**, *33*, 5978–5990. [CrossRef]
288. Pavletich, N.P.; Pabo, C.O. Zinc finger-DNA recognition: Crystal structure of a Zif268-DNA complex at 2.1 A. *Science* **1991**, *252*, 809–817. [CrossRef]
289. Liu, Q.; Segal, D.J.; Ghiara, J.B.; Barbas, C.F. Design of polydactyl zinc-finger proteins for unique addressing within complex genomes. *Proc. Natl. Acad. Sci. USA* **1997**, *94*, 5525–5530. [CrossRef]
290. Sharma, R.; Anguela, X.M.; Doyon, Y.; Wechsler, T.; DeKelver, R.C.; Sproul, S.; Paschon, D.E.; Miller, J.C.; Davidson, R.J.; Shivak, D.A.; et al. In vivo genome editing of the albumin locus as a platform for protein replacement therapy. *Blood* **2015**, *126*, 1777–1784. [CrossRef]
291. Ou, L.; DeKelver, R.C.; Rohde, M.; Tom, S.; Radeke, R.; Martin, S.J.S.; Santiago, Y.; Sproul, S.; Przybilla, M.J.; Koniar, B.L.; et al. ZFN-Mediated In Vivo Genome Editing Corrects Murine Hurler Syndrome. *Mol. Ther.* **2019**, *27*, 178–187. [CrossRef]
292. Laoharawee, K.; DeKelver, R.C.; Podetz-Pedersen, K.M.; Rohde, M.; Sproul, S.; Nguyen, H.-O.; Nguyen, T.; Martin, S.J.S.; Ou, L.; Tom, S.; et al. Dose-Dependent Prevention of Metabolic and Neurologic Disease in Murine MPS II by ZFN-Mediated In Vivo Genome Editing. *Mol. Ther.* **2018**, *26*, 1127–1136. [CrossRef]

293. Scholze, H.; Boch, J. TAL effectors are remote controls for gene activation. *Curr. Opin. Microbiol.* **2011**, *14*, 47–53. [CrossRef]
294. Christian, M.; Cermak, T.; Doyle, E.L.; Schmidt, C.; Zhang, F.; Hummel, A.; Bogdanove, A.J.; Voytas, D.F. Targeting DNA Double-Strand Breaks with TAL Effector Nucleases. *Genetics* **2010**, *186*, 757–761. [CrossRef]
295. Miller, J.C.; Tan, S.; Qiao, G.; Barlow, K.A.; Wang, J.; Xiangdong, M.; Meng, X.; Paschon, D.E.; Leung, E.; Hinkley, S.J.; et al. A TALE nuclease architecture for efficient genome editing. *Nat. Biotechnol.* **2010**, *29*, 143–148. [CrossRef]
296. Ramalingam, S.; Annaluru, N.; Kandavelou, K.; Chandrasegaran, S. TALEN-mediated generation and genetic correction of disease-specific human induced pluripotent stem cells. *Curr. Gene Ther.* **2014**, *14*, 461–472. [CrossRef]
297. Jinek, M.; Chylinski, K.; Fonfara, I.; Hauer, M.; Doudna, J.A.; Charpentier, E. A Programmable dual-RNA-guided DNA endonuclease in adaptive bacterial immunity. *Science* **2012**, *337*, 816–821. [CrossRef]
298. Broeders, M.; Herrero-Hernandez, P.; Ernst, M.P.; van der Ploeg, A.T.; Pijnappel, W.P. Sharpening the Molecular Scissors: Advances in Gene-Editing Technology. *iScience* **2020**, *23*, 100789. [CrossRef]
299. Ou, L.; Przybilla, M.J.; Ahlat, O.; Kim, S.; Overn, P.; Jarnes, J.; O'Sullivan, M.G.; Whitley, C.B. A Highly Efficacious PS Gene Editing System Corrects Metabolic and Neurological Complications of Mucopolysaccharidosis Type I. *Mol. Ther.* **2020**, *28*, 1442–1454. [CrossRef]
300. Ou, L.; Przybilla, M.J.; Tăbăran, A.-F.; Overn, P.; O'Sullivan, M.G.; Jiang, X.; Sidhu, R.; Kell, P.J.; Ory, D.S.; Whitley, C.B. A novel gene editing system to treat both Tay–Sachs and Sandhoff diseases. *Gene Ther.* **2020**, *27*, 226–236. [CrossRef]
301. Karumuthil-Melethil, S.; Kalburgi, S.N.; Thompson, P.; Tropak, M.; Kaytor, M.D.; Keimel, J.G.; Mark, B.L.; Mahuran, D.; Walia, J.S.; Gray, S.J. Novel Vector Design and Hexosaminidase Variant Enabling Self-Complementary Adeno-Associated Virus for the Treatment of Tay-Sachs Disease. *Hum. Gene Ther.* **2016**, *27*, 509–521. [CrossRef]
302. Osmon, K.J.; Woodley, E.; Thompson, P.; Ong, K.; Karumuthil-Melethil, S.; Keimel, J.G.; Mark, B.L.; Mahuran, D.; Gray, S.J.; Walia, J.S. Systemic Gene Transfer of a Hexosaminidase Variant Using an scAAV9.47 Vector Corrects GM2Gangliosidosis in Sandhoff Mice. *Hum. Gene Ther.* **2016**, *27*, 497–508. [CrossRef]
303. Schuh, R.S.; de Carvalho, T.G.; Giugliani, R.; Matte, U.; Baldo, G.; Teixeira, H.F. Gene editing of MPS I human fibroblasts by co-delivery of a CRISPR/Cas9 plasmid and a donor oligonucleotide using nanoemulsions as nonviral carriers. *Eur. J. Pharm. Biopharm.* **2018**, *122*, 158–166. [CrossRef]
304. Miki, T.; Vazquez, L.; Yanuaria, L.; Lopez, O.; Garcia, I.M.; Ohashi, K.; Rodriguez, N.S. Induced Pluripotent Stem Cell Derivation and Ex Vivo Gene Correction Using a Mucopolysaccharidosis Type 1 Disease Mouse Model. *Stem Cells Int.* **2019**, *2019*, 1–10. [CrossRef] [PubMed]
305. Komor, A.C.; Kim, Y.B.; Packer, M.S.; Zuris, J.A.; Liu, D.R. Programmable editing of a target base in genomic DNA without double-stranded DNA cleavage. *Nature* **2016**, *533*, 420–424. [CrossRef] [PubMed]
306. Gaudelli, N.M.; Komor, A.C.; Rees, H.A.; Packer, M.S.; Badran, A.H.; Bryson, D.I.; Liu, D.R. Programmable base editing of A•T to G•C in genomic DNA without DNA cleavage. *Nature* **2017**, *551*, 464–471. [CrossRef] [PubMed]
307. Levy, J.M.; Yeh, W.-H.; Pendse, N.; Davis, J.R.; Hennessey, E.; Butcher, R.; Koblan, L.W.; Comander, J.; Liu, Q.; Liu, D.R. Cytosine and adenine base editing of the brain, liver, retina, heart and skeletal muscle of mice via adeno-associated viruses. *Nat. Biomed. Eng.* **2020**, *4*, 97–110. [CrossRef]
308. Truong, D.-J.J.; Kühner, K.; Kühn, R.; Werfel, S.; Engelhardt, S.; Wurst, W.; Ortiz, O. Development of an intein-mediated split–Cas9 system for gene therapy. *Nucleic Acids Res.* **2015**, *43*, 6450–6458. [CrossRef]
309. Anzalone, A.V.; Randolph, P.B.; Davis, J.R.; Sousa, A.A.; Koblan, L.W.; Levy, J.M.; Chen, P.J.; Wilson, C.; Newby, G.A.; Raguram, A.; et al. Search-and-replace genome editing without double-strand breaks or donor DNA. *Nat. Cell Biol.* **2019**, *576*, 149–157. [CrossRef]

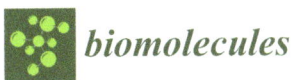

Article

Effect of Substrate Reduction Therapy in Comparison to Enzyme Replacement Therapy on Immune Aspects and Bone Involvement in Gaucher Disease

Renuka P. Limgala * and Ozlem Goker-Alpan

Lysosomal and Rare Disorders Research and Treatment Center (LDRTC), Fairfax, VA 22030, USA; ogoker-alpan@ldrtc.org
* Correspondence: rlimgala@ldrtc.org; Tel.: +1-703-261-6220

Received: 25 February 2020; Accepted: 27 March 2020; Published: 31 March 2020

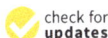

Abstract: Gaucher disease (GD) is caused by mutations in the *GBA* gene, leading to deficient activity of the lysosomal enzyme glucocerebrosidase. Among all the symptoms across various organ systems, bone disease is a major concern as it causes high morbidity and reduces quality of life. Enzyme replacement therapy (ERT) is the most accepted treatment; however, there are still unmet needs. As an alternative, substrate reduction therapy (SRT) was developed using glucosylceramide synthase inhibitors. In the current study, the effects of ERT vs. SRT were compared, particularly the immunological and bone remodeling aspects. GD subjects were divided into three cohorts based on their treatment at initial visit: ERT, SRT, and untreated (UT). Immunophenotyping showed no significant immune cell alterations between the cohorts. Expression of RANK/RANKL/Osteoprotegerin pathway components on immune cells and the secreted markers of bone turnover were analyzed. In the ERT cohort, no significant changes were observed in RANK, RANKL or serum biomarkers. RANKL on T lymphocytes, Osteopontin and MIP-1β decreased with SRT treatment indicating probable reduction in osteoclast activity. Other secreted factors, Osteocalcin and RANKL/Osteoprotegerin did not change with the treatment status. Insights from the study highlight personalized differences between subjects and possible use of RANK pathway components as markers for bone disease progression.

Keywords: Gaucher disease; bone involvement; enzyme replacement therapy; substrate reduction therapy; Osteoimmunology; RANK/RANKL; Osteopontin; MIP-1β

1. Introduction

Gaucher disease (GD) (OMIM ID: 230800) is the most prevalent lysosomal disorder, caused by pathogenic mutations in the *GBA* gene, leading to a deficient activity of the lysosomal enzyme β-glucocerebrosidase (GCase). Deficiency of GCase results in the accumulation of glycosphingolipids in various organ systems, most notably in cells of mononuclear phagocyte system. The effects of the glycolipid accumulation are manifested in multiple organ systems, resulting in major signs and symptoms that include enlargement of the liver and spleen (hepatosplenomegaly), lung disease and skeletal abnormalities [1]. Among all these symptoms, bone disease is a major matter of concern for physicians as it causes high morbidity and reduces quality of life. The main clinical manifestations of skeletal disease in GD may be classified into a) bone marrow disease resulting in thrombocytopenia (low number of platelets) and anemia (reduced red blood cells) and b) structural involvement. Structural complications can further be subclassified into (1) focal infarcts leading to avascular necrosis (osteonecrosis), sclerosis and osteolytic lesions, (2) generalized osteoporosis and osteopenia, which result in reduced bone density and frequent fractures, and (3) local manifestations that include structural deformities (Erlenmeyer flask deformities) and cortical thinning [2]. Such extensive involvement of complications encompassing multiple facets of the skeletal system occurs in very few cases as the inherent pathology of a medical condition, but rather as a result of the response to external factors such as exposure to long-term corticosteroid medications, radiation therapy, organ transplants etc. This could indicate immune system alterations resulting from such factors may play a significant role in causing these bone complications. Bone is a mineralized connective tissue, which contains embedded osteocytes, and is covered by bone lining cells, osteoclasts, reversal cells and osteoblasts. Furthermore, bone is a living organ in continuous remodeling. Bone remodeling is a highly complex process of resorption by osteoclasts and matrix formation by osteoblasts. Osteoclasts are multinucleated cells that derive from the fusion of cells of monocyte/macrophage lineage under the influence of various molecular mediators [3]. The term osteoimmunology was coined many years ago to describe the research field that investigates the cross-regulation between skeletal and immune systems. Several immune cell subtypes including T/B lymphocytes and dendritic cells (DC) along with secreted factors participate in bone-immune system cross talk affecting osteoblast/osteoclast related bone remodeling [4,5].

Studies using animal models of GD have shown the involvement of osteoblasts in the bone pathophysiology of the disease [6]. Therefore, bone alterations observed in GD patients could be explained, at least partially, by changes in bone generating cells. On the other hand, it has been demonstrated that GCase deficiency is associated with increased osteoclastogenesis and bone resorption both in in vitro models and patients' samples. In GD type 1, the number of cytotoxic T lymphocytes was found to be significantly lower in patients presenting bone involvement, and this correlated with higher levels of plasma tartrate resistant acid phosphatase (TRAP) activity, a putative marker of osteoclast cell activity [7–9]. Components of the RANKL/RANK/OPG pathway, consisting of the cytokine receptor activator of nuclear factor kappa-B ligand (RANKL), its signaling receptor, receptor activator of NF-κB (RANK), and the soluble decoy receptor osteoprotegerin (OPG) have been shown to be major effectors at multiple levels of the bone regeneration cycle and act as interfaces between immune and skeletal systems [10–12].

Macrophage-directed enzyme replacement therapy (ERT) has been the most accepted form of treatment for GD; however, there are still unmet needs in treating all aspects of the disease. As an alternative to ERT, substrate reduction therapy (SRT) was developed using glucosylceramide synthase inhibitors [13–17]. In the current internal review board (IRB) approved study (NCT02605603), we closely monitored and compared the effects of ERT vs. SRT, particularly the immunological aspects and secreted biomarkers involved in bone remodeling.

2. Materials and Methods

Subjects: Thirty-two patients with confirmed GD were enrolled into this active comparator study (NCT02605603). The handling of tissue samples and patient data was approved by the internal review board (Western IRB) including the procedure whereby all patients gave informed consent to participate in this study. Written informed consent was obtained using an IRB-approved informed consent form. At enrollment, a medical history was obtained and a detailed physical examination was performed. Medical records were reviewed as a part of the clinical evaluation and bone disease findings were assessed. All subjects were evaluated during three visits over a period of 12-18 months. Total subjects were divided into three cohorts based on their treatment at the time of initial visit: ERT, GD patients under long-term enzyme replacement therapy with velaglucerase alfa, (VPRIV®, Shire Human Genetic Therapies, Inc., MA, USA) or imiglucerase, (Cerezyme®, Sanofi Genzyme, Cambridge, MA) (n = 14, ERT-1 to ERT-14); SRT, GD patients who were switched to substrate reduction therapy with eliglustat (Cerdelga®, Sanofi Genzyme, Cambridge, MA, USA) during their first visit (n = 10, SRT-01-SRT-10); UT, GD subjects who were either untreated or had long interruption to treatments (n = 8, UT-01 to UT-08). Three subjects in the UT cohort (UT-01, UT-02 and UT-03) were started on SRT and one subject on ERT (UT-04) during subsequent visits. Only initial visit data from UT-07 were available as the subject discontinued participation and was not available for subsequent visits (Table 1).

Table 1. Basic characteristics of the subjects. Pathogenic mutations in *GBA* gene, treatment at initial and follow up visits are noted. M, Male; F, female; ERT, enzyme replacement therapy; SRT, Substrate reduction therapy; UT, Untreated. ERT ¶ -ERT with velaglucerase alfa (VPRIV®), ERT * - ERT with imiglucerase (Cerezyme®), SRT- eliglustat (Cerdelga®).

ID	Gender	Age (Years)	Genotype	Initial Visit	Follow-Up Visit
SRT-01	F	50	N370S/N370S	ERT ¶	SRT
SRT-02	M	59	N370S/N370S	ERT *	SRT
SRT-03	F	46	N370S/N370S	ERT *	SRT
SRT-04	F	57	N370S/N370S	ERT *	SRT
SRT-05	F	35	N370S/R463C	ERT *	SRT
SRT-06	F	37	N370S/R463C	ERT *	SRT
SRT-07	F	24	N370S/L444P	ERT *	SRT
SRT-08	F	62	N370S/R463C	ERT *	SRT
SRT-09	F	52	1448C/L444P	ERT ¶	SRT
SRT-10	F	47	N370S/N370S	ERT ¶	SRT
ERT-01	F	34	N370S/L444P	ERT ¶	ERT ¶
ERT-02	F	35	N370S/R120Q	ERT ¶	ERT ¶
ERT-03	F	45	N370S/N370S	ERT ¶	ERT ¶
ERT-04	F	61	N370S/L444P	ERT ¶	ERT ¶
ERT-05	F	20	L444P/L444P	ERT *	ERT *
ERT-06	M	18	L444P/L444P	ERT *	ERT *
ERT-07	F	10	L444P/L444P	ERT *	ERT *
ERT-08	F	27	N370S/L444P	ERT *	ERT *
ERT-09	F	42	N370S/L444P	ERT *	ERT *
ERT-10	M	50	N370S/L444P	ERT ¶	ERT ¶
ERT-11	M	76	N370S/N370S	ERT *	ERT *
ERT-12	M	14	L444P/L444P	ERT *	ERT *
ERT-13	F	40	L444P/R463C	ERT ¶	ERT ¶
ERT-14	F	23	N370S/W381X	ERT ¶	ERT ¶
UT-01	M	27	C677T/C677T	UT	SRT
UT-02	F	56	N370S/N370S	UT	SRT
UT-03	M	38	N370S/N370S	UT	SRT
UT-04	M	34	N370S/N370S	UT	ERT ¶
UT-05	F	36	N370S/N370S	UT	UT
UT-06	F	32	N370S/N370S	UT	UT
UT-07	F	61	N370S/N370S	UT	UT
UT-08	F	58	N370S/N370S	UT	UT

Immunophenotyping: Direct immunofluorescence with specific antibodies was performed on peripheral blood as previously described [18,19] with some modifications using the following antibodies: anti-IgG1 FITC, anti-CD5-FITC, anti-CD8-FITC, anti-CD14-FITC, anti-CD22-FITC, anti-CD34-FITC, anti-IgG1-PE, anti-CD3-FITC/CD16$^+$CD56-PE, anti-CD11C-PE, anti-CD21-PE, anti-CD27-PE, anti-CD183-PE, anti-CD194-PE, anti-CD20-PerCP and anti-HLA-DR-PerCP (BD Bioscience, San Jose, CA, USA). Anti-CD19-FITC, anti-IgA-FITC, anti-IgD-FITC, anti-CD8-PE, anti-CD19-PE, anti-IgG-PE, anti-IgG1-PerCP, anti-CD3-PerCP, anti-CD4-PerCP, anti-CD8-PerCP and anti-CD3-APC (Invitrogen, Carlsbad, CA, USA). Anti-Lineage-FITC (anti CD3/CD14/CD16/CD19/CD20/CD56), anti-CD196-PerCP, anti-IgM-PerCP and anti-CD45-APC (Biolegend, San Diego, CA, USA). Anti-CD4-FITC (eBioscience, San Diego, CA, USA), anti-CD45RO-FITC (Abcam, Cambridge, MA, USA) and anti-BDCA2-APC (Miltenyi Biotech, San Diego, CA, USA). Briefly, after washing the whole blood with PBS, 100 µl of blood was stained with the relevant cocktail of antibodies at 4 °C for 30 min followed by red blood cell lysis using BD FACS lysis solution (BD Bioscience, San Jose, CA, USA). Samples were acquired on Accuri C6 flow cytometer (BD Bioscience, San Jose, CA, USA) and analyzed using FCS express software (De Novo software, Glendale, CA, USA). During acquisition, a lymphocyte gate was assigned and 10,000 events were collected for the T cells and NK cells, and 25,000 events for the B cell analysis. For dendritic cells, a million ungated events were acquired.

Assessment of Bone biomarkers: Plasma samples were collected by centrifuging the whole blood within 12 h of collection and stored at −20 °C till use. Enzyme linked immunosorbent assays (ELISAs) were carried out using plasma samples for secreted factors—RANKL, OPG (Origene technologies, Rockville, MD, USA), osteocalcin, osteopontin, MIP-1β and CCL18 (Thermo Fisher Scientific, Waltham, MA, USA)—according to manufacturers' protocols.

Statistical analysis: All statistical analysis was performed using GraphPad Prism software (GraphPad Software, Inc., La Jolla, CA, USA) and graphs were generated as dot plots. Statistical evaluation of differences was performed using Wilcoxon signed-rank test for comparing results between visits for each cohort. P-values were indicated where found significant, *: $p < 0.05$; **: $p < 0.01$.

3. Results

Bone involvement was assessed with the presence of bone pain, pathological fractures, bone density and radiological changes (Erlenmeyer flask and cystic deformities), bone marrow infiltration, history of osteonecrosis and previous surgery (Table 2). At enrollment, 72% of subjects presented with radiological changes (23/32), and 59% reported bone pain (19/32). Five subjects had severe skeletal involvement (three in the SRT and two in the ERT cohort), and all of these were splenectomized. Among the subjects who had a history of osteonecrosis, half of them were splenectomized (4/8). There were eight untreated patients at presentation, and three with moderate to severe bone disease were started on SRT, and one was treated with ERT. All subjects had involvement of the bone marrow. Bone density changes were observed about 50% of the total subjects (16/32), and there were five subjects with osteoporosis in the SRT, six subjects in the ERT cohorts, and three among the untreated. Overall, skeletal manifestations were equally represented in each treatment group on presentation.

Table 2. Bone disease in subjects at the time of enrollment. Bone involvement for each subject is characterized by bone marrow infiltration, bone pain, EM-flask deformity, cystic/lytic lesions, osteoporosis, osteopenia and avascular necrosis. Subjects who have undergone splenectomy are indicated.

ID	Splenectomy	Bone Surgery	Bone Pain	Bone Marrow Infiltration	EM-Flask Deformity	Cystic/Lytic Lesions	Pathologic Fractures	Osteo Penia	Osteo Porosis	AVN
SRT-01	No	No	Moderate	Moderate dark marrow	No	No	No	No	No	No
SRT-02	No	No	Moderate	Patchy dark marrow	No	Yes	No	No	Yes	No
SRT-03	No	No	Moderate	Patchy dark marrow	Yes	No	No	Yes	No	No
SRT-04	No	No	Mild	Patchy dark marrow	Yes	Yes	No	No	Yes	No
SRT-05	No	No	Mild	Mild symmetric dark marrow	No	No	No	Yes	No	No
SRT-06	No	No	Mild	Mild symmetric dark marrow	No	No	No	No	No	No
SRT-07	No	No	No	Patchy dark marrow	Yes	No	No	No	No	No
SRT-08	Yes	Yes	Moderate	Extensive dark marrow	Yes	Yes	Yes	Yes	Yes	Yes
SRT-09	Yes	Yes	Moderate	Mild symmetric dark marrow	Yes	Yes	Yes	Yes	Yes	No
SRT-10	Yes	Yes	Severe	Marrow infarcts	Yes	Yes	No	Yes	Yes	Yes
ERT-01	No	No	No	Mild patchy dark marrow	Yes	No	No	No	No	No
ERT-02	No	No	Moderate	Patchy, hypo intense marrow	Yes	No	No	Yes	No	No
ERT-03	Yes	Yes	No	Heterogeneous dark marrow	Yes	Yes	No	Yes	Yes	No
ERT-04	Yes	Yes	Moderate	Marrow infarcts/patchy dark	Yes	Yes	Yes	Yes	Yes	Yes

Table 2. Cont.

ID	Splenectomy	Bone Surgery	Bone Pain	Bone Marrow Infiltration	EM-Flask Deformity	Cystic/Lytic Lesions	Pathologic Fractures	Osteo Penia	Osteo Porosis	AVN
ERT-05	No	No	No	Patchy dark marrow	Yes	No	No	No	No	No
ERT-06	No	No	No	Patchy dark marrow	No	No	No	No	No	No
ERT-07	No	No	No	Patchy dark marrow	No	No	No	No	No	No
ERT-08	No	No	No	Patchy dark marrow	Yes	No	No	Yes	Yes	No
ERT-09	No	Yes	Moderate	Marrow infarcts	Yes	Yes	No	Yes	No	Yes
ERT-10	No	No	No	Marrow infarcts	No	No	No	Yes	Yes	Yes
ERT-11	No	No	Moderate	Marrow infarcts	Yes	Yes	No	Yes	Yes	Yes
ERT-12	No	No	Moderate	Patchy dark marrow	Yes	No	No	No	No	No
ERT-13	Yes	Yes	Severe	Marrow infarcts	Yes	Yes	No	Yes	Yes	Yes
ERT-14	No	No	Mild	Symmetric dark marrow	Yes	No	No	Yes	No	No
UT-01	No	No	No	Patchy dark marrow	No	No	No	No	No	No
UT-02	No	Yes	Moderate	Marrow infarcts/dark marrow	Yes	No	No	Yes	No	Yes
UT-03	No	No	No	Confluent dark marrow	Yes	No	No	No	Yes	No
UT-04	Yes	No	No	Patchy dark marrow	Yes	No	No	No	No	No
UT-05	No	No	No	Symmetric dark marrow	Yes	No	No	No	Yes	No
UT-06	No	No	No	Symmetric dark marrow	Yes	No	No	Yes	No	No
UT-07	No	No	Moderate	Mild symmetric dark marrow	No	No	No	Yes	No	No
UT-08	No	No	Mild	Patchy dark marrow	Yes	No	No	Yes	Yes	No

At every visit, after the clinical evaluation of each subject, peripheral blood was drawn for in-depth immunophenotyping. Flow cytometry-based immune profiling analysis was performed to elaborate on T/B-lymphocytes, NK/NKT cells and dendritic cell fractions in peripheral blood. Overall percentages of T lymphocytes, T helper cells, and cytotoxic T cells were maintained between visits within each cohort. However, cytotoxic T cells were found to be higher in the UT cohort resulting in lower T helper to cytotoxic T cell ratio. In subjects UT-02, UT-03 and UT-04, an increase in T helper to cytotoxic T cell ratio was observed, most likely as a result of the initiation of treatment. When memory T cell subsets were analyzed using CD45RO, no significant differences were observed either between cohorts or between visits within each cohort (Figure 1A–F).

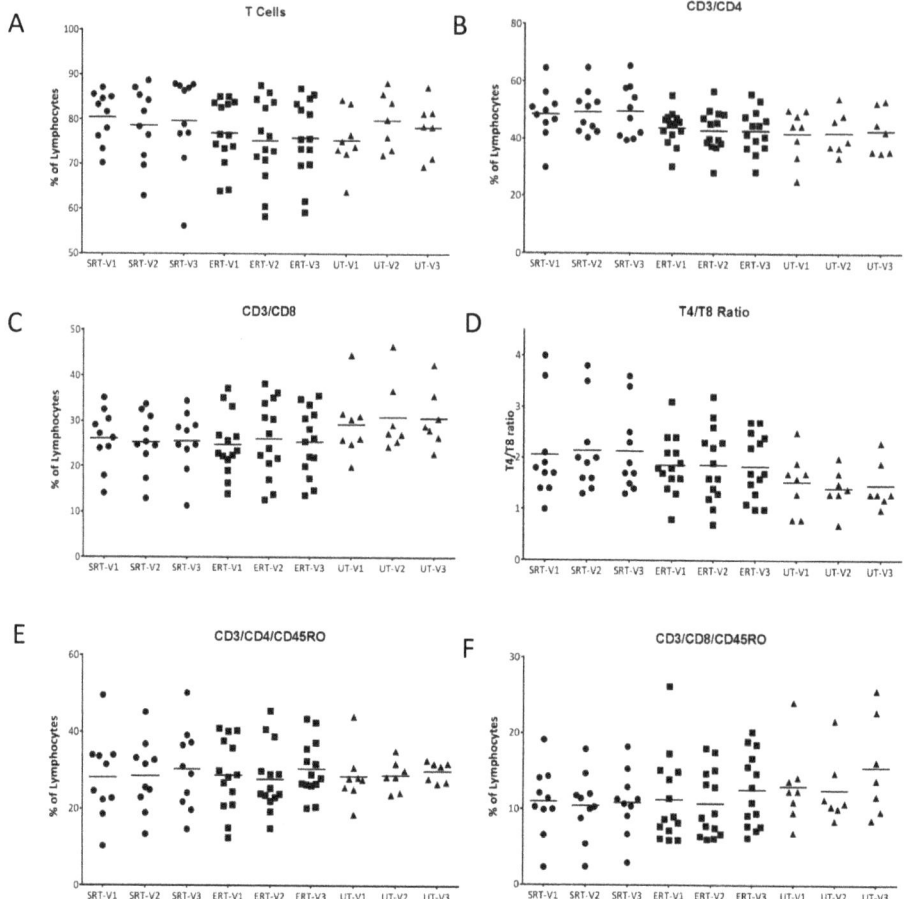

Figure 1. T-lymphocytes and subsets in GD patients. Percentages of T-lymphocytes (CD3+) from peripheral blood of GD patients at each visit were assessed using flow cytometry and plotted (**A**). T helper cells (CD3+/CD4+) (**B**) and cytotoxic T cells (CD3+/CD8+) (**C**) were calculated and a ratio of CD4 to CD8 cells was plotted (**D**). Similarly memory subsets of CD4 (CD3+/CD4+/CD45RO+) and CD8 T cells (CD3+/CD8+/CD45RO+) were calculated and plotted (**E,F**).

Other immune cell types, namely B lymphocytes, NK cells, NKT cells and dendritic cells, were quantified at each visit but no significant differences were found, indicating that treatment differences did not influence overall immune cell subsets in a significant manner (Figure 2A–D).

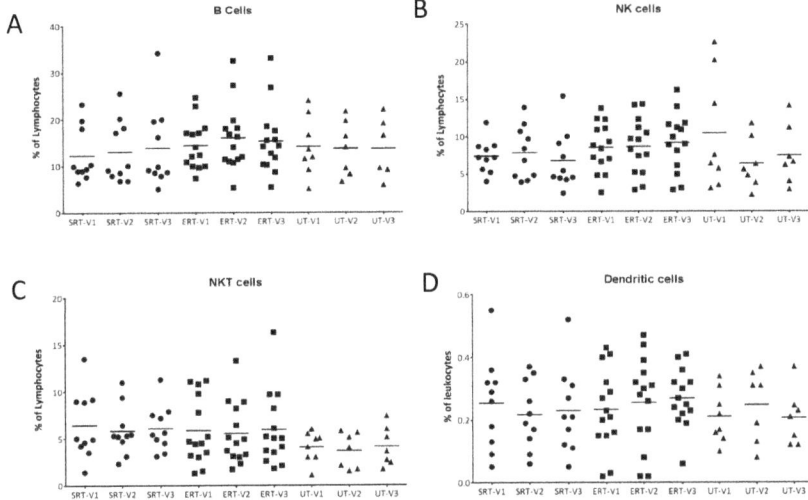

Figure 2. B-lymphocytes, NK, NKT and dendritic cells in GD patients. Percentage of B-lymphocytes (CD20+), NK cells (CD3-/CD16+ or CD56+), NKT cells (CD3+/CD16+ or CD56+) from peripheral blood of GD patients at each visit were assessed using flow cytometry and plotted (**A–C**). Dendritic cells were enumerated as Lin-/CD34-/HLA DR+ cells and plotted as a percentage of total leukocytes (**D**). • SRT cohort; ■ ERT cohort; ▲ UT cohort.

In GD patients, chemokine (C-C motif) ligand 18 (CCL18) is known to be secreted at elevated levels by activated macrophages and has been used as biomarker to study response to ERT. CCL18 was measured using ELISA from the plasma samples collected from all the subjects during each visit. As expected, CCL18 levels were markedly elevated at visit 1 in the UT cohort compared to the SRT and ERT (p value = 0.008 and 0.02 respectively). No significant differences were observed within the ERT cohort between visits as expected. In subjects UT-01 to UT-04 who had started treatment for GD, there was a decrease in CCL18 levels between visits 2 and 3 compared to visit 1 as a positive response to therapy. Interestingly, in the SRT cohort, subjects showed overall lower CCL18 in subsequent visits compared to visit 1 (p value = 0.027) (Figure 3A).

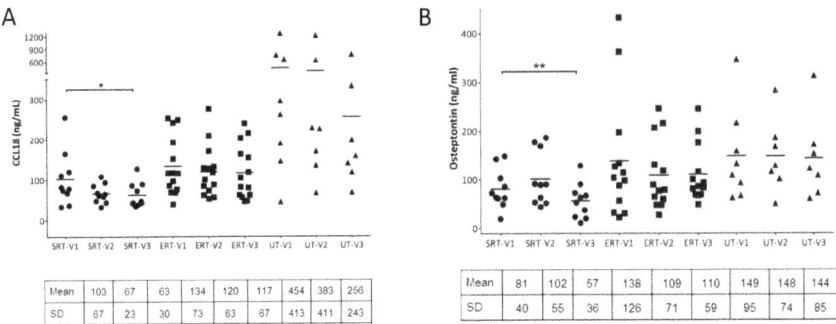

Figure 3. *Cont.*

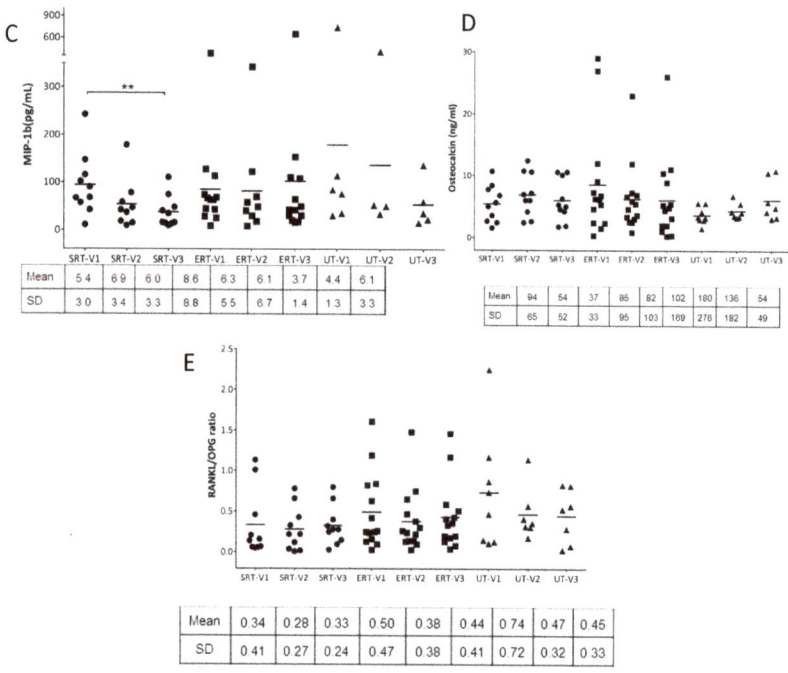

Figure 3. Analysis of secreted biomarkers from plasma: Macrophage activation marker, CCL18 was quantitated using ELISA from plasma samples at each visit and compared (A). Bone recycling biomarkers, osteopontin, osteocalcin, and bone disease markers, MIP-1β were quantified at each visit and plotted (B–D). Secreted RANKL and Osteoprotegerin (OPG) were quantified from plasma were plotted as RANKL to OPG ratio at each visit (E). Paired student's t-test was performed to calculate significance values and included in the plots where significant difference was observed. *: p < 0.05; **: p < 0.01. Mean and +/− SD values are noted below individual plots. ● SRT cohort; ■ ERT cohort; ▲ UT cohort.

Osteopontin (OPN) and osteocalcin (OC) are major non-collagenous proteins that play vital roles in bone remodeling and homeostasis. OPN is a multifunctional protein which promotes osteoclastogenesis and osteoclast activity as well as osteoclast survival and motility. OPN is also considered an atypical immune regulator and higher levels of OPN have been associated with inflammatory bone diseases. When OPN was measured from plasma samples from each cohort during multiple visits, OPN levels did not change between visits for the ERT and UT cohorts. In the SRT cohort, while OPN was found to be slightly elevated in seven out of 10 subjects, in all the subjects OPN levels were reduced by visit 3, especially compared to visit 1 (p value = 0.009) (Figure 3B). Osteocalcin, which is produced by osteoblasts, is widely regarded as a marker of bone formation and plasma concentrations of osteocalcin are used as markers of bone formation. In the current study, no significant differences in plasma OC levels were observed within the SRT and ERT cohort between visits. However, within the UT cohort, three UT subjects (UT-01, UT-03 and UT-04) showed increase in OC by visit 3 compared to visit 1, most likely as a result of treatment initiation (Figure 3C). Macrophage inflammatory protein-1 beta (MIP-1β) has been shown to be a marker for bone disease in GD [20]. Secreted MIP-1β level was significantly decreased by visit 3 in the SRT cohort compared to visit 1 (p value = 0.004) (Figure 3D). RANK/RANKL/OPG signaling has been shown to be critical in osteoclastogenesis and influencing bone remodeling. Serum concentrations of RANKL and OPG were analyzed for each subject at every visit and expressed as RANKL/OPG ratio. There were significant differences in RANKL/OPG ratio within the ERT cohort between visits. In the SRT cohort, four out of 10 subjects showed lower RANKL/OPG ratios due to an increase in OPG concentration. Within the UT cohort, three UT subjects (UT-01, UT-03 and UT-04) showed a decrease in RANKL/OPG ratio by visit 3 compared to visit 1, again as a likely result of treatment initiation (Figure 3E).

Cell surface expression of RANK on T and B lymphocytes and monocytes as well as RANKL expression on T lymphocytes was assessed using flow cytometry. In subjects within the ERT cohort, no major alterations were observed in surface expression of RANK or RANKL over the three visits. Within the SRT cohort, there was a marked increase at visit 2 in the expression of RANK on T cells and B cells (in four out of 10 subjects), and monocytes (in five out of 10 subjects). However, these alterations were seen to be reversed by visit 3. Overall cell surface expression of RANK was in fact significantly reduced on both T and B lymphocytes (p value = 0.019 and 0.012 respectively) at visit 3 compared to visit 1. RANKL expression on T lymphocytes at visit 3 was also significantly reduced in the SRT cohort compared to visit 1 (p value = 0.002) (Figure 4A–D).

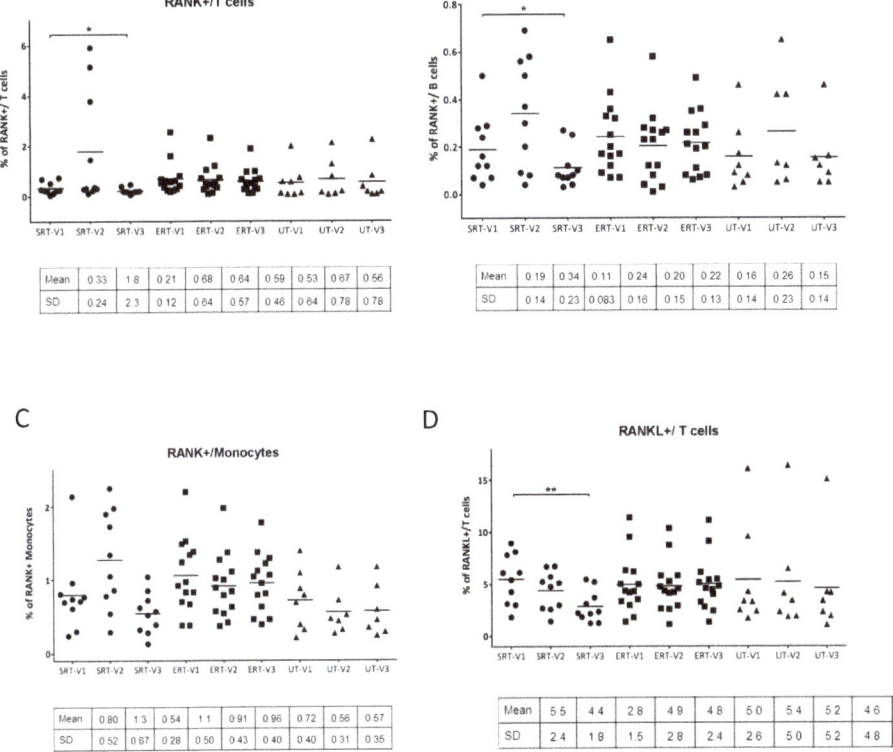

Figure 4. Analysis of RANK and RANKL on immune cell subsets: Percentage of RANK+ T-lymphocytes (CD45+/CD3+/RANK+), B-lymphocytes (CD45+/CD20+/RANK+) and monocytes (CD45+/CD14+/RANK+) and RANKL+ T-lymphocytes (CD45+/CD3+/RANKL+) at each visit quantitated using flow cytometry analysis from peripheral blood samples at each visit and compared (A-D). Paired student's t-test was performed to calculate significance values and included in the plots where significant difference was observed. *: $p < 0.05$; **: $p < 0.01$. Mean and +/− SD values are noted below individual plots. • SRT cohort; ■ ERT cohort; ▲ UT cohort.

4. Discussion

While GD affects multiple organ systems, skeletal complications are a common occurrence in majority of GD patients with debilitating consequences. Skeletal system involvement in GD includes growth retardation, structural distortions like Erlenmeyer flask deformities, lytic lesions, avascular necrosis, osteopenia, osteoporosis, bone marrow infiltration and bone crises. GD patients are also susceptible to fractures and bone surgery at higher rates. Furthermore, the severity of bone manifestations does not necessarily reflect the pathological involvement in other organ systems [2]. Such a wide array of complications in skeletal system points to a complex inter-linking of multiple pathways in bone development and bone remodeling over a time period. Since the hallmark of GD is the accumulation of sphingolipids including GL-1 and lyso GL-1, especially in the cells of monocyte/macrophage lineage, the effect of immune system modulation on bone development and remodeling is not trivial. It has been shown that although ERT is associated with improvement of bone crises and other bone complications over a period of time, not all symptoms are reversible. Moreover, it has been shown that certain GD patients continue to develop avascular necrosis (AVN) even after being on long-term ERT, especially if the treatment was delayed more than 2 y after diagnosis [21]. SRT was developed as alternate mode of treatment in adult GD patients with an aim to reduce accumulating glycosphingolipids by inhibiting their synthesis. SRT consists of small compounds that are taken orally and have the potential to rapidly diffuse into various tissues, with potential advantages of better prevention of bone complications due to drug delivery in the bone compartments. While certain components of bone disease see improvement with SRT, it is not possible to conclude with certainty as to superiority of SRT over ERT regarding bone complications [15–17,22–24]. Recent case reports demonstrate that judicious use of the SRT-ERT combination therapy may benefit in certain GD patients [25,26].

The skeletal system is a highly complex and dynamic structure with continuous turnover as a result of its constant remodeling cycle, essential for maintaining the integrity of the skeleton. Bone remodeling is a lifelong process consisting of three consecutive phases: bone resorption, during which osteoclasts digest the old bone; reversal, when mononuclear cells appear on the bone surface; and formation or ossification, when osteoblasts lay down new bone until the resorbed bone is completely replaced. In normal bone remodeling, there is no net change in bone mass and strength. However, the bone remodeling cycle may be derailed at multiple points, resulting in metabolic bone disorders [12]. In the current study, we investigated the influence of peripheral immune system on bone remodeling and whether bone remodeling defects could be assessed using the secreted markers of bone turnover including soluble RANKL (sRANKL), OPG, OPN, OC and MIP-1β. In addition, the expression of RANK/RANKL pathway components on relevant immune cell types was analyzed using flow cytometry. The results were then followed with their treatment status over a period of time. When major immune subsets were compared within the three cohorts, no significant differences were observed in overall fraction of lymphocytes, NK/NKT cells or dendritic cells. A decrease in the concentration of the chemokine CCL18 following SRT treatment in the SRT and UT cohorts indicated a reduction in macrophage inflammation in the subjects. Another cytokine, OPN, is known to play multiple roles in bone remodeling and acts as a positive regulator of osteoclastogenesis. It has also been indicated that OPN could be a bridge between bone and the immune system. In the SRT cohort, OPN and MIP-1β concentrations were found to be significantly lower at visit 3, indicating a probable reduction in osteoclast activity that could result in lower bone resorption. Other secreted factors, OC and RANKL/OPG did not change over time with the treatment status.

RANK is a member of the TNF family and its ligand, RANKL, was initially identified to be expressed on T cells and enhance dendritic cell survival. Later it was shown that RANKL-expressing T cells can also activate RANK-expressing osteoclasts, thereby mimicking RANKL-expressing osteoblasts and explaining the crosstalk of immune cells and bone. This crosstalk was found to be a causative factor for the bone loss observed in patients with a chronically activated immune system which induces osteoclastogenesis, thereby shifting the balance in favor of bone resorption over bone deposition [3,10,11,27]. In order to study the expression of RANK and RANKL on immune cell subsets, cell surface expression of these molecules was studied using flow cytometry. In a subset of the SRT cohort, there was a marked increase in expression of RANK on T and B lymphocytes as well as monocytes (Figure 4A–C). This effect was not only reversed by visit 3, but the overall RANK expression was reduced in the whole cohort. The results indicate that the cell-surface changes observed in the SRT cohort at visit 2 could be a result of initial reaction to the SRT treatment which did not have long term effects as seen by normalization or improvement by visit 3. RANKL expression on T cells was also significantly reduced in the SRT cohort by visit 3. Taken together these results indicate the reduction in osteoclastogenic biomarkers in the SRT cohort compared to the ERT cohort. One of the limitations of the study was inclusion of a higher ratio of females to males (24F/8M) which resulted from unbiased recruiting given our center's patient population. However, the distribution of bone disease was comparable between females and males in the study subjects as seen in Tables 1 and 2. Another limitation of the study was the brief period of study, as a result of which the correlation of the findings to the improvement of clinical symptoms has not been performed since that requires a longer follow up. However, insights from the study highlight personalized differences between subjects with different treatment modalities.

Author Contributions: Conceptualization, R.P.L.; Formal analysis, R.P.L.; Funding acquisition, O.G.-A.; Investigation, R.P.L.; Methodology, R.P.L.; Project administration, R.P.L.; Supervision, O.G.-A.; Writing—original draft, R.P.L.; Writing—review & editing, R.P.L. and O.G.-A. All authors have read and agreed to the published version of the manuscript.

Funding: This study was supported by an investigator-initiated research grant from Sanofi-Genzyme (GZ-2014-11295). We thank Dr. Ravi S. Kamath (Fairfax Radiological consultants, Fairfax, VA, USA) for imaging of skeletal manifestations of GD patients. We appreciate Miriam Lopez and Chidima Ioanou (O&O Alpan, LLC, Fairfax, VA, USA) for their support in coordinating collection of samples.

Conflicts of Interest: This study was funded by an investigator initiated research grant to OGA from Sanofi-Genzyme (GZ-2014-11295). The authors declare no conflict of interest.

References

1. Nagral, A. Gaucher disease. *J. Clin. Exp. Hepatol.* **2014**, *4*, 37–50. [CrossRef]
2. Goker-Alpan, O. Therapeutic approaches to bone pathology in Gaucher disease: Past, present and future. *Mol. Genet. Metab.* **2011**, *104*, 438–447. [CrossRef]
3. Feng, X.; McDonald, J.M. Disorders of bone remodeling. *Annu. Rev. Pathol.* **2011**, *6*, 121–145. [CrossRef]
4. Srivastava, R.K.; Dar, H.Y.; Mishra, P.K. Immunoporosis: Immunology of Osteoporosis-Role of T Cells. *Front. Immunol.* **2018**, *9*, 657. [CrossRef]
5. Ponzetti, M.; Rucci, N. Updates on Osteoimmunology: What's New on the Cross-Talk Between Bone and Immune System. *Front. Endocrinol.* **2019**, *10*, 236. [CrossRef]
6. Mistry, P.K.; Liu, J.; Yang, M.; Nottoli, T.; McGrath, J.; Jain, D.; Zhang, K.; Keutzer, J.; Chuang, W.L.; Mehal, W.Z.; et al. Glucocerebrosidase gene-deficient mouse recapitulates Gaucher disease displaying cellular and molecular dysregulation beyond the macrophage. *Proc. Natl. Acad. Sci. USA* **2010**, *107*, 19473–19478. [CrossRef]
7. Mucci, J.M.; Rozenfeld, P. Pathogenesis of Bone Alterations in Gaucher Disease: The Role of Immune System. *J. Immunol. Res.* **2015**, *2015*, 192761. [CrossRef]
8. Pandey, M.K.; Grabowski, G.A. Immunological cells and functions in Gaucher disease. *Crit. Rev. Oncog.* **2013**, *18*, 197–220. [CrossRef]
9. Lacerda, L.; Arosa, F.A.; Lacerda, R.; Cabeda, J.; Porto, G.; Amaral, O.; Fortuna, A.; Pinto, R.; Oliveira, P.; McLaren, C.E.; et al. T cell numbers relate to bone involvement in Gaucher disease. *Blood Cellsmolecules Dis.* **1999**, *25*, 130–138. [CrossRef]
10. Atkins, G.J.; Kostakis, P.; Vincent, C.; Farrugia, A.N.; Houchins, J.P.; Findlay, D.M.; Evdokiou, A.; Zannettino, A.C. RANK Expression as a cell surface marker of human osteoclast precursors in peripheral blood, bone marrow, and giant cell tumors of bone. *J. Bone Miner. Res.: Off. J. Am. Soc. Bone Miner. Res.* **2006**, *21*, 1339–1349. [CrossRef]

11. Leibbrandt, A.; Penninger, J.M. Novel functions of RANK(L) signaling in the immune system. *Adv. Exp. Med. Biol.* **2010**, *658*, 77–94. [CrossRef] [PubMed]
12. Weitzmann, M.N. Bone and the Immune System. *Toxicol. Pathol.* **2017**, *45*, 911–924. [CrossRef] [PubMed]
13. Bennett, L.L.; Mohan, D. Gaucher disease and its treatment options. *Ann. Pharmacother.* **2013**, *47*, 1182–1193. [CrossRef] [PubMed]
14. Charrow, J.; Scott, C.R. Long-term treatment outcomes in Gaucher disease. *Am. J. Hematol.* **2015**, *90*, S19–S24. [CrossRef]
15. Goker-Alpan, O. Optimal therapy in Gaucher disease. *Clin. Risk Manag* **2010**, *6*, 315–323. [CrossRef]
16. Van Rossum, A.; Holsopple, M. Enzyme Replacement or Substrate Reduction? A Review of Gaucher Disease Treatment Options. *Hosp. Pharm.* **2016**, *51*, 553–563. [CrossRef]
17. Zimran, A.; Elstein, D. Management of Gaucher disease: Enzyme replacement therapy. *Pediatric Endocrinol. Rev.: Per* **2014**, *12*, 82–87.
18. Limgala, R.P.; Ioanou, C.; Plassmeyer, M.; Ryherd, M.; Kozhaya, L.; Austin, L.; Abidoglu, C.; Unutmaz, D.; Alpan, O.; Goker-Alpan, O. Time of Initiating Enzyme Replacement Therapy Affects Immune Abnormalities and Disease Severity in Patients with Gaucher Disease. *PLoS ONE* **2016**, *11*, e0168135. [CrossRef]
19. Sonder, S.U.; Limgala, R.P.; Ivanova, M.M.; Ioanou, C.; Plassmeyer, M.; Marti, G.E.; Alpan, O.; Goker-Alpan, O. Persistent immune alterations and comorbidities in splenectomized patients with Gaucher disease. *Blood Cellsmolecules Dis.* **2016**, *59*, 8–15. [CrossRef]
20. Van Breemen, M.J.; de Fost, M.; Voerman, J.S.; Laman, J.D.; Boot, R.G.; Maas, M.; Hollak, C.E.; Aerts, J.M.; Rezaee, F. Increased plasma macrophage inflammatory protein (MIP)-1alpha and MIP-1beta levels in type 1 Gaucher disease. *Biochim. Biophys. Acta* **2007**, *1772*, 788–796. [CrossRef]
21. Mistry, P.K.; Deegan, P.; Vellodi, A.; Cole, J.A.; Yeh, M.; Weinreb, N.J. Timing of initiation of enzyme replacement therapy after diagnosis of type 1 Gaucher disease: Effect on incidence of avascular necrosis. *Br. J. Haematol.* **2009**, *147*, 561–570. [CrossRef] [PubMed]
22. Van Dussen, L.; Biegstraaten, M.; Dijkgraaf, M.G.; Hollak, C.E. Modelling Gaucher disease progression: Long-term enzyme replacement therapy reduces the incidence of splenectomy and bone complications. *Orphanet J. Rare Dis.* **2014**, *9*, 112. [CrossRef]
23. Weinreb, N.; Taylor, J.; Cox, T.; Yee, J.; vom Dahl, S. A benchmark analysis of the achievement of therapeutic goals for type 1 Gaucher disease patients treated with imiglucerase. *Am. J. Hematol.* **2008**, *83*, 890–895. [CrossRef]
24. Smid, B.E.; Ferraz, M.J.; Verhoek, M.; Mirzaian, M.; Wisse, P.; Overkleeft, H.S.; Hollak, C.E.; Aerts, J.M. Biochemical response to substrate reduction therapy versus enzyme replacement therapy in Gaucher disease type 1 patients. *Orphanet J. Rare Dis.* **2016**, *11*, 28. [CrossRef] [PubMed]
25. Ceravolo, F.; Grisolia, M.; Sestito, S.; Falvo, F.; Moricca, M.T.; Concolino, D. Combination therapy in a patient with chronic neuronopathic Gaucher disease: A case report. *J. Med. Case Rep.* **2017**, *11*, 19. [CrossRef] [PubMed]
26. Amato, D.; Patterson, M.A. Combined miglustat and enzyme replacement therapy in two patients with type 1 Gaucher disease: Two case reports. *J. Med. Case Rep.* **2018**, *12*, 19. [CrossRef] [PubMed]
27. Gravallese, E.M. Osteopontin: A bridge between bone and the immune system. *J. Clin. Investig.* **2003**, *112*, 147–149. [CrossRef] [PubMed]

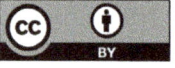

© 2020 by the authors. Licensee MDPI, Basel, Switzerland. This article is an open access article distributed under the terms and conditions of the Creative Commons Attribution (CC BY) license (http://creativecommons.org/licenses/by/4.0/).

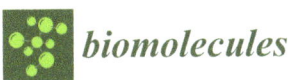

Article

Elevated Dkk1 Mediates Downregulation of the Canonical Wnt Pathway and Lysosomal Loss in an iPSC Model of Neuronopathic Gaucher Disease

Manasa P. Srikanth and Ricardo A. Feldman *

Department of Microbiology and Immunology, School of Medicine, University of Maryland, Baltimore, MD 21201, USA; MSrikanth@som.umaryland.edu
* Correspondence: rfeldman@som.umaryland.edu; Tel.: +1-(410)-706-4198

Received: 13 November 2020; Accepted: 30 November 2020; Published: 3 December 2020

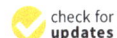

Abstract: Gaucher Disease (GD), which is the most common lysosomal storage disorder, is caused by bi-allelic mutations in *GBA1*—a gene that encodes the lysosomal hydrolase β-glucocerebrosidase (GCase). The neuronopathic forms of GD (nGD) are characterized by severe neurological abnormalities that arise during gestation or early in infancy. Using GD-induced pluripotent stem cell (iPSC)-derived neuronal progenitor cells (NPCs), we have previously reported that neuronal cells have neurodevelopmental defects associated with the downregulation of canonical Wnt signaling. In this study, we report that GD NPCs display elevated levels of Dkk1, which is a secreted Wnt antagonist that prevents receptor activation. Dkk1 upregulation in mutant NPCs resulted in an increased degradation of β-catenin, and there was a concomitant reduction in lysosomal numbers. Consistent with these results, incubation of the mutant NPCs with recombinant Wnt3a (rWnt3a) was able to outcompete the excess Dkk1, increasing β-catenin levels and rescuing lysosomal numbers. Furthermore, the incubation of WT NPCs with recombinant Dkk1 (rDkk1) phenocopied the mutant phenotype, recapitulating the decrease in β-catenin levels and lysosomal depletion seen in nGD NPCs. This study provides evidence that downregulation of the Wnt/β-catenin pathway in nGD neuronal cells involves the upregulation of Dkk1. As Dkk1 is an extracellular Wnt antagonist, our results suggest that the deleterious effects of Wnt/β-catenin downregulation in nGD may be ameliorated by the prevention of Dkk1 binding to the Wnt co-receptor LRP6, pointing to Dkk1 as a potential therapeutic target for *GBA1*-associated neurodegeneration.

Keywords: Gaucher Disease; Wnt/β-catenin; Dkk1; Wnt3a; lysosomes; iPSC; neuronopathy

1. Introduction

Gaucher Disease (GD) is an autosomal recessive disease caused by monogenic mutations in the *GBA1* gene. *GBA1* encodes β-glucocerebrosidase (GCase), which is a 60 KDa lysosomal hydrolase that breaks down glucosylceramide (GlcCer). Mutations in *GBA1* affect GCase protein folding, resulting in endoplasmic reticulum retention and subsequent degradation [1,2]. The decreased enzyme activity in GD results in an accumulation of its lipid substrate GlcCer and its metabolite glucosylsphingosine in different organs, including the spleen, liver, bone marrow, and nervous system [3–6]. GD patients have varied onsets and severities of clinical manifestations, with a poor correlation between the genotype and phenotype [6,7]. Patients with neuronopathic subtypes (type 2 and type 3 GD) display severe neurological manifestations, including neurodegeneration, neuronal loss, ataxia, myoclonic seizures, and other abnormalities [8–15]. The rapid progression of the disease in type 2 GD (GD2) patients results in death within two years of age, while patients with type 3 GD (GD3) exhibit a slower clinical course [16–18]. Additionally, mutations in *GBA1* are the most common genetic risk factor for

Parkinson's disease (PD), with a 5–20 fold increased risk of developing PD in GD patients or carriers of *GBA1* mutations [19–24].

Neurodegeneration in neuronopathic GD (nGD) has been associated with dysfunction in the autophagy and lysosomal (ALP) pathway, which is essential for the survival of post-mitotic neurons [25,26]. Many studies have shown that *GBA1* mutations cause lysosomal abnormalities, defects in autophagic clearance, and the accumulation of protein aggregates in neurons [21,27–29]. Using an induced pluripotent stem cell (iPSC) model of GD, we have recently shown that ALP dysfunction was associated with a mammalian target of rapamycin (mTOR) hyperactivation, which resulted in transcription factor EB (TFEB) degradation [27,30]. TFEB is the master regulator of lysosomal biogenesis and autophagy [31,32]. Furthermore, Taelman et al. and others have shown a connection between the endo-lysosomal system and the Wnt/β-catenin pathway [33–35], suggesting that the ALP plays a role in the regulation of signal transduction networks essential for neuronal development.

The Wnt pathway is an important regulator of biological phenomena such as gastrulation, cell fate decisions, cell polarity, embryonic patterning, organogenesis, and the maintenance of stem cell pluripotency [36–39]. In addition, it also plays a vital role in early patterning of the central nervous system, as well as higher functions, such as memory, synaptic maintenance, and plasticity in the adult brain [40–42]. Due to the multi-faceted role of this signaling pathway in developmental and adult processes, its deregulation often leads to detrimental effects that have been linked to cancer, osteoporosis, and neurodegenerative disorders such as Alzheimer's disease (AD) and PD [43–47]. The Wnt signaling pathway is highly regulated and complex, consisting of numerous *Wnt* genes, receptors, cofactors, and regulators. Among the different Wnt signaling mechanisms identified, the "canonical" Wnt pathway is the most studied and well-characterized. This signaling cascade begins with the interaction between Wnt ligands (secreted glycoproteins) and the receptor complex, consisting of Frizzled (Fz) seven-pass transmembrane receptor and single pass low density lipoprotein receptor-related protein 5/6 (LRP5/6) co-receptors [48]. This interaction facilitates the stabilization of β-catenin in the cytoplasm by preventing its association with the destruction complex consisting of glycogen synthase kinase 3β (GSK3β), casein kinase 1 alpha (CK1α), the adaptor axis inhibition protein (AXIN), and adenomatosis polyposis coli (APC). In particular, GSK3β directly controls β-catenin levels by phosphorylating it at three residues (Ser33, Ser37, and Thr41), which leads to its degradation by the proteasome [39,49,50]. Activation of the canonical Wnt pathway results in the sequestration of GSK3β into the endo-lysosomal compartment, thereby preventing the phosphorylation and degradation of β-catenin. The resulting accumulation of β-catenin in the cytoplasm triggers its translocation to the nucleus, where it modulates gene transcription by interacting with members of the T-cell factor/lymphoid enhancer-binding factor (TCF/LEF) class of transcription factors [48].

Wnt signaling can be modulated both intracellularly and extracellularly. Various extracellular antagonists of the canonical Wnt pathway have been identified, such as the secreted frizzled-related protein (sFRP), Wnt inhibitory factor 1 (Wif1), and Dickkopf (Dkk) family of secreted proteins. Dickkopf-1 (Dkk1), which is one of the four known Dkk family members, is a negative regulator of the Wnt pathway. Dkk1 inhibits Wnt signaling by binding to the co-receptor LRP6, thereby disrupting the LRP6-Fz complex and promoting LRP6 receptor internalization, hence limiting the availability of the receptor complex to Wnt ligands [51,52]. It has been hypothesized that Wnt antagonists such as Dkk1 could play a role in the pathogenesis of a number of diseases, making them important therapeutic targets [52,53]. For instance, Dkk1 has been implicated in AD [54]. Brains from AD patients and mouse models of AD display Amyloid beta (Aβ) and Tau aggregates, which induce the upregulation of Dkk1 [46,55]. Dkk1 is also elevated in GD; Lecourt et al. reported increased Dkk1 secretion by patient-derived mesenchymal stem cells [56], and Zancan et al. have shown increased *DKK1* gene expression in fibroblasts from type 1 GD patients [57]. However, a potential role of Dkk1 in nGD pathogenesis has not yet been explored.

Using GD patient-derived iPSCs, we previously showed that this in vitro system recapitulated pathological hallmarks of the disease in all of the cell types that we tested [58]. GD-macrophages have severe defects in clearing phagocytosed red blood cells, mimicking a pathological hallmark of GD [59]. Furthermore, GD-iPSC-derived hematopoietic progenitors showed decreased erythropoiesis and aberrant myelopoesis, reflecting cytopenias in GD patients [60]. Lastly GD-iPSC-derived neuronal cells display defects in the ALP and the downregulation of canonical Wnt signaling, contributing to neurodegeneration [27,30,61]. In this study, we utilized nGD iPSC-derived neuronal progenitor cells (NPCs) to investigate whether Dkk1 was involved in nGD pathogenesis. We found that nGD NPCs exhibit an elevation in Dkk1 mRNA and protein levels, which were responsible for suppressing activation of the Wnt co-receptor LRP6, increasing GSK3β activity, destabilizing β-catenin, and reducing lysosomal numbers. We also observed that the incubation of nGD NPCs with recombinant Wnt3a (rWnt3a) was able to override the effects of elevated Dkk1, showing that exogenous Wnt agonists are capable of reversing the phenotypic abnormalities of nGD neuronal cells. Our study reports, for the first time, increased Dkk1 expression in GD iPSC-derived NPCs, uncovers a novel link between elevated Dkk1 and deregulation of the lysosomal compartment, and suggests that Dkk1 may be a therapeutic target for nGD.

2. Materials and Methods

2.1. Generation of iPSC-Derived Neuronal Progenitor Cells (NPCs)

The nGD and control (MJ) iPSC lines utilized in this study have been previously described [58,59]. The nGD iPSC lines were derived from one type 2 GD patient (GD2; genotype: W184R/D409H) and one type 3 GD patient (GD3; genotype: L444P/L444P). We used two different iPSC clones from each nGD patient. NPCs were derived from iPSCs as previously described [27]. Briefly, iPSCs cultured on irradiated mouse embryo fibroblasts (MEFs) were detached using 0.2% dispase and transferred to a 6-well ultra-low attachment plate (Costar) to generate embryoid bodies (EBs). The EBs were conditioned for neuronal induction through dual SMAD inhibition using 5 μM dorsomorphin (DM) and 10 μM SB431542 (SB) (Sigma–Aldrich, St. Louis, MO, USA). The iPSC-derived EBs were transferred to Petri dishes coated with Matrigel (Corning) and maintained in Dulbecco's modified Eagle's medium/F12 media (Life Technologies, Grand Island, NE, USA) containing 1X (v/v) N2 supplement (Life Technologies) and 20 ng/mL basic fibroblast growth factor (bFGF) (Peprotech, Rocky Hill, NJ, USA). The EBs adhered to the Matrigel and started the formation of neuronal rosettes within 7–10 days in culture. The rosettes were manually picked and expanded as NPCs in Neurobasal Medium (Life Technologies) containing 1X (v/v) GlutaMAX (Life Technologies), 1X (v/v) non-essential amino acids (Life Technologies), 1X (v/v) B27 supplement (Life Technologies), 1X (v/v) Pen/Strep, and 20 ng/mL bFGF (Peprotech), with a change of media every other day. The work with the human iPSC lines used in this study is considered non-human research; these iPSC lines are exempt under 45 CFR Part 46. This work was approved by the University of Maryland School of Medicine Institutional Review Board (IRB) on 15 July 2009 (HP-42545).

2.2. Chemical Reagents and Treatments

rWnt3a (5036-WN) and rDkk1 (5439-DK) were purchased from R&D Systems (Minneapolis, MN, USA) and reconstituted as per the manufacturer's instructions. Stocks of rWnt3a (200 μg/mL) and rDkk1 (100 μg/mL) were prepared in sterile PBS containing 0.2% bovine serum albumin. The final concentration used for both recombinant proteins was 100 ng/mL.

2.3. Quantitative PCR (qPCR)

To analyze gene expression in NPCs, mRNA was isolated using an RNA isolation kit (Qiagen, Germantown, MD, USA), and cDNA was synthesized using the iScript kit (Bio-Rad, Hercules, CA, USA). Utilizing SYBR Green PCR Master Mix (Thermo Fisher Scientific, Waltham, MA, USA), the gene

expression was determined by qPCR (7500 Fast Real-time PCR System, Applied Biosystems, Foster City, CA, USA) in duplicate or triplicate wells. The mRNA expression for every gene was normalized to the corresponding values of GAPDH and the relative gene expression was calculated using the $2^{(-\Delta\Delta Ct)}$ method. The primer sequences used in this study were as follows:
CYCD1
Forward: 5'- CCG TCC ATG CGG AAG ATC- 3'
Reverse: 5'- GAA GAC CTC CTC CTC GCA CT- 3'
AXIN2
Forward: 5'- AGT GTG AGG TCC ACG GAA AC- 3'
Reverse: 5'- TGG CTG GTG CAA AGA CAT AG- 3'
DKK1
Forward: 5'- GAT CAT AGC ACC TTG GAT GGG- 3'
Reverse: 5'- GGC ACA GTC TGA TGA CCG G- 3'
GAPDH
Forward: 5'- CAA GAT CAT CAC GAA TGC CTC- 3'
Reverse: 5'- GCA TGG ACT GTG GTC ATG AGT C- 3'

2.4. Immunocytochemistry/Immunofluorescence

NPCs were plated in 8-well chamber slides (Thermo Fisher Scientific) and cultured as described above. When the slides were ready to be stained, media were aspirated from the chambers and the cells were washed once with Dulbecco's Phosphate-Buffered Saline (DPBS) (Life Technologies, Waltham, MA, USA). The cells were then fixed with 4% (v/v) paraformaldehyde (Santa Cruz, Santa Cruz, CA, USA) for 15 min, washed thrice with DPBS, and blocked in Buffer A (PBS containing 8% FBS (v/v)) for 30 min at room temperature. Primary antibodies were prepared in Buffer B (Buffer A with 2 mg/mL saponin) and incubated for 1–2 h at room temperature or overnight at 4 °C. The cells were then incubated with the appropriate fluorochrome-conjugated secondary antibodies for 1 h at room temperature. Nuclei were labeled using 4',6-diamidino-2-phenylindole (DAPI)-containing mounting medium (Vector Laboratories, H-1200, Burlingame, CA, USA).

Lysotracker staining was performed by adding 1 µM Lysotracker Red DND-99 (ThermoFisher Scientific) directly to cell culture medium and incubating it for 45 min to 1 h at 37 °C. The cells were then processed as described above. The following antibodies were used in this study: Primary antibodies; Cell Signaling Technology (Danvers, MA, USA): pLRP6 (Ser1490) (#2568), non-phospho (Active) β-catenin (#8814), and pGSK-3β (Ser9) (#9323); U. Iowa Developmental Hybridoma Bank (Iowa City, IA, USA): LAMP1 (H4A3); Santa Cruz: Dkk1 (sc-374574) and total β-catenin (sc-7199). Additionally, the secondary antibodies were Goat anti-rabbit Alexa Fluor 488 and Donkey anti-mouse Cy3 (Jackson ImmunoResearch Laboratories, West Grove, PA, USA).

2.5. Image Acquisition and Analysis

Confocal immunofluorescence images were taken using an inverted Nikon Eclipse Ti2 microscope attached to a spinning disk unit (CSU-W1, Yokogawa, Melville, NY, USA) and Hamamatsu sCMOS camera (Hamamatsu City, Japan). A Nikon oil immersion objective (Plan Fluor 40X, NA 1.30) was used for all imaging experiments. The excitation wavelengths used were 405, 488, and 561 nm for blue, green, and red fluorophores, respectively. Further image processing and analysis was conducted using Fiji software (version 2.1.0/1.53c, open source). The fluorescence intensity of the respective signal or Lysotracker counts was obtained from at least three independent replicates (3–5 different fields/replicate). The mean fluorescence intensity (MFI) and average puncti count were calculated accordingly.

2.6. Western Blot Analysis

NPCs were cultured in 12-well plates (Corning, Corning, NY, USA) and treated as indicated in the text. The cells were lysed directly in SDS sample buffer, sonicated, and denatured by heating at 95 °C for 5 min. The samples were then loaded onto 4–20% SDS/polyacrylamide gels (Bio-Rad, Hercules, CA, USA), and electrophoresis was performed at 100 V for 2 h. This was followed by the transfer of protein onto a nitrocellulose membrane, blocking with 5% milk in Tris-buffered saline Tween (TBS-T), and incubation with the indicated primary antibodies overnight at 4 °C. Anti-mouse or anti-rabbit HRP-conjugated secondary antibodies were added to the membrane for 1 h at room temperature. Membranes were developed with SuperSignal West Femto Maximum Sensitivity Substrate (ThermoFisher Scientific), and imaged using the Chemidoc system and Imagelab software (BioRad). Densitometry analysis was conducted using the Imagelab software (BioRad) and all proteins were normalized to β-actin.

2.7. Statistical Analysis

Data were analyzed using Prism software version 7.0a (GraphPad Software, San Diego, CA, USA). Significance was assessed using two-tailed unpaired Student's *t*-tests for comparing two groups with a confidence interval of 95%. Results are expressed as the mean ± standard error of the mean (SEM).

3. Results

3.1. Upregulation of Dkk1 mRNA and Protein Levels in Neuronopathic GD NPCs

We have previously shown that *GBA1* mutations downregulate the Wnt/β-catenin pathway in nGD iPSC-derived NPCs. In this system, the level of β-catenin, which is the main mediator of canonical Wnt signaling, was lower in nGD NPCs when compared to wild-type (WT) cells. This was attributed to the destabilization of β-catenin through proteasomal degradation since treatment with a proteasomal inhibitor was able to rescue the levels of both total and active (non-phosphorylated) β-catenin [61]. In accordance with our previous report, GD2 and GD3 NPCs exhibited reduced immunofluorescence staining of total β-catenin compared to control NPCs (Figure 1A). Additionally, when we analyzed the expression of two transcriptional targets of β-catenin, namely *AXIN2* and *CYCD1* by qRT-PCR analysis, there was a significant reduction in *AXIN2* and *CYCD1* transcript levels in the mutant NPCs, consistent with reduced β-catenin activity in these cells (Figure 1B,C).

We then investigated whether Dkk1 is involved in deregulation of the canonical Wnt pathway in nGD. To examine this question, we performed a qRT-PCR analysis of *DKK1* mRNA expression in WT and nGD NPCs. As shown in Figure 1D, both GD2 and GD3 NPCs displayed a significant elevation in *DKK1* expression relative to the control. Similarly, immunofluorescence staining revealed higher levels of Dkk1 protein in GD2 NPCs (Figure 1E). Taken together, we conclude that mutations in *GBA1* downregulate the Wnt/β-catenin pathway with concomitant upregulation of the Wnt antagonist Dkk1.

3.2. Recombinant Dkk1 Downregulates the Wnt/β-Catenin Pathway and Disrupts the Lysosomal Compartment in WT NPCs

Dkk1 is a Wnt antagonist that binds the Wnt co-receptor LRP6 and prevents formation of the LRP6-Fz receptor complex, thus suppressing the canonical Wnt pathway [52]. To investigate the mechanism of action of Dkk1, we treated control WT iPSC-derived NPCs with exogenous rDkk1 and analyzed the levels of various Wnt components. Firstly, incubation with rDkk1 decreased the activation of co-receptor LRP6, as shown by reduced levels of phosphorylated LRP6 (Ser1490) (pLRP6) (Figure 2A). As LRP6 is phosphorylated at several residues, including Ser1490, upon Wnt activation, our results suggest that rDkk1 was able to bind LRP6 and limit its availability to activating Wnt ligands. This was translated into the destabilization of β-catenin, as shown by lower levels of the non-phosphorylated, active form of β-catenin, following rDkk1 treatment (Figure 2A).

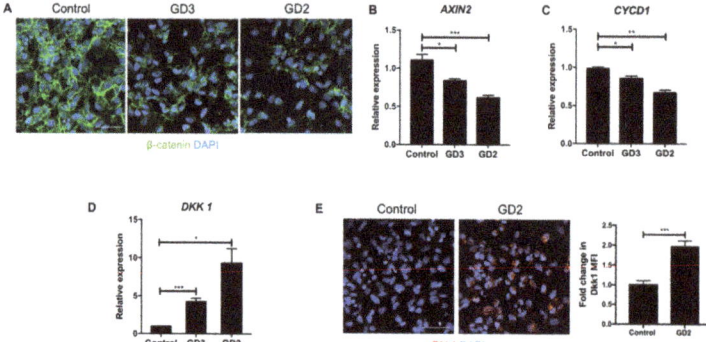

Figure 1. Downregulation of canonical Wnt signaling with a concomitant elevation of Dkk1 in neuronopathic forms of Gaucher Disease (nGD) neuronal progenitor cells (NPCs). (**A**) Representative confocal immunofluorescence images of control (WT) and nGD (GD2 and GD3) NPCs stained with antibodies to total β-catenin (green). Nuclei were stained with DAPI (blue). Scale bar: 50 μm. (**B–D**) qRT-PCR analysis of AXIN2, CYCD1, and DKK1 gene expression in control, GD2, and GD3 NPCs. The data are presented as the mean ± S.E.M (standard error of the mean). For AXIN2, $n = 3$ for control, $n = 5$ for GD2 (data were pooled from two clones derived from the same GD2 patient), and $n = 3$ for GD3 (data were pooled from two clones derived from the same GD3 patient). For CYCD1, $n = 3$ for control, $n = 3$ for GD2 (data pooled from two GD2 clones), and $n = 2$ for GD3 (data were obtained from one clone of GD3). For DKK1, $n = 4$ for control, $n = 8$ for GD2 (data were pooled from two GD2 clones), and $n = 5$ for GD3 (data were pooled from two GD3 clones). * $p < 0.05$, ** $p < 0.01$, and *** $p < 0.001$ between the indicated groups, as assessed by an unpaired Student's t-test. (**E**) Representative immunofluorescence images of endogenous Dkk1 staining (red) in control and GD2 NPCs. Nuclei were stained with DAPI (blue). Scale bar: 50 μm. Quantitation of the mean fluorescence intensity (MFI) of Dkk1 is plotted to the right of the images. Results are expressed as the mean ± S.E.M ($n = 3$, *** $p < 0.001$, unpaired Student's t-test).

GSK3β is a constitutively active kinase that acts as a negative regulator of the Wnt pathway by phosphorylating β-catenin, causing its degradation by the proteasome. GSK3β activity is negatively regulated by phosphorylation at Ser 9 [49,62]. We previously reported that in nGD NPCs, there is a decrease in the levels of pGSK3β (Ser9), with no significant difference in the levels of total GSK3β [61]. To investigate whether rDkk1 had an effect on GSK3β activity, we examined the levels of pGSK3β (Ser9) in WT NPCs treated with rDkk1. As shown in Figure 2B, rDkk1 treatment lowered the levels of pGSK3β (Ser9) in WT NPCs, as determined by immunofluorescence staining. Therefore, treatment with rDkk1 recapitulated the decrease in levels of pGSK3β that we observed in nGD NPCs [61].

We and others have previously shown that the endo-lysosomal system positively modulates the canonical Wnt pathway by sequestering GSK3β into endo-lysosomal vesicles, thus stabilizing β-catenin levels [35,61,63,64]. We also showed that nGD NPCs exhibit severe lysosomal depletion and a reduced co-localization of pGSK3β with the lysosomal marker LAMP1 [61]. Hence, we wanted to determine whether rDkk1 treatment would also cause lysosomal depletion and alter the localization of pGSK3β. As shown in Figure 2B–D, rDkk1 treatment of WT NPCs resulted in deregulation of the lysosomal compartment. There were decreased levels of the lysosomal marker LAMP1, as determined by immunoblotting (Figure 2C) and immunofluorescence staining (Figure 2B), and a reduction in Lysotracker staining (Figure 2D). When we overlaid the pGSK3β signal with that of LAMP1 in untreated WT NPCs, there was almost complete co-localization of pGSK3β with LAMP1. On the other hand, after the incubation of WT NPCs with rDkk1, there was a considerable reduction in pGSK3β co-localization with LAMP1 (Figure 2B).

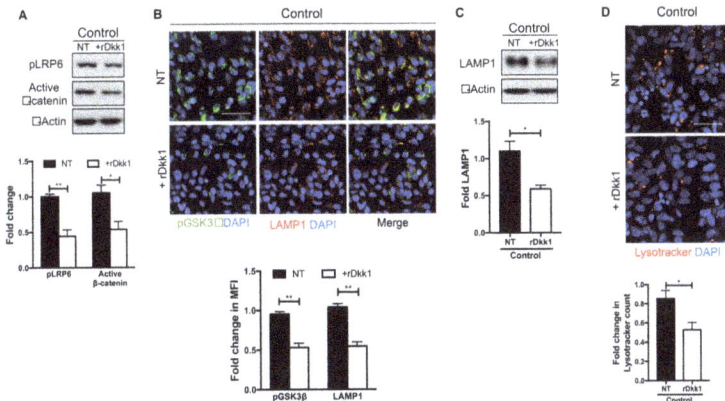

Figure 2. Treatment of WT control NPCs with recombinant Dkk1 mimics the phenotypes observed in nGD NPCs. (**A**) Western blot showing the expression of phosphorylated LRP6 (pLRP6) and (non-phospho) active β-catenin in control (WT) NPCs that were either left untreated (NT) or were treated with 100 ng/mL rDkk1 (+rDkk1) for 24 h. The proteins were normalized to β-actin, and fold-change was calculated with respect to NT WT. (**B**) Immunofluorescence staining of pGSK3β (Ser9) (green) and the lysosomal marker LAMP1 (red) in control NPCs that were either left untreated (NT, top panel) or were treated with rDkk1 (+rDkk1, bottom panel), as in A. The nuclei are labeled with DAPI (blue). Scale bar: 50 μm. The fold-change in mean fluorescence intensity (MFI) is plotted below the images. (**C**) Representative Western blot showing LAMP1 expression in control NPCs treated as in A. The bands were normalized to β-actin, and the plot below the WB shows fold-change. (**D**) Control cells were either left untreated (NT, top panel) or were treated with rDkk1 (+rDkk1, bottom panel). Untreated and treated cells were stained with Lysotracker (red) and imaged. Scale bar: 50 μm. The fold-change in Lysotracker count is plotted below the images. * $p < 0.05$ and ** $p < 0.01$ ($n = 3$, mean ± S.E.M, unpaired Student's t-test).

We can conclude from these results that the treatment of WT NPCs with exogenous Dkk1 was able to phenocopy the reduction in active β-catenin, lysosomal depletion, and alterations in the activity and subcellular distribution of GSK3β that we observed in nGD NPCs. These results lend strong support to the idea that Dkk1 is a key mediator of canonical Wnt downregulation in nGD neuronal cells.

3.3. Recombinant Wnt3a Treatment of nGD NPCs Rescues Wnt/β-Catenin Signaling and Restores the Lysosomal Compartments

As our results implicated Dkk1 in suppression of the canonical Wnt pathway, we wanted to determine whether exogenous Wnt3a would be able to abrogate the effects of excess Dkk1 in nGD NPCs. To this end, we incubated control and mutant NPCs with rWnt3a for 3 or 24 h, and analyzed its effect on different components of the Wnt/β-catenin pathway. As shown in Figure 3A, immunoblot analysis demonstrated that rWnt3a triggered the engagement and activation of the receptor complex, as determined by an increase in pLRP6 levels. rWnt3a stimulated a robust response at 3 h, which returned to basal levels within 24 h. Similar results were obtained in GD2 and GD3 cells; under non-treated conditions, the mutant NPCs had significantly lower levels of pLRP6 when compared to WT NPCs, but rWnt3a was able to stabilize and increase pLRP6 levels. Importantly, rWnt3a treatment for 3 h also caused an increase in the levels of active β-catenin in GD2 and GD3 NPCs (Figure 3B), showing that this ligand was able to restore canonical Wnt signaling and overcome the inhibitory effect of elevated Dkk1 in the mutant NPCs.

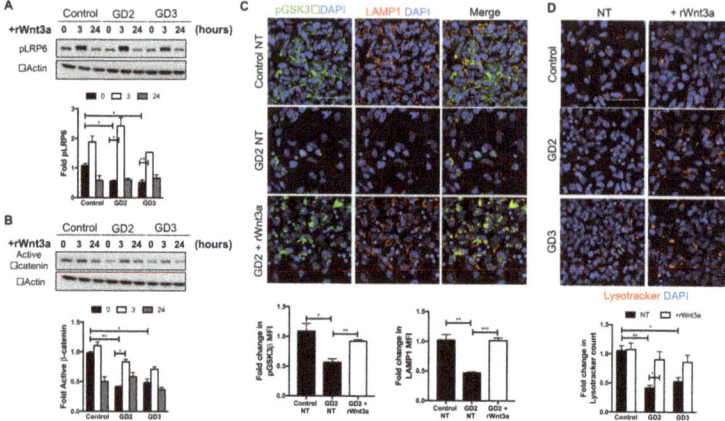

Figure 3. Exogenous addition of recombinant Wnt3a reverses the abnormal phenotype of nGD NPCs. (**A**,**B**) Western blots showing the levels of pLRP6 (**A**) and active β-catenin (**B**) in control, GD2, and GD3 NPCs treated with 100 ng/mL rWnt3a for 0, 3, and 24 h. The proteins were normalized to β-actin, and fold-change was calculated based on control (0 h). * $p < 0.05$ and ** $p < 0.01$ ($n = 2$, mean ± S.E.M, unpaired Student's t-test between the indicated groups). (**C**) Immunofluorescence staining of pGSK3β (Ser9) (green) and LAMP1 (red) in untreated control NPCs and GD2 NPCs that were either left untreated (NT) or were treated with 100 ng/mL rWnt3a (+rWnt3a) for 3 h. Nuclei were stained with DAPI (blue). Scale bar: 50 μm. The fold-change in MFI is plotted below the images. * $p < 0.05$, ** $p < 0.01$, and *** $p < 0.001$ ($n = 3$, mean ± S.E.M, unpaired Student's t-test). (**D**) Control, GD2, and GD3 NPCs were either left untreated (NT) or were incubated with rWnt3a as in B. The treated and untreated cells were stained with Lysotracker (red) and imaged. Nuclei were stained with DAPI (blue). Scale bar: 50 μm. The fold change in Lysotracker count is plotted below the images. * $p < 0.05$ and ** $p < 0.01$ ($n = 4$, mean ± S.E.M, unpaired Student's t-test).

We next investigated whether rWnt3a had any effect on pGSK3β (Ser9) and the lysosomal compartment. Figure 3C shows that the incubation of GD2 NPCs with rWnt3a for 3 h resulted in increased pGSK3β (Ser9) and LAMP1 staining, and lysosomal colocalization of these two proteins similar to control cells. Lysotracker staining also showed that rWnt3a prevented lysosomal depletion in GD2 and GD3 NPCs (Figure 3D). These results suggest that exogenous Wnt3a stabilized β-catenin through an increased sequestration of GSK3β into the endo-lysosomal compartment, and that lysosomal numbers also increased following treatment with the recombinant Wnt ligand. These results may suggest the existence of a bi-directional feedback mechanism between the canonical Wnt signaling network and the lysosome.

4. Discussion

In this study, we report that Dkk1 plays a key role in downregulation of the canonical Wnt pathway in nGD iPSC-derived NPCs, and that Wnt downregulation interferes with the lysosomal function. Dkk1 elevation in the mutant cells led to lysosomal depletion, reducing the sequestration of GSK3β into these organelles, thereby facilitating the phosphorylation and subsequent degradation of β-catenin. A critical role of Dkk1 in this process was confirmed by demonstrating that the addition of rDkk1 to WT NPCs recapitulated the mutant phenotype. Importantly, the phenotypic abnormalities of the nGD neuronal cells were reversed by incubation with rWnt3a. The addition of this ligand to mutant NPCs outcompeted the elevated levels of endogenous Dkk1, enabling GSK3β sequestration into the lysosomal compartment, protecting β-catenin from degradation, and preventing lysosomal depletion.

The Dkk family consists of four secreted proteins (Dkk1-4). Although Dkk2 has been shown to activate Wnt signaling, the other members of the family play mostly inhibitory roles [52]. Dkk1 was identified as a Wnt pathway antagonist that is essential for induction of the head in Xenopus during early embryogenesis [65]. Dkk1 exerts its action by interacting with the extracellular domains of Wnt co-receptors LRP5/6, in order to competitively inhibit the binding of Wnt1 and Wnt3 classes of ligands. Dkk1 deregulation has been implicated in human disease. Excess Dkk1 produced by myeloma cells suppresses osteoblast differentiation, resulting in lytic bone lesions in multiple myeloma [66,67]. Similarly, increased Dkk1 expression has been associated with the apoptosis of bone cells in femoral head osteonecrosis [68], with a low bone mineral density in children and adolescents with type 1 diabetes mellitus [69]. Additionally, elevated levels of Dkk1 have been observed in brains from AD patients and mouse models of AD and PD [45–47,55]. Furthermore, Dkk1 increases after NMDA excitotoxicity [70], and pharmacological inhibition of the NMDA receptor reduces the neurological manifestations in mouse models of nGD [71]. Therefore, Dkk1 elevation may play a wide role in neurodegeneration. The excess secretion of Dkk1 has also been reported in bone marrow-derived mesenchymal stem cells from GD patients [56], and Zancan et al. reported a higher *DKK1* mRNA expression in type 1 GD patient fibroblasts [57]. It will be interesting to determine whether Dkk1 is also elevated in nGD patient brains, and if there are increased levels of Dkk1 in serum or cerebrospinal fluid (CSF), which might then suggest the consideration of Dkk1 as a potential marker for nGD.

We have previously shown that in nGD NPCs, a loss of GCase activity downregulates the canonical Wnt pathway, leading to an increased degradation of β-catenin [61]. This was attributed to reduced lysosomal sequestration of GSK3β, which resulted in increased phosphorylation of β-catenin, thereby reducing its stability [61]. In the present study, we found that these alterations were likely mediated by an increased production of the Wnt antagonist Dkk1. Not only was Dkk1 elevated in the mutant NPCs, but the treatment of WT NPCs with exogenous rDkk1 resulted in diminished Wnt signaling due to interference with ligand binding to the LRP6 co-receptor. Remarkably, rDkk1 treatment also phenocopied the lysosomal depletion we observed in nGD cells (Figure 2). Therefore, Dkk1 appears to be an important mediator of the phenotypic abnormalities caused by GCase deficiency.

When nGD NPCs were treated with rWnt3a, the mutant phenotype was reversed, showing that this extracellular ligand was capable of overcoming the inhibitory effects of elevated, endogenous Dkk1. There was an increased activation of LRP6, β-catenin stabilization through GSK3β lysosomal sequestration, and an increase in lysosome numbers. The strong link between the Wnt and ALP pathways we observed suggests the existence of a bi-directional feedback loop, so that alterations in one pathway may affect the other. This idea is in line with other reports on the ability of the endo-lysosomal system to modulate Wnt signaling and in turn, the Wnt pathway regulating the lysosomal compartment [35,61,63,72–75]. Albrecht et al. reported an increase in both endocytosis and the lysosomal degradation of extracellular proteins within minutes of the addition of Wnt3a in NIH-3T3 fibroblasts. Additionally, Wnt3a treatment or inhibition of GSK3β in HeLa and HCC Alexander cells increased Lysotracker staining, and Cathepsin D and GCase activity [75]. A neuroprotective effect of Wnt ligands in vivo has also been reported [76–80]. The intranasal delivery of rWnt3a has been shown to modulate autophagy and regenerative pathways in a traumatic brain injury mouse model [79], and to have anti-apoptotic effects in a rat model of stroke [80]. Future studies will determine whether modulating the canonical Wnt pathway can help to ameliorate or prevent nGD neuronopathy.

As Wnt agonists (e.g., Wnt3a) and antagonists (e.g., Dkk1 and Sclerostin) act extracellularly, these are important pharmacological targets. For instance, the inhibition of Dkk1 and sclerostin using a bi-specific antibody has been shown to stimulate bone formation, increase the bone mass density and strength, and improve fracture healing in pre-clinical models of bone disease [81]. Similarly, a Dkk1 neutralizing antibody (BHQ880A, Novartis) has shown striking effects in multiple myeloma by increasing bone formation and inhibiting tumor growth both in vitro and in vivo [82,83]. Additionally, there are currently three ongoing clinical trials using a Dkk1-neutralizing monoclonal antibody (DKN-01, Leap therapeutics) for advanced biliary tract cancer (NCT04057365), prostate cancer (NCT03837353), and locally advanced or metastatic gastric or gastroesophageal junction adenocarcinoma (NCT04363801). Similarly, NCI8642 is a small molecule that was designed to displace Dkk1 from LRP5/6 and block the inhibitory effect of Dkk1 on Wnt signaling [84]. Derivatives of NCI8642 were found to lower Dkk1-induced Tau phosphorylation in SH-SY5Y cells [85]. Future studies will determine whether Wnt modulators have therapeutic potential to treat GD abnormalities, including the Wnt-related neurodevelopmental defects we reported in nGD [61] and bone abnormalities caused by defective Wnt signaling [57,86].

In conclusion, this study suggests that the elevation of Dkk1 observed in nGD NPCs is responsible for downregulation of the canonical Wnt pathway and deregulation of the lysosomal compartment. We also found that exogenous rWnt3a was able to outcompete the deleterious effects of elevated Dkk1 in the mutant cells. This study implicates Dkk1 in *GBA1*-associated neuropathology, and suggests that the canonical Wnt pathway is a potential therapeutic target for *GBA1*-associated neurodegeneration.

Author Contributions: M.P.S. planned and conducted all of the experiments, analyzed the data, and wrote the manuscript. R.A.F. directed the project, helped plan experiments, analyzed data, and edited the manuscript. All authors have read and agreed to the published version of the manuscript.

Funding: This work was supported by grants from the Maryland Stem Cell Research Fund (MSCRF) 2015-MSCRFI-1662 and 2018-MSCRFD-4246, and by a grant from the Children's Gaucher Research Fund.

Conflicts of Interest: The authors declare no conflict of interest.

References

1. Schmitz, M.; Alfalah, M.; Aerts, J.M.; Naim, H.Y.; Zimmer, K.P. Impaired trafficking of mutants of lysosomal glucocerebrosidase in gaucher's disease. *Int. J. Biochem. Cell. Biol.* **2005**, *37*, 2310–2320. [CrossRef] [PubMed]
2. Bendikov-Bar, I.; Ron, I.; Filocamo, M.; Horowitz, M. Characterization of the erad process of the l444p mutant glucocerebrosidase variant. *Blood Cells Mol. Dis.* **2011**, *46*, 4–10. [CrossRef] [PubMed]
3. Chen, M.; Wang, J. Gaucher disease: Review of the literature. *Arch. Pathol. Lab. Med* **2008**, *132*, 851–853. [PubMed]
4. Cox, T.M. Gaucher disease: Clinical profile and therapeutic developments. *Biologics* **2010**, *4*, 299–313. [CrossRef]
5. Grabowski, G.A.; Golembo, M.; Shaaltiel, Y. Taliglucerase alfa: An enzyme replacement therapy using plant cell expression technology. *Mol. Genet. Metab.* **2014**, *112*, 1–8. [CrossRef]
6. Sidransky, E. Gaucher disease: Insights from a rare mendelian disorder. *Discov. Med.* **2012**, *14*, 273–281.
7. Dandana, A.; Ben Khelifa, S.; Chahed, H.; Miled, A.; Ferchichi, S. Gaucher disease: Clinical, biological and therapeutic aspects. *Pathobiology* **2016**, *83*, 13–23. [CrossRef]
8. Alaei, M.R.; Tabrizi, A.; Jafari, N.; Mozafari, H. Gaucher disease: New expanded classification emphasizing neurological features. *Iran. J. Child. Neurol.* **2019**, *13*, 7–24.
9. Eblan, M.J.; Goker-Alpan, O.; Sidransky, E. Perinatal lethal gaucher disease: A distinct phenotype along the neuronopathic continuum. *Fetal Pediatr. Pathol.* **2005**, *24*, 205–222. [CrossRef]
10. Kaplan, P.; Andersson, H.C.; Kacena, K.A.; Yee, J.D. The clinical and demographic characteristics of nonneuronopathic gaucher disease in 887 children at diagnosis. *Arch. Pediatr. Adolesc. Med.* **2006**, *160*, 603–608. [CrossRef]
11. Pastores, G.M. Neuropathic gaucher disease. *Wien. Med. Wochenschr.* **2010**, *160*, 605–608. [CrossRef]
12. Roshan Lal, T.; Sidransky, E. The spectrum of neurological manifestations associated with gaucher disease. *Diseases* **2017**, *5*, 10. [CrossRef] [PubMed]
13. Vellodi, A.; Tylki-Szymanska, A.; Davies, E.H.; Kolodny, E.; Bembi, B.; Collin-Histed, T.; Mengel, E.; Erikson, A.; Schiffmann, R. Management of neuronopathic gaucher disease: Revised recommendations. *J. Inherit. Metab. Dis.* **2009**, *32*, 660–664. [CrossRef] [PubMed]
14. Vitner, E.B.; Futerman, A.H. Neuronal forms of gaucher disease. *Handb. Exp. Pharmacol.* **2013**, *216*, 405–419.
15. Wong, K.; Sidransky, E.; Verma, A.; Mixon, T.; Sandberg, G.D.; Wakefield, L.K.; Morrison, A.; Lwin, A.; Colegial, C.; Allman, J.M.; et al. Neuropathology provides clues to the pathophysiology of gaucher disease. *Mol. Genet. Metab.* **2004**, *82*, 192–207. [CrossRef]
16. Stone, D.L.; Tayebi, N.; Orvisky, E.; Stubblefield, B.; Madike, V.; Sidransky, E. Glucocerebrosidase gene mutations in patients with type 2 gaucher disease. *Hum. Mutat.* **2000**, *15*, 181–188. [CrossRef]

17. Orvisky, E.; Sidransky, E.; McKinney, C.E.; Lamarca, M.E.; Samimi, R.; Krasnewich, D.; Martin, B.M.; Ginns, E.I. Glucosylsphingosine accumulation in mice and patients with type 2 gaucher disease begins early in gestation. *Pediatr. Res.* **2000**, *48*, 233–237. [CrossRef]
18. Weiss, K.; Gonzalez, A.; Lopez, G.; Pedoeim, L.; Groden, C.; Sidransky, E. The clinical management of type 2 gaucher disease. *Mol. Genet. Metab.* **2015**, *114*, 110–122. [CrossRef]
19. Lwin, A.; Orvisky, E.; Goker-Alpan, O.; LaMarca, M.E.; Sidransky, E. Glucocerebrosidase mutations in subjects with parkinsonism. *Mol. Genet. Metab.* **2004**, *81*, 70–73. [CrossRef]
20. Maor, G.; Cabasso, O.; Krivoruk, O.; Rodriguez, J.; Steller, H.; Segal, D.; Horowitz, M. The contribution of mutant gba to the development of parkinson disease in drosophila. *Hum. Mol. Genet.* **2016**, *25*, 2712–2727.
21. Mazzulli, J.R.; Xu, Y.H.; Sun, Y.; Knight, A.L.; McLean, P.J.; Caldwell, G.A.; Sidransky, E.; Grabowski, G.A.; Krainc, D. Gaucher disease glucocerebrosidase and alpha-synuclein form a bidirectional pathogenic loop in synucleinopathies. *Cell* **2011**, *146*, 37–52. [CrossRef] [PubMed]
22. Mazzulli, J.R.; Zunke, F.; Tsunemi, T.; Toker, N.J.; Jeon, S.; Burbulla, L.F.; Patnaik, S.; Sidransky, E.; Marugan, J.J.; Sue, C.M.; et al. Activation of beta-glucocerebrosidase reduces pathological alpha-synuclein and restores lysosomal function in parkinson's patient midbrain neurons. *J. Neurosci.* **2016**, *36*, 7693–7706. [CrossRef] [PubMed]
23. Moors, T.; Paciotti, S.; Chiasserini, D.; Calabresi, P.; Parnetti, L.; Beccari, T.; van de Berg, W.D. Lysosomal dysfunction and alpha-synuclein aggregation in parkinson's disease: Diagnostic links. *Mov. Disord.* **2016**, *31*, 791–801. [CrossRef] [PubMed]
24. Taguchi, Y.V.; Liu, J.; Ruan, J.; Pacheco, J.; Zhang, X.; Abbasi, J.; Keutzer, J.; Mistry, P.K.; Chandra, S.S. Glucosylsphingosine promotes alpha-synuclein pathology in mutant gba-associated parkinson's disease. *J. Neurosci.* **2017**, *37*, 9617–9631. [CrossRef]
25. Sun, Y.; Grabowski, G.A. Impaired autophagosomes and lysosomes in neuronopathic gaucher disease. *Autophagy* **2010**, *6*, 648–649. [CrossRef] [PubMed]
26. Sun, Y.; Liou, B.; Ran, H.; Skelton, M.R.; Williams, M.T.; Vorhees, C.V.; Kitatani, K.; Hannun, Y.A.; Witte, D.P.; Xu, Y.H.; et al. Neuronopathic gaucher disease in the mouse: Viable combined selective saposin c deficiency and mutant glucocerebrosidase (v394l) mice with glucosylsphingosine and glucosylceramide accumulation and progressive neurological deficits. *Hum. Mol. Genet.* **2010**, *19*, 1088–1097. [CrossRef]
27. Awad, O.; Sarkar, C.; Panicker, L.M.; Miller, D.; Zeng, X.; Sgambato, J.A.; Lipinski, M.M.; Feldman, R.A. Altered tfeb-mediated lysosomal biogenesis in gaucher disease ipsc-derived neuronal cells. *Hum. Mol. Genet.* **2015**, *24*, 5775–5788. [CrossRef]
28. Du, T.T.; Wang, L.; Duan, C.L.; Lu, L.L.; Zhang, J.L.; Gao, G.; Qiu, X.B.; Wang, X.M.; Yang, H. Gba deficiency promotes snca/alpha-synuclein accumulation through autophagic inhibition by inactivated ppp2a. *Autophagy* **2015**, *11*, 1803–1820. [CrossRef]
29. Schondorf, D.C.; Aureli, M.; McAllister, F.E.; Hindley, C.J.; Mayer, F.; Schmid, B.; Sardi, S.P.; Valsecchi, M.; Hoffmann, S.; Schwarz, L.K.; et al. Ipsc-derived neurons from gba1-associated parkinson's disease patients show autophagic defects and impaired calcium homeostasis. *Nat. Commun.* **2014**, *5*, 4028. [CrossRef]
30. Brown, R.A.; Voit, A.; Srikanth, M.P.; Thayer, J.A.; Kingsbury, T.J.; Jacobson, M.A.; Lipinski, M.M.; Feldman, R.A.; Awad, O. Mtor hyperactivity mediates lysosomal dysfunction in gaucher's disease ipsc-neuronal cells. *Dis. Model. Mech.* **2019**, *12*. [CrossRef]
31. Settembre, C.; Di Malta, C.; Polito, V.A.; Garcia Arencibia, M.; Vetrini, F.; Erdin, S.; Erdin, S.U.; Huynh, T.; Medina, D.; Colella, P.; et al. Tfeb links autophagy to lysosomal biogenesis. *Science* **2011**, *332*, 1429–1433. [CrossRef]
32. Settembre, C.; Zoncu, R.; Medina, D.L.; Vetrini, F.; Erdin, S.; Erdin, S.; Huynh, T.; Ferron, M.; Karsenty, G.; Vellard, M.C.; et al. A lysosome-to-nucleus signalling mechanism senses and regulates the lysosome via mtor and tfeb. *Embo. J.* **2012**, *31*, 1095–1108. [CrossRef]
33. Dobrowolski, R.; Vick, P.; Ploper, D.; Gumper, I.; Snitkin, H.; Sabatini, D.D.; De Robertis, E.M. Presenilin deficiency or lysosomal inhibition enhances wnt signaling through relocalization of gsk3 to the late-endosomal compartment. *Cell Rep.* **2012**, *2*, 1316–1328. [CrossRef] [PubMed]
34. Bilić, J.; Huang, Y.-L.; Davidson, G.; Zimmermann, T.; Cruciat, C.-M.; Bienz, M.; Niehrs, C. Wnt induces lrp6 signalosomes and promotes dishevelled-dependent lrp6 phosphorylation. *Science* **2007**, *316*, 1619–1622. [CrossRef] [PubMed]

35. Taelman, V.F.; Dobrowolski, R.; Plouhinec, J.-L.; Fuentealba, L.C.; Vorwald, P.P.; Gumper, I.; Sabatini, D.D.; De Robertis, E.M. Wnt signaling requires sequestration of glycogen synthase kinase 3 inside multivesicular endosomes. *Cell* **2010**, *143*, 1136–1148. [CrossRef] [PubMed]
36. Diehl, J.A.; Cheng, M.; Roussel, M.F.; Sherr, C.J. Glycogen synthase kinase-3beta regulates cyclin d1 proteolysis and subcellular localization. *Genes Dev.* **1998**, *12*, 3499–3511. [CrossRef] [PubMed]
37. Nusse, R.; Varmus, H. Three decades of wnts: A personal perspective on how a scientific field developed. *Embo. J.* **2012**, *31*, 2670–2684. [CrossRef] [PubMed]
38. Inestrosa, N.C.; Arenas, E. Emerging roles of wnts in the adult nervous system. *Nat. Rev. Neurosci.* **2010**, *11*, 77–86. [CrossRef]
39. Nusse, R.; Clevers, H. Wnt/β-catenin signaling, disease, and emerging therapeutic modalities. *Cell* **2017**, *169*, 985–999. [CrossRef]
40. Maguschak, K.A.; Ressler, K.J. Wnt signaling in amygdala-dependent learning and memory. *J. Neurosci.* **2011**, *31*, 13057–13067. [CrossRef]
41. Marzo, A.; Galli, S.; Lopes, D.; McLeod, F.; Podpolny, M.; Segovia-Roldan, M.; Ciani, L.; Purro, S.; Cacucci, F.; Gibb, A.; et al. Reversal of synapse degeneration by restoring wnt signaling in the adult hippocampus. *Curr. Biol.* **2016**, *26*, 2551–2561. [CrossRef] [PubMed]
42. McLeod, F.; Salinas, P.C. Wnt proteins as modulators of synaptic plasticity. *Curr. Opin. Neurobiol.* **2018**, *53*, 90–95. [CrossRef] [PubMed]
43. Inestrosa, N.C.; Toledo, E.M. The role of wnt signaling in neuronal dysfunction in alzheimer's disease. *Mol. Neurodegener.* **2008**, *3*, 9. [CrossRef] [PubMed]
44. Stephano, F.; Nolte, S.; Hoffmann, J.; El-Kholy, S.; von Frieling, J.; Bruchhaus, I.; Fink, C.; Roeder, T. Impaired wnt signaling in dopamine containing neurons is associated with pathogenesis in a rotenone triggered drosophila parkinson's disease model. *Sci. Rep.* **2018**, *8*, 2372. [CrossRef]
45. Dun, Y.; Li, G.; Yang, Y.; Xiong, Z.; Feng, M.; Wang, M.; Zhang, Y.; Xiang, J.; Ma, R. Inhibition of the canonical wnt pathway by dickkopf-1 contributes to the neurodegeneration in 6-ohda-lesioned rats. *Neurosci. Lett.* **2012**, *525*, 83–88. [CrossRef]
46. Caricasole, A.; Copani, A.; Caraci, F.; Aronica, E.; Rozemuller, A.J.; Caruso, A.; Storto, M.; Gaviraghi, G.; Terstappen, G.C.; Nicoletti, F. Induction of dickkopf-1, a negative modulator of the wnt pathway, is associated with neuronal degeneration in alzheimer's brain. *J. Neurosci.* **2004**, *24*, 6021–6027. [CrossRef]
47. L'Episcopo, F.; Tirolo, C.; Testa, N.; Caniglia, S.; Morale, M.C.; Cossetti, C.; D'Adamo, P.; Zardini, E.; Andreoni, L.; Ihekwaba, A.E.; et al. Reactive astrocytes and wnt/β-catenin signaling link nigrostriatal injury to repair in 1-methyl-4-phenyl-1,2,3,6-tetrahydropyridine model of parkinson's disease. *Neurobiol. Dis.* **2011**, *41*, 508–527. [CrossRef]
48. Mikels, A.J.; Nusse, R. Wnts as ligands: Processing, secretion and reception. *Oncogene* **2006**, *25*, 7461–7468. [CrossRef]
49. Verheyen, E.M.; Gottardi, C.J. Regulation of wnt/beta-catenin signaling by protein kinases. *Dev. Dyn.* **2010**, *239*, 34–44.
50. Willert, K.; Nusse, R. Beta-catenin: A key mediator of wnt signaling. *Curr. Opin. Genet. Dev.* **1998**, *8*, 95–102. [CrossRef]
51. Mao, B.; Wu, W.; Li, Y.; Hoppe, D.; Stannek, P.; Glinka, A.; Niehrs, C. Ldl-receptor-related protein 6 is a receptor for dickkopf proteins. *Nature* **2001**, *411*, 321–325. [CrossRef] [PubMed]
52. Niehrs, C. Function and biological roles of the dickkopf family of wnt modulators. *Oncogene* **2006**, *25*, 7469–7481. [CrossRef] [PubMed]
53. Huang, Y.; Liu, L.; Liu, A. Dickkopf-1: Current knowledge and related diseases. *Life Sci.* **2018**, *209*, 249–254. [CrossRef] [PubMed]
54. Apostolova, L.G. Alzheimer disease. *Continuum* **2016**, *22*, 419–434. [CrossRef]
55. Rosi, M.C.; Luccarini, I.; Grossi, C.; Fiorentini, A.; Spillantini, M.G.; Prisco, A.; Scali, C.; Gianfriddo, M.; Caricasole, A.; Terstappen, G.C.; et al. Increased dickkopf-1 expression in transgenic mouse models of neurodegenerative disease. *J. Neurochem.* **2010**, *112*, 1539–1551. [CrossRef]
56. Lecourt, S.; Mouly, E.; Freida, D.; Cras, A.; Ceccaldi, R.; Heraoui, D.; Chomienne, C.; Marolleau, J.-P.; Arnulf, B.; Porcher, R.; et al. A prospective study of bone marrow hematopoietic and mesenchymal stem cells in type 1 gaucher disease patients. *PLoS ONE* **2013**, *8*, e69293. [CrossRef]

57. Zancan, I.; Bellesso, S.; Costa, R.; Salvalaio, M.; Stroppiano, M.; Hammond, C.; Argenton, F.; Filocamo, M.; Moro, E. Glucocerebrosidase deficiency in zebrafish affects primary bone ossification through increased oxidative stress and reduced wnt/beta-catenin signaling. *Hum. Mol. Genet.* **2015**, *24*, 1280–1294. [CrossRef]
58. Panicker, L.M.; Miller, D.; Park, T.S.; Patel, B.; Azevedo, J.L.; Awad, O.; Masood, M.A.; Veenstra, T.D.; Goldin, E.; Stubblefield, B.K.; et al. Induced pluripotent stem cell model recapitulates pathologic hallmarks of gaucher disease. *Proc. Natl. Acad. Sci. USA* **2012**, *109*, 18054–18059. [CrossRef]
59. Panicker, L.M.; Miller, D.; Awad, O.; Bose, V.; Lun, Y.; Park, T.S.; Zambidis, E.T.; Sgambato, J.A.; Feldman, R.A. Gaucher ipsc-derived macrophages produce elevated levels of inflammatory mediators and serve as a new platform for therapeutic development. *Stem Cells* **2014**, *32*, 2338–2349. [CrossRef]
60. Sgambato, J.A.; Park, T.S.; Miller, D.; Panicker, L.M.; Sidransky, E.; Lun, Y.; Awad, O.; Bentzen, S.M.; Zambidis, E.T.; Feldman, R.A. Gaucher disease-induced pluripotent stem cells display decreased erythroid potential and aberrant myelopoiesis. *Stem Cells Transl. Med.* **2015**, *4*, 878–886. [CrossRef]
61. Awad, O.; Panicker, L.M.; Deranieh, R.M.; Srikanth, M.P.; Brown, R.A.; Voit, A.; Peesay, T.; Park, T.S.; Zambidis, E.T.; Feldman, R.A. Altered differentiation potential of gaucher's disease ipsc neuronal progenitors due to wnt/beta-catenin downregulation. *Stem Cell Rep.* **2017**, *9*, 1853–1867. [CrossRef]
62. Doble, B.W.; Woodgett, J.R. Gsk-3: Tricks of the trade for a multi-tasking kinase. *J. Cell. Sci.* **2003**, *116*, 1175–1186. [CrossRef] [PubMed]
63. Niehrs, C.; Acebron, S.P. Wnt signaling: Multivesicular bodies hold gsk3 captive. *Cell* **2010**, *143*, 1044–1046. [CrossRef] [PubMed]
64. Young, N.P.; Kamireddy, A.; Van Nostrand, J.L.; Eichner, L.J.; Shokhirev, M.N.; Dayn, Y.; Shaw, R.J. Ampk governs lineage specification through tfeb-dependent regulation of lysosomes. *Genes. Dev.* **2016**, *30*, 535–552. [CrossRef] [PubMed]
65. Glinka, A.; Wu, W.; Delius, H.; Monaghan, A.P.; Blumenstock, C.; Niehrs, C. Dickkopf-1 is a member of a new family of secreted proteins and functions in head induction. *Nature* **1998**, *391*, 357–362. [CrossRef]
66. Haaber, J.; Abildgaard, N.; Knudsen, L.M.; Dahl, I.M.; Lodahl, M.; Thomassen, M.; Kerndrup, G.B.; Rasmussen, T. Myeloma cell expression of 10 candidate genes for osteolytic bone disease. Only overexpression of dkk1 correlates with clinical bone involvement at diagnosis. *Br. J. Haematol.* **2008**, *140*, 25–35. [CrossRef]
67. Tian, E.; Zhan, F.; Walker, R.; Rasmussen, E.; Ma, Y.; Barlogie, B.; Shaughnessy, J.D., Jr. The role of the wnt-signaling antagonist dkk1 in the development of osteolytic lesions in multiple myeloma. *N. Engl. J. Med.* **2003**, *349*, 2483–2494. [CrossRef]
68. Ko, J.-Y.; Wang, F.-S.; Wang, C.-J.; Wong, T.; Chou, W.-Y.; Tseng, S.-L. Increased dickkopf-1 expression accelerates bone cell apoptosis in femoral head osteonecrosis. *Bone* **2010**, *46*, 584–591. [CrossRef]
69. Tsentidis, C.; Gourgiotis, D.; Kossiva, L.; Marmarinos, A.; Doulgeraki, A.; Karavanaki, K. Increased levels of dickkopf-1 are indicative of wnt/β-catenin downregulation and lower osteoblast signaling in children and adolescents with type 1 diabetes mellitus, contributing to lower bone mineral density. *Osteoporos. Int.* **2017**, *28*, 945–953. [CrossRef]
70. Cappuccio, I.; Calderone, A.; Busceti, C.L.; Biagioni, F.; Pontarelli, F.; Bruno, V.; Storto, M.; Terstappen, G.T.; Gaviraghi, G.; Fornai, F.; et al. Induction of dickkopf-1, a negative modulator of the wnt pathway, is required for the development of ischemic neuronal death. *J. Neurosci.* **2005**, *25*, 2647–2657. [CrossRef]
71. Klein, A.D.; Ferreira, N.S.; Ben-Dor, S.; Duan, J.; Hardy, J.; Cox, T.M.; Merrill, A.H., Jr.; Futerman, A.H. Identification of modifier genes in a mouse model of gaucher disease. *Cell Rep.* **2016**, *16*, 2546–2553. [CrossRef] [PubMed]
72. Albrecht, L.V.; Ploper, D.; Tejeda-Muñoz, N.; De Robertis, E.M. Arginine methylation is required for canonical wnt signaling and endolysosomal trafficking. *Proc. Natl. Acad. Sci. USA* **2018**, *115*, E5317–E5325. [CrossRef] [PubMed]
73. Redelman-Sidi, G.; Binyamin, A.; Gaeta, I.; Palm, W.; Thompson, C.B.; Romesser, P.B.; Lowe, S.W.; Bagul, M.; Doench, J.G.; Root, D.E.; et al. The canonical wnt pathway drives macropinocytosis in cancer. *Cancer Res.* **2018**, *78*, 4658–4670. [CrossRef] [PubMed]
74. Saito-Diaz, K.; Benchabane, H.; Tiwari, A.; Tian, A.; Li, B.; Thompson, J.J.; Hyde, A.S.; Sawyer, L.M.; Jodoin, J.N.; Santos, E.; et al. Apc inhibits ligand-independent wnt signaling by the clathrin endocytic pathway. *Dev. Cell* **2018**, *44*, 566–581.e568. [CrossRef] [PubMed]

75. Albrecht, L.V.; Tejeda-Muñoz, N.; Bui, M.H.; Cicchetto, A.C.; Di Biagio, D.; Colozza, G.; Schmid, E.; Piccolo, S.; Christofk, H.R.; De Robertis, E.M. Gsk3 inhibits macropinocytosis and lysosomal activity through the wnt destruction complex machinery. *Cell Rep.* **2020**, *32*, 107973. [CrossRef]
76. Park, J.H.; Min, J.; Baek, S.R.; Kim, S.W.; Kwon, I.K.; Jeon, S.R. Enhanced neuroregenerative effects by scaffold for the treatment of a rat spinal cord injury with wnt3a-secreting fibroblasts. *Acta. Neurochir.* **2013**, *155*, 809–816. [CrossRef]
77. Gao, K.; Wang, Y.S.; Yuan, Y.J.; Wan, Z.H.; Yao, T.C.; Li, H.H.; Tang, P.F.; Mei, X.F. Neuroprotective effect of rapamycin on spinal cord injury via activation of the wnt/β-catenin signaling pathway. *Neural. Regen. Res.* **2015**, *10*, 951–957.
78. González-Fernández, C.; Fernández-Martos, C.M.; Shields, S.D.; Arenas, E.; Javier Rodríguez, F. Wnts are expressed in the spinal cord of adult mice and are differentially induced after injury. *J. Neurotrauma* **2014**, *31*, 565–581. [CrossRef]
79. Zhang, J.Y.; Lee, J.H.; Gu, X.; Wei, Z.Z.; Harris, M.J.; Yu, S.P.; Wei, L. Intranasally delivered wnt3a improves functional recovery after traumatic brain injury by modulating autophagic, apoptotic, and regenerative pathways in the mouse brain. *J. Neurotrauma* **2018**, *35*, 802–813. [CrossRef]
80. Matei, N.; Camara, J.; McBride, D.; Camara, R.; Xu, N.; Tang, J.; Zhang, J.H. Intranasal wnt3a attenuates neuronal apoptosis through frz1/piwil1a/foxm1 pathway in mcao rats. *J. Neurosci.* **2018**, *38*, 6787–6801. [CrossRef]
81. Ke, H.Z.; Richards, W.G.; Li, X.; Ominsky, M.S. Sclerostin and dickkopf-1 as therapeutic targets in bone diseases. *Endocr. Rev.* **2012**, *33*, 747–783. [CrossRef] [PubMed]
82. Fulciniti, M.; Tassone, P.; Hideshima, T.; Vallet, S.; Nanjappa, P.; Ettenberg, S.A.; Shen, Z.; Patel, N.; Tai, Y.T.; Chauhan, D.; et al. Anti-dkk1 mab (bhq880) as a potential therapeutic agent for multiple myeloma. *Blood* **2009**, *114*, 371–379. [CrossRef] [PubMed]
83. Iyer, S.P.; Beck, J.T.; Stewart, A.K.; Shah, J.; Kelly, K.R.; Isaacs, R.; Bilic, S.; Sen, S.; Munshi, N.C. A phase ib multicentre dose-determination study of bhq880 in combination with anti-myeloma therapy and zoledronic acid in patients with relapsed or refractory multiple myeloma and prior skeletal-related events. *Br. J. Haematol.* **2014**, *167*, 366–375. [CrossRef]
84. Iozzi, S.; Remelli, R.; Lelli, B.; Diamanti, D.; Pileri, S.; Bracci, L.; Roncarati, R.; Caricasole, A.; Bernocco, S. Functional characterization of a small-molecule inhibitor of the dkk1-lrp6 interaction. *ISRN Mol. Biol.* **2012**, *2012*, 823875. [CrossRef] [PubMed]
85. Thysiadis, S.; Katsamakas, S.; Mpousis, S.; Avramidis, N.; Efthimiopoulos, S.; Sarli, V. Design and synthesis of gallocyanine inhibitors of dkk1/lrp6 interactions for treatment of alzheimer's disease. *Bioorg. Chem.* **2018**, *80*, 230–244. [CrossRef] [PubMed]
86. Panicker, L.M.; Srikanth, M.P.; Castro-Gomes, T.; Miller, D.; Andrews, N.W.; Feldman, R.A. Gaucher disease ipsc-derived osteoblasts have developmental and lysosomal defects that impair bone matrix deposition. *Hum. Mol. Genet.* **2018**, *27*, 811–822. [CrossRef] [PubMed]

Publisher's Note: MDPI stays neutral with regard to jurisdictional claims in published maps and institutional affiliations.

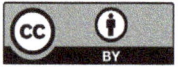

© 2020 by the authors. Licensee MDPI, Basel, Switzerland. This article is an open access article distributed under the terms and conditions of the Creative Commons Attribution (CC BY) license (http://creativecommons.org/licenses/by/4.0/).

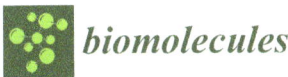

Article

Rapid Clathrin-Mediated Uptake of Recombinant α-Gal-A to Lysosome Activates Autophagy

Margarita M. Ivanova *, Julia Dao, Neil Kasaci, Benjamin Adewale, Jacqueline Fikry and Ozlem Goker-Alpan

Lysosomal and Rare Disorders Research and Treatment Center, Fairfax, VA 22030, USA; jdao@ldrtc.org (J.D.); neilkass@gmail.com (N.K.); adewalejr.ben@gmail.com (B.A.); jfikry@ldrtc.org (J.F.); ogoker-alpan@ldrtc.org (O.G.-A.)
* Correspondence: mivanova@ldrtc.org

Received: 19 March 2020; Accepted: 28 May 2020; Published: 30 May 2020

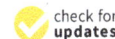

Abstract: Enzyme replacement therapy (ERT) with recombinant alpha-galactosidase A (rh-α-Gal A) is the standard treatment for Fabry disease (FD). ERT has shown a significant impact on patients; however, there is still morbidity and mortality in FD, resulting in progressive cardiac, renal, and cerebrovascular pathology. The main pathway for delivery of rh-α-Gal A to lysosome is cation-independent mannose-6-phosphate receptor (CI-M6PR) endocytosis, also known as insulin-like growth factor 2 receptor (IGF2R) endocytosis. This study aims to investigate the mechanisms of uptake of rh-α-Gal-A in different cell types, with the exploration of clathrin-dependent and caveolin assisted receptor-mediated endocytosis and the dynamics of autophagy-lysosomal functions. rh-α-Gal-A uptake was evaluated in primary fibroblasts, urine originated kidney epithelial cells, and peripheral blood mononuclear cells derived from Fabry patients and healthy controls, and in cell lines HEK293, HTP1, and HUVEC. Uptake of rh-α-Gal-A was more efficient in the cells with the lowest endogenous enzyme activity. Chloroquine and monensin significantly blocked the uptake of rh-α-Gal-A, indicating that the clathrin-mediated endocytosis is involved in recombinant enzyme delivery. Alternative caveolae-mediated endocytosis coexists with clathrin-mediated endocytosis. However, clathrin-dependent endocytosis is a dominant mechanism for enzyme uptake in all cell lines. These results show that the uptake of rh-α-Gal-A occurs rapidly and activates the autophagy-lysosomal pathway.

Keywords: Fabry disease; enzyme replacement therapy; alpha-galactosidase A; endocytosis; lysosome; IGF2R/M6P; clathrin; chloroquine

---

1. Introduction

The past two decades have been highlighted by impressive progress in the treatment of lysosomal storage disorders (LSD) with the development of innovative therapies, including enzyme replacement therapy (ERT) [1]. The success of ERT in Gaucher disease stimulated the expansion of targeted enzyme replacement for other LSD. Currently, ERT is the first specific treatment for several LSD, including Anderson–Fabry disease (FD) [2]. FD is an X-linked disorder that results from a mutation of the gene (*GLA*) that encodes the lysosomal enzyme α-Galactosidase A (α -Gal-A).

The symptoms of FD are heterogeneous and include renal failure, cardiovascular disease, cerebrovascular complications, dermatologic manifestations, ocular and hearing complications, auditory, and neurologic complications [3–5]. Cardiovascular pathology and end-stage renal disease are the leading causes of death in male FD. The involvement of the central nervous system in FD increases the incidence of ischemic strokes and causes a significant decrease in lifespan in Fabry patients. The life expectancy of male patients with FD, if untreated, is approximately 40–42 years. Heterozygous females have higher residual α–Gal A activities. However, females develop clinical manifestations of varying severity and also have a reduced life span [6].

The α-Gal-A deficiency leads to the accumulation of globotriasylceramide (Gb3) in lysosomes of many cell types, including neurons, cardiomyocytes, and renal cells. ERT is effective in reducing glycolipid substrate accumulation in cells and appears to slow the progression of the FD [2,3]. Not all organs or tissues equally benefit from ERT. In general, the effectiveness of ERT becomes limited when treatment is started in adults. ERT can stabilize kidney function in patients with stage 1 or 2 chronic kidney disease; however, ERT is not effective with advanced kidney pathology, glomerular fibrosis, and sclerosis [7–9]. Additionally, ERT preserves the cardiac structure and heart function if treatment is initiated before the development of significant cardiac involvement. However, many patients with cellular hypertrophy in cardiomyocytes and vascular smooth muscle cells associated with tissue fibrosis still experience progressive cardio complications [10,11].

Intravenously-administered recombinant enzyme uptakes by cells through the cell surface receptor IGF2R/M6P. It is shown that, in most ERT, the IGF2R/M6P-mediated endocytosis is crucial for efficient enzyme delivery [12–14]. IGF2R/M6P is a bifunctional receptor that mediates binding and endocytosis of proteins via the clathrin-associated pathway [15,16]. IGF2R/M6P is essential for several cell signaling processes, including lysosomal enzyme trafficking from trans-Golgi apparatus, clearance, activation of growth factors, endocytosis-mediated delivery of macromolecules to the lysosomes [16]. IGF2R/M6P is expressed in most tissues, with relatively higher expression in kidneys and lungs, which makes this receptor attractive for the development of intracellular drug delivery. The function of IGF2R/M6P is to bind and transport the M6P enzyme to lysosomes and has been utilized for the therapeutic applications of ERT. For FD disease, two rh-α-gal-A enzymes, agalsidase beta and agalsidase alfa, are used for ERT, and both enzymes contain M6P [17,18].

The current challenge of ERT is that treatment does not produce satisfactory results when initiated in patients with advanced stages of the disease. A better understanding of the mechanism of enzymatic uptake in different tissues and cell types is needed to improve the therapeutic outcome of ERT for FD. In this study, we compared the enzyme uptake efficiency in primary cells derived from different tissue sources—PBMC, fibroblasts, kidney epithelial cells derived from FD patients—with cell lines of different origin—HEK293, HUVEC, and HTP1 cells.

We demonstrated that uptake and transport of recombinant enzyme to lysosome is the immediate activation of autophagy. Efficiency and the maximum capacity of uptake rh-α-Gal-A is time- and cell type-specific. The FD fibroblasts demonstrated maximum enzyme uptake and HUVEC cells—the lowest enzyme uptake efficiency. IGF2R/M6P plays an essential role in the delivery of rh-α-Gal-A to the lysosome via clathrin- and, to a lesser extent, caveolae-mediated endocytosis.

2. Materials and Methods

2.1. Chemicals

Genistein, chloroquine, monensin, nocodazole (cat no. 1228) were purchased from Tocris Bioscience (Bristol, UK). The recombinant rh-α-Gal-A enzyme was from commercial source: "Fabrazyme" from Sanofi/Genzyme Corporation (Cambridge, MA, USA). Biochemical and pharmacological characteristics of commercial rh-α-Gal-A described [18]. We used rh-α-Gal-A from leftover vials after reconstitution for patient use.

2.2. Subjects

Primary cells derived from FD patients have been used for the study. The diagnosis of FD was confirmed by clinical presentations and enzyme, and molecular analysis. All patients gave a written informed consent form for the collection and analysis of their data. The clinical protocol was approved by the ethics committees and data protection agencies (WIBR l #20131424).

2.3. Cell Lines

HEK293, HUVEC, THP-1, and wild-type primary dermal fibroblast cells were purchased from American Type Tissue Collection (ATCC; Manassas, VA, USA). Primary Dermal Fibroblasts cells were grown in Media 106 with the addition of LSGS kit (S-003-10) (ThermoFisher, Rockford, IL, USA) and used between passage 4-10. HEK293 cells were maintained in 5% FBS with Improved Minimum Essential Medium (IMEM) (ThermoFisher, Rockford, IL, USA), THP-1 cells were grown in RPMI (ThermoFisher, Rockford, IL, USA) with 10% FBS following the manufacturer's recommendation. HUVEC cells were grown in vascular cell basal medium with the addition of VEGF endothelial cell growth kit (ATCC; Manassas, VA, USA), and used between passages 3 and 8.

2.4. Isolation and Growth of Primary Skin Fibroblasts

Tissue samples were obtained from two patients carrying V269E and Y134D mutations in the *GLA* gene (Table S1). Skin biopsies were placed into a 50 mL conical tube and washed in PBS with 1% penicillin/streptomycin solution (ThermoFisher Scientific, Rockford, IL, USA). Skin fibroblasts were cultured as per standard methodology with complete Media 106 (Media 106, Low Serum Growth Supplement Kit and normocin, ATCC) [19]. LSGS specifically designed for the growth of dermal fibroblasts and endothelial cells. Fibroblast cells were sub-cultured at a split ratio 1:4 and used between passages 4 and 10. Cells were not immortalized.

2.5. Isolation, Purification, and Growth of Urine-Derived Kidney Cells

Fresh 25–50 mL of midstream urine samples were collected from two male patients with FD carrying deletion mutation c.194+1/195-1 and C2233Y mutations in the *GLA* gene and healthy controls (Table S1) The samples were processed immediately followed the protocol [19]. Briefly, urine samples were centrifuged at $400 \times g$ for 10 min, washed with PBS containing 1% ampicillin/streptomycin, and cell pellets were collected. Then, cells were plated in a 24-well dish with renal epithelial cell basal media supplemented with renal epithelial cell growth kit (ATCC) specifically designed for the growth of renal epithelial cells and mixed of antibiotics, normocin (InvivoGen, San Diego, CA, USA). While most cells from urine failed to attach, kidney epithelial cells attached to plate surfaces. The culture media was changed every 2–3 days until cells formed colonies. The cells were split using 0.05% Trypsin when culture cells reached the formation of large colonies. After the first passages, kidney epithelial cells (UKEC) were continuously grown in complete renal epithelial cell basal media. The cell culture subsets of composition and characteristics were analyzed. As expected, we detected a significant decrease of α-Gal A activity in patient samples compared to controls (Table S1). RT-PCR reveals the presence of epithelial markers E-cadherin (CDH1) and epithelial cell adhesion molecule (EPCAM) and the absence of podocyte markers: Podocin (NPHS2) and Nephrin (NPHS1) [20]. The maximum passage number was used 6–8 passages, or until cells were unable to reach confluence and started to undergo apoptosis. Cells were not immortalized.

2.6. Isolation, Purification, and Culture of Peripheral Blood Monocytes (PBMC)

PBMC were purified from blood samples from patients with Fabry disease using Lymphoprep™ reagent and SepMate™ tubes (Stemcell Technologies, Vancouver, BC, Canada) following the manufacturer's protocol. Lymphoprep™ was added to the lower compartment of the SepMate tube. Blood was mixed with PBS + 2% FBS in a 1:1 ratio, then layered on top of Lymphoprep™ following the company protocol. Samples were centrifuged at $800 \times g$ for 20 min at 18 °C with the brake off. The upper plasma layer was discarded. The PBMCs layer was removed carefully, then washed with PBS and centrifuged at $300 \times g$ for 8 min at room temperature between each wash. Isolated PBMC were treated in 5% CO_2 in phenol red-free RPMI media with 10% FBS. PBMC always was used fresh following the experiments.

2.7. Treatment of Cells with rh-α-Gal-A and Other Chemicals

The cells were split, and cultures using the recommended media for specific cell lines were established 24 h before the treatments. DMSO was used as the vehicle control for experiments with inhibitors. Cells were treated with various concentrations of rh-α-Gal-A enzymes, as shownd in the figures. For the indicated experiments, cells were pretreated with 50 µg/mL nocodazole, 200 µM chloroquine, 50 ng monensin for 30 min, and 100 µM genistein for 1 h before rh-α-Gal-A treatment.

2.8. Uptake rh-α-Gal-A via an Alexa Fluor^{TM} Protein Labeling Kit

Rh-α-Gal-A protein conjugates containing the Alexa Fluor dyes (488 or 555) were prepared following the manufacture's protocol (ThermoFisher, Rockford, IL, USA). We titrated the range of enzyme activity pre- and post-labeling towards the artificial substrate 4-MUI in different volumes (Figure S1A). The log IC50 = −4.6 for unlabeled enzyme and log IC50 = −3.4 for labeled enzyme indicates that approximately 76% of the enzyme was recovered. Intracellular uptake of Alexa-Fluor-α-Gal-A was further verified qualitatively by a confocal microscope (Figure S1B). Fluorescence clusters were confirmed in fibroblast cells cultured with Alexa-Fluor-α-Gal-A conjugates and the absence of a fluorescence signal in cells cultured with free dye. Validation of uptake was investigating using co-incubating live cells with Alexa-Fluor-α-Gal-A conjugates for 1 and 3 h. LysoTracker or autophagy dyes were added 30 min prior to stop the reaction. Then cells were washed with PBS three times. Cells were visualized by fluorescent microscopy, where co-localization of green-(488)-labeled α-Gal-A protein with red-labeled lysosomes appears yellow in color-merged images. Green-labeled autophagy vesicles were co-stained with red-(550)-labeled α-Gal-A protein.

2.9. α-Galactosidase A Activity Assay

Cells were washed with cold PBS three times and lysed in cold H_2O after the treatments as described above. Protein concentration was determined by the Pierce BCA protein assay kit (ThermoFisher, Rockford, IL, USA) according to the manufacturer's manual. An activity was fluorometrically determined by incubating 10 µg/mL of samples with 5 mM 4-Methylumbelliferyl α-D-galactopyranoside and in 0.06 M phosphate citrate buffer (pH 4.7) for 1 h (Santa Cruz Biotechnology, Dallas, TX, USA). Enzyme activity was measured as described previously and is expressed as the nmol 4-MU/mg protein/time incubation or as a relative level to control, untreated samples [21,22].

2.10. Protein Isolation and Western Blot Analysis

Antibodies were purchased as follows: IGF-II Receptor/CI-M6PR (D3V8C) and β-actin (# 8H10D10) (Cell Signaling Technology, Danvers, MA, USA), α-Gal-A (#GTX101178) (GeneTex, Irvine, CA, USA). Whole-cell extracts (WCEs) were prepared in radioimmunoprecipitation (RIPA) buffer. Protein concentrations were determined using the BCA Protein Assay Kit (ThermoFisher, Rockford, IL, USA). Thirty micrograms (30 µg) of WCE were separated on mini protein TGX stain-free gel (Bio-Rad, Hercules, CA, USA) and electroblotted using the Trans-Blot® Turbo™ Midi PVDF Transfer Packs (Bio-Rad, Hercules, CA, USA). Membranes were diluted with antibodies (1:1000 dilutions) in 5% BSA, 1 × TBS, 0.1% Tween20, and gently shaking overnight at +4 °C. The ChemiDoc™ MP Imaging system (Bio-Rad) was used to visualize and quantitate optical density (IOD). The IODs of bands of interest were normalized to the loading control actin used in the same blot [8], and the normalized value of the controls was set to 1 for a comparison between separate experiments.

2.11. Autophagy Assay

The DALgreen Autophagy detection kit (Dojindo Laboratories, Kumamoto, Japan) was used according to the manufacture's protocol to quantify autophagic vesicle formation and Hoechst 33342 dye as an index of the nucleus. The resulting fluorescence was visualized by fluorescent microscopy (Evos^R digital microscope, Evos, Hatfield, PA, USA).

2.12. Measurement of Lysosome Levels

The LysoTracker Red (LifeTechnology, ThermoFisher, Rockford, IL, USA) assay was used as briefly described. LysoTracker (50 nM) was added to the cells as a fluorescent acidophilic probe for the labeling of the acidic organelles. After 30 min staining, cells were stained with Hoechst, and washed three times with PBS. The resulting fluorescence was visualized by fluorescent microscopy (Evos^R Digital microscope, Evos, Hatfield, PA, USA).

2.13. RNA Isolation and Quantitative Real-Time-PCR (qPCR)

RNA was extracted from cells using the Quick-RNA kit (Zymo Research, Irvine, CA, USA). The Luna® Universal Probe One-Step RT-qPCR Kit was used to reverse-transcribe RNA using random hexamers primers. Individual samples were run in triplicate, and mRNA levels were compared to the loading control, GADPH, using StepOnePlus™ Real-time PCR System (ThermoFisher Scientific, Rockford, IL, USA). The E-cadherin primers [23], EpCAM [24], and two pairs of IGF2R/M6P [24,25] primers were purchased from Eurofins Genomics. Analyses and fold differences were determined using the comparative CT method. Fold change was calculated from the ΔΔCT values with the formula $2^{-\Delta\Delta CT}$ relative to mRNA expression in the untreated control.

2.14. Immunofluorescence Microscopy Analysis

Scatter plots, Person's correlation coefficient, and colocalization threshold were obtained using ImageJ-win64 plug-in intensity correlation analysis. The image and statistical analysis of colocalization was performed with Coloc 2 Fiji's plugin and colocalization threshold (Figure S3). In a scatter plot, the intensity distribution of the two channels are plotted (X vs. Y) and a diagonal line indicates proportional co-distribution, where $R^2 = 1$ is a perfect positive linear relationship between two fluorescence intensities.

2.15. Interactive 3D Surface Plots Analysis

ImageJ plugins (NIH, Bethesda, MD, USA) with the option of 3D surface plot techniques of image data was used to analyze the intensity projection (Z coordinates) of autophagy staining. Pixels with higher intensity values lay higher on the Z axis. Parameters of the surface are plotted as 100% of the polygon multiplier, drawn in wireframe, shaded, and drawn on the axis.

3. Results

3.1. The Efficiency of Enzyme Uptake Is Cell Type-Specific

To test the hypothesis that the efficiency of rh-α-Gal-A uptake is cell type-specific, seven cell lines of different origins were examined (Table S1). HEK293, primary fibroblasts derived from healthy controls, and FD patients were selected because these cells are prevalent for studies of molecular mechanisms of drug delivery, including FD [26]. Since FD notably affects the vascular endothelium [27], human umbilical vein endothelial cells (HUVEC) were selected as a vascular model to study the delivery of the recombinant enzyme. Monocyte cell lines derived from a patient with acute monocytic leukemia (THP-1), PBMC derived from control, and FD patients were selected as models of the hematopoietic system. Since FD affects the kidney in almost all males and many females, the kidney epithelial cells isolated from urine were selected to study the mechanism of enzyme uptake. Cell lines and primary cells were treated for 1 h using a range of rh-α-Gal-A enzyme: from 0.05 g/mL to 500 g/mL (Figure 1). It appears that the efficiency of recombinant enzyme uptake was cell-type dependent (Figure 1A–C). In UKEC derived from two FD patients, the maximum uptake capacity differed greatly between patients with different *GLA* genotypes. The robust, but different, amplitude of the dose-dependent response was demonstrated in HEK293, PBMC, THP-1, fibroblasts, and UKEC cells. The rh-α-Gal-A enzyme uptake was less efficient in HUVEC cells (Figure 1A). Under this condition, our results demonstrated that enzyme activity reached a plateau at a concentration of 50 ug/mL in HUVEC, THP-1, fibroblasts, and UKEC-FD-2 cells (Figure 1C). The highest level of α-Gal-A activity approximated 1200–1600 nmol/mg/h and was observed in HEK293, control PBMC, and THP-1 cells. Medium level in the range of 330–800 nmol/mg/h of α-Gal-A activity was observed in primary fibroblasts and UKEC (Figure 1E). The lowest level was observed in HUVEC cells. Based on the fact that different cells have the different activity of endogenous α-Gal-A, the relative enzyme uptake was calculated as the percentage of treated vs. untreated cells for each cell line (Figure 1F). PBMC, FD derived fibroblasts, and UKEC cells showed greater than 3000-fold increase in α-Gal-A activity level compared with untreated cells (Figure 1F). Since the uptake of rh-α-Gal-A less efficient in cells with high endogenous α-Gal-A activity, we analyzed the correlation between endogenous enzyme activity and enzyme uptake efficiency. Uptake of rh-α-Gal-A was higher in cells with the lowest endogenous enzyme activity. Conversely, cells with high endogenous α-Gal-A activity demonstrated less effective uptake of the recombinant enzyme (Figure 1G). Moreover, HUVEC cells showed the lowest response to rh-α-Gal-A treatment (Figure 1A,D,G).

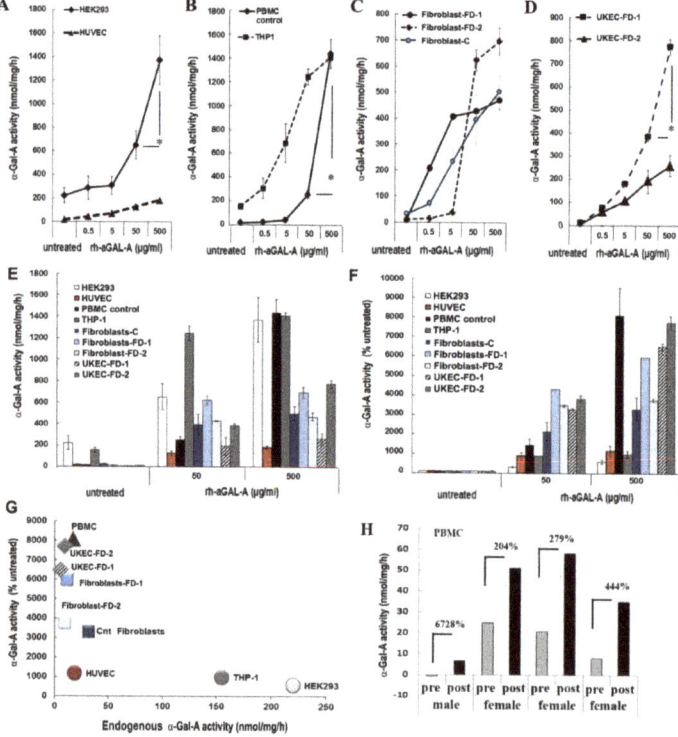

Figure 1. The efficiency of the delivery of recombinant α-Gal A enzyme (rh-α-Gal A). (**A**) HEK293 and HUVEC, (**B**) THP1 and control PBMC, (**C**) fibroblasts, and (**D**) UKEC cells were treated with increasing concentration of rh-α-Gal A for 1 h. A total α-Gal A enzyme activity level was determined using 4-MU. * $p < 0.05$ 50 vs. 500 µg/mL of α-Gal A treatment (**E,D**) Comparing the total absolute (**E**) and relative (**D**) enzyme activity levels. Measurements performed at the concentrations of 50 and 500 µg/mL were compared with the enzyme activity in untreated samples. (**G**) Correlation analysis between endogenous enzyme concentration and enzyme uptake efficiency. (**H**) α-Gal A activity was measured immediately following ERT treatment. Blood was collected before (pre) and after (post) ERT infusion and PBMCs were isolated from FD patients, one male, and three females. Values represent 4-MU pre- and post-infusion levels. Samples were measured in triplicate.

Next, we assessed ERT efficiency in the in vivo model. Immediately before and after ERT infusion, blood was collected from four FD patients (one male and three females), and α-Gal-A activity was measured. Plasma rh-α-Gal-A activity after ERT infusion was very similar among the four subjects and averaged 4502 ± 404 nmol/mL/h for all samples. In contrast, enzyme uptake efficiency into PBMC differed significantly among patients. The highest percentages of enzyme uptake were observed in PBMC derived from FD male with zero enzyme activity and female with the lowest endogenous α-Gal-A activity (Figure 1H). However, the highest total α-Gal-A activity was observed in cells from patients with the highest endogenous enzyme activity (Figure 1H).

3.2. The Uptake of rh-α-Gal-A Occurs On a Minute to Hours' Time Scale

Significant increases in α-Gal-A activity were detected within 1 h of treatment with the recombinant enzyme in all cell lines, including cells derived from FD patients. After 1 h, the α-Gal-A activity did not change drastically within 3h of treatment in HEK293 and control fibroblasts; however, the maximum uptake was observed within 6 h of treatment (Figure 2A,B). FD fibroblasts showed the maximum level of rh-α-Gal-A activity with 3 h treatment (Figure 2B,C). Significant increases in α-Gal-A activity were observed in control, and FD derived UKEC after 1h treatment with increased uptake after 3 h treatment (Figure 2C). Interestingly, both control and FD UKEC cells showed similar enzyme activity of α-Gal-A after 1 h and 3 h treatment with the recombinant enzyme (Figure 2D). Thus, this result indicates that the maximum α-Gal-A capacity for control and FD UKEC are similar.

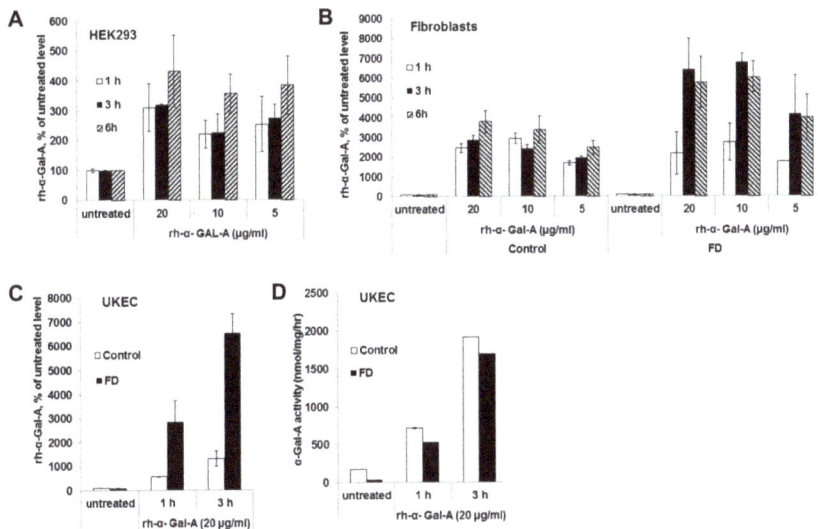

Figure 2. The rapid uptake of rh-α-Gal A. HEK293 (**A**), fibroblasts (**B**), and UKEC (**C**,**D**) cells were treated with the indicated concentration of rh-α-Gal A in a time-dependent manner. The enzyme assay was performed to determine the relative α-Gal A enzyme level. FD fibroblasts and UKEC cells represent data from FD-1 and FD-2 cell lines respectably. Values are average ±STDEV of minimum three experiments. * $p < 0.01$ vs. untreated control.

3.3. IGF2R/M6P Increase in HEK293 After Six Hours of Enzyme Uptake

Effectiveness of ERT with rh-α-Gal-A is dependent on recognition of mannose 6-phosphate (M6P) residues on the enzyme by the widely distributed IGF2R/M6P receptor [13,17]. The half-life of IGF2R/M6P is approximately $t_{\frac{1}{2}} \sim 20$ h, while the receptor cycles between trans-Golgi network, endosomes and the plasma membrane where it loads and unloads ligands [28]. The molecular mechanism of the cycle includes packaged enzymes into lysosomes, whereas the "free" IGF2R returns to the Golgi apparatus or move to the plasma membrane. To test the IGF2R/M6P cycling during uptake of rh-α-Gal-A, HEK293 cells were treated for 1, 3, and 6 h with increasing concentration of rh-α-Gal-A (Figure 3). The highest rh-α-Gal-A uptake was detected after 6h treatment without toxicity effect (Figure 3A,B, Figure S1C). Treatment HEK293 cells with Alexa-Fluor-α-Gal-A conjugates confirmed the highest rh-α-Gal-A uptake after 6h treatment (Figure 3D). Interestingly, the increasing level of IGF2R/M6P protein was detected after 6h treatment (Figure 3C). Accordingly, 6 h treatment with an increasing concentration of rh-α-Gal-A increased IGF2R/M6P expression of mRNA (Figure S2).

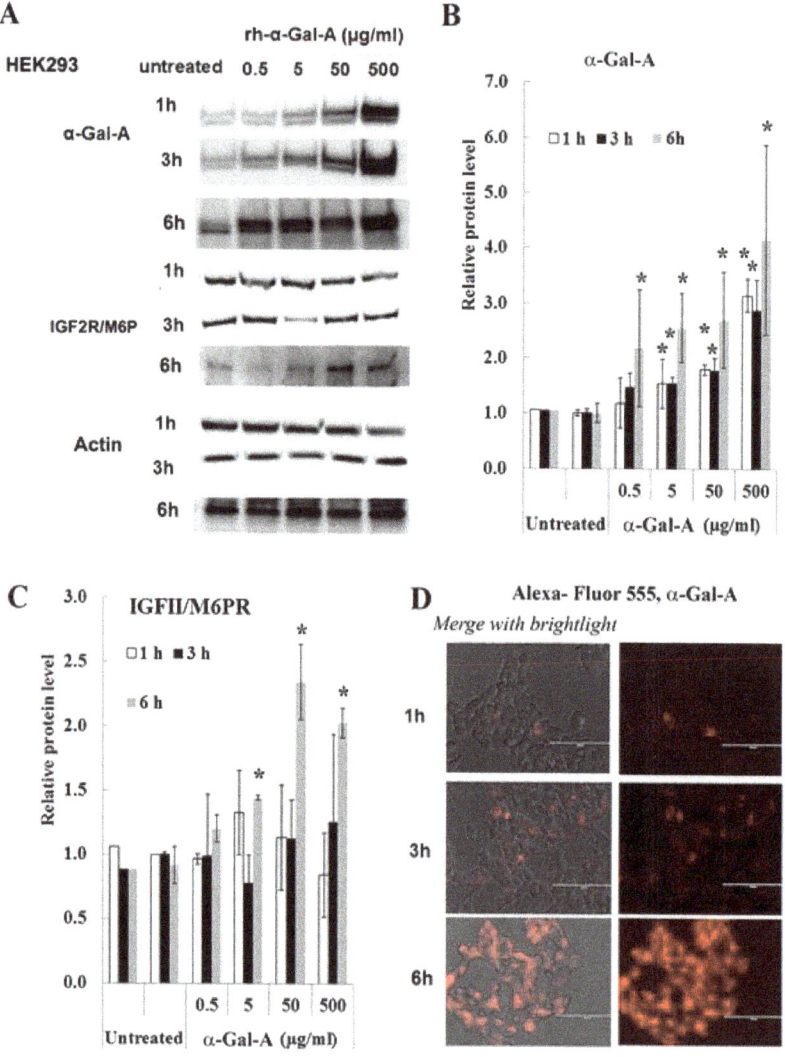

Figure 3. IGF2R/M6P decreases during rapid uptake of rh-α-Gal A. HEK293 cells were treated with the indicated concentrations of rh-α-Gal A for 1, 3, and 6 h. (**A**) Western blot (30 µg WCE) shows that uptake of rh-α-Gal A protein increases in concentration- and time-dependent manners. IGF2R/M6P increased after 6 h treatment. Membranes were reprobed for actin for normalization. (**B**) Quantitation of the relative level of α-Gal A. (**C**) Quantitation of relative level IGF2R/M6P. (**D**)) Immunofluorescence images of time course treated HEK293 cells with Alexa-Fluor-α-Gal-A conjugates. Bars: 100 µm.

3.4. Transport of rh-α-Gal-A Is Achieved by Clathrin and Caveolae-Mediated Endocytosis in a Cell Type-Specific Manner

Endocytosis, followed by lysosomal transport, support numerous cellular functions and has been used for intracellular delivery of recombinant enzymes. For the majority of cells, clathrin-coated and caveolae-mediated endocytosis are the most common uptake mechanisms [29]. However, the contribution of clathrin and caveolar pathways to endocytosis has been shown to differ between cell types and tissues, and that can contribute to the failure to efficiently deliver the recombinant enzyme to some organs [30]. We evaluated potential changes in the trafficking of the recombinant enzyme via clathrin and caveolae endocytosis. For this purpose, clathrin inhibitors (chloroquine and monensin) and caveolae inhibitor (genistein) have been used. HEK293, HUVEC, primary fibroblasts, and UKEC cells were pretreated with 100 μM of genistein, 100 μM of chloroquine, and 50 μM of monensin for 1h. The following pretreatment cells were incubated with 20 μg/mL rh-α-Gal-A plus inhibitors for 3h. Chloroquine and monensin blocked uptake of recombinant enzyme, indicating that the clathrin-mediated endocytosis is involved in recombinant enzyme delivery (Figure 4A–D and Figure 5A). Genistein (caveolae inhibitor) partially suppressed transport of rh-α-Gal-A in fibroblasts and UKEC cells, indicating that the caveolae-mediated endocytosis is partially involved in enzyme delivery (Figure 4A–D and Figure 5A).

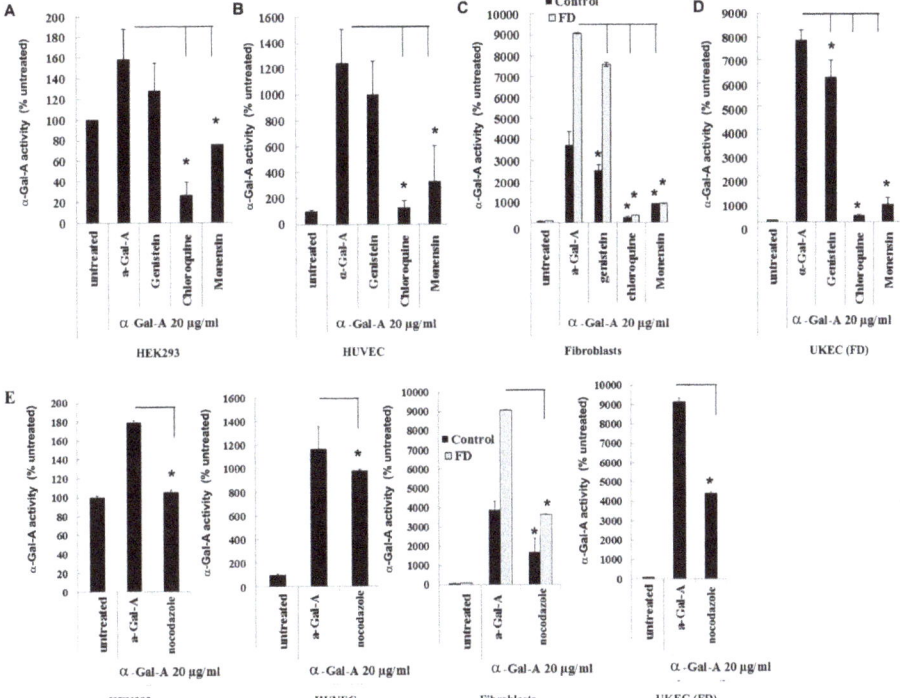

Figure 4. The rapid uptake of rh-α-Gal-A is achieved by clathrin and caveolae-mediated endocytosis. HEK293 (**A**), HUVEC (**B**), fibroblasts (**C**), and UKEC (**D**) cells were co-treated with the indicated concentration of rh-α-Gal A and inhibitors genistein, chloroquine, and monensin for 1 h. The enzyme assay was performed to determine the relative α-Gal A enzyme level. (**E**) HEK293, HUVEC, fibroblast, and UKEC cells were treated with the microtubule inhibitor, nocodazole. The enzyme assay was performed to determine the relative α-Gal A enzyme level. Values are average ±STDEV of minimum three experiments. * $p < 0.01$ vs. untreated control.

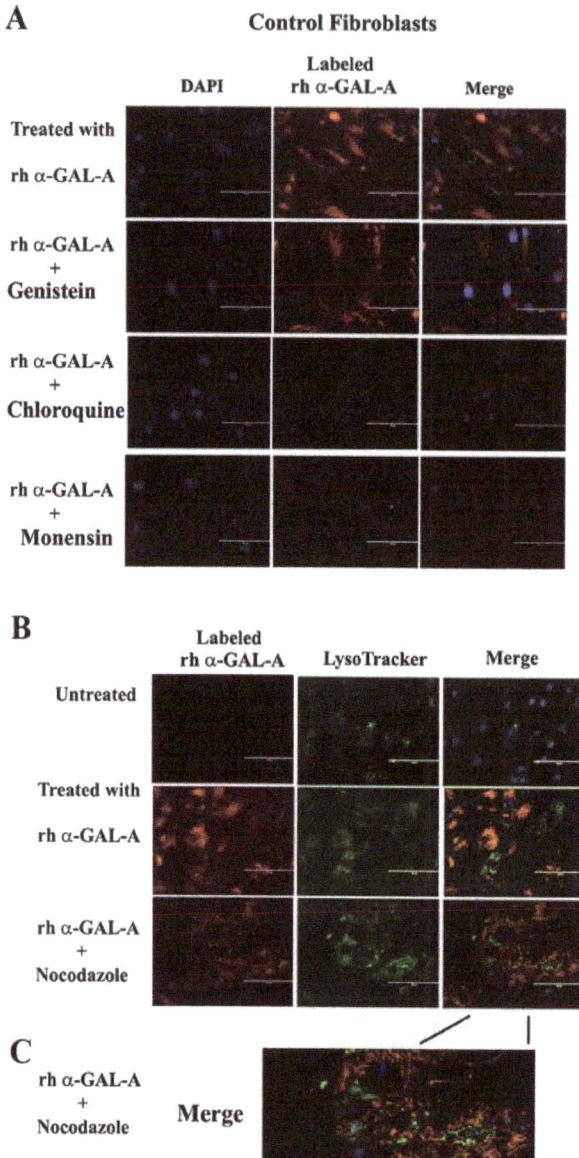

Figure 5. The trafficking of the recombinant enzyme is inhibited in the presence of chloroquine, monensin, and nocodazole. Control fibroblasts were co-treated with fluorescence-labeled rh-α-Gal-A and inhibitors genistein, chloroquine, monensin, and nocodazole. (**A**) Immunofluorescence images of control fibroblasts treated with fluorescence-labeled rh-α-Gal-A (red). Bars: 200 μm. (**B**) Immunofluorescence images of control fibroblasts treated with fluorescence-labeled rh-α-Gal-A (red) and stained with LysoTracker (green). Bars: 200 μm. (**C**). The magnified merge image of cells with Alexa-Fluor-α-Gal-A (red) and LysoTracker (green) after nocodazole treatment.

3.5. Activator of Microtubule Depolymerization, Nocodazole, Blocked rh-α-Gal-A Uptake

Since microtubule-based active transport is crucial for trafficking clathrin-coated vesicles and plays a role in the relocation and distribution of lysosomes [31], it should play an essential role in the transport of recombinant enzyme to the lysosomes. To investigate the role of microtubules in the transport of recombinant enzyme, we depolymerized the microtubule cytoskeleton by treating cells with 50 ng/mL of nocodazole. After 30 min of pretreatment, cells were treated with 20 µg/mL rh-α-Gal-A. Nocodazole inhibits the increase in α-Gal-A activity after 3h treatment with the recombinant enzyme, indicating that the microtubule cytoskeleton plays a vital role in the enzyme uptake (Figure 4E). Additionally, intracellular trafficking of Alexa Fluor tagged rh-α-Gal-A (red) to lysosomes in the presence of nocodazole was examined by immunofluorescence microscopy. The colocalization between rh-α-Gal-A and lysosomes was analyzed using Coloc 2 Fiji's plugin and colocalization threshold (ImageJ-win64) methods. Coloc 2 plugin analysis showed a reduction of that α-Gal-A colocalization with the lysosome marker after nocadozole treatment, with Pearson's coefficient of 0.62 (untreated cells) and 0.47 (nocodazole treated cells) (Figure S3). Colocalization threshold analysis showed decreasing areas of colocalization α-Gal-A with the lysosomes in presence of nocodazole (Figure S3). Analysis of the lysosomal staining (LysoTracker, green) merged with rh-α-Gal-A (red) demonstrated that nocodazole partially inhibited the transport of the recombinant enzyme to the lysosomal compartment (Figure 5B,C, Figure S3).

3.6. Robust Uptake of rh-α-Gal-A to the Lysosomes Increases Autophagy

The final destination of rh-α-Gal-A is the lysosomes, where enzyme catalyzes the removal of terminal α-galactose residues. Intracellular trafficking of rh-α-Gal-A was examined by fluorescence microscopy to assess co-localization of the recombinant enzyme with lysosomes. Fibroblasts and UKEC derived from FD patients were treated with rh-α-Gal-A labeled with the Alexa Fluor dyes (488) (Figure 6A). After treatment, live cells were stained with LysoTracker and visualized under the microscope. Co-localization of Fluor-488-α-Gal-A (green color) and LysoTracker appears as the yellow-orange color after the merging of images (Figure 6A). The distinct yellow-orange color of lysosomes demonstrates that rh-α-Gal-A traffics to lysosomes in a relatively short period of time in both cell lines. Figure 6B shows an enlarged image of 1-h treated fibroblasts and UKEC cells incubated with a combination of labeled Fluor-488-α-Gal-A and LysoTracker.

The disruption of the autophagy has been documented in fibroblasts, podocytes, and in PBMC derived from FD patients [20,32–34]. Next, we investigated the effect of rh-α-Gal-A on autophagy activation (Figures 7 and 8). Fibroblasts and UKEC cells from healthy controls and FD patients were treated with rh-α-Gal-A labeled with the Alexa Fluor dye (550) (Figure 7). After 3 h treatment, live cells were stained with a DALGreen autophagy detection kit to visualize autolysosomes, a unique acidic compartment in autophagy [35]. The level of autolysosomes was increased after 3 h treatment with Alexa-Fluor-α-Gal-A conjugates in all cells (Figure 7). The interactive surface plot analysis visualized DALGreen autophagy stain configuration in 3D format. The detailed observation of maximum intensity projection (Z coordinates) showed increasing levels of autolysosomes in α-Gal-A treated cells (Figure 8). Merge analysis of autophagy staining (green) with rh-α-Gal-A (red) demonstrated that the recombinant enzyme partially co-localizes with the autolysosomal compartment (Figure 7).

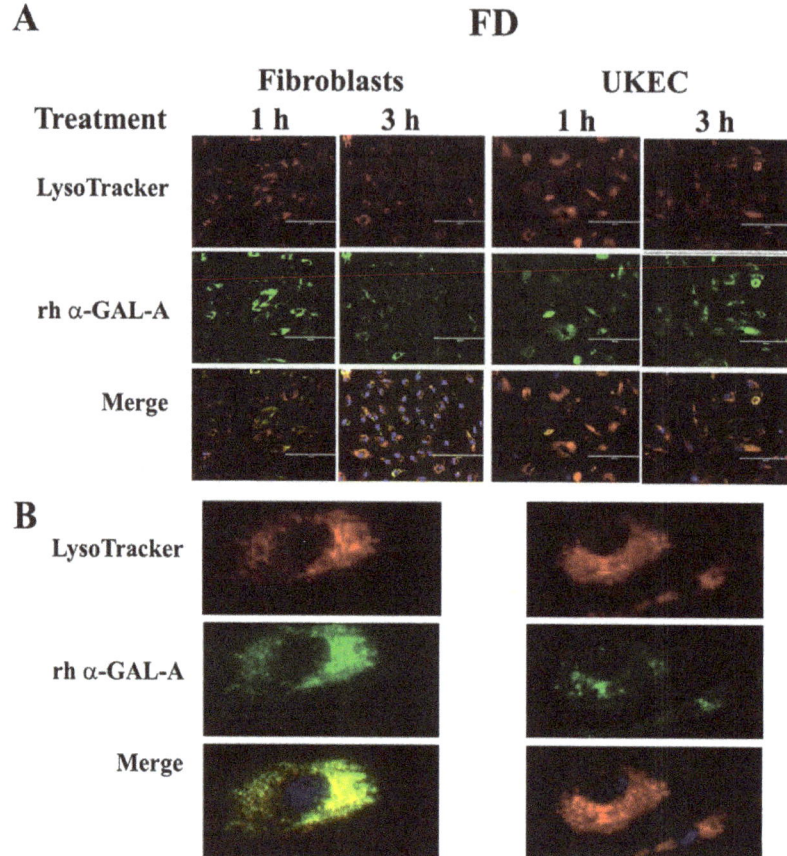

Figure 6. Immediate transport of rh-α-Gal-A to the lysosome. (**A**) Immunofluorescence images of FD fibroblasts and UKEC cells treated with fluorescence-labeled rh-α-Gal-A (green) and stained with LysoTracker (red). Bars: 200 μm. (**B**) Magnified image of cells with 1 h Alexa-Fluor-α-Gal-A conjugate treatment.

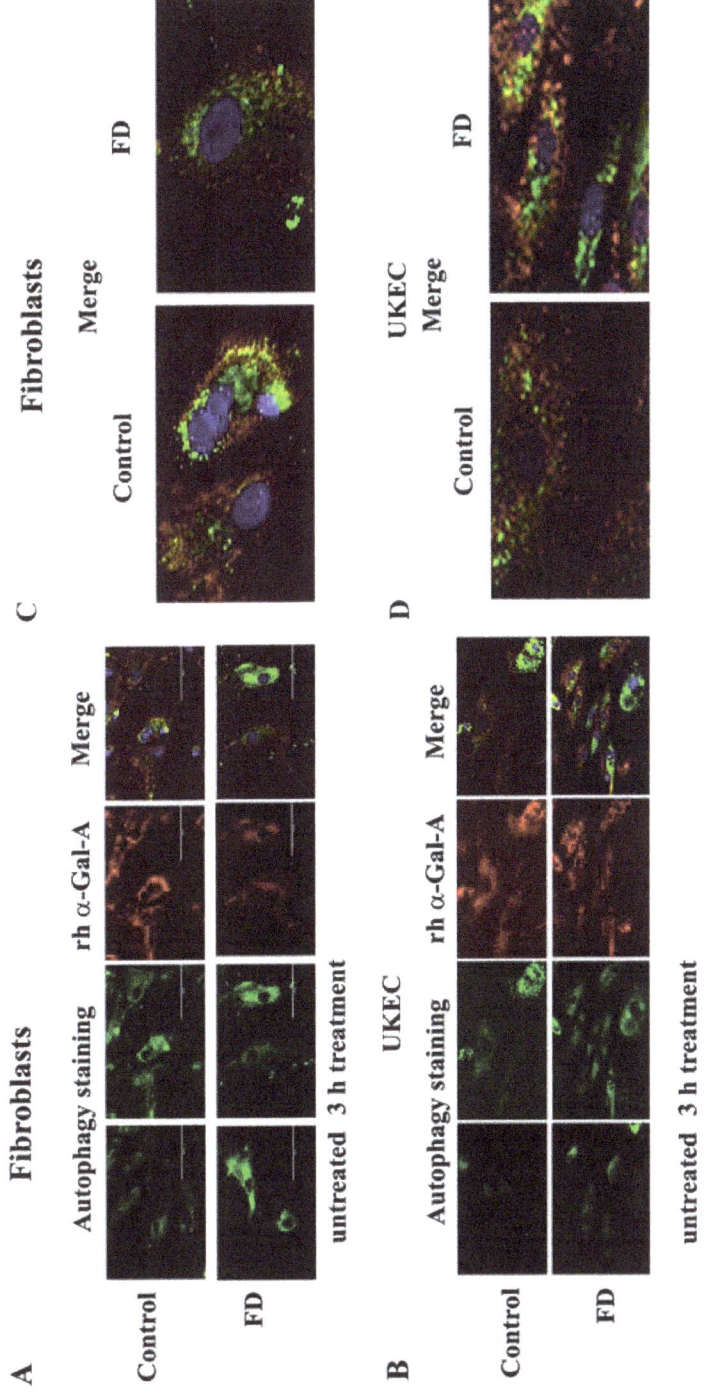

Figure 7. rh-α-Gal-A enhanced autolysosomal compartment. (**A**) Immunofluorescence images of control and FD fibroblasts treated with fluorescence-labeled rh-α-Gal-A (red) and stained with autophagy dye (DALgreen, green). Bar: 100 μm. (**B**). Representative images of control and FD UKEC treated with fluorescence-labeled rh-α-Gal-A (red) and stained with DALgreen (green). (**C, D**). Merge images of control and FD fibroblasts (**C**) and UKEC cells (**D**) treated with fluorescence-labeled rh-α-Gal-A (red) and stained with autophagy dye (DALgreen, green).

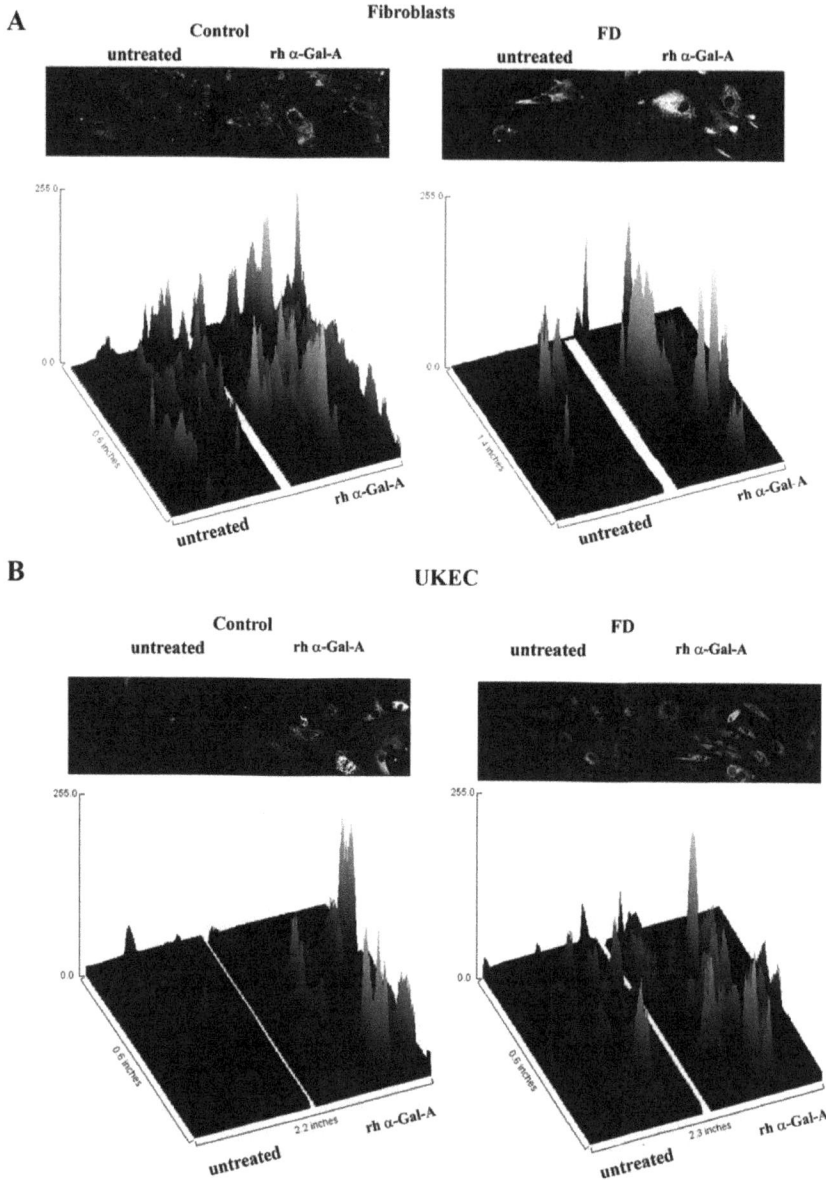

Figure 8. The interactive 3D surface plots displayed a three-dimensional graph of the intensities of pixels (Z) of autophagy in grayscale images. Immunofluorescence images of control vs. FD fibroblasts (**A**) and UKEC cells (**B**) treated with fluorescence-labeled rh-α-Gal-A were stained with DALgreen autophagy dye. The autophagy images used in Figure 7 were converted to 2D gray color images, and then interactive 3D surface plots were built using the ImageJ program. 2D and 3D images of control and FD fibroblast are displayed.

4. Discussion

ERT has been shown to be less effective in patients who have initiated treatment at a later age and/or with advanced renal, cardiovascular, and cerebrovascular involvement. The continued accumulation of Lyso-Gb3 in the vascular endothelium and smooth muscle cells was suggested to contribute to renal failure and strokes despite ERT [36]. The mechanisms of enzyme delivery in vascular or renal cells were not fully understood. Studies of enzyme delivery or small molecules therapy in FD mostly relied on in vitro observations using HEK293 cells and fibroblasts with wild-type GLA [13,26,37]. However, molecular mechanisms of enzyme delivery to lysosomes may vary depending on the type/origin of cells.

In the present study, we show that the efficient delivery of rh-α-Gal-A is cell-type specific. Moreover, the efficiency of rh-α-Gal-A uptake is determined by endogenous enzyme activity in cells. Treated HEK293, PBMC, and THP1 cells demonstrated the highest level of α-Gal-A enzyme activity (combined endogenous and recombinant enzyme activity) without a visual toxicity effect. The calculation of uptake efficiency in different cells showed that HEK293 cells have the lowest uptake due to high concentrations of endogenous α-Gal-A. Opposite to HEK293 cells, cells with low endogenous enzyme activity, including cells derived from FD patients, showed the most efficient uptake of the recombinant enzyme. A negative correlation between the level of endogenous α-Gal-A enzyme activity and the uptake efficiency indicates that the enzyme becomes saturated in cells and that different types of cells have a different maximum capacity for α-Gal-A uptake. The only vascular type of cells, HUVEC, did not show the same trend; these cells demonstrated the lowest enzyme uptake efficiency in the presence of low endogenous α-Gal-A activity. Our study indicates that the transport of recombinant enzyme was rapid in all cell lines leading to a significant increase in α-Gal-A activity. That transport reached the maximum capacity after 1-h treatment in HEK293 and control fibroblasts. There is continued enzyme uptake thereafter in FD fibroblasts, and UKEC cells. The time course shows that the dynamics of α-Gal-A uptake are cell type-specific.

For ERT to be successful, the proteins in different tissues must be correctly targeted to the lysosome. The IGF2R/M6P was selected for ERT because IGF2R/M6P mediated endocytosis transports M6P-bearing recombinant enzyme to lysosomes [12]. The effective transport of recombinant α-Gal-A depends on the variation in glycosylation of M6P residues, recognized by the IGF2R/M6P receptor located on the cytoplasmic membrane (Figure 9) [18,38]. The activation of IGF2R/M6P-mediated endocytosis is the key factor responsible for efficient enzyme uptake, which also depends on the distribution of the IGF2R/M6P receptor in different cells/tissues, and the mechanism of the shuttling of the receptor between cellular membrane, Golgi complex, and lysosomes in different cells/tissues.

IGF2R/M6P receptor is localized mostly in the Golgi and endosomal compartments with less than 10% on the plasma membrane. The receptor always shuttles between intracellular compartments and cytoplasmic membrane during endocytosis (Figure 9) [14,16]. The IGF2R/M6P mediated endocytosis has been very well characterized; however, the mechanisms of IGF2R/M6P shuttle between membrane-Golgi-lysosome during rapid delivery of rh-α-Gal A to lysosomes, is unknown. HEK293 cells were used to test IGF2R/M6P cycling during rh-α-Gal-A uptake. The data verified that rapid uptake of rh-α-Gal-A is associated with increasing IGF2R/M6P level after 6 h treatment.

Although it is clear that IGF2R/M6P receptor-mediated endocytosis plays a key role in the delivery of the recombinant enzyme to the cells, the mechanisms mediating the endocytosis remain undefined and are likely to be multi-faceted. For example, in the human podocyte cell line, three endocytic receptors, IGF2R/M6P, megalin, and sortilin are responsible for the α-Gal A uptake [13]. The design of the delivery of the recombinant enzyme relies on the nature of the IGF2R/M6P membrane receptor; however, the whole complex of endocytosis machinery is involved in this process. Normally, secreted pro-enzymes are taken up by the IGF2R/M6P receptor, formed pro-enzyme/ IGF2R/M6P complexes are then internalized through clathrin-mediated endocytosis (Figure 9) [39]. Monensin and chloroquine have been used to inhibit the initial step of clathrin-dependent endocytosis: formation of the clathrin-coated pit to the clathrin-coated vesicles [40]. We showed that inhibition of initiation of clathrin-coated vesicles resulted in a significant blockade of the transport of recombinant enzyme to HEK293, HUVEC, fibroblasts, and UKEC cells. This result highlights the universal role of clathrin in the delivery of recombinant enzyme through IGF2R/M6P receptor-mediated endocytosis.

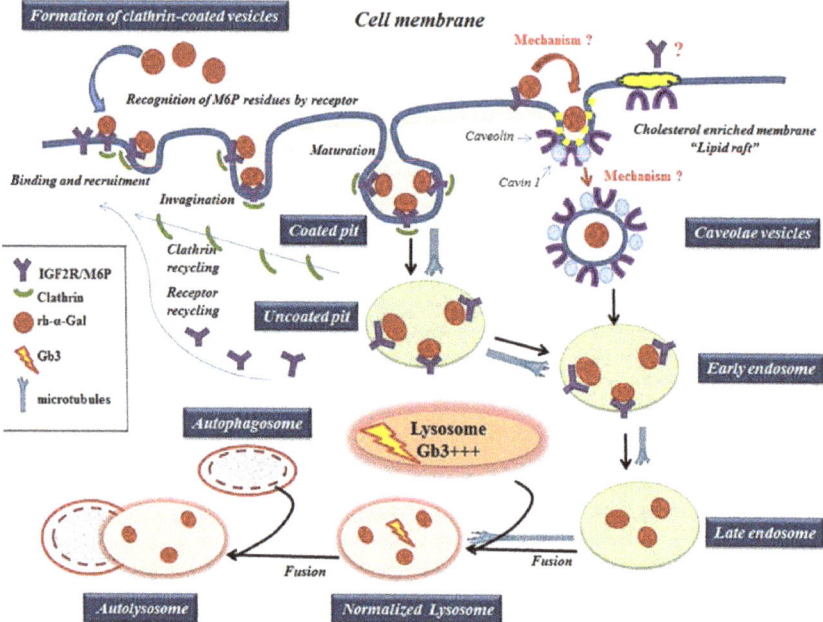

Figure 9. A working model of rh-α-Gal A uptake through clathrin- and caveolae-mediated endocytosis. The rh-α-Gal A contains terminal mannose residues for which conferring the high affinity for IGF2R/M6P on cells. The model proposes that the IGF2R/M6P internalizes the majority of the rh-α-Gal A through clathrin-mediated endocytosis. A small portion of IGF2R/M6P—rh-α-Gal A complex can also be uptake by caveolae-endocytic mechanisms. The microtubule cytoskeleton is involved in rh-α-Gal A endocytosis and transport enzyme to lysosomes. Early endosomes are containing recombinant enzyme mature into late endosomes, while IGF2R/M6P is recycling back to the cellular membrane. Late endosomal fuses with lysosome and delivers the therapeutic enzyme to the lysosome, which subsequently normalized Gb3 level. Normalized lysosomes fused with autophagosomes and form autolysosomes.

Does clathrin-dependent endocytosis provide the optimal mechanism for enzyme delivery in the FD cells? The phenomenon of decreased uptake through IGF2R/M6P endocytosis has been documented for several lysosomal storage disorders, such as in fibroblasts from Pompe and Niemann Pick patients [41–43]. A fluid-phase uptake study demonstrated reduced dextran uptake in Gaucher and FD fibroblasts due to the alteration of clathrin-mediated endocytosis [44]. Deficits in neurotransmitter recycling via clathrin-coated pits have been shown in mouse models of Gaucher and Batten disease [45]. Clathrin is a part of the trafficking pathway of lysosomal enzymes, and lysosomal abnormalities could be a contributing factor for inhibition of clathrin-mediated endocytosis.

Caveolar endocytosis is suggested not to be involved in endogenous lysosomal enzyme trafficking; therefore, it is less likely to be affected by lysosomal alterations [46]. The caveolae is a lipid raft that contains a high level of caveolin proteins [47]. The lipid rafts stabilize the membrane structure and contain not only lipids, but also various signaling proteins, and growth factor receptors [48]. For example, clathrin- and caveolae-dependent endocytosis controls IGF1R endocytosis [49]. We hypothesized that IGF2R/M6P could be set off via a clathrin and/or caveolae related mechanism. (Figure 9). In our study, we have shown that an alternative IGF2R/M6P-caveolar mediated endocytosis coexist with clathrin-mediated endocytosis. However, clathrin-dependent endocytosis is a dominant mechanism for enzyme uptake in all cell lines including cell lines derived from FD patients.

Lysosomes are the final destination of the recombinant enzyme. We confirmed that the trafficking of the recombinant enzyme to the lysosome is a rapid process, with significant accumulation of rh-α-Gal A within the lysosomes after 1-h treatment. Formation of the clathrin-coated vesicles and the fusion of vesicles with the lysosomes is coordinated by actin cytoskeleton and microtubules. The microtubule-depolymerizing agent, nocodazole, blocked the transport of recombinant enzyme to the lysosome. Dysfunctional lysosomes due to Gb3 accumulation can impair the trafficking of the recombinant enzyme to the lysosomes, and initiate a cascade of events that lead to autophagy abnormality in Fabry disease [32,34]. In this study, we observed that the delivery of wild type α-Gal A enzyme immediately induces the activation of autophagy in fibroblasts and UKEC cells derived from FD patients.

5. Conclusions

The rapid uptake and delivery of rh-α-Gal-A to the lysosome via clathrin- and, to a lesser extent, caveolae-mediated endocytosis activates autophagy in Fabry disease.

Supplementary Materials: The following are available online at http://www.mdpi.com/2218-273X/10/6/837/s1, Figure S1: (A) The titration of rh-α-Gal-A enzyme activity pre- and post-labeling towards the artificial substrate 4-MUI. (B) Immunofluorescence images of fibroblasts treated with Alexa-Fluor 488- fluorescent dye alone and 488-fluorescence-labeled rh-α-Gal-A (green) for 1h and stained with LysoTracker (red). (C) Effects of rh-α-Gal-A on cell viability. HEK293 cells were treated with different concentrations of unlabeled rh-α-Gal-A fro 6h. The CCK-8 assay was performed to measure cell viability; Figure S2: HEK293 cells were treated 6 h with the indicated concentrations of rh-α-Gal-A, or vehicle control (untreated), and real-time-PCR analysis of IGFII/M6PR was performed: three separate experiments; Figure S3: Colocalization analysis of immunofluorescence images (Figure 5B) of control fibroblasts treated with fluorescence-labeled rh-α-Gal-A (red) and stained with LysoTracker (green) with and without nocodazole treatment. (A) Immunofluorescence images of untreated fibroblasts: fluorescence-labeled rh-α-Gal-A (left top panel), LysoTracker (left bottom panel), merge red and green images using ImageJ-win64 (right top panel) and image of co-localization areas (yellow) (right bottom panel). (B) 2D intensity histogram of the red and green pixels in the images labeled rh-α-Gal-A (channel 1, red) and LysoTracker staining (channel 2, green) for cells shown in (A). Fluorescence intensity analysis between the signal corresponding to rh-α-Gal-A and the signal corresponding to LysoTracker staining showing good correlation with a Pearson's coefficient (R2) for the colocalization volume $R^2 = 0.62$. (C) The table represents the measurement of areas of colocalization pixels vs. total cells area (image A, co-localization regions, yellow color). (D) Immunofluorescence images of nocodazole treated fibroblasts: fluorescence-labeled rh-α-Gal-A (left top panel), LysoTracker (left bottom panel), merge red and green images using ImageJ-win64 (right top panel) and image of co-localization areas (yellow) (right bottom panel). (E) 2D intensity histogram analysis between the signal corresponding to rh-α-Gal-A and the signal corresponding to LysoTracker showing low correlation with a Pearson's coefficient (R2) for the colocalization volume $R^2 = 0.62$. (F) The table represents the measurement of areas of colocolized pixels and all cells areas (image D, co-localization regions, yellow color); Table S1: Characteristics of cells used in this study and summary of a-Gal enzyme activity.

Author Contributions: Conceptualization, M.M.I. and O.G.-A.; methodology, J.D., N.K., B.A., J.F.; software, M.M.I.; validation, M.M.I., J.D. and B.A.; formal analysis, M.M.I. and J.D.; investigation, M.M.I.; resources, O.G.-A.; data curation, M.M.I.; writing—original draft preparation, M.M.I.; writing—review and editing, M.M.I. and O.G.-A.; visualization, M.M.I.; supervision, M.M.I.; project administration, O.G.-A.; funding acquisition, O.G.-A. All authors have read and agreed to the published version of the manuscript.

Funding: This research did not receive any specific grant from funding agencies in the public, commercial, or not-for-profit sectors.

Acknowledgments: The authors gratefully acknowledge and thank the effort of the study coordinators and nursing staff in LDRTC center, including Loren Noll, Eva Permaul.

Conflicts of Interest: The authors declare no conflict of interest.

References

1. Desnick, R.J. Enzyme replacement and enhancement therapies for lysosomal diseases. *J. Inherit. Metab. Dis.* **2004**, *27*, 385–410. [CrossRef] [PubMed]

2. Germain, D.P.; Elliott, P.M.; Falissard, B.; Fomin, V.V.; Hilz, M.J.; Jovanovic, A.; Kantola, I.; Linhart, A.; Mignani, R.; Namdar, M.; et al. The effect of enzyme replacement therapy on clinical outcomes in male patients with Fabry disease: A systematic literature review by a European panel of experts. *Mol. Genet. Metab. Rep.* **2019**, *19*, 1–20. [CrossRef] [PubMed]
3. Desnick, R.J.; Brady, R.; Barranger, J.; Collins, A.J.; Germain, D.P.; Goldman, M.; Grabowski, G.; Packman, S.; Wilcox, W.R. Fabry disease, an under-recognized multisystemic disorder: Expert recommendations for diagnosis, management, and enzyme replacement therapy. *Ann. Intern. Med.* **2003**, *138*, 338–346. [CrossRef] [PubMed]
4. Zarate, Y.A.; Hopkin, R. Fabry's disease. *Lancet* **2008**, *372*, 1427–1435. [CrossRef]
5. Waldek, S.; Giannini, E.; Mehta, A.; Hilz, M.; Beck, M.; Bichet, D.; Brady, R.; West, M.; Germain, D.; Wanner, C.; et al. 140. A validated disease severity scoring system for Fabry disease. *Mol. Genet. Metab.* **2010**, *99*, S37. [CrossRef]
6. MacDermot, K.D.; Holmes, A.; Miners, A.H. Anderson-Fabry disease: Clinical manifestations and impact of disease in a cohort of 60 obligate carrier females. *J. Med. Genet.* **2001**, *38*, 769–775. [CrossRef]
7. Lenders, M.; Schmitz, B.; Stypmann, J.; Duning, T.; Brand, S.-M.; Kurschat, C.; Brand, E. Renal function predicts long-term outcome on enzyme replacement therapy in patients with Fabry disease. *Nephrol. Dial. Transplant.* **2016**, *32*, 2090–2097. [CrossRef]
8. Najafian, B.; Tøndel, C.; Svarstad, E.; Sokolovkiy, A.; Smith, K.; Mauer, M. One Year of Enzyme Replacement Therapy Reduces Globotriaosylceramide Inclusions in Podocytes in Male Adult Patients with Fabry Disease. *PLoS ONE* **2016**, *11*, e0152812. [CrossRef]
9. Waldek, S.; Feriozzi, S. Fabry nephropathy: A review – how can we optimize the management of Fabry nephropathy? *BMC Nephrol.* **2014**, *15*, 72–91. [CrossRef]
10. Sheng, S.; Wu, L.; Nalleballe, K.; Sharma, R.; Brown, A.; Ranabothu, S.; Kapoor, N.; Onteddu, S. Fabry's disease and stroke: Effectiveness of enzyme replacement therapy (ERT) in stroke prevention, a review with meta-analysis. *J. Clin. Neurosci.* **2019**, *65*, 83–86. [CrossRef]
11. Hughes, D.; Elliott, P.M.; Shah, J.; Zuckerman, J.; Coghlan, G.; Brookes, J.; Mehta, A.B. Effects of enzyme replacement therapy on the cardiomyopathy of Anderson Fabry disease: A randomised, double-blind, placebo-controlled clinical trial of agalsidase alfa. *Heart* **2008**, *94*, 153–158. [CrossRef] [PubMed]
12. Gary-Bobo, M.; Nirdé, P.; Jeanjean, A.; Morère, A.; Garcia, M. Mannose 6-phosphate receptor targeting and its applications in human diseases. *Curr. Med. Chem.* **2007**, *14*, 2945–2953. [CrossRef] [PubMed]
13. Prabakaran, T.; Nielsen, R.; Larsen, J.V.; Sørensen, S.S.; Rasmussen, U.F.-; Saleem, M.A.; Petersen, C.M.; Verroust, P.J.; Christensen, E.I. Receptor-Mediated Endocytosis of α-Galactosidase A in Human Podocytes in Fabry Disease. *PLoS ONE* **2011**, *6*, e025065. [CrossRef]
14. Prabakaran, T.; Nielsen, R.; Satchell, S.C.; Mathieson, P.W.; Feldt-Rasmussen, U.; Sørensen, S.S.; Christensen, E.I. Mannose 6-Phosphate Receptor and Sortilin Mediated Endocytosis of α-Galactosidase A in Kidney Endothelial Cells. *PLoS ONE* **2012**, *7*, e039975. [CrossRef] [PubMed]
15. Ansar, M.; Serrano, D.; Papademetriou, I.; Bhowmick, T.K.; Muro, S. Biological Functionalization of Drug Delivery Carriers To Bypass Size Restrictions of Receptor-Mediated Endocytosis Independently from Receptor Targeting. *ACS Nano* **2013**, *7*, 10597–10611. [CrossRef]
16. Wang, Y.; Macdonald, R.; Thinakaran, G.; Kar, S. Insulin-Like Growth Factor-II/Cation-Independent Mannose 6-Phosphate Receptor in Neurodegenerative Diseases. *Mol. Neurobiol.* **2016**, *54*, 2636–2658. [CrossRef]
17. Dahms, N.M.; Lobel, P.; Kornfeld, S. Mannose 6-phosphate receptors and lysosomal enzyme targeting. *J. Boil. Chem.* **1989**, *264*, 12115–12118.
18. Lee, K.; Jin, X.; Zhang, K.; Copertino, L.; Andrews, L.; Baker-Malcolm, J.; Geagan, L.; Qiu, H.; Seiger, K.; Barngrover, D.; et al. A biochemical and pharmacological comparison of enzyme replacement therapies for the glycolipid storage disorder Fabry disease. *Glycobiology* **2003**, *13*, 305–313. [CrossRef]
19. Ivanova, M.; Changsila, E.; Göker-Alpan, Ö. Individualized screening for chaperone activity in Gaucher disease using multiple patient derived primary cell lines. *Mol. Genet. Metab.* **2018**, *123*, S69. [CrossRef]
20. Slaats, G.G.; Braun, F.; Hoehne, M.; Frech, L.E.; Blomberg, L.; Benzing, T.; Schermer, B.; Rinschen, M.M.; Kurschat, C. Urine-derived cells: A promising diagnostic tool in Fabry disease patients. *Sci. Rep.* **2018**, *8*, 11042–11053. [CrossRef]

21. Bishop, D.F.; Desnick, R.J. Affinity purification of alpha-galactosidase A from human spleen, placenta, and plasma with elimination of pyrogen contamination. Properties of the purified splenic enzyme compared to other forms. *J. Boil. Chem.* **1981**, *256*, 1307–1316.
22. Ishii, S.; Chang, H.-H.; Kawasaki, K.; Yasuda, K.; Wu, H.-L.; Garman, S.C.; Fan, J.-Q. Mutant α-galactosidase A enzymes identified in Fabry disease patients with residual enzyme activity: Biochemical characterization and restoration of normal intracellular processing by 1-deoxygalactonojirimycin. *Biochem. J.* **2007**, *406*, 285–295. [CrossRef] [PubMed]
23. Hichino, A.; Okamoto, M.; Taga, S.; Akizuki, R.; Endo, S.; Matsunaga, T.; Ikari, A. Down-regulation of Claudin-2 Expression and Proliferation by Epigenetic Inhibitors in Human Lung Adenocarcinoma A549 Cells*. *J. Boil. Chem.* **2017**, *292*, 2411–2421. [CrossRef] [PubMed]
24. Tveito, S.; Andersen, K.; Kåresen, R.; Fodstad, Ø. Analysis of EpCAM positive cells isolated from sentinel lymph nodes of breast cancer patients identifies subpopulations of cells with distinct transcription profiles. *Breast Cancer Res.* **2011**, *13*, 75–91. [CrossRef] [PubMed]
25. Ou, J.-M.; Lian, W.-S.; Qiu, M.-K.; Dai, Y.-X.; Dong, Q.; Shen, J.; Dong, P.; Wang, X.-F.; Liu, Y.; Quan, Z.-W.; et al. Knockdown of IGF2R suppresses proliferation and induces apoptosis in hemangioma cells in vitro and in vivo. *Int. J. Oncol.* **2014**, *45*, 1241–1249. [CrossRef] [PubMed]
26. Benjamin, E.R.; Della Valle, M.C.; Wu, X.; Katz, E.; Pruthi, F.; Bond, S.; Bronfin, B.; Williams, H.; Yu, J.; Bichet, D.G.; et al. The validation of pharmacogenetics for the identification of Fabry patients to be treated with migalastat. *Genet. Med.* **2016**, *19*, 430–438. [CrossRef]
27. Altarescu, G.; Moore, D.F.; Pursley, R.; Campia, U.; Goldstein, S.; Bryant, M.; Panza, J.A.; Schiffmann, R. Enhanced Endothelium-Dependent Vasodilation in Fabry Disease. *Stroke* **2001**, *32*, 1559–1562. [CrossRef]
28. Dahms, N.M.; Olson, L.J.; Kim, J.-J.P. Strategies for carbohydrate recognition by the mannose 6-phosphate receptors. *Glycobiology* **2008**, *18*, 664–678. [CrossRef]
29. Bareford, L.M.; Swaan, P. Endocytic mechanisms for targeted drug delivery. *Adv. Drug Deliv. Rev.* **2007**, *59*, 748–758. [CrossRef]
30. Miaczynska, M.; Stenmark, H. Mechanisms and functions of endocytosis. *J. Cell Boil.* **2008**, *180*, 7–11. [CrossRef]
31. Granger, E.; McNee, G.; Allan, V.J.; Woodman, P.G. The role of the cytoskeleton and molecular motors in endosomal dynamics. *Semin. Cell Dev. Boil.* **2014**, *31*, 20–29. [CrossRef] [PubMed]
32. Liebau, M.C.; Braun, F.; Höpker, K.; Weitbrecht, C.; Bartels, V.; Müller, R.-U.; Brodesser, S.; Saleem, M.A.; Benzing, T.; Schermer, B.; et al. Dysregulated Autophagy Contributes to Podocyte Damage in Fabry's Disease. *PLoS ONE* **2013**, *8*, e063506. [CrossRef] [PubMed]
33. Nelson, M.P.; Tonia, E.T.; O'Quinn, D.B.; Percival, S.M.; Jaimes, E.A.; Warnock, D.G.; Shacka, J.J. Autophagy-lysosome pathway associated neuropathology and axonal degeneration in the brains of alpha-galactosidase A-deficient mice. *Acta Neuropathol. Commun.* **2014**, *2*, 20–35. [CrossRef] [PubMed]
34. Ivanova, M.M.; Changsila, E.; Iaonou, C.; Goker-Alpan, O. Impaired autophagic and mitochondrial functions are partially restored by ERT in Gaucher and Fabry diseases. *PLoS ONE* **2019**, *14*, e0210617. [CrossRef] [PubMed]
35. Iwashita, H.; Sakurai, H.T.; Nagahora, N.; Ishiyama, M.; Shioji, K.; Sasamoto, K.; Okuma, K.; Shimizu, S.; Ueno, Y. Small fluorescent molecules for monitoring autophagic flux. *FEBS Lett.* **2018**, *592*, 559–567. [CrossRef]
36. Aerts, J.M.F.G.; Groener, J.E.; Kuiper, S.; Donker-Koopman, W.E.; Strijland, A.; Ottenhoff, R.; Van Roomen, C.; Mirzaian, M.; Wijburg, F.A.; Linthorst, G.E.; et al. Elevated globotriaosylsphingosine is a hallmark of Fabry disease. *Proc. Natl. Acad. Sci. USA* **2018**, *105*, 2812–2817.
37. Ebrahim, H.Y.; Baker, R.J.; Mehta, A.; Hughes, D. Functional analysis of variant lysosomal acid glycosidases of Anderson-Fabry and Pompe disease in a human embryonic kidney epithelial cell line (HEK 293 T). *J. Inherit. Metab. Dis.* **2011**, *35*, 325–334. [CrossRef]
38. Marchesan, D.; Cox, T.M.; Deegan, P.B. Lysosomal delivery of therapeutic enzymes in cell models of Fabry disease. *J. Inherit. Metab. Dis.* **2012**, *35*, 1107–1117. [CrossRef]
39. Tortorella, L.L.; Schapiro, F.B.; Maxfield, F.R. Role of an Acidic Cluster/Dileucine Motif in Cation-Independent Mannose 6-Phosphate Receptor Traffic. *Traffic* **2007**, *8*, 402–413. [CrossRef]
40. Wang, H. Endocytosis and membrane receptor internalization implication of F-BAR protein Carom. *Front. Biosci.* **2017**, *22*, 1439–1457. [CrossRef] [PubMed]

41. Dhami, R.; Schuchman, E.H. Mannose 6-Phosphate Receptor-mediated Uptake Is Defective in Acid Sphingomyelinase-deficient Macrophages. *J. Boil. Chem.* **2003**, *279*, 1526–1532. [CrossRef]
42. Rappaport, J.; Manthe, R.L.; Garnacho, C.; Muro, S. Altered Clathrin-Independent Endocytosis in Type A Niemann-Pick Disease Cells and Rescue by ICAM-1-Targeted Enzyme Delivery. *Mol. Pharm.* **2015**, *12*, 1366–1376. [CrossRef] [PubMed]
43. Cardone, M.; Porto, C.; Tarallo, A.; Vicinanza, M.; Rossi, B.; Polishchuk, E.; Donaudy, F.; Andria, G.; De Matteis, M.A.; Parenti, G. Abnormal mannose-6-phosphate receptor trafficking impairs recombinant alpha-glucosidase uptake in Pompe disease fibroblasts. *Pathogenetics* **2008**, *1*, 6–28. [CrossRef] [PubMed]
44. Rappaport, J.; Manthe, R.L.; Solomon, M.; Garnacho, C.; Muro, S. A Comparative Study on the Alterations of Endocytic Pathways in Multiple Lysosomal Storage Disorders. *Mol. Pharm.* **2016**, *13*, 357–368. [CrossRef] [PubMed]
45. Ginns, E.I.; Mak, S.K.-K.; Ko, N.; Karlgren, J.; Akbarian, S.; Chou, V.P.; Guo, Y.; Lim, A.; Samuelsson, S.; Lamarca, M.L.; et al. Neuroinflammation and α-synuclein accumulation in response to glucocerebrosidase deficiency are accompanied by synaptic dysfunction. *Mol. Genet. Metab.* **2014**, *111*, 152–162. [CrossRef] [PubMed]
46. Pelkmans, L. Secrets of caveolae- and lipid raft-mediated endocytosis revealed by mammalian viruses. *BBA Bioenerg.* **2005**, *1746*, 295–304. [CrossRef] [PubMed]
47. Gong, Q.; Huntsman, C.; Ma, D. Clathrin-independent internalization and recycling. *J. Cell. Mol. Med.* **2007**, *12*, 126–144. [CrossRef] [PubMed]
48. Pelkmans, L.; Bürli, T.; Zerial, M.; Helenius, A. Caveolin-Stabilized Membrane Domains as Multifunctional Transport and Sorting Devices in Endocytic Membrane Traffic. *Cell* **2004**, *118*, 767–780. [CrossRef]
49. Martins, A.S.; Ordóñez, J.L.; Amaral, A.T.; Prins, F.; Floris, G.; Debiec-Rychter, M.; Hogendoorn, P.C.W.; Álava, E. IGF1R Signaling in Ewing Sarcoma Is Shaped by Clathrin-/Caveolin-Dependent Endocytosis. *PLoS ONE* **2011**, *6*, e019846. [CrossRef]

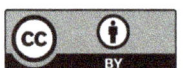

© 2020 by the authors. Licensee MDPI, Basel, Switzerland. This article is an open access article distributed under the terms and conditions of the Creative Commons Attribution (CC BY) license (http://creativecommons.org/licenses/by/4.0/).

MDPI
St. Alban-Anlage 66
4052 Basel
Switzerland
Tel. +41 61 683 77 34
Fax +41 61 302 89 18
www.mdpi.com

Biomolecules Editorial Office
E-mail: biomolecules@mdpi.com
www.mdpi.com/journal/biomolecules

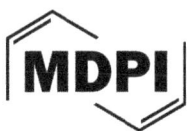

www.ingramcontent.com/pod-product-compliance
Lightning Source LLC
LaVergne TN
LVHW070206100526
838202LV00015B/2009